D0718658

Essentials of Engineering Mathematics

WORKED EXAMPLES AND PROBLEMS

Alan Jeffrey

Professor of Engineering Mathematics
University of Newcastle upon Tyne

CHAPMAN & HALL

University and Professional Division

London · Glasgow · New York · Tokyo · Melbourne · Madras

Published by Chapman & Hall, 2-6 Boundary Row, London SE1 8HN, UK

Chapman & Hall, 2-6 Boundary Row, London SE1 8HN, UK

Blackie Academic & Professional, Wester Cleddens Road, Bishopbriggs, Glasgow G64 2NZ, UK

Chapman & Hall GmbH, Pappelallee 3, 69469 Weinheim, Germany

Chapman & Hall USA, One Penn Plaza, 41st Floor, New York, NY10119, USA

Chapman & Hall Japan, ITP - Japan, Kyowa Building, 3F, 2-2-1 Hirakawacho, Chiyoda-ku, Tokyo 102, Japan

Chapman & Hall Australia, Thomas Nelson Australia, 102 Dodds Street, South Melbourne, Victoria 3205, Australia

Chapman & Hall India, R. Seshadri, 32 Second Main Road, CIT East, Madras 600 035, India

First edition 1992
Reprinted 1994, 1995

© 1992 Alan Jeffrey

Typeset in 10/12pt Times by Puretech Corporation, India
Printed and bound in Singapore

ISBN   0 412 39680 7

Apart from any fair dealing for the purposes of research or private study, or criticism or review, as permitted under the UK Copyright Designs and Patents Act, 1988, this publication may not be reproduced, stored, or transmitted, in any form or by any means, without the prior permission in writing of the publishers, or in the case of reprographic reproduction only in accordance with the terms of the licences issued by the Copyright Licensing Agency in the UK, or in accordance with the terms of licences issued by the appropriate Reproduction Rights Organization outside the UK. Enquiries concerning reproduction outside the terms stated here should be sent to the publishers at the London address printed on this page.

The publisher makes no representation, express or implied, with regard to the accuracy of the information contained in this book and cannot accept any legal responsibility or liability for any errors or omissions that may be made.

A Catalogue record for this book is available from the British Library

Library of Congress Cataloging-in-Publication Data available

Contents

Preface

Preface

This book presents the essentials of first year engineering mathematics as simply as possible. It has evolved from lectures given in Newcastle over many years, and it is intended that the book should be suitable both as a text to supplement a lecture course, and also for private study. Unlike standard texts, instead of comprising broadly based chapters, the book is divided into short sections, each of which discusses a specific topic. This enables the contents to be identified easily, and topics of interest to be studied separately with the minimum of background reading.

Each section is written in a straightforward manner and illustrated by many detailed worked examples, always prefaced by an outline of the underlying theory. Formal proofs are kept to a minimum, and are only included when they are considered to be absolutely essential for a proper understanding of a topic. The problem sets at the end of each section form an integral part of the text. A selection of problems from each problem set must be worked if the subject matter is to be properly understood. To help the reader, an answer to almost every problem is given at the end of the book, and they are given in far greater detail than is usual in a text.

For ease of reference, a list of mathematical formulae, standard integrals and Laplace transform pairs is to be found at the end of the book. The reader should learn to take full advantage of this material, after first understanding how it has been derived.

I am grateful to the many students who, through their reactions to lectures and by their questions in tutorials, have done much to influence the content and style of this book. Finally, thanks are due to both the publisher for readily accepting my proposal for a different type of engineering mathematics book, and to Mrs Lynn Kelly for her expert typing of the manuscript and for the uncomplaining way in which she accepted my many revisions.

Alan Jeffrey
Newcastle upon Tyne

Real numbers, inequalities and intervals 1

The study of the calculus and its many applications depends crucially on the properties of real numbers. The set of all real numbers is often represented symbolically by writing either $\mathbb{R}$ or $\mathbf{R}$. If x is a real number this is often shown by writing $x \in \mathbb{R}$ or $x \in \mathbf{R}$. Here the symbol $\in$ is to be read 'belongs to'. The formal mathematical name for this symbol is the **set membership relation** symbol. There are three different types of real numbers:

1. the **positive integers** or **natural numbers** 1, 2, 3, ...;
2. the **rational numbers** (fractions) of the form p/q with p, q integers with no common factor, such as 1/3, 27/5, − 5/16, ...;
3. the **irrational numbers** – numbers such as $\sqrt{2}$ which cannot be expressed as a rational number.

Calculations with real numbers depend on what are called the **field axioms** for real numbers which determine how real numbers may be combined.

Field axioms

1. Real numbers **commute** with respect to the operations of addition and subtraction, in the sense that if x, y are real numbers, then

$$x + y = y + x \quad \text{and} \quad xy = yx$$

Thus, **commutativity** means that the order in which real numbers are added or multiplied is immaterial.

2. Real numbers are **associative** with respect to the operations of addition and subtraction, in the sense that if x, y, z are real numbers, then

$$x + (y + z) = (x + y) + z \quad \text{and} \quad x(yz) = (xy)z.$$

Thus **associativity** means that the order in which real numbers are grouped when performing additions or multiplications is immaterial.

3. Real numbers are **distributive** with respect to multiplication, in the sense that if x, y, z are real numbers, then

$$x(y + z) = xy + xz.$$

Thus the **distributivity** means that the product of a number and a sum is equal to the sum of the respective products.

4 Real numbers 0 and 1 exist, called **identity elements** with respect to addition and multiplication, and they have the property that if x is a real number, then

$$x + 0 = x \quad \text{and} \quad 1 \cdot x = x.$$

Thus adding zero to a real number leaves it unchanged, as does multiplying it by unity.

5 For every real number x there is a number y, with the property that

$$x + y = 0.$$

Thus associated with every real number x there is another real number y which is its **negative**. Only when $x = 0$ does the negative of x equal x.

6 For every real number $x \neq 0$ (the symbol $\neq$ is to be read 'is not equal to') there exists a real number y, called the **reciprocal** of x, with property that

$$xy = 1.$$

7 If x and y are real numbers, then $x + y$ and xy are also real numbers. This is called the **closure axiom**, and it says that adding or multiplying two real numbers can only produce another real number (it cannot produce a different type of number – say a complex number).

ORDER PROPERTY OF REAL NUMBERS

There is a **natural order** amongst the real numbers which always makes it possible to say which of two different numbers is the larger. If x and y are two distinct (different) real numbers, with x **greater than** y, we write

$$x > y.$$

This is to be interpreted to mean that x is **greater** than y if $x - y$ is positive, written

$$x - y > 0.$$

If $x - y$ is negative, we write

$$x < y$$

and say x is **less than** y.

The signs $>, <$ (respectively read 'greater than' and 'less than') are called **inequality signs**. The obvious modifications

$$x \geqslant y \quad \text{and} \quad x \leqslant y$$

mean, respectively, that x is **greater than or equal** to y and x is **less than or equal to** y.

Extensive use is made of inequalities throughout mathematics and its many applications. Although they are largely self-evident, the following elementary inequalities arise sufficiently frequently for it to be worth while listing them for future reference.

Elementary inequalities

1   If $a > b$ and $c \geqslant d$, then $a + c > b + d$.

2   If $a > b \geqslant 0$ and $c \geqslant d > 0$, then $ac > bd$.

3   If $k > 0$ and $a > b$, then $ka > kb$; and if $k < 0$ and $a > b$, then $ka > kb$.

4   If $0 < a < b$, then $a^2 < b^2$ and if $a < b < 0$, then $a^2 > b^2$.

5   If $a < 0$ or $a > 0$, then $a^2 > 0$.

6   If $a > b$, then $-a < -b$.

7   If $a < 0, b > 0$, then $ab < 0$, while if $a < 0, b < 0$, then $ab > 0$.

8   If $a > 0$, then $1/a > 0$, while if $a < 0$, then $1/a < 0$.

9   If $a > b > 0$, then $1/b > 1/a > 0$, while if $a < b < 0$, $1/b < 1/a < 0$.

When working with real numbers it is necessary to have a measure of the magnitude (size) of a real number without regard to it sign. This measure is provided by the **absolute value** of the number which is defined as follows.

If a is a real number, then its absolute value, written $|a|$, is defined as

$$|a| = \begin{cases} a & \text{if } a \geqslant 0 \\ -a & \text{if } a < 0. \end{cases}$$

Thus $|a|$ is a non-negative number (i.e. positive or zero, but never negative) which measures the magnitude of a. For example $|-25| = 25$, $|7| = 7$, $|-2\pi| = 2\pi$ and $|4/3| = 4/3$.

Two important and useful properties of the absolute value are that if a and b are real numbers,

$$|ab| = |a||b| \quad \text{and} \quad \left|\frac{a}{b}\right| = \frac{|a|}{|b|}, \text{ provided } b \neq 0.$$

See Example 1.1 which now follows for a proof of these results.

Example 1.1

Prove that if a, k are real numbers:

(i) $|ka| = |k||a|$;

(ii) $\left|\dfrac{a}{k}\right| = \dfrac{|a|}{|k|}$ provided $k \neq 0$;

(iii) $|a|^2 = a^2$;

(iv)   find the value of x such that
$$-\tfrac{1}{2} < x < 4 \quad \text{and} \quad |2x + 1| = |x - 4|.$$

Solution

(i)   We consider each case.

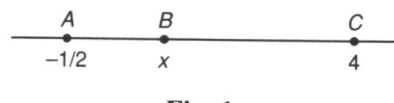

Fig. 1

1 If either k or a (or both) is zero, then $|ka| = 0 = |k||a|$.

2 If $k > 0, a > 0$, then $|ka| = ka$, but $|k||a| = ka$, so $|ka| = |k||a|$.

3 If $k < 0, a > 0$, then $|ka| = -ka$, but $|k||a| = (-k)a = -ka$, so $|ka| = |k||a|$. The same from of argument shows the result to be true if $k > 0$ and $a < 0$.

4 If $k < 0$ and $a < 0$, then $|ka| = ka$, while $|k||a| = (-k)(-a) = ka$, so that $|ka| = |k||a|$. The result is proved.

(ii) This result follows directly from (i) by setting $K = 1/k$ and using the fact that $|Ka| = |K||a|$.

(iii) If $a > 0$, then $|a| = a$, so $|a|^2 = a^2$.

If $a < 0$, then $|a| = -a$, and $|a|^2 = (-a)^2 = a^2$.

If $a = 0$, then $|a| = 0 = a$ and again $|a|^2 = a^2$, so the result is proved.

(iv) This equation is best solved using the interpretation of $|a - b|$ as the **distance** between a and b, and plotting points on the x-axis. We say more about such geometrical representations after this problem. Using (i) we may write

$$|2x + 1| = 2|x + \tfrac{1}{2}|,$$

so the equation becomes

$$2|x + \tfrac{1}{2}| = |x - 4|.$$

This says the distance of x from 4 is twice the distance of x from $-1/2$. Thus, in terms of Fig. 1 in which x is at the point B, we see that $BC = 2AB$. However, $AC = 9/2$ and $AC = AB + BC$, so

$$9/2 = AB + 2AB = 3AB$$

and thus $AB = 3/2$. Hence

$$x = -1/2 + AB = -1/2 + 3/2 = 1. \qquad \blacktriangle$$

The order property of real numbers allows them to be represented by points on a straight line. To do this we take a point on the line as an origin 0, a unit of length to represent the integer 1, and use the convention that distances to the right of 0 are positive and those to the left are negative. Then, for example, the number 2.9 is represented by the point distant 2.9 length units to the right of 0, while the number -1.3 is represented by the point 1.3 length units to the left of 0, as shown in Fig. 2. The set of all real numbers **R** is called the **real line**, and the numbers 2.9 and -1.3 are two particular numbers belonging to

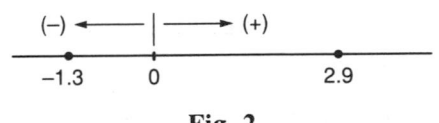

Fig. 2

R, so that $2.9 \in$ **R** and $-1.3 \in$ **R**. As numbers and point are equivalent in such a representation, the terms 'number' and 'point' are used interchangeably.

Inequalities are useful for identifying **intervals on a line**, and these are necessary when working with functions, and elsewhere. An interval on the real line **R** is the set of all points (numbers) between two specified (end) points on the real line. An interval may be **open**, **closed** or **half-open**, depending on whether both end points are excluded from the intervals, both are included, or one is included and the other excluded. Graphically, an end point excluded from an interval is shown as a small circle on the line and one which is included as a solid dot.

Equivalent notations for intervals

1 Open interval

  $a < x < b; \quad (a, b)$.

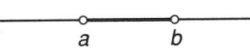

2 Closed interval

  $a \leqslant x \leqslant b; \quad [a, b]$.

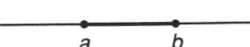

3 Half-open interval

  $a < x \leqslant b; \quad (a, b]$,

  $a \leqslant x < b; \quad [a, b)$.

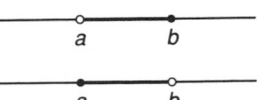

4 Semi-infinite intervals

  $a < x < \infty; \quad (a, \infty)$,

  $a \leqslant x < \infty; \quad [a, \infty)$,

  $-\infty < x < a; \quad (-\infty, a)$,

  $-\infty < x \leqslant a; \quad (-\infty, a]$.

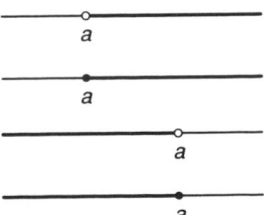

Infinity (∞) is a limiting operation, and **not** a number, so when it occurs at the end of an interval, by convention this is regarded as an open end.

5   Infinite interval

$-\infty < x < \infty;\quad (-\infty, \infty).$

Entire real line

When using the absolute value to define an interval, it is helpful to interpret $|a-b|$ as the **distance** between the points representing a and b on the real line, with the distance regarded as a non-negative quantity as in Example 1.1(iv).

Example 1.2

Show graphically the intervals
(i) $2 < x < 5$;
(ii) $x \leqslant 3, x > 4$;
(iii) $|x - 3| < 1$;
(iv) $0 < |x - 3| < 1$.

Solution
(i)

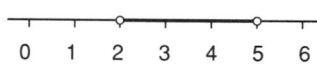

(ii)

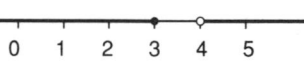

(iii) *Method 1*
Let us use the interpretation of the absolute value as a distance. The inequality $|x - 3| < 1$ then says that the interval contains all the points (numbers) whose distance from the fixed point 3 is strictly less than 1. Thus the interval in question is $3 - 1 < x < 3 + 1$, or $2 < x < 4$:

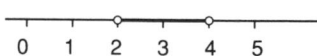

Method 2
Let us use the definition of the absolute value,

$$|x - 3| = x - 3$$

if $x - 3 \geqslant 0$, which is equivalent to $x \geqslant 3$; while

$$|x - 3| = -(x - 3) = 3 - x$$

if $x - 3 < 0$, which is equivalent to $x < 3$.
Thus if $x \geqslant 3$,

$$|x - 3| < 1 \quad \text{is equivalent to } x - 3 < 1, \text{ or to } x < 4,$$

while if $x < 3$

$$|x - 3| < 1 \text{ is equivalent to } 3 - x < 1, \text{ or to } 2 < x.$$

Combining results we have

$$2 < x < 4.$$

Method 3

In this method we make use of the fact that $|a|^2 = a^2$ so that, in particular, $|x-3|^2 = (x-3)^2$. Squaring both sides of the inequality and using elementary inequality property 4 we have

$$(x-3)^2 < 1 \quad \text{and so} \quad x^2 - 6x + 8 < 0.$$

As $x^2 - 6x + 8 = (x-2)(x-4)$ this is equivalent to

$$(x-2)(x-4) < 0.$$

For this product to be negative, one factor must be positive and the other negative. This is only possible for x in the interval

$$2 < x < 4,$$

so again we arrive at the same inequality.

(iv) The inequality $0 < |x-3| < 1$ says that the distance of x from the fixed point 3 must be greater than zero and strictly less than 1. Thus this case only differs from the situation in (iii) above by the exclusion of the single point $x = 3$ from the open interval $2 < x < 4$. Hence the inequality $0 < |x-3| < 1$ defines the points in the open intervals $2 < x < 3$ and $3 < x < 4$. Graphically, these inequalities correspond to the situation shown in Fig. 3.

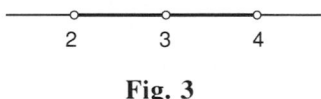

Fig. 3   ▲

Example 1.3

For what values of x is the following inequality satisfied?

$$\frac{x+2}{x-1} > \frac{x}{x+2}.$$

Solution

If $(x-1)(x+2) > 0$ we may multiply the original inequality by this product and leave the sign > **unchanged** to obtain

$$(x+2)^2 > x(x-1) \quad \text{or} \quad x^2 + 4x + 4 > x^2 - x,$$

which is equivalent to

$$5x > -4, \quad \text{or to} \quad x > -4/5.$$

However, $(x-1)(x+2)$ will be positive if either $x > 1$ and $x > -2$ (both factors are positive) or if $x < 1$ and $x < -2$ (both factors are negative).

Case (i)

The conditions $x > 1, x > -2$ and $x > -4/5$ will all be satisfied simultaneously if $x > 1$.

Case (ii)

The conditions $x < 1$, $x < -2$ and $x > -4/5$ can **never** all be satisfied simultaneously, so we conclude that when $(x-1)(x+2) > 0$ the original inequality is satisfied if $x > 1$.

If, however, $(x-1)(x+2) < 0$, after multiplying the original inequality by this product we must **reverse** the sign $>$ to $<$ to obtain

$$(x+2)^2 < x(x-1)$$

so that now $x < -4/5$. However, $(x-1)(x+2)$ will be negative if its factors have different signs, so that either $x > 1$ and $x < -2$, or $x < 1$ and $x > -2$.

Case (iii) .

The conditions $x > 1$, $x < -2$ and $x < -4/5$ can **never** all be satisfied simultaneously.

Case (iv)

The conditions $x < 1, x > -2$ and $x < -4/5$ are all satified simultaneously for $-2 < x < -4/5$, so the original inequality is satisfied when x lies in this interval.

Combining cases (i) and (iv) we see that

$$\frac{x+2}{x-1} > \frac{x}{x+2}$$

for $-2 < x < -4/5$ and $x > 1$. ▲

The next example proves two important and useful inequalities involving the absolute value. The first is called the **triangle inequality**, for reasons which will become clear when complex numbers and vectors are studied. The second inequality is derived from the triangle inequality.

Example 1.4

Prove that if a, b are any two real numbers, then

(i) $|a+b| \leq |a| + |b|$ (**triangle inequality**)

(ii) $||a| - |b|| \leq |a-b|$.

Solution

(i)   We have

$$|a+b|^2 = (a+b)^2$$
$$= a^2 + 2ab + b^2$$
$$= |a|^2 + 2ab + |b|^2$$

Also

$$(|a| + |b|)^2 = |a|^2 + 2|a||b| + |b|^2,$$

but $ab \leq |a||b|$, so

$$|a+b|^2 \leq (|a| + |b|)^2,$$

and hence

$$|a+b| \leq |a| + |b|.$$

(ii) Writing $a = (a-b) + b$, it follows from the triangle inequality that

$$|a| \leq |a-b| + |b|,$$

and so

$$|a| - |b| \leq |a-b|.$$

Also $b = (b-a) + a$, so from the triangle inequality we have

$$|b| \leq |b-a| + |a|,$$

or

$$-|b-a| \leq |a| - |b|.$$

However, $|a-b| = |b-a|$, so the result show that

$$-|a-b| \leq |a| - |b| \leq |a-b|.$$

Thus $|a| - |b|$ lies in the interval $[-|a-b|, |a-b|]$ which is equivalent to writing

$$||a| - |b|| \leq |a-b|. \qquad \blacktriangle$$

Example 1.5

Find a positive number M such that $|x^3 - 5x^2 + 3| \leq M$ for x in the interval $-3 \leq x \leq 2$.

Solution

$$x^3 - 5x^2 + 3 = x^3 + (-5x^2 + 3),$$

so by the triangle inequaltiy

$$|x^3 - 5x^2 + 3| \leq |x^3| + |-5x^2 + 3|.$$

After a further application of the triangle inequality to the last term this becomes

$$|x^3 - 5x^2 + 3| \leq |x^3| + |-5x^2| + |3|$$

$$= |x|^3 + 5|x|^2 + |3|.$$

Now the largest value of $|x|$ in the interval $-3 \leq x \leq 2$ is 3, and so

$$\left| x^3 - 5x^2 + 3 \right| \leq 3^3 + 5 \cdot 3^2 + 3 = 75$$

and thus we may set $M = 75$.

A more careful examination shows the smallest possible value of M to be 69 (prove this). ▲

PROBLEMS 1

Mark on a line the points satisfying the following inequalities, using a circle to indicate an end point which is omitted from an interval and a dot to indicate an end point which is included.

1. $x < 3$, $x \geq -1$.
2. $2 < x \leq 4$.
3. $x \leq -1$, $x \geq 2$.
4. $-2 \leq x < 1$ and $1 < x \leq 3$.

Show graphically on a line, and also using inequalities, the values of x for which the following inequalities are true.

5. $(x + 2)(x - 3) > 0$.
6. $(x + 2)(x - 3) \leq 0$.
7. $(x - 1)(x - 2) > 0$.
8. $(x - 1)(x - 2) < 0$.
9. $x > 1$ and $x^2 \leq 9$.
10. $-9 < x < 1$ and $x^2 < 4$.
11. $-16 \leq x \leq 6$ and $x^2 \geq 4$.
12. $-4 < x \leq 2$ and $(x + 1)^2 \geq 4$.
13. Show that if $a < b$, then

$$a < \frac{a + b}{2} < b$$

14. If $a > b > 0$ and $k > 0$, show by considering the differences

$$\frac{b + k}{a + k} - \frac{b}{a} \quad \text{and} \quad 1 - \frac{b + k}{a + k}$$

that

$$\frac{b}{a} < \frac{b + k}{a + k} < 1.$$

15. If $a > b > 0$ and $k > 0$, show by considering the differences

$$\frac{a}{b} - \frac{a + k}{b + k} \quad \text{and} \quad \frac{a + k}{b + k} - 1$$

that

$$1 < \frac{a + k}{b + k} < \frac{a}{b}.$$

16. Verify inequalities (i) and (ii) in Example 1.4 when
    (a) $a = 3, b = -4$;   (b) $a = 4, b = 1$;
    (c) $a = -3, b = -5$;   (d) $a = -1, b = 1$.

17. Prove that for a, b any real numbers such that $a \neq b$,

$$\frac{1}{|a| + |b|} \leq \left| \frac{1}{a+b} \right| \leq \frac{1}{||a| - |b||}$$

18. Find a positive number M such that $|x^3 - 4x - 6| \leq M$ for $-1 \leq x \leq 3$.

19. Find a positive number M such that $|x^4 - 2x^3 + 1| \leq M$ for $-2 \leq x \leq 2$.

20. What is the value of $\dfrac{a + |a|}{a\,|a|}$ when (a) $a > 0$ and (b) $a < 0$?

21. Let $\{a_1, a_2, ..., a_n\}$, $\{b_1, b_2, ..., b_n\}$ and $\{k_n, k_2, ..., k_n\}$ be any three sets of n positive numbers, with m the smallest of the n numbers k_i and M the largest, then

$$m \left[\frac{a_1 + a_2 + ... + a_n}{b_1 + b_2 + ... + b_n} \right] \leq \frac{k_1 a_1 + k_2 a_2 + ... + k_n a_n}{b_1 + b_2 + ... + b_n} \leq M \left[\frac{a_1 + a_2 + ... + a_n}{b_1 + b_2 + ... + b_n} \right].$$

22. Let a and b be any two non-negative numbers (they may be positive or zero, but not negative) and p, q be positive integers. By considering the product $(a^p - b^p)(a^q - b^q)$, prove that

$$a^{p+q} + b^{p+q} \geq a^p b^q + a^q b^p.$$

23. If $a > 0, b > 0$ show by considering $(a + b)^2 - (a - b)^2$ that

$$\frac{a+b}{2} \geq \sqrt{ab}.$$

24. This problem outlines a proof by contradiction that $\sqrt{2}$ is **irrational**. Suppose, if possible, the converse is true and $\sqrt{2}$ is rational, and thus can be expressed in the from m/n, with m and n integers with no common factor. By squaring both sides of the expression $\sqrt{2} = m/n$ show that m and n must have a common factor, thereby contradicting the original assumption. Conclude from the contradiction that $\sqrt{2}$ cannot be expressed in the form m/n and so is not rational (it is *irrational*).

2   Function, domain and range

A simple and typical example of a function is

$$y = 1 + \sin x \quad \text{for} \quad -\pi \leqslant x \leqslant 3\pi/4.$$

In this example the **function** is the rule that says 'to each number x in the interval $-\pi \leqslant x \leqslant 3\pi/4$, associate a number y obtained by first finding $\sin x$ and then adding the result to unity'. The interval $-\pi \leqslant x \leqslant 3\pi/4$ is called the **domain of definition** (**domain** for short) of the function, and the interval $0 \leqslant y \leqslant 2$ over which y ranges for all x in the domain is called the **range** of the function. The graph of this function, together with its domain and range is shown in Fig. 4.

The general definition of a function is that it is a rule (usually a formula), which assigns to **every** number in the domain of the function a **unique** number in the range of the function.

A function is usually denoted by a symbol such as f, an arbitrary number in its domain by x, often called the **independent variable**, and the corresponding number in its range by y, often called the **dependent variable**. Thus when we write a general function in the form

$$y = f(x),$$

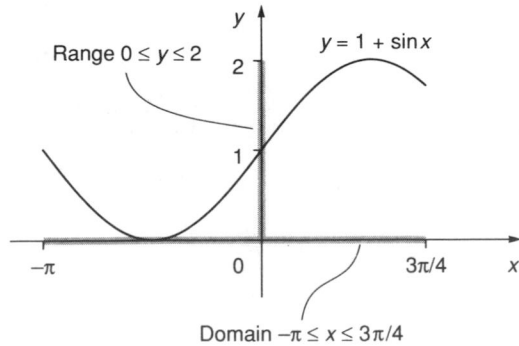

Fig. 4

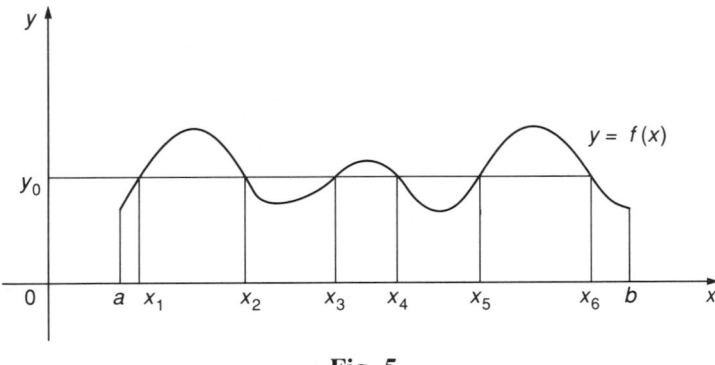

Fig. 5

f is the function, x is the independent variable and y is the dependent variable. The domain and range are an essential part of the definition of a function. If the domain is not specified, it is to be understood to be the largest interval containing x for which the function is defined.

The graph in Fig. 5 shows a function which is said to be a **many–one** function, in the sense that to **one** value of y there correspond **many** (more than one) values of x. In this case, in the interval $a \leqslant x \leqslant b$ the values $x_1, x_2, ..., x_6$ of x all correspond to the same value y_0. The two graphs in Fig. 6 show

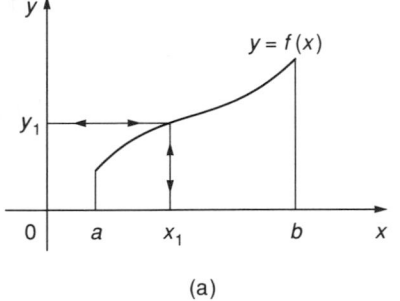

(a)

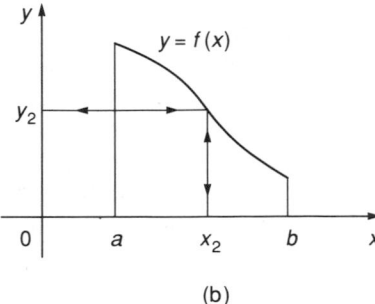

(b)

Fig. 6

functions which are said to be **one–one** or **monotonic** functions. These are functions which either increase or decrease steadily in a given interval. The graph in Fig. 6(a) shows a **monotonic increasing** function, and the one in Fig. 6(b) a **monotonic decreasing function**. In these cases one x corresponds to one y and, conversely, one y corresponds to one x.

The graph in Fig. 7 does not represent a function, because to one x there correspond more than one y. This is called a **one–many mapping**. It can be represented as a set of functions by dividing it up into several different monotonic functions, as shown, each with its own domain and range. In this case it may be represented as the three monotonic functions:

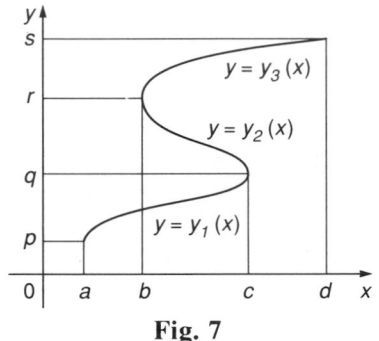

Fig. 7

1 $y = y_1(x)$, monotonic increasing with domain $a \leqslant x \leqslant c$ and range $p \leqslant y \leqslant q$;

2 $y = y_2(x)$, monotonic decreasing with domain $b \leqslant x \leqslant c$ and range $q \leqslant y \leqslant r$;

3 $y = y_3(x)$, monotonic increasing with domain $b \leqslant x \leqslant d$ and range $r \leqslant y \leqslant s$.

The most elementary and familiar example of a one–many mapping is provided by the square root function $\sqrt{x}$, because to any one $x > 0$ there correspond a positive and a negative square root. The graph of $y = 1 + \sqrt{x}$ is shown in Fig. 8, from which it is clear that it represents a one–many mapping and **not** a function.

If we regard $x^{1/2}$ as denoting the positive square root, Fig. 8 is seen to be described by the two monotonic functions:

1 $y_+ = 1 + x^{1/2}$, monotonic increasing with domain $x \geqslant 0$ and range $y_+ \geqslant 1$;

2 $y_- = 1 - x^{1/2}$, monotonic decreasing with domain $x \geqslant 0$ and range $y_- \leqslant 1$.

Notice that y_+ and y_- both have the same domain, but different ranges, so they are different (monotonic) functions.

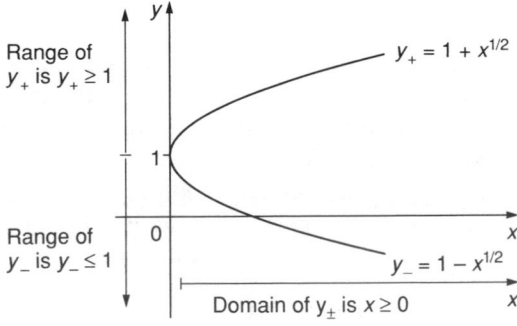

Fig. 8

Example 2.1

Find the largest possible domain and corresponding range for each of the following functions:

(i) $y = \sin x$;

(ii) $y = (3 - x)^{1/2}$, where the positive square root is taken;

(iii) $y = -(1 - x^2)^{1/2}$, where the positive square root is taken;

(iv) $y = |1 - x|^{1/2}$, where the positive square root is taken.

Solution

(i) $\sin x$ is defined for all x (it is periodic with period 2π) so the largest possible domain is the infinite interval $-\infty < x < \infty$, and the range is then the closed interval $-1 \leqslant y \leqslant 1$.

(ii) $(3 - x)^{1/2}$ is only real when $3 - x \geqslant 0$. Thus the largest possible domain is the semi-infinite interval $x \leqslant 3$, and the corresponding range is then the semi-infinite interval $0 \leqslant y < \infty$.

(iii) $(1 - x^2)^{1/2}$ is only real when $x^2 \leqslant 1$, corresponding to $-1 \leqslant x \leqslant 1$. Thus the largest possible domain is the closed interval $-1 \leqslant x \leqslant 1$, from which it follows that $-(1 - x^2)^{1/2}$ then has for its range the closed interval $-1 \leqslant y \leqslant 0$.

(iv) $|1 - x| \geqslant 0$ for all x, so $|1 - x|^{1/2}$ is defined for all x. Thus the largest possible domain is the infinite interval $-\infty < x < \infty$, and the corresponding range is then the semi-infinite interval $y \geqslant 0$.

PROBLEMS 2

Find the range of each of the following functions.

1. $y = x^3 + 2$ for $-1 \leqslant x \leqslant 2$.
2. $y = x^2 + 1$ for $-2 \leqslant x \leqslant 3$.
3. $y = 3 + \cos x$ for $0 \leqslant x \leqslant 3\pi/4$.
4. $y = 3 + \cos x$ for $\pi/4 \leqslant x \leqslant 3\pi/4$.
5. $y = \tan x$ for $-\pi/4 \leqslant x < \pi/2$.
6. $y = \sin^2 x$ for $-\pi/4 \leqslant x \leqslant \pi$.
7. $y = |x^3|$ for $-1 \leqslant x \leqslant 2$.
8. $y = \dfrac{1}{2} + |\cos x|$ for $0 \leqslant x \leqslant 3\pi/4$.

Clarify the following realtionships as one–one functions, may–one functions or one–many mappings.

9. $y = \sin x$ for $-\pi/2 \leqslant x \leqslant \pi/2$.
10. $y = \sin x$ for $-\pi/2 \leqslant x \leqslant 2\pi$.
11. $y = |\sqrt{x}|$ for $x \geqslant 0$.

12. $y = \cos x$ for $0 \leqslant x \leqslant \pi$.

13. $y = \sqrt{(x-1)}$ for $x \geqslant 1$.

14. $y = x + \sqrt{(x^2 - 1)}$ for $x \geqslant 1$

15. $y = x^3$ for $-3 \leqslant x \leqslant 4$.

16. $y = x |x^3|$ for $-1 \leqslant x \leqslant 2$.

17. $y = x^4$ for $-1 \leqslant x \leqslant 2$.

18. $y = 1/(1 + x^2)$ for $x \geqslant 0$.

Find the largest possible domain and the corresponding range for each of the following functions.

19. $y = 1 + x + x^2$

20. $y = 3 |\sin x|$.

21. $y = \sin \{ |1 - x|^{1/2} \}$, where the positive square root is to be taken.

22. $y = \sin \{ |1 - x|^{1/2} \}$, where the positive square root is to be taken.

Basic coordinate geometry 3

The most common graphical representation of a function involves the use of **rectangular cartesian coordinates**. These involve two mutually perpendicular axes on each of which (unless otherwise stated) the same length scale is used to represent real numbers. The horizontal axis is the x-axis with positive x to the right of the point of intersection of the two axes which is taken as the origin, and negative x to the left. The vertical axis is the y-axis, with positive y above the origin and negative y below it.

A typical point P in the (x, y)-plane shown in Fig. 9 is identified by its x-coordinate a and its y-coordinate b, with a the number of length units P is distant from the y-axis, and b the number of length units P is distant from the x-axis, with due regard to sign. Thus Q is the point $(2, 1)$ and R is the point $(-3, -2)$. The number pair (a, b) is called an **ordered pair** because the order in which a and b appear is important. Interchanging a and b in the ordered pair (a, b) to give (b, a) changes the point represented by this notation.

The distance AB between points $A(x_1, y_1)$ and $B(x_2, y_2)$ in Fig. 9 is the length of the straight line AB so, by Pythagoras' theorem,

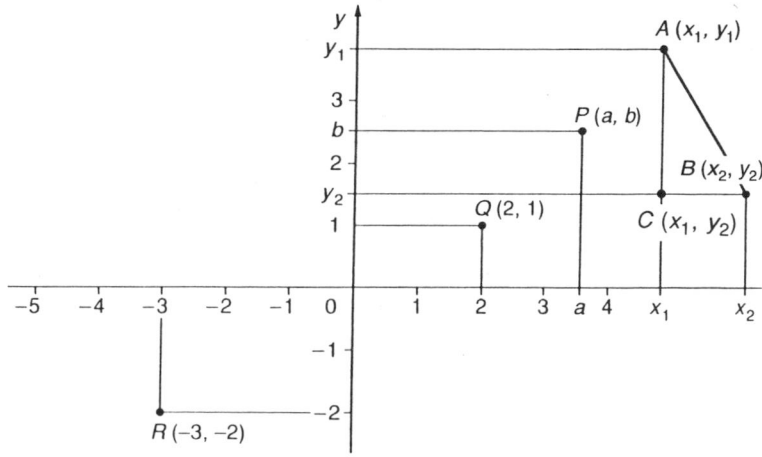

Fig. 9

$$(AB)^2 = (CB)^2 + (AC)^2$$

$$= \left| x_2 - x_1 \right|^2 + \left| y_2 - y_1 \right|^2$$

and hence

$$AB = \sqrt{[(x_2 - x_1)^2 + (y_2 - y_1)^2]}.$$

Thus, by way of example, the distance QR in Fig. 9 is

$$QR = \sqrt{[(2 - (-3))^2 + (1 - (-2))^2]} = \sqrt{34}.$$

THE STRAIGHT LINE $y = mx + c$

The graph of

$$y = mx + c$$

is the straight line shown in Fig. 10. The number m is called the gradient (slope) of the line and $\tan \theta = m$, where θ is the angle between the line and the x-axis, as measured in Fig. 10. The number c is the intercept of the line on the y-axis. If $m > 0$ the line $y = mx + c$ is a monotonic increasing function, and if $m < 0$ it is a monotonic decreasing function. When $m = 0$ the equation of the line reduces to the constant function $y = c$, whose graph is the dashed line in the figure parallel to the x-axis and passing through the point c on the y-axis. Lines parallel to the y-axis are of the form $x = c$, where c is a constant.

A straight line is completely specified if:

1 m and c are given.
2 m is given together with a point $P(x_1, y_1)$ on the line,
3 two points $P(x_1, y_1)$ and $Q(x_2, y_2)$ on the line are given.

Case 1
If m and c are given, the equation of the straight line

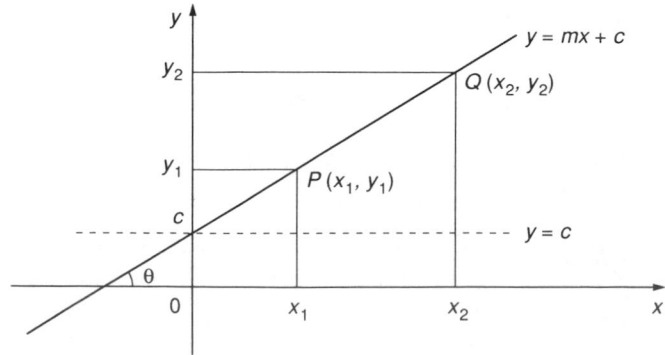

Fig. 10

$$y = mx + c$$

can be written down immediately.

Case 2
If m and $P(x_1, y_1)$ are given, only the constant c in the equation

$$y = mx + c$$

needs to be determined. As the line passes through the point $P(x_1, y_1)$ it follows that $y = y_1$ when $x = x_1$, so substituting into the equation we have

$$y_1 = mx_1 + c, \text{ or } c = y_1 - mx_1.$$

Thus the equation of the straight line becomes

$$y = mx + y_1 - mx_1$$

or

$$y = m(x - x_1) + y_1.$$

Case 3
If the line passes through $P(x_1, y_1)$ and $Q(x_2, y_2)$, the gradient m of the line is

$$m = \frac{y_2 - y_1}{x_2 - x_1}.$$

Substituting this value for m into $y = mx + c$ and using the fact that the line passes through $P(x_1, y_1)$ (or $Q(x_2, y_2)$) determines c and leads to the equation of the line in the form

$$y - y_1 = \left(\frac{y_2 - y_1}{x_2 - x_1} \right)(x - x_1)$$

or, equivalently, to

$$y - y_2 = \left(\frac{y_2 - y_1}{x_2 - x_1} \right)(x - x_2).$$

SHIFT OF ORIGIN

The change of variable

$$X = x - \alpha, \ Y = y - \beta$$

represents a **shift** of every point in the (x, y)-plane by an amount α in the x-direction and β in the y-direction. This is called a **shift of origin without scaling or rotation**, because distances between points are unaltered and no rotation occurs. Thus any graph of a function in the (x, y)-plane is simply shifted (translated) without scaling or rotation to the (X, Y)-plane in which the origin corresponds to the point (α, β) in the (x, y)-plane:

An important application of this simple transformation is the proof of the result that two straight lines

$$y = m_1 x + c_1 \text{ and } y = m_2 x + c_2$$

are **orthogonal** (mutually perpendicular) if

$$m_1 m_2 = -1.$$

To prove this result it will suffice for us to consider the two orthogonal lines $L_1(y = m_1 x)$ and $L_2(y = m_2 x)$ through the origin in Fig. 11. This follows because if they intersect at the point (α, β) instead of at the origin, a change of variable will reduce them to this case. The line $x = 1$ intersects L_1 at $(1, m_1)$ and L_2 at $(1, m_2)$, so by Pythogoras' theorem

$$(AB)^2 = (OA)^2 + (OB)^2$$

thus

$$(1 - 1)^2 + (m_2 - m_1)^2 = (1 + m_1^2) + (1 + m_2^2),$$

and after simplification this reduces to

$$m_1 m_2 = -1.$$

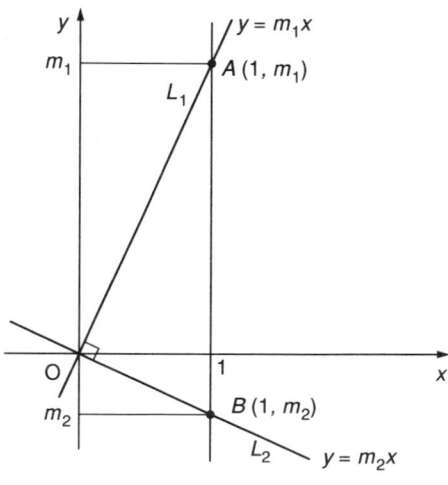

Fig. 11

Example 3.1

Find the equation of the straight line $y = mx + c$ such that:
(i) $m = 2$ and the line passes through the point $(1, -3)$;
(ii) the line passes through the points $(-1, 2)$ and $(3, 4)$;
(iii) it is the line through the point $(2, -5)$ orthogonal to $y = 3x - 11$.

Solution

(i) This is case 2 in which $m = 2$, $x_1 = 1$ and $y_1 = -3$. Thus the equation of the line is

$$y = 2(x - 1) - 3 \quad \text{or} \quad y = 2x - 5.$$

(ii) This is case 3 in which $x_1 = -1$, $y_1 = 2$, $x_2 = 3$ and $y_2 = 4$. Thus the equation of the line is

$$y = 2 + \left(\frac{4-2}{3-(-1)} \right)(x - (-1)) \text{ or } y = \frac{1}{2}(x + 5).$$

(iii) The gradient of the given line is 3, so the gradient of the orthogonal straight line must be $-1/3$ (so that $m_1 m_2 = -1$). Thus the required line is of the form $y = -\frac{1}{3}x + c$. As the line must pass through $(2, -5)$ it follows that $-5 = -\frac{1}{3} \times 2 + c$, so $c = -13/3$. Hence the required line has the equation

$$y = -(x + 13)/3. \qquad \blacktriangle$$

The equation of a straight line is an example of a polynomial in x of degree 1, also called a **linear function** of x. A **polynomial** $P_n(x)$ in x is an expression of the form

$$P_n(x) = a_0 x^n + a_1 x^{n-1} + a_2 x^{n-2} + \ldots + a_{n-1}x + a_n,$$

in which the numbers $a_0, a_1, \ldots, a_n$ are called the **coefficients** of the polynomial, and the number n (the highest power of x in $P_n(x)$) is called the **degree** of the polynomial. A polynomial is defined for all x.

When n is small the corresponding polynomials are named as follows:

$n = 0$: a constant function (degree zero);
$n = 1$: a linear polynomial (degree 1);
$n = 2$: a quadratic polynomial (degree 2);
$n = 3$: a cubic polynomial (degree 3);
$n = 4$: a quartic polynomial (degree 4);
$n = 5$: a quintic polynomial (degree 5).

THE CIRCLE

The circle of radius R with its centre at the point (α, β) shown in Fig. 12 has the equation

$$(x - \alpha)^2 + (y - \beta)^2 = R^2.$$

This is called the standard form of the equation of the circle, and the equation is derived by applying Pythagoras' theorem to the triangle ABP where $AB = x - \alpha$, $PB = y - \beta$ and $AP = R$.

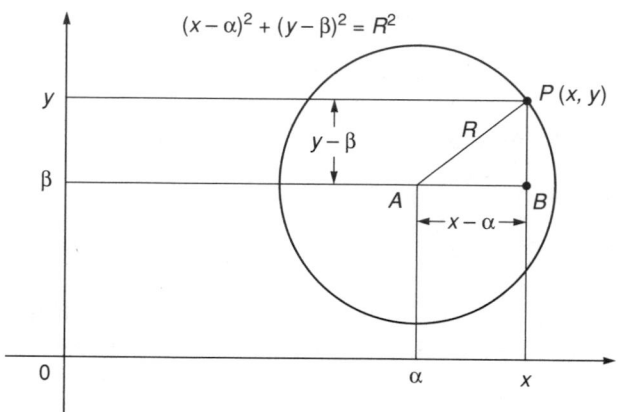

Fig. 12

An equation of the form

$$x^2 + y^2 + ax + by + c = 0$$

is the equation of a circle with its centre at (α, β) where

$$\alpha = -\frac{1}{2}a \quad \text{and} \quad \beta = -\frac{1}{2}b,$$

provided $a^2 + b^2 - 4c > 0$, and then its radius is

$$R = \left[\frac{1}{4}(a^2 + b^2) - c\right]^{1/2}.$$

THE ELLIPSE

The ellipse is a symmetrical closed curve of the form shown in Fig. 13, and it is characterized geometrically by the fact that the sum of the distances from two points F_1 and F_2 called the **foci** to any point P on the ellipse is a constant, so

$$d_1 + d_2 = \text{const.}$$

The longest chord AB of length $2a$ is called the **major axis** of the ellipse and the shortest chord CD, which is perpendicular to AB, is called the **minor axis** and it is of length $2b$, with $a > b$. The points A and B are called the **vertices** of the ellipse and point Q the **centre** of the ellipse.

The number

$$e = c/a,$$

where $c^2 = a^2 - b^2$ is called the **eccentricity** of the ellipse. The eccentricity is

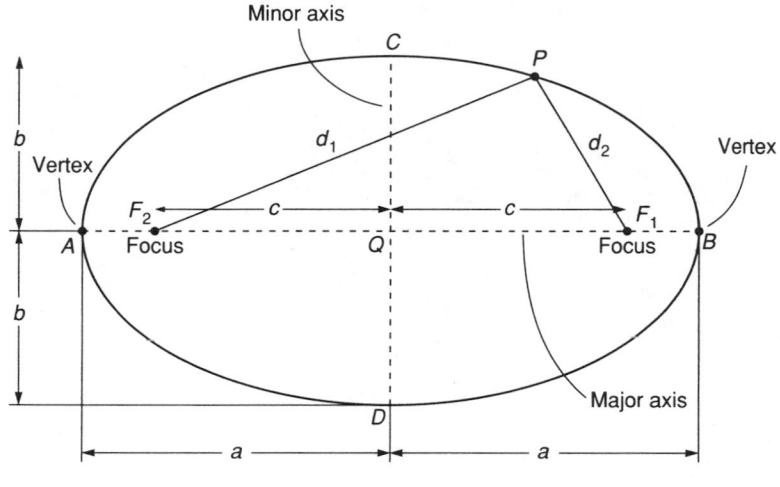

Fig. 13

such that $0 \leqslant e < 1$, and when e is small the ellipse is nearly circular, but when it is close to 1 the ellipse is very elongated.

The **standard equation** of an ellipse with its major axis **horizontal** and its centre at the point (α, β) is

$$\frac{(x - \alpha)^2}{a^2} + \frac{(y - \beta)^2}{b^2} = 1, \text{ with } a > b.$$

The corresponding form of the standard equation of an ellipse when its major axis is vertical is

$$\frac{(x - \alpha)^2}{b^2} + \frac{(y - \beta)^2}{a^2} = 1, \text{ with } a > b.$$

THE HYPERBOLA

The **hyperbola** is the curve shown in Fig. 14, and it is characterized geometrically by the fact that every point on the hyperbola is such that the difference of its distances from two fixed points F_1 and F_2 called the **foci** is a constant. The line on which F_1 and F_2 lie is called the **transverse axis** of the hyperbola, and the line perpendicular to the transverse axis which passes through the mid-point Q of $F_1 F_2$ is called the **directrix**. The point Q is called the **centre**, and the points A and B the **vertices** of the hyperbola. The distance of the vertices from either side of the centre Q is a,

The **standard form** of the equation of the hyperbola with its centre at (α, β) and its transverse axis **horizontal** is

$$\frac{(x - \alpha)^2}{a^2} - \frac{(y - \beta)^2}{b^2} = 1 .$$

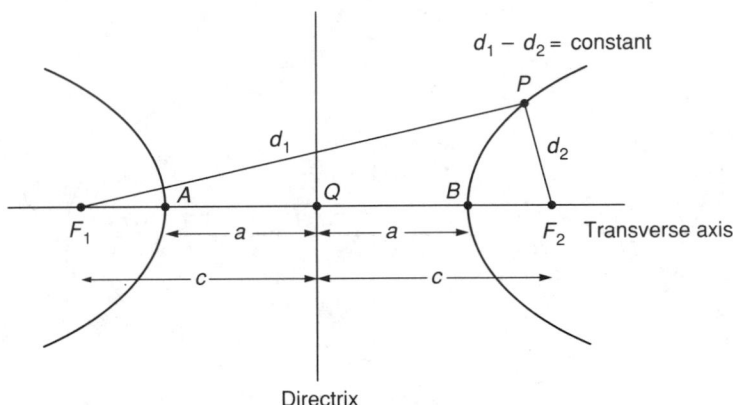

Fig. 14

Similarly, the standard form of the equation of the hyperbola with its centre at (α, β) and its transverse axis **vertical** is

$$\frac{(y - \beta)^2}{a^2} - \frac{(x - \alpha)^2}{b^2} = 1,$$

The distance c of the foci from either side of the centre Q is given by

$$c^2 = a^2 + b^2.$$

A straight line tangent to a curve at infinity is called an **asymptote**. The asymptotes to the hyperbola with its centre at (α, β) and its transverse axis **horizontal** are

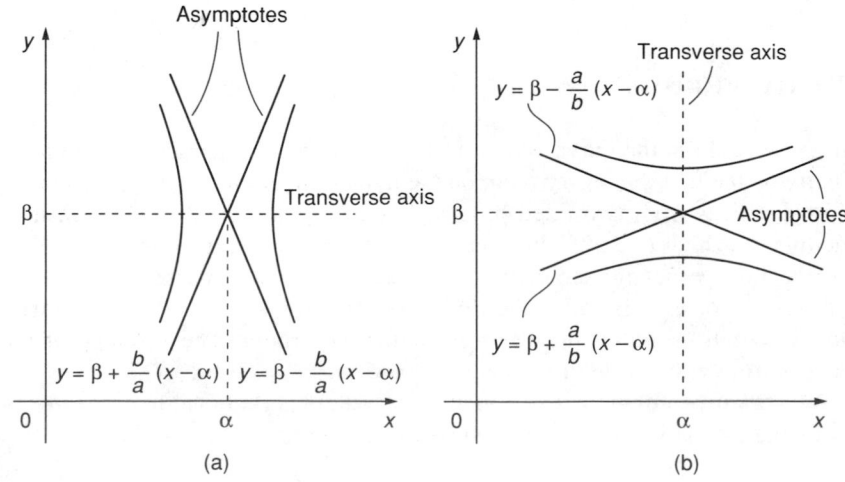

Fig. 15

$$y = \beta \pm \frac{b}{a}(x - \alpha);$$

the asymptotes to the hyperbola with its centre at (α, β) and its transverse axis **vertical** are

$$y = \beta \pm \frac{a}{b}(x - \alpha).$$

These asymptotes are shown in Fig. 15.

THE PARABOLA

The **parabola** is a curve of the type shown in Fig. 16. It is characterized geometrically by the fact that points on a parabola are such that their distance from a fixed point F called the **focus** equals their perpendicular distance from a fixed straight line called the **directrix**. The point A on the parabola closest to the directrix is called the **vertex** and the line through A perpendicular to the diretrix is called **axis**.

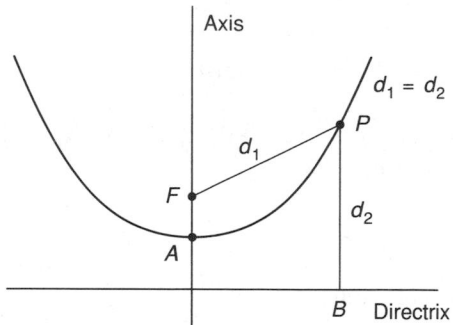

Fig. 16

The **standard form** of the equation of a parabola with its axis **vertical**, its vertex at the point (α, β), its focus at the point $(\alpha, \beta + a)$ and its directrix along the line $y = \beta - a$ is

$$(x - \alpha)^2 = 4a(y - \beta).$$

The vertex of this parabola will be at the bottom (**concave-up**) if $a > 0$ and at the top (**concave-down**) if $a < 0$. The corresponding **standard form** of the equation of a parabola with its axis **horizontal**, its vertex at the point (α, β), its focus at the point $(\alpha + a, \beta)$ and its directrix along the line $x = \alpha - a$ is

$$(y - \beta)^2 = 4a(x - \alpha).$$

The vertex of this parabola will lie to the left (**concave to the right**) if $a > 0$

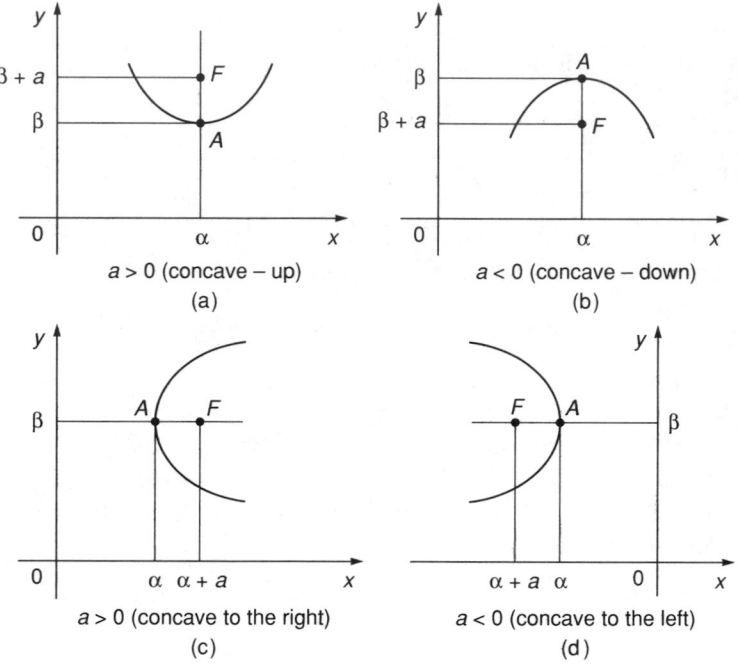

Fig. 17

and to the right (**concave to the left**) if $a < 0$. Typical examples of these parabolas are shown in Fig. 17.

Example 3.2

(i)   Show that the equation

$$x^2 + y^2 - 4x + 6y + 9 = 0$$

represents a circle, and find its centre and radius.

(ii) Find the centre and semi-major and minor axes of the ellipse with the equation

$$4x^2 + y^2 + 8x + 4y - 8 = 0.$$

(iii) Find the centre of the hyperbola with the equation

$$9x^2 - 4y^2 - 18x - 8y - 31 = 0$$

Determine whether its axis is horizontal or vertical, write its equation in standard form and determine its asymptotes.

(iv) Determine whether the axis of the parabola with equation

$$x^2 - 6x - 8y + 17 = 0$$

is horizontal or vertical. Write down the standard form of the equation, and hence find the location of its vertex and focus.

Solution

(i)   Using our previous notation we see that $a = -4$, $b = 6$ and $c = 9$.
Now

$$a^2 + b^2 - 4c = 16 + 36 - 36 = 16 > 0,$$

so this is the equation of a circle. Its centre lies at (α, β) where

$$\alpha = -\frac{1}{2}(-4) = 2 \text{ and } \beta = -\frac{1}{2}(6) = -3.$$

The radius

$$R = \left[\frac{1}{4}(a^2 + b^2) - 4c\right]^{1/2} = 2.$$

(ii)   To find the centre at point (α, β) and the positive constants a and b we start by expanding the standard equation for an ellipse with its major axis **horizontal**

$$\frac{(x - \alpha)^2}{a^2} + \frac{(y - \beta)^2}{b^2} = 1$$

to obtain as our reference equation

$$x^2 + \left[\frac{a^2}{b^2}\right]y^2 - 2\alpha x - 2\beta\left(\frac{a^2}{b^2}\right)y + \alpha^2 + \beta^2\left(\frac{a^2}{b^2}\right) - a^2 = 0.$$

If it turns out that the major axis of the ellipse in question is **vertical** we will find that $b > a$.

If necessary, we now rewrite the given equation in the same form as the reference equation, making the coefficient of x^2 equal to 1. We will then compare corresponding coefficients in both the reference equation and the given equation.

As the coefficient of x^2 is 4, we divide the equation by 4 to obtain

$$x^2 + \frac{1}{4}y^2 + 2x + y - 2 - 0.$$

A comparison of corresponding coefficients gives

coefficient of y^2 : $\dfrac{a^2}{b^2} = \dfrac{1}{4}$,   (A)

coefficient of x : $-2\alpha = 2$,   (B)

coefficient of y : $-2\beta\left(\dfrac{a^2}{b^2}\right) = 1$,   (C)

constants: $\alpha^2 + \beta^2\left(\dfrac{a^2}{b^2}\right) - a^2 = -2$.   (D)

From (B) we find $\alpha = -1$; from (A) and (C) we find $\beta = -2$, and from (D) we find

$$(-1)^2 + (-2)^2 \left(\frac{1}{4}\right) - a^2 = -2 \text{ or } a^2 = 4.$$

As the semi-axes are both positive, it follows from this that $a = 2$, and after combining this result with (A), that $b = 4$

Thus the ellipse has its centre at $(-1, -2)$, and when written in standard form its equation is

$$\frac{(x+1)^2}{2^2} + \frac{(y+2)^2}{4^2} = 1.$$

By convention, the semi-major axis is greater than the semi-minor axis, so the equation is seen to be in the second standard form, corresponding to the case in which the major axis is vertical. Thus the semi-major axis is of length 4 and the semi-minor axis is of length 2.

(iii) We start, as in (ii), by expanding the standard equation of a hyperbola with its axis horizontal

$$\frac{(x-\alpha)^2}{a^2} - \frac{(y-\beta)^2}{b^2} = 1$$

in the form

$$x^2 - \left(\frac{a^2}{b^2}\right)y^2 - 2\alpha x + 2\beta \left(\frac{a^2}{b^2}\right)y + \alpha^2 - \beta^2 \left(\frac{a^2}{b^2}\right) - a^2 = 0.$$

This is now our reference equation. If a^2 and b^2 turn out to have opposite signs (which is in reality impossible), the above reference equation must be replaced by the corresponding one derived from the standard equation of a hyperbola with its axis vertical.

As in the given equation the coefficient of x^2 is 9, we must first divide the equation by 9 to bring it into the form of the reference equation in which the coefficient of x^2 is 1, and as a result obtain

$$x^2 - \frac{4}{9}y^2 - 2x - \frac{8}{9}y - \frac{31}{9} = 0.$$

A comparison of the coefficients of corresponding terms then gives

coefficient of $y^2 : \dfrac{a^2}{b^2} = \dfrac{4}{9}$,   (E)

coefficient of $x : -2\alpha = -2$,   (F)

coefficient of $y : 2\beta \left(\dfrac{a^2}{b^2}\right) = -\dfrac{8}{9}$,   (G)

constants: $\alpha^2 + \beta^2 \left(\dfrac{a^2}{b^2}\right) - a^2 = -\dfrac{31}{9}$.   (H)

From (F) we have $\alpha = 1$; from (E) and (G) we find $\beta = -1$, and from (H) we find

$$1^2 - (-1)^2 \frac{4}{9} - a^2 = -\frac{31}{9}, \text{ or } a^2 = 4,$$

and after combining this result with (E) we see that $b^2 = 9$. The signs of a^2 and b^2 are the same, so the axis of the hyperbola is horizontal. As, by convention, a and b are positive, it follows that $a = 2$ and $b = 3$. The standard form of the equation is thus

$$\frac{(x-1)^2}{4} - \frac{(y+1)^2}{9} = 1,$$

and substituting for a and b in the equations for the asymptotes to a hyperbola with its axis horizontal gives

$$y = -1 \pm \frac{3}{2}(x-1).$$

(iv) A parabola with its axis vertical will contain a term in x^2 and one with its axis horizontal a term in y^2. As the equation in question is quadratic in x the axis must be vertical.

Expanding the standard form of the equation of a parabola with its axis vertical

$$(x - \alpha)^2 = 4a(y - \beta),$$

we obtain

$$x^2 - 2\alpha x - 4ay + \alpha^2 + 4a\beta = 0.$$

Comparing corresponding coefficients in this equation and in

$$x^2 - 6x - 8y + 17 = 0$$

(we can do this since the coefficient of x^2 is 1 in both cases) gives

coefficients of x : $-2\alpha = -6$,   (I)

coefficients of y : $-4a = -8$,   (J)

constants: $\alpha^2 + 4a\beta = 17$.   (K)

From (I) we find $\alpha = 3$; from (J) $a = 2$, and from (K) $\beta = 1$, so the standard form of the equation of the parabola is

$$(x - 3)^2 = 8(y - 1).$$

As $\alpha = 3$ and $\beta = 1$ the vertex is at (3, 1), and as $a = 3$ the focus is at (3, 4). The parabola is concave-up because the axis is vertical and $a = 3 > 0$

▲

ASYMPTOTES

As already stated, an **asymptote** is a straight line which is tangent to a curve at infinity. Not all curves have asymptotes, but some of the simplest ones to find belong to rational functions.

A function of the form

$$y = \frac{P(x)}{Q(x)},$$

where $P(x)$, $Q(x)$ are polynomials, is called a **rational function**.

1 A rational function will have a **vertical asymptote** at any point $x = c$ for which $Q(c) = 0$ but $P(c) \neq 0$. Thus c is a **zero** of $Q(x)$ or, equivalently, a **root** of $Q(x) = 0$.

2 A rational function will have a **horizontal asymptote** if $P(x)/Q(x)$ tends to a constant value as x becomes large.

3 A rational function will have an **oblique asymptote** of the form $y = mx + c$, with m finite and non-zero, if the degree of $P(x)$ exceeds the degree of $Q(x)$ by 1. Oblique asymptotes of rational functions are best found by long division.

Example 3.3

Find the asymptotes of

(i) $y = \dfrac{3}{x^2 + x - 2}$;

(ii) $y = \dfrac{4x - 1}{2x + 3}$;

(iii) $y = \dfrac{2 + x + 2x^2 - x^3}{x^2 + x}$.

Solution

(i) $y = \dfrac{3}{x^2 + x - 2} = \dfrac{3}{(x + 2)(x - 1)}$.

The denominator vanishes for $x = -2$ and $x = 1$, but the numerator is non-zero at these points (it is constant), so $x = -2$ and $x = 1$ are vertical asymptotes to the graph of this function. As y approaches the value zero when x is large and positive or large and negative, it follows that the line $y = 0$ is a horizontal asymptote to the graph of this function. Figure 18(a) shows both the graph of this function and its asymptotes.

(ii)   The denominator of

$$y = \frac{4x - 1}{2x + 3}$$

vanishes when $x = -3/2$, at which point the numerator becomes -7. Thus $x = -3/2$ is a vertical asymptote to the graph of this function. Rewriting the function in the form

$$y = \frac{4 - (1/x)}{2 + (3/x)}$$

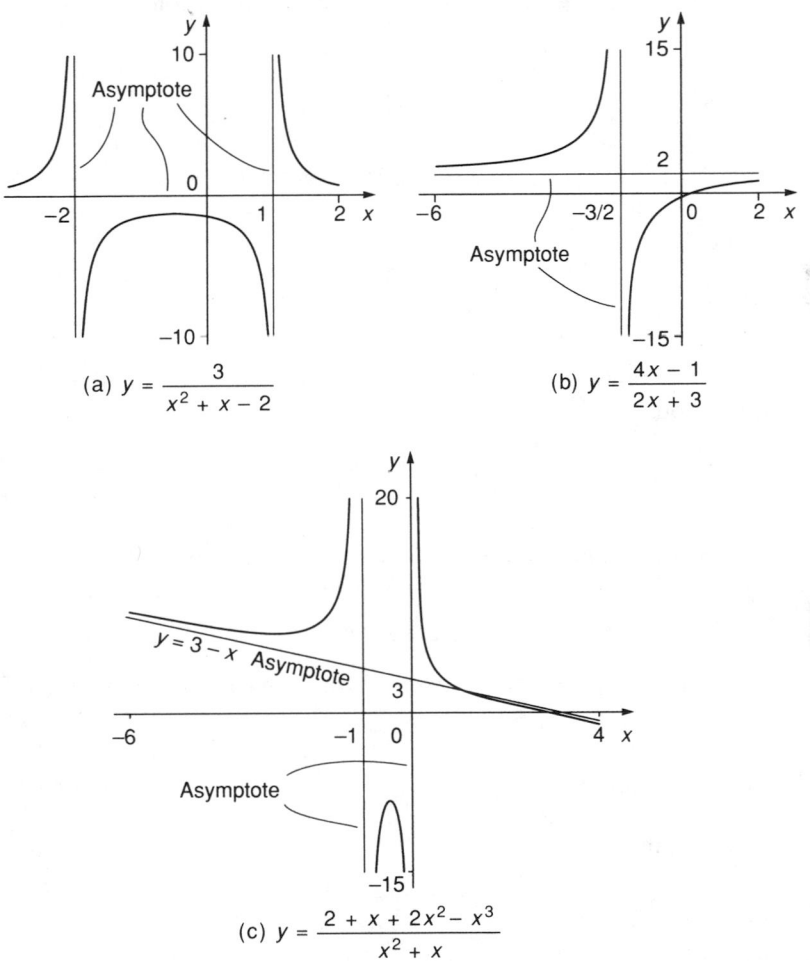

(a) $y = \dfrac{3}{x^2 + x - 2}$

(b) $y = \dfrac{4x - 1}{2x + 3}$

(c) $y = \dfrac{2 + x + 2x^2 - x^3}{x^2 + x}$

Fig. 18

shows that y approaches the value 2 as x becomes large and positive or large and negative. Thus this function has the line $y = 2$ as a horizontal asymptote. The graph of this function together with its asymptotes is shown in Fig. 18(b)

(iii) Writing the function in the form

$$y = \frac{2 + x + 2x^2 - x^3}{x(x + 1)}$$

shows the denominator vanishes when $x = 0$ and when $x = -1$; these are vertical asymptotes to the graph of this function.

The degree of the numerator is 3 and that of the denominator is 2, so there will also be an oblique asymptote.

Dividing the denominator into the numerator using long division gives

$$
\begin{array}{r}
-x+3 \\
x^2 + x \overline{\smash{\big)}\ -x^3 + 2x^2 + x + 2} \\
\underline{-x^3 - x^2} \\
3x^2 + x \\
\underline{3x^2 + 3x} \\
-2x + 2
\end{array}
$$

and so

$$y = -x + 3 - \frac{2(x-1)}{x^2 + x}.$$

When the numerator and denominator of the last term are divided by x^2 this becomes

$$y = -x + 3 - \frac{2[(1/x) - (1/x^2)]}{1 + (1/x)}.$$

We see from this that when x becomes large and positive or large and negative the last term tends to zero, and so the oblique asymptote is

$$y = -x + 3.$$

The graph of this function together with its asymptotes is shown in Fig. 18(c). ▲

Example 3.4

Find the asymptotes of

$$y = \frac{2x^2 + 4x + 5}{|x|}.$$

Solution
The denominator vanishes when $x = 0$, for which value the numerator becomes 5, so $x = 0$ is a *vertical asymptote* to the graph of this function. The degree of the numerator exceeds the degree of the denominator by 1, so there will be an oblique asymptote.
If $x > 0$, then $|x| = x$, so after division by x we see that

$$y = 2x + 4 + \frac{5}{x}.$$

The oblique asymptote for large positive x is thus

$$y = 2x + 4.$$

If $x < 0$, then $|x| = -x$, so after division by $-x$ we see that

$$y = -2x - 4 - \frac{5}{x}.$$

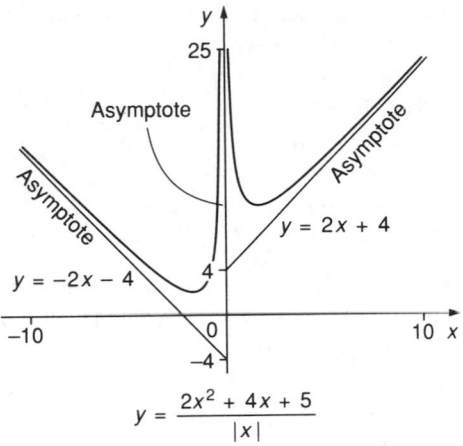

$$y = \frac{2x^2 + 4x + 5}{|x|}$$

Fig. 19

The oblique asymptote for large negative x is seen to be

$$y = -2x - 4.$$

This is an example of a function with different oblique asymptotes for positive and negative x. The graph of the function together with its asymptotes is shown in Fig. 19. ▲

PROBLEMS 3

Find the centre and radius of each of the following circles and write its equation in standard form
1. $x^2 + y^2 + 6x - 6y + 2 = 0$.
2. $x^2 + y - 4x - 8y + 16 = 0$.
3. $x^2 + y^2 - 4x - 8y + 11 = 0$.
4. $x^2 + y^2 + 4x + 6y + 4 = 0$.
5. $x^2 + y^2 - 8x + 2y + 16 = 0$.
6. $x^2 + y^2 + 4x - 6y - 12 = 0$.

Find the centre of each of the following ellipses, the semi-major and minor axes, write its equation in standard form and determine whether the major axis is horizontal or vertical.
7. $9x^2 + 4y^2 - 36x + 8y + 4 = 0$.
8. $x^2 + 4y^2 + 2x - 16y + 1 = 0$.
9. $x^2 + 9y^2 + 54y + 80 = 0$.
10. $x^2 + 4y^2 - 2x + 16y + 13 = 0$.
11. $16x^2 + 9y^2 - 32x + 36y - 92 = 0$.
12. $4x^2 + y^2 + 32x + 4y + 60 = 0$.

Find the centre of each of the following hyperbolas, write its equation in standard form, determine whether its axis is horizontal or vertical and write down the equations of its asymptotes.

13. $9x^2 - 4y^2 - 18x - 16y - 43 = 0$.

14. $9x^2 - y^2 + 36x - 2y + 26 = 0$.

15. $4x^2 - 9y^2 + 8x + 54y - 41 = 0$.

16. $4x^2 - y^2 + 24x + 2y + 51 = 0$.

17. $4x^2 - 9y^2 - 16x - 72y - 164 = 0$.

18. $4x^2 - y^2 + 8x - 2y + 7 = 0$.

Find whether the axis of each of the following parabolas is horizontal or vertical, write its equation in standard form, locate its vertex and focus and state the direction in which it is concave.

19. $x^2 - 4x + 8y + 20 = 0$.

20. $y^2 - 12x - 6y + 21 = 0$.

21. $y^2 + 4x + 8y + 24 = 0$.

22. $x^2 - 6x - 12y + 69 = 0$.

23. $x^2 + 6x + 8y + 1 = 0$.

24. $y^2 - 12x - 6y + 9 = 0$.

Find the asymptotes associated with each of the following functions.

25. $y = \dfrac{1 - 4x}{1 + 2x}$.

26. $y = \dfrac{4x - 3x^3}{2x^2 + 5}$.

27. $y = \dfrac{x^2}{x + 1}$.

28. $y = \dfrac{5x + 3}{3 - 2x}$.

29. $y = \dfrac{x^3}{x^4 - 6x^2 + 8}$.

30. $y = x + \dfrac{x^2}{x^2 - 1}$.

31. $y = \dfrac{2x^2}{1 + |x|}$.

Polar coordinates   4

The **plane polar coordinates** (r, θ) identify the position of a point P in the plane by giving its **radial distance** r from a fixed **origin** O (the **pole**), and the **angle** θ measured anticlockwise in radians from a fixed reference line through O called the **polar axis**, to the radial line joining the origin to point P. The polar coordinate system is shown in Fig. 20. This figure shows also that the polar angle θ is not unique, because for any given r and θ, the point $P(r, \theta)$ will be the same as the points $P(r, \theta \pm 2n\pi)$ for $n = 0, 1, 2, \dots$. To remove this ambiguity it is usual to confine θ to the interval $0 \leqslant \theta \leqslant 2\pi$.

The radial distance r is, by convention, taken to be **positive**. Thus the polar coordinate system identifies the location of a point in the plane by means of circles centred on O on which $r =$ constant but around which θ varies from 0 to 2π, and radial lines through O on which $\theta =$ constant but $r > 0$ varies. This

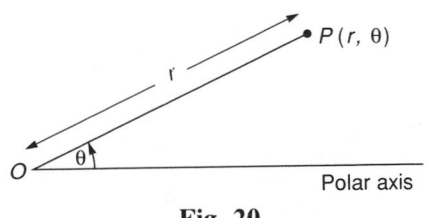

Fig. 20

coordinate system of concentric circles and radial lines is shown in Fig. 21, on which the point $P(3, \pi/4)$ is seen to lie in the first quadrant, the point $Q(2, 4\pi/3)$ in the third quadrant and the point $R(4, 7\pi/4)$ in the fourth quadrant.

As the **positive** sense of increase of θ is **anticlockwise**, angles measured **clockwise** from the polar axis must be regarded as **negative**. Thus in Fig. 21 the point $R(4, 7\pi/4)$ in the fourth quadrant is also the point $R(4, -\pi/4)$.

It is often necessary to convert between polar and Cartesian coordinates. This is accomplished by making the origins in both planes coincide and aligning the polar axis with the x-axis. The connection between the point $P(x, y)$ in Cartesian coordinates and the same point $P(r, \theta)$ in plane polar coordinates, and conversely, can be seen from Fig. 22.

Polar coordinates to Cartesian coordinates:

$$x = r \cos \theta, \quad y = r \sin \theta.$$

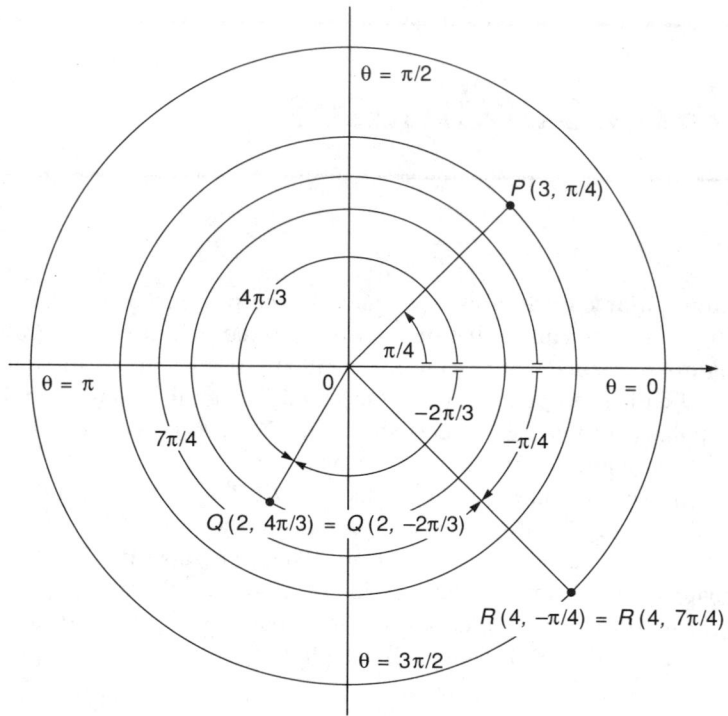

Fig. 21

Cartesian coordinates to polar coordinates:

$$r^2 = x^2 + y^2, \quad \tan \theta = \frac{y}{x}.$$

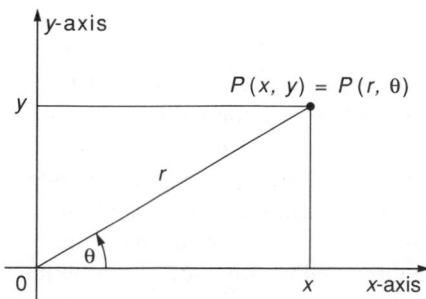

Fig. 22

When determining θ the signs of x and y must be taken into account to ensure that the angle is assigned to the correct quadrant.

Example 4.1

(i)   Find the Cartesian coordinates of the point with the polar coordinates $(3, 5\pi/6)$.

(ii) Find the Cartesian coordinates of the point with the polar coordinates $(7, -\pi/4)$.

(iii) Find the polar coordinates of the point with the Cartesian coordinates $(4, 4\sqrt{3})$.

(iv) Find the polar coordinates of the point with the Cartesian coordinates $(2\sqrt{3}, -2)$.

Solution

(i) $x = 3 \cos \dfrac{5\pi}{6} = -\dfrac{3\sqrt{3}}{2}, \quad y = 3 \sin \dfrac{5\pi}{6} = \dfrac{3}{2}.$

(ii) $x = 7 \cos \left[\dfrac{-\pi}{4} \right] = \dfrac{7}{\sqrt{2}}, \quad y = 7 \sin \left[\dfrac{-\pi}{4} \right] = \dfrac{-7}{\sqrt{2}}.$

(iii) $r^2 = 4^2 + (4\sqrt{3})^2$ so $r = 8$. Both x and y are positive, so the angle lies in the first quadrant hence

$$\tan \theta = \frac{y}{x} = \frac{4\sqrt{3}}{4} = \sqrt{3},$$

so that

$$\theta = \pi/3.$$

The point with Cartesian coordinates $(4, 4\sqrt{3})$ is thus seen to have the polar coordinates $(8, \pi/3)$.

(iv) $r^2 = (2\sqrt{3})^2 + (-2)^2$, so $r = 4$. In this case x is positive and y is negative, so the angle must lie in the fourth quadrant. Thus

$$\tan \theta = \frac{(-2)}{2\sqrt{3}} \quad \text{and so} \quad \tan \theta = -\frac{1}{\sqrt{3}},$$

from which it follows that $\theta = -\pi/6$ or, equivalently, $\theta = 11\pi/6$.   ▲

Sometimes the polar representation of a function is more convenient when drawing its graph than the Cartesian representation. This is illustrated by the next example.

Example 4.2

Use polar coordinates to draw the graph of the **lemniscate**
$$(x^2 + y^2)^2 = a^2(x^2 - y^2).$$

Solution

Setting $x = r \cos \theta$ and $y = r \sin \theta$ the equation becomes
$$(r^2)^2 = a^2 \, | \, r^2 \cos^2 \theta - r^2 \sin^2 \theta \, |$$

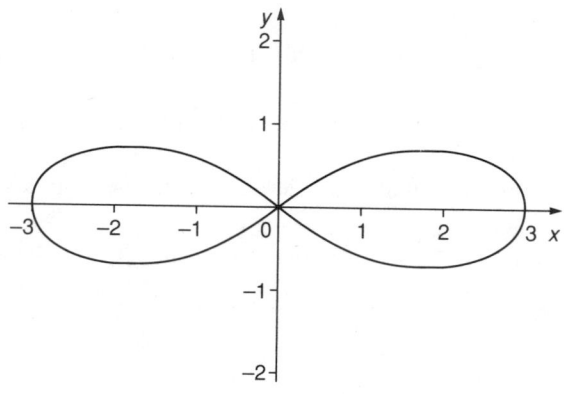

Fig. 23

or

$$r^2 = a^2 |\cos^2 \theta - \sin^2 \theta|,$$

where the absolute value is necessary because the left-hand side is non-negative. This can be further simplified by using the trigonometric identity $\cos 2\theta = \cos^2 \theta - \sin^2 \theta$, for it then reduces to

$$r^2 = a^2 |\cos 2\theta|.$$

The graph of a lemniscate for which $a = 3$ is shown in Fig. 23.   ▲

PROBLEMS 4

1. Find the Cartesian coordinates of the following points with the polar coordinates

   (a) $\left[3, \dfrac{\pi}{4} \right]$; (b) $\left[3, \dfrac{3\pi}{2} \right]$; (c) $\left[3.5, \dfrac{5\pi}{6} \right]$;

   (d) $\left[6, \dfrac{15\pi}{8} \right]$.

2. Find the polar coordinates of the following points with the Cartesian coordinates

   (a) $(4.8446, -1.2370)$; (b) $(1.75, 3.0311)$;

   (c) $(-1.8478, 0.7654)$; (d) $(-2.7716, -1.1481)$.

   Find the Cartesian forms of the following polar representations of curves.

3. $r \cos \theta = a$.

4. $r = 2a \sin \theta$.

5. $r^2 \sin 2\theta = 2k$.

6. $r \sin\left[\theta + \dfrac{\pi}{4}\right] = a\sqrt{2}.$

7. $r = a(1 + \cos\theta).$

8. $r = \dfrac{9}{5 - 4\cos\theta}.$

9. $r = \dfrac{9}{4 - 5\cos\theta}.$

10. $r = \dfrac{3}{1 - \cos\theta}.$

11. Sketch the **cardioid** with the polar representation
$$r = a(1 - \cos\theta).$$

12. Sketch the **spiral of Archimedes** with the polar representation
$$r = k\theta \quad (k > 0).$$

13. Sketch the **parabolic spiral** with the polar representation
$$r^2 = \theta .$$

14. Sketch the **four petal rose** with the polar representation
$$r = \sin 4\theta .$$

5   Mathematical induction

The name **mathematical induction** is given to a method used to show that a mathematical proposition which depends only on an integer n is either true or false. If we denote the proposition by P_n, mathematical induction involves the following steps.

1. Show, if possible, that P_n is true for some integer n, say n_0. This step is carried out by substituting $n = n_0$ into the proposition P_n and showing P_{n_0} to be true.
2. Show, if possible, that if P_n is assumed to be true for an arbitrary integer $n = k > n_0$, then it follows that P_{n+1} is also true. This is the difficult step when using mathematical induction.
3. If it has been shown in step 2 that property P_{n+1} follows from P_n, then since P_{n_0} is true, it follows that P_n is true for all $n \geqslant n_0$.
4. If in step 2 it can be shown that property P_{n+1} does not follow from property P_n, then the proposition P_n is false.

Example 5.1

Prove by mathematical induction that
$$3 + 5 + 7 + 9 + \ldots + (2n + 1) = n(n + 2).$$

Solution
The proposition P_n is that the sum of the n numbers $3, 5, 7, 9, \ldots, 2n + 1$ is equal to $n(n + 2)$.
Step 1
     The first of the sequence of n numbers to be summed is 3, and setting $n = 1$ in P_n, that is in the expression $n(n + 2)$, gives 3. Thus P_n is true for $n = 1$. Hence the 'sum' of the first of the sequence of numbers is given by the formula $n(n + 2)$ by setting $n = 1$, so in step 1 we may set $n_0 = 1$.
Step 2
     In this step we must prove that if P_n is true for $n = k > 1$, then P_{n+1} is also true. If P_k is true the sum of the first $k + 1$ terms is
$$\underbrace{\frac{k(k + 2)}{\text{sum of first } k \text{ terms}}} + \underbrace{\frac{(2k + 3)}{(k + 1)\text{th term}}} = k^2 + 4k + 3 = (k + 1)(k + 3).$$

However, if we replace k by $k + 1$ in P_k, the sum of the first $k + 1$ terms is seen to be $(k + 1)(k + 3)$ in agreement with the result just obtained by adding the $(k + 1)$th term to the sum of the first k terms. Thus, if proposition P_k is true, it implies the truth of proposition P_{k+1}, and so the truth of step 2 has been established.

Step 3

As proposition P_1 is true, and the truth of proposition P_n implies the truth of proposition P_{n+1}, it follows that P_n is true for $n = 1, 2, 3, \ldots$, and the result is established for all positive integers n.   ▲

Example 5.2

Prove by mathematical induction that for any positive integer n the number $2^{n+2} \times 3^n + 5n - 4$ is divisible by 25.

Solution

The proposition P_n is equivalent to the statement that $2^{n+2} \times 3^n + 5n - 4$ contains a factor 25 for $n = 1, 2, \ldots$.

Step 1

Setting $n = 1$ we have

$$2^3 \times 3 + 5 - 4 = 25,$$

so the expression is divisible by 25 when $n = 1$, and hence we may set $n_0 = 1$.

Step 2

If we assume P_n to be true for some $n = k > 1$, we need to show that it implies P_{n+1} is also true (i.e. contains a factor 25). Replacing k by $k + 1$ to find the form of P_{k+1} we have

$$2^{(k+1)+2} \times 3^{k+1} + 5(k+1) - 4 = 6 \times 2^{k+2} \times 3^k + 5k + 1.$$

To relate this result to P_k we use the standard device of adding a convenient quantity and then subtracting it again. In this case we add and then subtract the number $25k - 24$ to obtain

$$6 \times 2^{k+2} \times 3^k + 5k + 1 + (25k - 24) - (25k - 24)$$

$$= 6(2^{k+2} \times 3^k + 5k - 4) - 25(k - 1).$$

However, by hypothesis the bracketed expression in the first term is divisible by 25, and the second term is obviously divisible by 25, so their sum is also divisible by 25, and hence proposition P_{k+1} is also true.

Step 3

As proposition P_1 is true, and proposition P_n implies proposition P_{n+1}, the result is true for $n = 1, 2, \ldots$.   ▲

Example 5.3

Prove by mathematical induction that for some n_0 and all integers $n \geqslant n_0$

$$3^n > 6n + 1.$$

Solution

Proposition P_n is equivalent to the assertion that for $n \geqslant n_0$ the inequality $3^n - 6n - 1 > 0$ holds.

Step 1

Direct substitution into the inequality shows it to be false for $n = 1$ and $n = 2$, but to be true for $n = 3$. Thus if we set $n_0 = 3$, proposition P_3 is true.

Step 2

We now assume P_n is true for some $n = k > 3$, so that

$$3^k - 6k - 1 > 0.$$

Consider the expression

$$D = 3^{k+1} - 6(k + 1) - 1.$$

This may be rewritten as

$$D = 3 \times 3^k - 6k - 7,$$

and by adding and subtracting $4 - 12k$ this becomes

$$D = 3[3^k - 6k - 1] + 12k - 4.$$

Now if P_k is true, the first term in D is positive. The other terms are also positive because $k \geqslant 3$, and so

$$D = 3^{k+1} - 6(k + 1) - 1 > 0.$$

However, this is simply proposition P_{k+1} so we have established that P_k implies P_{k+1}, but P_3 is true so the proposition is true for every integer $n \geqslant 3$.   ▲

Example 5.4

Use mathematical induction to prove the **generalized triangle inequality**

$$\left| a_1 + a_2 + \ldots + a_n \right| \leqslant \left| a_1 \right| + \left| a_2 \right| + \ldots + \left| a_n \right|,$$

with $a_1, a_2, \ldots, a_n$ any n real numbers.

Solution

We take the proposition P_n to be that

$$\left| a_1 + a_2 + \ldots + a_n \right| \leqslant \left| a_1 \right| + \left| a_2 \right| + \ldots + \left| a_n \right|.$$

Step 1

We know from the triangle inequality that

$$\left| a_1 + a_2 \right| \leqslant \left| a_1 \right| + \left| a_2 \right|,$$

so P_2 is true and we may set $n_0 = 2$.

Step 2

Assume P_n to be true for $n = k > 2$, so that

$$\left| a_1 + a_2 + \ldots + a_n \right| \leqslant \left| a_1 \right| + \left| a_2 \right| + \ldots + \left| a_k \right|.$$

We must now prove that this remains true when k is replaced by $k + 1$. Setting $a_1 + a_2 + \ldots + a_k = b$ we know from the triangle inequality that

$$\left| b + a_{k+1} \right| \leq |b| + \left| a_{k+1} \right|,$$

but as P_k is true

$$|b| \leq \left| a_1 \right| + \left| a_2 \right| + \ldots + \left| a_k \right|,$$

so

$$\left| a_1 + a_2 + \ldots + a_k + a_{k+1} \right| \leq \left| a_1 \right| + \left| a_2 \right| + \ldots + \left| a_k \right| + \left| a_{k+1} \right|.$$

This establishes the fact that P_k implies P_{k+1}.

Step 3

As proposition P_2 is true, and proposition P_n implies proposition P_{n+1}, it follows that P_n is true for $n \geq 2$.   ▲

PROBLEMS 5

Prove each of the following results by means of mathematical induction.

1. $1 + 3 + 5 + 7 + \ldots + (2n - 1) = n^2$.

2. $1 \cdot 2 + 2 \cdot 5 + 3 \cdot 8 + \ldots + n(3n - 1) = n^2(n + 1)$.

3. $1^3 + 2^3 + 3^3 + \ldots + n^3 = \left[\dfrac{n(n + 1)}{2} \right]^2$.

4. $\dfrac{1}{1 \cdot 3} + \dfrac{1}{3 \cdot 5} + \dfrac{1}{5 \cdot 7} + \ldots + \dfrac{1}{(2n - 1)(2n + 1)} = \dfrac{n}{2n + 1}$.

5. $\dfrac{1}{1 \cdot 4} + \dfrac{1}{4 \cdot 7} + \dfrac{1}{7 \cdot 10} + \ldots + \dfrac{1}{(3n - 2)(3n + 1)} = \dfrac{n}{3n + 1}$.

6. $\dfrac{1}{1 \cdot 6} + \dfrac{1}{6 \cdot 11} + \dfrac{1}{11 \cdot 16} + \ldots + \dfrac{1}{(5n - 4)(5n + 1)} = \dfrac{n}{5n + 1}$.

7. $1 + \dfrac{1}{3} + \dfrac{1}{3^2} + \dfrac{1}{3^3} + \ldots + \dfrac{1}{3^n} = \dfrac{3^{n+1} - 1}{2 \times 3^n}$.

8. Prove by mathematical induction that $6^{2n} - 1$ is divisible by 35.

9. Prove by mathematical induction that $6^{2n} + 3^{n+2} + 3^n$ is divisible by 11.

10. Prove by mathematical induction that $3^{2n+1} + 40n - 67$ is divisible by 64.

11. Prove by mathematical induction that

$$\left[1 - \frac{1}{2} \right]\left[1 - \frac{1}{3} \right]\left[1 - \frac{1}{4} \right] \ldots \left[1 + \frac{1}{n + 1} \right] = \frac{1}{n + 1}.$$

12. Prove by mathematical induction that

$$\left[1 - \frac{1}{4} \right]\left[1 - \frac{1}{9} \right]\left[1 - \frac{1}{10} \right] \ldots \left[1 - \frac{1}{(n + 1)^2} \right] = \frac{n + 2}{2n + 2}.$$

6   Binomial theorem

The **binomial theorem** is the name given to the expansion

$$(a + b)^\alpha = a^\alpha + \alpha a^{\alpha - 1}b + \frac{\alpha(\alpha - 1)}{2!}\, a^{\alpha - 2}b^2 + \frac{\alpha(\alpha - 1)(\alpha - 2)}{3!}\, a^{\alpha - 3}b^3 + \ldots ,$$

where α, a and b are real numbers with $a > 0$, and the number $n!$ $= 1 \cdot 2 \cdot 3 \ldots n$ is called **factorial** n. Thus $1! = 1$, $2! = 1 \times 2 = 2$, $3! = 1 \times 2 \times 3$ $= 6$, $4! = 1 \times 2 \times 3 \times 4 = 24$, and for convenience we define $0! = 1$.

When $\alpha = n$ is a positive integer this expansion is finite and contains $n + 1$ terms, and it takes the form

$$(a + b)^n = a^n + na^{n - 1}b + \frac{n(n - 1)}{2!}\, a^{n - 2}b^2 + \frac{n(n - 1)(n - 2)}{2!}\, a^{n - 3}b^3 + \ldots + b^n.$$

This is also written as

$$(a + b)^n = a^n + \binom{n}{1}a^{n - 1}b + \binom{n}{2}a^{n - 2}b^2 + \binom{n}{3}a^{n - 3}b^3 + \ldots + b^n$$

where the numbers

$$\binom{n}{r} = \frac{n!}{(n - r)!\, r!}$$

are called **binomial coefficients**; Table 1 gives some binomial coefficients.

Table 1   Binomial coefficients $\binom{n}{r}$

n	0	1	2	3	4	5	6
0	1						
1	1	1					
2	1	2	1				
3	1	3	3	1			
4	1	4	6	4	1		
5	1	5	10	10	5	1	
6	1	6	15	20	15	6	1

Using the **summation symbol** Σ this last result becomes

$$(a + b)^n = \sum_{r=0}^{n} \binom{n}{r} a^{n-r} b^r$$

where $\displaystyle\sum_{r=0}^{n}$ signifies that the terms which follow are to be added (summed) starting with $r = 0$ and ending with $r = n$. Thus, for example,

$$(a + b)^4 = \sum_{r=0}^{4} \binom{4}{r} a^{4-r} b^r$$

$$= \binom{4}{0} a^4 + \binom{4}{1} a^3 b + \binom{4}{2} a^2 b^2 + \binom{4}{3} ab^3 + \binom{4}{4} b^4,$$

so

$$(a + b)^4 = a^4 + 4a^3 b + 6a^2 b^2 + 4ab^3 + b^4,$$

where use has been made of the entries corresponding to $n = 4$ in the above table.

If k is any other real number, either positive or negative, the expansion of $(a + b)^k$ will not terminate after a finite number of terms and so will become an **infinite series**. Under these circumstances the expansion is only valid provided $|b/a| < 1$.

It is often more convenient to rewrite $(a + b)^k$ as

$$(a + b)^k = a^k (1 + b/a)^k,$$

to set $c = b/a$ and to expand $(1 + c)^k$ to obtain the result

$$(a + b)^k = a^k \left[1 + kc + \frac{k(k-1)}{2!} c^2 + \frac{k(k-1)(k-2)}{3!} c^3 + \dots \right],$$

after which the substitution $c = b/a$ is made, yielding

$$(a + b)^k = a^k \left[1 + k\left(\frac{b}{a}\right) + \frac{k(k-1)}{2!} \left(\frac{b}{a}\right)^2 + \frac{k(k-1)(k-2)}{3!} \left(\frac{b}{a}\right)^3 + \dots \right].$$

If the numerical constant b in $(a + b)^k$ is replaced by the variable x the binomial expansion provides a **power series** expansion of the function $(a + x)^k$ valid for $|x/a| < 1$.

Example 6.1

Expand

(i) $(1 + x)^{-1}$;

(ii) $(1 - x)^{-1}$;

(iii) $(1 + x)^{-1/2}$;

(iv) $(2 - x)^{1/2}$.

Solution

(i) $(1 + x)^{-1} = 1 - x + x^2 - x^3 + ...,$ for $|x| < 1$.

(ii) $(1 - x)^{-1} = 1 + x + x^2 + x^3 + ...,$ for $|x| < 1$.

(iii) $(1 + x)^{-1/2} = 1 - \dfrac{1}{2}x + \dfrac{1 \cdot 3}{2 \cdot 4}x^2 - \dfrac{1 \cdot 3 \cdot 5}{2 \cdot 4 \cdot 6}x^3 + ...,$ for $|x| < 1$.

(iv) $(2 - x)^{1/2} = 2^{1/2}\left[1 - \dfrac{x}{2}\right]^{1/2} = 2^{1/2}\left[1 - \dfrac{x}{4} - \dfrac{x^2}{32} - \dfrac{x^3}{128} - \dfrac{5}{2048}x^4 - ...\right]$ for

$|x/2| < 1.$ ▲

Binomial expansions may be added, subtracted, multiplied and divided to obtain the expansion of the corresponding combined function.

Example 6.2

Find the binomial expansion of

$$(1 + x)^{1/2} \quad \text{and} \quad (1 + 2x)^{1/2},$$

and hence find the expansion of

(i) $(1 + x)^{1/2} + (1 + 2x)^{1/2}$;

(ii) $(1 + x)^{1/2} - (1 + 2x)^{1/2}$;

(iii) $\dfrac{(1 + x)^{1/2}}{1 - x}$;

(iv) $(1 + x)^{1/2}(1 + 2x)^{1/2}$;

(v) $\dfrac{(1 + 2x)^{1/2} - 1}{3x}$

Solution

$$(1 + x)^{1/2} = 1 + \frac{x}{2} - \frac{x^2}{8} + \frac{x^3}{16} - \frac{5x^4}{128} + \frac{7x^5}{256} - ..., \quad \text{for} \quad |x| < 1.$$

$$(1 + 2x)^{1/2} = 1 + x - \frac{x^2}{2} + \frac{x^3}{2} - \frac{5x^4}{8} + \frac{7x^5}{8} - ..., \quad \text{for} \quad |x| < 1/2.$$

Notice that this second expansion could have been deduced from the first one by replacing x by $2x$.

(i) Adding corresponding terms gives

$$(1 + x)^{1/2} + (1 + 2x)^{1/2} = 2 + \frac{3x}{2} - \frac{5x^2}{8} + \frac{9x^3}{16} - \frac{85x^4}{128} + \frac{231x^5}{236} ..., \quad \text{for} \quad |x| < 1/2$$

Notice that the values of x for which this is true are obtained by finding the values of x common to both $|x| < 1$ and $|x| < 1/2$.

(ii)   Subtracting corresponding terms gives

$$(1+x)^{1/2} - (1+2x)^{1/2} = -\frac{x}{2} + \frac{3x^2}{8} - \frac{7x^3}{16} + \frac{75x^4}{128} - \frac{217x^5}{256} \dots, \quad \text{for} \quad |x| < 1/2.$$

(iii) To evaluate this we write it as the product

$$\frac{(1+x)^{1/2}}{1-x} = (1+x)^{1/2}(1-x)^{-1}$$

and multiply the two series on the right together taking the expansion of $(1-x)^{-1}$ from Example 6.1(ii) to obtain

$$(1+x)^{1/2}(1-x)^{-1} = \left[1 + \frac{x}{2} - \frac{x^2}{8} + \frac{x^3}{16} - \dots\right](1 + x + x^2 + x^3 + \dots).$$

Grouping terms we find

$$(1+x)^{1/2}(1-x)^{-1} = 1 + \left[1 + \frac{1}{2}\right]x + \left[1 + \frac{1}{2} - \frac{1}{8}\right]x^2 + \left[1 + \frac{1}{2} - \frac{1}{8} + \frac{1}{16}\right]x^3 + \dots,$$

and so

$$\frac{(1+x)^{1/2}}{1-x} = 1 + \frac{3}{2}x + \frac{11}{8}x^2 + \frac{23}{16}x^3 + \dots, \quad \text{for} \quad |x| < 1.$$

Here each series is valid for $|x| < 1$, so this is the condition on x for the product of the series.

(iv) Multiplying the series and grouping terms gives

$$(1+x)^{1/2}(1+2x)^{1/2} = \left[1 + \frac{x}{2} - \frac{x^2}{8} + \frac{x^3}{16} - \dots\right]\left[1 + x - \frac{x^2}{2} - \frac{x^3}{2} - \dots\right]$$

$$= 1 + \left[1 + \frac{1}{2}\right]x + \left[-\frac{1}{2} + \frac{1}{2} - \frac{1}{8}\right]x^2$$

$$+ \left[\frac{1}{2} - \frac{1}{4} - \frac{1}{8} + \frac{1}{16}\right]x^3 + \dots,$$

$$= 1 + \frac{3}{2}x - \frac{1}{8}x^2 + \frac{3}{16}x^3 + \dots, \quad \text{for} \quad |x| < 1/2.$$

(v) $$\frac{(1+2x)^{1/2} - 1}{3x} = \frac{\left[1 + x - \frac{x^2}{2} + \frac{x^3}{2} - \frac{5x^4}{8} + \dots\right] - 1}{3x}$$

$$= \frac{1}{3} - \frac{1}{6}x + \frac{1}{6}x^2 - \frac{5}{24}x^3 + \dots, \quad \text{for} \quad |x| < 1/2$$

▲

PROBLEMS 6

1. Verify by direct multiplication that
$$(1 + k)^5 = 1 + 5k + 10k^2 + 10k^3 + 5k^4 + k^5.$$

2. Verify that
$$\binom{7}{2} = 21, \quad \binom{8}{3} = 56, \quad \binom{5}{4} = 5, \quad \binom{9}{3} = 84.$$

3. Find the coefficients of the terms a^2b^7 and a^3b^6 in the expansion $(a - b)^9$.

4. Find the coefficients of the terms a^2b^6 and a^4b^4 in the expansion of $(a + b)^8$.

Verify the following binomial expansions.

5. $(1 - x)^{-1/2} = 1 + \dfrac{x}{2} + \dfrac{3x^2}{8} + \dfrac{5x^3}{16} + \dfrac{35x^4}{128} + \dots,$ for $|x| < 1$.

6. $\left(1 + \dfrac{1}{4} x^2\right)^{1/2} = 1 + \dfrac{x^2}{8} - \dfrac{x^4}{128} + \dfrac{x^6}{1024} - \dfrac{5x^8}{32\,768} + \dots,$ for $|x| < 2$.

7. $\left(1 + \dfrac{1}{2} x\right)^{-1/2} = 1 - \dfrac{x}{4} + \dfrac{3x^2}{32} - \dfrac{5x^3}{128} + \dfrac{35x^4}{2048} - \dots,$ for $|x| < 2$.

8. $\left(1 - \dfrac{1}{2} x^2\right)^{1/2} = 1 - \dfrac{x^2}{4} - \dfrac{x^4}{32} - \dfrac{x^6}{128} - \dfrac{5x^8}{2048} - \dots,$ for $|x| < \sqrt{2}$.

9. $\left(1 - \dfrac{3}{4} x\right)^{1/2} = 1 - \dfrac{3}{8} x - \dfrac{9}{128} x^2 - \dfrac{27}{1024} x^3 - \dfrac{405}{32\,768} x^4 - \dots,$ for $|x| < 4/3$.

10. $\left(1 - \dfrac{3}{2} x\right)^{3/4} = 1 - \dfrac{9}{8} x - \dfrac{27}{128} x^2 - \dfrac{135}{1024} x^3 - \dfrac{3645}{32\,768} x^4 - \dots,$ for $|x| < 2/3$.

11. $(2 - x)^{-1/2} = 2^{1/2} \left[\dfrac{1}{2} + \dfrac{x}{8} + \dfrac{3x^2}{64} + \dfrac{5x^3}{256} + \dots \right],$ for $|x| < 2$.

12. $(3 + 2x)^{-1/3} = 3^{2/3} \left[\dfrac{1}{3} - \dfrac{2x}{27} + \dfrac{8x^2}{243} - \dfrac{112x^3}{6561} + \dots \right],$ for $|x| < 3/2$.

13. $(2 - 5x)^{1/4} = 2^{1/4} \left[1 - \dfrac{5x}{8} - \dfrac{75x^2}{128} - \dfrac{875x^3}{1024} - \dots \right],$ for $|x| < 2/5$.

14. $(5 + x)^{-1/2} = \sqrt{5} \left[\dfrac{1}{5} - \dfrac{x}{50} + \dfrac{3x^2}{1000} - \dfrac{x^3}{2000} + \dfrac{7x^4}{80\,000} - \dots \right],$ for $|x| < 5$.

15. $(2 + 3x)^{-1} = \dfrac{1}{2} - \dfrac{3x}{4} + \dfrac{9x^2}{8} - \dfrac{27x^3}{16} + \dfrac{81x^4}{32} - \dots,$ for $|x| < 2/3$.

Verify the following results by means of a suitable combination of the appropriate binomial expansions.

16. $(1+x)^{1/2} - (1-x)^{1/2} = x + \dfrac{x^3}{8} + \dfrac{7x^2}{128} + \dots,$ for $|x| < 1.$

17. $(1-x^2)^{1/2} - (1-x)^{-1/2} = -\dfrac{x}{2} - \dfrac{7x^2}{8} - \dfrac{5x^3}{16} - \dfrac{51x^4}{128}.$

18. $(1-x)^{1/2}(1+x)^{-1/2} = 1 - x + \dfrac{x^2}{2} - \dfrac{x^3}{2} + \dfrac{3x^4}{8} - \dots,$ for $|x| < 1.$

19. $\left(1 + \dfrac{1}{2}x\right)^{1/4}(1+x)^{-1} = 1 - \dfrac{7x}{8} + \dfrac{109}{128}x^2 - \dfrac{865}{1024}x^3 + \dots,$ for $|x| < 1.$

20. $\dfrac{x^2}{(1+x)^{1/2}} = x^2 - \dfrac{x^3}{3} + \dfrac{3x^4}{8} - \dfrac{5x^5}{16} + \dots,$ for $|x| < 1.$

21. $\left[\dfrac{1+x}{1-x}\right]^{1/2} = 1 + x + \dfrac{x^2}{2} + \dfrac{x^3}{2} + \dots,$ for $|x| < 1.$

22. $\dfrac{(1-x^2)^{1/2}}{1+x} = 1 - x + \dfrac{x^2}{2} - \dfrac{x^3}{2} + \dots,$ for $|x| < 1.$

23. $\dfrac{(1+x)^{1/2} - 1}{x} = \dfrac{1}{2} - \dfrac{1}{8}x + \dfrac{1}{16}x^2 - \dfrac{5}{128}x^3 + \dots,$ for $|x| < 1.$

24. $\dfrac{(1-x^2)^{1/2} - 1}{x^2} = -\dfrac{1}{2} - \dfrac{1}{8}x^2 - \dfrac{1}{16}x^4 - \dots,$ for $|x| < 1.$

7   Combination of functions

New functions are often formed from simpler ones, say $f(x)$ and $g(x)$, by the algebraic processes of addition, subtraction, multiplication and division. When such functions are formed their domains of definition comprise those values of x which are common to the domain of definition (a, b) associated with $f(x)$ and the domain of definition (α, β) associated with $g(x)$. The domain of definition of the combined functions is illustrated diagrammatically in Fig. 24.

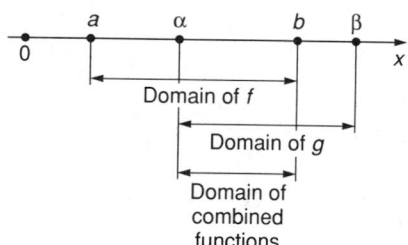

Sum: $f(x) + g(x)$

Difference: $f(x) - g(x)$

Product: $f(x)\, g(x)$

Quotient: $f(x)/g(x),\ g(x) \neq 0$

Fig. 24

Example 7.1

Given

$$f(x) = 4x^2 + 1,$$

$$g(x) = \sqrt{(9 - x^2)},$$

where each function is defined on the largest possible domain of definition, find

(i) $f(x) \pm g(x)$;

(ii) $f(x)\, g(x)$;

(iii) $f(x)/g(x)$,

stating in each case the domain of definition and range of the combined function.

Solution

Domain of $f(x)$ is $(-\infty, \infty)$.

Range of $f(x)$ is $[1, \infty)$.
Domain of $g(x)$ is $[-3, 3]$.
Range of $g(x)$ is $[0, 3]$.

(i)   Sum:

$$f(x) + g(x) = 4x^2 + 1 + \sqrt{(9 - x^2)}.$$

Domain $[-3, 3]$; because although $f(x)$ is defined for all x, $g(x)$ is only defined for $[-3, 3]$.

Range $[4, 37]$; this is most easily seen by graphing the function which has a parabola shape with the minimum value of 4 when $x = 0$ and a maximum value of 37 when $x = -3$ and $x = 3$.

Difference:

$$f(x) - g(x) = 4x^2 + 1 - \sqrt{(9 - x^2)}.$$

Domain $[-3, 3]$; for the reason given in (i).

Range $[-2, 3]$; this is most easily seen by graphing the function which has a parabola shape with the minimum value of -2 when $x = 0$ and a maximum value of 37 when $x = -3$ and $x = 3$.

(ii)   Product:

$$f(x)\, g(x) = (4x^2 + 1)\, \sqrt{(9 - x^2)}.$$

Domain $[-3, 3]$; for the reason given in (i).

Range $[0, 43]$; this is the approximate range estimated from the graph of $y = f(x)\, g(x)$ shown in Fig. 25(a).

(iii)   Quotient:

$$\frac{f(x)}{g(x)} = \frac{4x^2 + 1}{\sqrt{(9 - x^2)}}.$$

Domain $(-3, 3)$; for the reason given in (i).

Range $[1/3, \infty)$; this follows by examining the graph of $f(x)/g(x)$ shown in Fig. 25(b). The minimum value of $f(x)$ occurs at $x = 0$ when $f(0) = 1$ and the maximum value of $g(x)$ occurs at $x = 0$ when $g(0) = 3$, so $f(0)/g(0) = 1/3$. The lines $x = \pm 3$ are vertical asymptotes because $f(3) = f(-3) = 37$, but $g(3) = g(-3) = 0$.

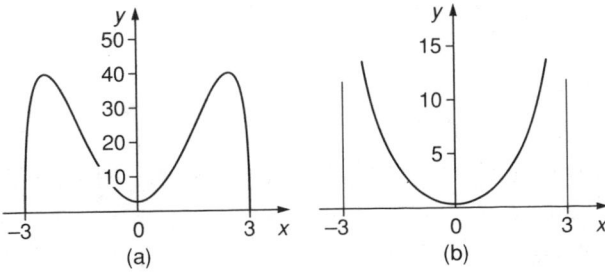

(a)   (b)

Fig. 25

A different and important way of combining functions is by replacing the independent variable x in $f(x)$ by the function $g(x)$ to form the function $f(g(x))$. This is loosely called a **function of a function**, but in stricter mathematical language it is called the **composition** of function f with g and it is then written

$$(f \circ g)(x),$$

with the same meaning as the more suggestive $f(g(x))$. The domain of $f(g(x))$ comprises all the x in the domain of g which cause $g(x)$ to lie in the domain of $f(x)$. Thus $f(g(x))$ can be formed provided the range of $g(x)$ lies in the domain of $f(x)$.

In general $f(g(x)) \neq g(f(x))$ and, indeed, when one of these functions of a function can be defined, the other may not even exist.

Example 7.2

Given that $f(x) = 3x - 1$ and $g(x) = x^2$, both defined for all real x, find $f(g(x))$ and $g(f(x))$.

Solution

$$f(g(x)) = 3(x^2) - 1 = 3x^2 - 1,$$

$$g(f(x)) = (3x - 1)^2 = 9x^2 - 6x + 1.$$

Both of these functions of a function (composite functions) are defined for all x, but

$$f(g(x)) \neq g(f(x)). \qquad \blacktriangle$$

Example 7.3

Consider $f(g(x))$ and $g(f(x))$ when

$$f(x) = x^2, \quad g(x) = \sqrt{(1 - x)},$$

and each function is defined on the largest possible domain.

Solution
$f(x)$ has domain $(-\infty, \infty)$ and range $[0, \infty)$, $g(x)$ has domain $(-\infty, 1]$ and range $[0, \infty)$. As the range of g is contained in the domain of f the function of a function $f(g(x))$ may be constructed to give

$$f(g(x)) = [\sqrt{(1 - x)}]^2 = 1 - x.$$

Thus $f(g(x))$ has domain $(-\infty, 1]$ and range $[0, \infty)$.

When considering $f(g(x))$ we see that the range of f is not contained in the domain of g, so $g(f(x))$ is not defined (see Fig. 26).

There is, however, an interval $[0, 1]$ which belongs to both the range of f and the domain of g, so if f is restricted so that its range lies in this interval it will be possible to construct a composite function. To do this we require $0 \leq x^2 \leq 1$, which defines the interval $-1 \leq x \leq 1$. Thus defining a new function

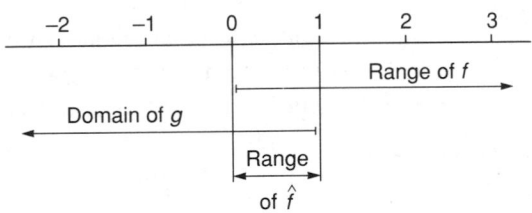

Fig. 26

$$\hat{f}(x) = x^2$$

with domain $[-1, 1]$ and range $[0, 1]$, we see that $g(\hat{f}(x))$ is defined, and we have

$$g(\hat{f}(x)) = \sqrt{(1 - x^2)},$$

with domain $[-1, 1]$ and range $[0, 1]$.   ▲

PROBLEMS 7

In problems 1 to 8 find $f(x) + g(x)$, $f(x) - g(x)$, $f(x)g(x)$ and $f(x)/g(x)$, giving the domain of definition of the combined function in each case.

1. $f(x) = 2 + \sin x$, $g(x) = 2x$, both defined on the domain $(-\infty, \infty)$.

2. $f(x) = 1 + x^2$, $g(x) = 2 + x^2$, both defined on the domain $(-\infty, \infty)$.

3. $f(x) = \sin^2 x$, $g(x) = \sin x$, both defined on the domain $(-\infty, \infty)$.

4. $f(x) = \sin x$, $g(x) = \sin^2 x$, both defined on the domain $(-\infty, \infty)$.

5. $f(x) = \sin x^2$, $g(x) = \dfrac{1}{1 + x^2}$, both defined on the domain $(-\infty, \infty)$.

6. $f(x) = \cos x^2$, $g(x) = \dfrac{1}{1 - x^2}$, both defined on the domain $(-\infty, \infty)$ but with $x \neq \pm 1$ in $g(x)$.

7. $f(x) = x^2$, $g(x) = \sqrt{(4 - x)}$, with $f(x)$ defined for $(-\infty, \infty)$ and $g(x)$ for $x \leqslant 4$.

8. $f(x) = \sqrt{(|1 - x|)}$, $g(x) = x$, both defined on the domain $(-\infty, \infty)$.

In problems 9 to 15 find $f(g(x))$ and $g(f(x))$ (when they exist) and determine whether $f(g(x)) = g(f(x))$.

9. $f(x) = x - 1$, $g(x) = 2x^3 + 1$, both defined on the domain $(-\infty, \infty)$.

10. $f(x) = x^2$, $g(x) = \sqrt{|2x + 1|}$, both defined on the domain $(-\infty, \infty)$.

11. $f(x) = 5x - 3$, $g(x) = (x + 3)/5$, both defined on the domain $(-\infty, \infty)$.

12. $f(x) = \sqrt{(9 - x)}$, $g(x) = x^2 - 2$, both defined in the largest possible domain.

13. $f(x) = \dfrac{4x - 1}{2 + x}$, $g(x) = \dfrac{2x + 1}{4 - x}$, both defined in the largest possible domain.

14. $f(x) = |x| + 3$, $g(x) = x^2$, both defined on the domain $(-\infty, \infty)$.

15. $f(x) = 1/(x - 1)$, $g(x) = 2/x$.

Symmetry in functions and graphs
8

Many functions exhibit some form of **symmetry** with respect to their argument. The most important forms of symmetry can be interpreted geometrically in terms of a straight line acting as though it were a mirror and 'reflecting' the graph of a function in the line.

EVEN FUNCTIONS

A function $f(x)$ is said to be an **even** function if $f(-x) = f(x)$. Thus since in an even function changing the sign of the argument does not change the function, the y-axis acts as a line in which the function for $x > 0$ is reflected to produce the function for $x < 0$. Examples of even functions are

$$1, \quad x^2, \quad \cos x, \quad a + bx^2 + cx^4, \quad (1 + x^2)\cos 2x.$$

The graph of a typical even function is shown in Fig. 27. An even function is said to be **symmetric** with respect to x.

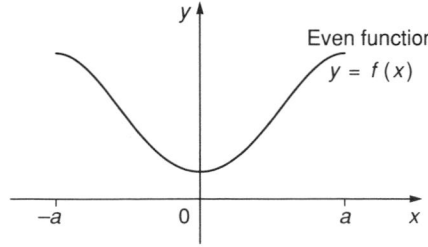

Fig. 27

ODD FUNCTIONS

A function $f(x)$ is said to be an **odd** function if $f(-x) = -f(x)$. Thus changing the sign of the argument of an odd function leaves its magnitude unchanged, but changes its sign. This corresponds to two reflections, in which the function

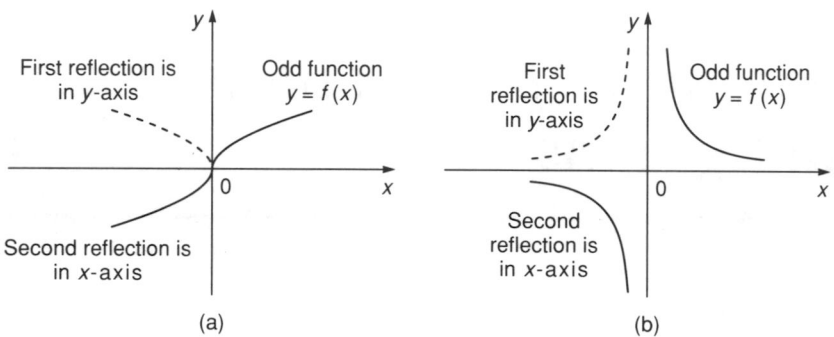

First reflection is in y-axis

Odd function
y = f(x)

Second reflection is in x-axis

(a)

First reflection is in y-axis

Odd function
y = f(x)

Second reflection is in x-axis

(b)

Fig. 28

for $x > 0$ is first reflected in the y-axis, and then the reflection itself is reflected in the x-axis, to produce the function for $x < 0$. Examples of odd functions are

$$x, \quad x^3, \quad \sin x, \quad x \cos x, \quad x^2 \sin 2x.$$

If an odd function $f(x)$ is finite at the origin then $f(0) = 0$, because $f(0) = -f(0)$. If an odd function is not finite at the origin, the y-axis will be an asymptote. An odd function is said to be **skew-symmetric** with respect to x. Graphs of typical odd functions are shown in Fig. 28.

Simple properties of even and odd functions
1   The product of two even functions is an even function.
2   The product of two odd functions is an even function.
3   The product of an even and an odd function is an odd function.
4   A function which is neither even nor odd can be represented as the sum of an even function and an odd function.

Example 8.1

Show that

$$f(x) = 4 + x(1 - x^2) + \sin^2 x + |x|$$

is neither even nor odd and represent it as the sum of an even function and an odd function.

Solution

$$f(-x) = 4 - x(1 - x^2) + \sin^2 x + |x|,$$

but $f(-x) \neq f(x)$ and $f(-x) \neq -f(x)$, so $f(x)$ is neither even nor odd.
   The function

$$g(x) = 4 + \sin^2 x + |x|$$

is an even function, because

$$g(-x) = 4 + [\sin(-x)]^2 + |-x|$$
$$= 4 + [-\sin x]^2 + |x|$$
$$= 4 + \sin^2 x + |x| = g(x).$$

The function

$$h(x) = x(1 - x^2)$$

is an odd function, because

$$h(-x) = -x(1 - (-x)^2) = -x(1 - x^2) = -h(x).$$

Thus we may write

$$f(x) = g(x) + h(x),$$

with $g(x)$ even and $h(x)$ odd.   ▲

Also of importance is the case where the line in which the function is 'reflected' is the line $y = x$. This is illustrated in Fig. 29 for the case of the function $y = 3x + 4$ and its reflection which is the line $y = (x-4)/3$. In the next section it will be seen that this property is of importance when discussing inverse functions.

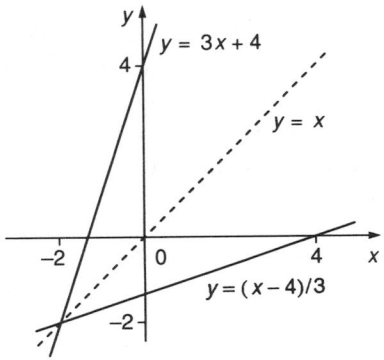

Fig. 29

Example 8.2

Find the equation of the line produced by $y = 2x - 3$ when it is reflected in the line $y = x$,

Solution
As $y = 2x - 3$ and its reflection $y = mx + c$ are symmetrical about the line $y = x$ it follows that:
1 both lines pass through the same point on the line $y = x$;
2 the intercept of $y = 2x - 3$ on the y-axis must equal the intercept of $y = mx + c$ on the x-axis.

From 1, setting $y = x$ in $y = 2x - 3$ shows that $x = 3$, and hence $y = 3$. Thus the line $y = 2x - 3$ passes through the point $(3, 3)$ on the line $y = x$, as does the line $y = mx + c$. Substitution of $(3, 3)$ into $y = mx + c$ gives $3 = 3m + c$. From 2, the intercept of $y = 2x - 3$ on the y-axis is $- 3$, so the intercept of $y = mx + c$ on the x-axis must be $- 3$, showing that the line $y = mx + c$ must pass through the point $(- 3, 0)$. Substituting $(- 3, 0)$ into $y = mx + c$ gives

$$0 = - 3m + c.$$

Solving the simultaneous equations $3 = 3m + c$ and $0 = - 3m + c$ gives $m = 1/2$, $c = 3/2$, and so the reflected line has the equation

$$y = (x + 3)/2. \qquad \blacktriangle$$

A different type of symmetry is exhibited by functions which are periodic, and these may or may not be even or odd functions. A function $f(x)$ is said to be **periodic** with **period** X if

$$f(x + X) = f(X),$$

and X is the smallest number for which the result is true. Familiar examples of periodic functions are

$$\sin x, \quad \cos x, \quad \text{with period} \quad 2\pi,$$

and

$$\sin 3x, \quad \cos 3x, \quad \text{with period} \quad 2\pi/3.$$

The function $\sin x$ is an odd periodic function and $\cos 3x$ an even periodic function. The function $f(x) = 2 - \sin x$ is neither even nor odd, but it is still periodic with period 2π.

The graph of a typical periodic function which is neither even nor odd is shown in Fig. 30.

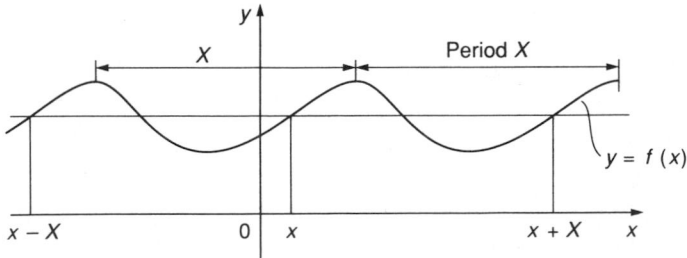

Fig. 30

PROBLEMS 8

Classify the functions in problems 1 to 10 as even, odd or neither.
1. $x + \sin 3x.$
2. $x^3 + x^2 + 1.$

3. $x^2 \cos x.$

4. $(x+1)^2.$

5. $(x^2+1)^2.$

6. $(x^3+1)^3.$

7. $x^3 + x \cos x.$

8. $1 + |x| + x^2.$

9. $x |x| + \sin 4x.$

10. $x + 2 |x|.$

11. Prove that if $f(x)$ and $g(x)$ are even functions, the product $f(x) \, g(x)$ is an even function.

12. Prove that if $f(x)$ and $g(x)$ are odd functions, the product $f(x) \, g(x)$ is an even function.

13. Prove that if $f(x)$ is an even function and $g(x)$ an odd function, the product $f(x)g(x)$ is an odd function.

In problems 14 to 18 find the equation of the straight line obtained when the given line is reflected in $y = x$.

14. $y = 4 - 2x.$

15. $y = 5x + 11.$

16. $y = x + 2.$

17. $y = 3x - 1.$

18. $y = 6 - 4x.$

19. Find the period of $f(x) = \sin x + \sin 2x.$

20. Find the period of $f(x) = \cos \dfrac{x}{2} + 2 \sin \dfrac{x}{2}.$

21. Find the period of $f(x) = 3 + \sin x + \sin \dfrac{3x}{2}.$

22. Find the period of $f(x) = \cos \dfrac{x}{2} + \sin \dfrac{3x}{2} - 1.$

23. Find the period of $f(x) = \sin \dfrac{x}{3} + \sin \dfrac{2x}{3}.$

24. Find the period of $f(x) = 2 \sin \dfrac{x}{4} + 5 \cos \dfrac{x}{2}.$

25. Find the period of $f(x) = 1 + 3 \sin 2x + \cos \dfrac{x}{2}.$

9 Inverse functions

A one–one (monotonic) function $f(x)$ is, by definition, a function with the property that to one x there corresponds one value of $f(x)$ and, conversely, to each value of $f(x)$ there corresponds only one x. The graph $y = f(x)$ of a typical one–one function is shown in Fig. 31. The one–one property can be expressed by saying that no two of the ordered pairs $(x, f(x))$ which describe the graph $f(x)$ have the same second component $f(x)$ with different first components x.

Because of this property another one–one function $f^{-1}(x)$ can be defined, called the **inverse function** of f. The inverse function f^{-1} is derived from f by interchanging the two components in the ordered pairs defining f. So, in the inverse function, $f(x)$ becomes the independent variable and x the dependent variable. We then see that the connection between f and f^{-1} can be expressed by saying that if $y = f(x)$, then $x = f^{-1}(y)$.

Let us now consider f^{-1} as a function in its own right, and forget for the moment that it originated from the function f. Then, since by convention x denotes the independent variable and y the dependent variable, it is appropriate to represent the inverse function by writing

$$y = f^{-1}(x).$$

Remember, this means that if $y = f^{-1}(x)$, then $x = f(y)$.

The important and useful geometrical interpretation of the relationship between f and f^{-1} can be seen when $y = f(x)$ and $y = f^{-1}(x)$ are both shown on the same graph, as in Fig. 32. Each function is seen to be the 'reflection' of the other in the line $y = x$. A basic property of the inverse function is that

$$f(f^{-1}(x)) = x \quad \text{and} \quad f^{-1}(f(x)) = x.$$

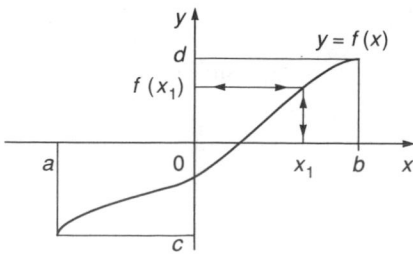

Fig. 31

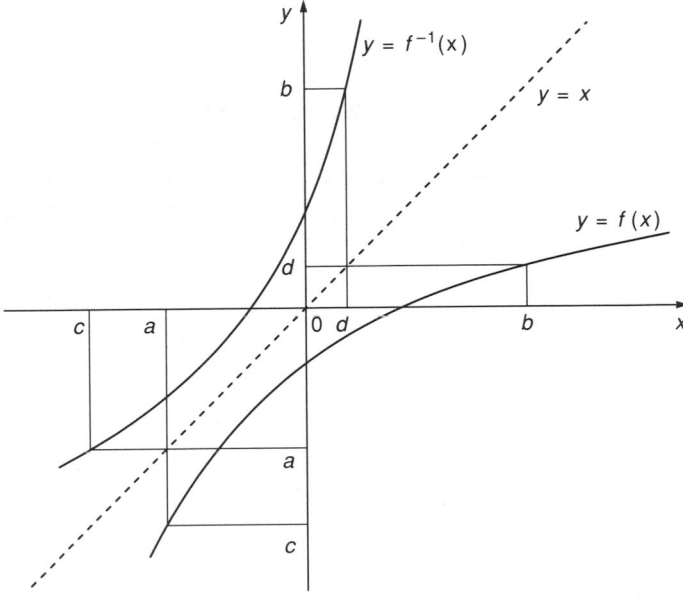

Fig. 32

The idea underlying Fig. 32 is clarified if we consider the case of the linear function

$$y = 2x - 3 \qquad (y = f(x)).$$

Solving for x we find the inverse function

$$x = (y + 3)/2 \qquad (x = f^{-1}(y)).$$

Interchanging x and y in the inverse function then gives

$$y = (x + 3)/2 \qquad (y = f^{-1}(x)).$$

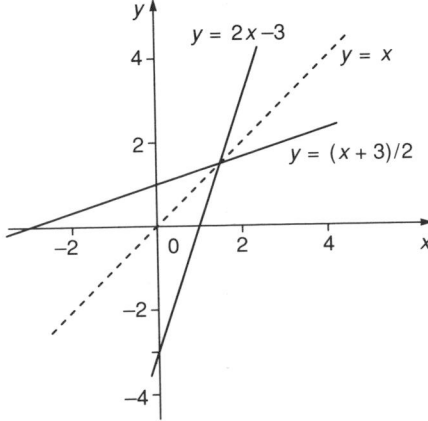

Fig. 33

The graphs of $y = f(x)$ and $y = f^{-1}(x)$ corresponding to Fig. 32 are shown in Fig. 33, together with the line $y = x$.

INVERSE TRIGONOMETRICAL FUNCTIONS

The trigonometrical functions sin x, cos x and tan x are many–one functions because of their periodicity. However, if their domains are suitably restricted they become one–one functions, as shown in Fig. 34.

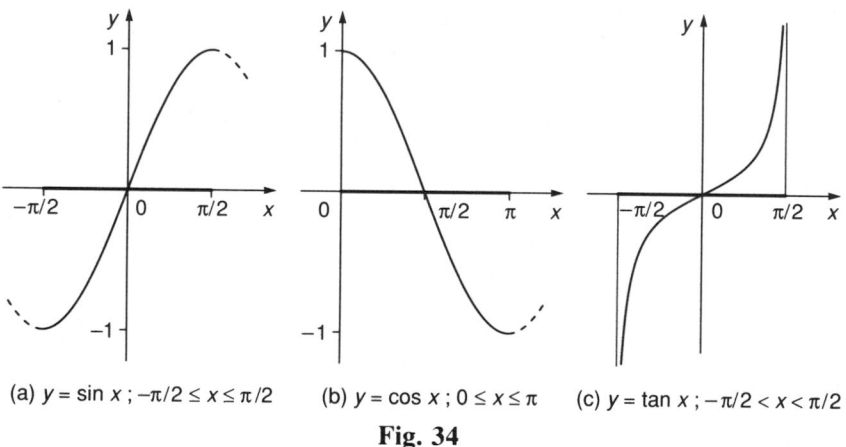

(a) $y = \sin x$; $-\pi/2 \le x \le \pi/2$ (b) $y = \cos x$; $0 \le x \le \pi$ (c) $y = \tan x$; $-\pi/2 < x < \pi/2$

Fig. 34

The corresponding inverse trigonometric functions which can be defined are denoted by arcsin x, arccos x and arctan x or, alternatively, by $\sin^{-1} x$, $\cos^{-1} x$, and $\tan^{-1} x$. These functions are defined as follows:

$$y = \arcsin x \text{ if } \sin y = x; \text{ domain } -1 \le x \le 1, \text{ range } -\frac{\pi}{2} \le y \le \frac{\pi}{2};$$

$$y = \arccos x \quad \text{if } \cos y = x; \text{ domain } -1 \le x \le 1, \text{ range } 0 \le y \le \pi;$$

$$y = \arctan x \text{ if } \tan y = x; \text{ domain } -\infty < x < \infty, \text{ range } -\frac{\pi}{2} < y < \frac{\pi}{2}.$$

Graphs of these functions are shown in Fig. 35. When y lies in the interval $-\pi/2 \le y \le \pi/2$, $0 \le y \le \pi$ and $-\pi/2 < y < \pi/2$ for the respective functions

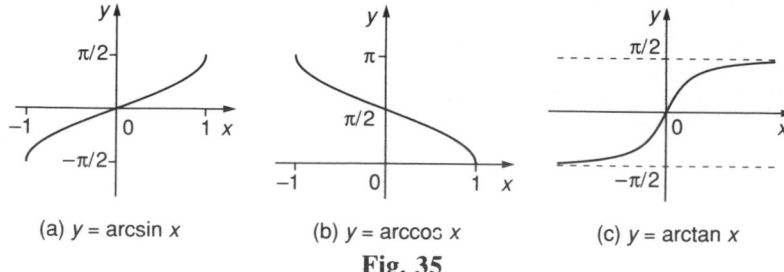

(a) $y = \arcsin x$ (b) $y = \arccos x$ (c) $y = \arctan x$

Fig. 35

arcsin x, arccos x and arctan x, it is called the **principal value** of the inverse function.

Example 9.1

Evaluate

(i)   arcsin $[-\sqrt{3}/2]$;

(ii)   arctan 1;

(iii)   arccos 0;

(iv)   arccos $[-1/\sqrt{2}]$;

(v)   arccos $(\cos 3\pi/2)$.

Solution

(i) $y = \arcsin[-\sqrt{3}/2]$ means $\sin y = -\sqrt{3}/2$, with y confined to the interval $-\pi/2 \leqslant y \leqslant \pi/2$. It then follows that the principal value is

$$\arcsin[-\sqrt{3}/2] = -\pi/3.$$

(ii) $y = \arctan 1$ means $\tan y = 1$, with y confined to the interval $-\pi/2 \leqslant y < \pi/2$. It then follows that the principal value is

$$\arctan 1 = \pi/4.$$

(iii) $y = \arccos 0$ means $\cos y = 0$, with y confined to the interval $0 \leqslant y \leqslant \pi$. It then follows that the principal value is

$$\arccos 0 = \pi/2.$$

(iv) $y = \arccos[-1/\sqrt{2}]$ means $\cos y = -1/\sqrt{2}$, with y confined to the interval $0 \leqslant y \leqslant \pi$. It then follows that the principal value is

$$\arccos[-1/\sqrt{2}] = 3\pi/4.$$

(v)   The basic property of inverse functions that $f^{-1}(f(x)) = x$ does not apply when the argument lies outside the domain of definition of $f(x)$. Here the domain of definition of arccos x is $[0, \pi]$, so it does not contain $3\pi/2$, and thus

$$\arccos(\cos 3\pi/2) \neq 3\pi/2.$$

However, $\cos 3\pi/2 = 0$, so

$$\arccos\left[\cos \frac{3\pi}{2}\right] = \arccos 0 = \pi/2. \qquad \blacktriangle$$

Example 9.2

Find x given that

(i) $\arcsin(3x - 2) = -\pi/3$;

(ii) $\arccos(2x + 1) = \pi/4$;

(iii) $2\arctan(4x - 5) = -1/\sqrt{3}$.

Solution

(i) $\arcsin(3x - 2) = -\pi/3$ means that

$$3x - 2 = \sin(-\pi/3) = -\frac{\sqrt{3}}{2},$$

so solving for x gives

$$x = \frac{2}{3} - \frac{\sqrt{3}}{6}.$$

(ii) $\arccos(2x + 1) = \pi/4$ means that

$$2x + 1 = \cos(\pi/4) = \frac{1}{\sqrt{2}},$$

so solving for x gives

$$x = \frac{1}{2\sqrt{2}} - \frac{1}{2}.$$

(ii) $2\arctan(4x = 5) = -1/\sqrt{3}$ means that

$$4x - 5 = \tan\left[-\frac{1}{2\sqrt{3}}\right] = -0.29697,$$

so solving for x gives

$$x = 1.17576. \qquad\qquad\qquad \blacktriangle$$

PROBLEMS 9

In problems 1 to 8, given the function $f(x)$ find $f^{-1}(x)$, graph $y = f(x)$ and $y = f^{-1}(x)$, and check that each is the reflection of the other in the line $y = x$.

1. $f(x) = 3x + 16$.

2. $f(x) = -(x + 2)$.

3. $f(x) = \sqrt{(9 - x)}$.

4. $f(x) = \sqrt{(x - 4)}$.

5. $f(x) = 1/x$, for $-\infty < x < \infty, x \neq 0$.

6. $f(x) = 1/(1 - x)$, $x \neq 0$.

7. $f(x) = 2x/(1 + x)$, $x \neq -1$.

8. $f(x) = (x + 2)/(3 - x)$, $x \neq 3$.

9. Find $\arcsin(-1/\sqrt{2})$.

10.   Find arctan $(-\sqrt{3})$.

11.   Find arccos 0.3.

12.   Find arctan 2.

13.   Find x given that arctan $(2x + 5) = \pi/4$.

14.   Find x given that arccos $(3 - 4x) = 3\pi/4$.

15.   Find x given that arcsin $(2x - 1) = -\pi/4$.

16.   Find x given that arccos $(3x + 1) = 0.7$.

Complex numbers:
10   real and imaginary forms

The real number system is such that not every equation can be solved in terms of real numbers. Thus the simple algebraic equation

$$x^2 + 1 = 0$$

has no solution in terms of real numbers. To overcome this limitation the real number system is **extended** to become the **complex number** system, and this is accomplished by introducing the **unit imaginary element** i defined as

$$i = \sqrt{(-1)}.$$

In terms of this so-called imaginary element, the equation $x^2 + 1 = 0$, which may be written as

$$x^2 = -1, \quad \text{or as} \quad x = \pm \sqrt{(-1)},$$

is seen to have the solutions $x = \pm i$. Similarly, the equation $x^2 + 16 = 0$ may be rewritten as

$$x^2 = -16, \quad \text{or as} \quad x = \pm \sqrt{(-16)}.$$

If we write $-16 = 16 \times (-1)$, this last result becomes

$$x = \pm \sqrt{16} \sqrt{(-1)} = \pm 4i,$$

and so the equation is seen to have the two **imaginary** solutions $x = 4i$ and $x = -4i$.

Numbers like i, 4i, $-3i$ are called **purely imaginary** numbers, and they represent special cases of the general **complex number**

$$a + ib$$

in which a, b are **real** numbers. It is the convention that a general complex number is denoted by z, so hereafter we set

$$z = a + ib.$$

The real number a is called the **real part** of the complex number z, and its relationship to z is shown by writing

$$a = \text{Re}\{z\}.$$

The real number b is called the **imaginary part** of the complex number z, and its relationship to z is shown by writing

$$b = \text{Im}\{z\}.$$

Thus $3 + 2i$, -4, $2 - 7i$ and $16i$ are all special cases of complex numbers. The complex number $z = a + ib$ is **purely real** (an ordinary real number) if $b = 0$ and it is **purely** imaginary if $a = 0$.
The general quadratic equation

$$ax^2 + bx + c = 0$$

can now be solved by the quadratic formula

$$x = \frac{-b \pm \sqrt{(b^2 - 4ac)}}{2a}$$

for any real a, b and c, and not simply those for which $b^2 - 4ac \geqslant 0$. Thus if $b^2 - 4ac < 0$ the solution becomes

$$x = \frac{-b \pm i\sqrt{(4ac - b^2)}}{2a}$$

Example 10.1

Solve

$$3x^2 - x + 4 = 0.$$

Solution
Applying the quadratic formula with $a = 3$, $b = -1$ and $c = 3$ gives

$$x = \frac{1 \pm \sqrt{[(-1)^2 - 4 \cdot 3 \cdot 4]}}{6} = \frac{1 \pm \sqrt{-47}}{6} = \frac{1 \pm i\sqrt{47}}{6}.$$

Thus the solutions are $x = (1 + i\sqrt{47})/6$ and $x = (1 - i\sqrt{47})/6$.   ▲

Example 10.2

Find by inspection a root of

$$x^3 + 2x^2 + 2x + 1 = 0,$$

and hence find the other two roots.

Solution
Inspection shows that $x = -1$ is a root of this equation, so $(x + 1)$ must be a factor. Dividing $x^3 + 2x^2 + 2x + 1$ by $x + 1$ gives

$$
\begin{array}{r}
x^2 + x + 1 \\
\hline
x + 1 \, \big|\, x^3 + 2x^2 + 2x + 1 \\
\underline{x^3 + x^2} \\
x^2 + 2x + 1 \\
\underline{x^2 + x} \\
x + 1 \\
\end{array}
$$

and so

$$x^3 + 2x^2 + 2x + 1 = (x + 1)(x^2 + x + 1).$$

Thus the original equation can be written

$$(x+1)(x^2+x+1)=0,$$

and this is satisfied if $x+1=0$, which yields the root $x=-1$ found by inspection, and also if $x^2+x+1=0$. Thus the two remaining roots follow by solving

$$x^2+x+1=0.$$

Applying the quadratic formula with $a=b=c=1$ we find that

$$x=\frac{-1\pm\sqrt{(1-4)}}{6}=(-1\pm i\sqrt{3})/2.$$

Thus the three roots of

$$x^3+2x^2+2x+1=0$$

are

$$x=-1,\quad x=(-1+i\sqrt{3})/2\quad\text{and}\quad x=(-1-i\sqrt{3})/2.\qquad\blacktriangle$$

BASIC ALGEBRAIC RULES FOR COMPLEX NUMBERS

Sum and difference

If $z_1=a+ib$ and $z_2=c+id$ are any two complex numbers, then their **sum** is

$$z_1+z_2=(a+c)+i(b+d),$$

and their **difference** is

$$z_1-z_2=(a-c)+i(b-d).$$

Thus when adding or subtracting complex numbers their real and imaginary parts are added or subtracted separately.

Example 10.3

Find z_1+z_2 and z_1-z_2 if

$$z_1=3-4i$$

and

$$z_2=-4+7i.$$

Solution

$$z_1+z_2=(3-4i)+(-4+7i)=(3-4)+(-4+7)i=-1+3i,$$
$$z_1-z_2=(3-4i)-(-4+7i)=(3-(-4))+(-4-7)i=7-11i.\qquad\blacktriangle$$

Product

If $z_1=a+ib$ and $z_2=c+id$ are any two complex numbers, then their **product** is

$$z_1z_2=(ac-bd)+i(ad+bc).$$

This is the formal definition of the product $z_1 z_2$, but when working with complex numbers, instead of using this definition it is simpler to multiply $(a + ib)$ and $(c + id)$ together in the usual way and then use the fact that $i^2 = -1$ to simplify the result.

It is an immediate consequence of the definition of a product that if k is a real number and $z = a + ib$, then

$$kz = k(a + ib) = ka + ikb.$$

Example 10.4

If $z_1 = 2 - 3i$ and $z_2 = -1 + i$, find

(i) $z_1 z_2$;   and

(ii) $z_1(2z_2 + 1)$.

Solution

(i) $z_1 z_2 = (2 - 3i)(-1 + i)$

$\qquad = -2 + 2i + 3i - 3i^2$

$\qquad = -2 + 5i - 3i^2,$

but $i^2 = -1$, so

$$z_1 z_2 = -2 + 5i - 3(-1) = 1 + 5i.$$

(ii) $z_1(2z_2 + 1) = (2 - 3i)[2(-1 + i) + 1]$

$\qquad = (2 - 3i)(-2 + 2i + 1)$

$\qquad = (2 - 3i)(-1 + 2i) = -2 + 4i + 3i - 6i^2$

$\qquad = -2 + 7i - 6(-1) = 4 + 7i.$ ▲

Complex conjugate

To any complex number $a + ib$ there corresponds a complex number $a - ib$, obtained by changing the sign of b. The complex number $a - ib$ is called the **complex conjugate** of the complex number $a + ib$ (conversely, $a + ib$ is the complex conjugate of $a - ib$). The complex conjugate of the complex number z is denoted by placing a bar over z to obtain $\bar{z}$, thus if

$$z = a + ib,$$

then

$$\bar{z} = a - ib.$$

The product

$$z\bar{z} = a^2 + b^2$$

is a purely real number. We also have the useful results that

$$\mathrm{Re}\{z\} = \frac{1}{2}(z + \bar{z}) \quad \text{and} \quad \mathrm{Im}\{z\} = \frac{1}{2i}(z - \bar{z}).$$

Example 10.5

Find $\bar{z}$ and $z\bar{z}$ if $z = 2 - i$.

Solution

$$z = 2 - i, \quad \text{so} \quad \bar{z} = 2 + i.$$

$$z\bar{z} = (2 - i)(2 + i) = 4 + 2i - 2i - i^2 = 4 - i^2 = 4 - (-1) = 5. \quad \blacktriangle$$

Quotient

If $z_1 = a + ib$ and $z_2 = c + id$, the quotient

$$\frac{z_1}{z_2} = \frac{ac + bd}{c^2 + d^2} + i\,\frac{(bc - ad)}{c^2 + d^2}.$$

This is the formal definition of the quotient z_1/z_2, but when working with complex numbers, instead of using this definition it is simpler to use the result that

$$\frac{z_1}{z_2} = \frac{z_1\,\bar{z}_2}{z_2\,\bar{z}_2} = \frac{z_1\,\bar{z}_2}{c^2 + d^2}.$$

Example 10.6

Find z_1/z_2 if $z_1 = 3 + 2i$ and $z_2 = 1 - 3i$, and hence determine $\mathrm{Re}\{z_1/z_2\}$ and $\mathrm{Im}\{z_1/z_2\}$.

Solution

$$\frac{z_1}{z_2} = \frac{3 + 2i}{1 - 3i} = \frac{(3 + 2i)(1 + 3i)}{(1 - 3i)(1 + 3i)}$$

$$= \frac{(3 + 2i)(1 + 3i)}{1^2 + 3^2}$$

$$= \frac{1}{10}[3 + 9i + 2i + 6i^2]$$

$$= \frac{1}{10}[3 + 11i + 6(-1)]$$

$$= \frac{-3 + 11i}{10} = -\frac{3}{10} + \frac{11i}{10}$$

Thus

$$\mathrm{Re}\{z_1/z_2\} = -\frac{3}{10}, \quad \mathrm{Im}\{z_1/z_2\} = \frac{11}{10}. \quad \blacktriangle$$

EQUALITY OF COMPLEX NUMBERS

If two complex numbers z_1 and z_2 are equal, then

$$\text{Re}\{z_1\} = \text{Re}\{z_2\} \quad \text{and} \quad \text{Im}\{z_1\} = \text{Im}\{z_2\}.$$

Thus equality of complex numbers means equality of their real parts and equality of their imaginary parts.

Example 10.7

Examine the possibility of equality between

$$z_1 = 1 - 2i, \quad z_2 = 1 + i \quad \text{and} \quad z_3 = 1 + ki,$$

with k an arbitrary real number.

Solution
$\text{Re}\{z_1\} = 1$, $\text{Im}\{z_1\} = -2$, $\text{Re}\{z_2\} = 1$, $\text{Im}\{z_2\} = 1$, $\text{Re}\{z_3\} = 1$ and $\text{Im}\{z_3\} = k$.

Clearly $z_1 \neq z_2$, because although $\text{Re}\{z_1\} = \text{Re}\{z_2\}$, $\text{Im}\{z_1\} \neq \text{Im}\{z_2\}$.

As $\text{Re}\{z_1\} = \text{Re}\{z_3\}$, we can only have $z_1 = z_3$ if $\text{Im}\{z_1\} = \text{Im}\{z_3\}$, which only occurs when $k = -2$.

As $\text{Re}\{z_2\} = \text{Re}\{z_3\}$, we can only have $z_2 = z_3$ if $\text{Im}\{z_2\} = \text{Im}\{z_3\}$, which only occurs when $k = 1$.   ▲

Zero complex number

The **zero** complex number is the number $0 + 0i$, and so it has zero real and imaginary parts. For simplicity it is written 0, but with the above meaning.

Example 10.8

Find the real numbers α, β such that $z_1 + z_2 = 0$, given that $z_1 = 3 + \alpha i$ and $z_2 = \beta - 5i$.

Solution

$$z_1 + z_2 = 3 + \alpha i + \beta - 5i = (3 + \beta) + (\alpha - 5)i.$$

Now if $z_1 + z_2 = 0$, then $\text{Re}\{z_1 + z_2\} = 0$ and $\text{Im}\{z_1 + z_2\} = 0$. Thus $3 + \beta = 0$, so $\beta = -3$ and $\alpha - 5 = 0$, so $\alpha = 5$.   ▲

The above results are consequences of the following general algebraic properties of complex numbers which are recorded here for reference.

Commutative property

If z_1 and z_2 are any two complex numbers, then

$$z_1 + z_2 = z_2 + z_1,$$

and

$$z_1 z_2 = z_2 z_1.$$

Thus the **order** in which addition or multiplication is performed is immaterial.

Associative property

If z_1, z_2 and z_3 are any three complex numbers, then

$$(z_1 + z_2) + z_3 = z_1 + (z_2 + z_3),$$

and

$$(z_1 z_2)z_3 = z_1(z_2 z_3).$$

Thus the way in which complex numbers are **grouped** together for addition or multiplication is immaterial.

Distributive property

If z_1, z_2 and z_3 are any three complex numbers, then

$$z_1(z_2 + z_3) = z_1 z_2 + z_1 z_3.$$

Multiplication is said to be **distributive** with respect to addition.

Powers of a complex number

If z is any complex number, then
$$z^n = \underbrace{z \cdot z \ldots z}_{n \text{ times}}, \quad z^{-n} = 1/z^n, \quad z^m z^n = z^{m+n}, \quad (z^n)^m = z^{nm},$$

and if z_1, z_2 are any two complex numbers

$$(z_1 z_2)^n = z_1^n z_2^n.$$

Example 10.9

Given $z = 1 + i$, $z_1 = 1 - 2i$, $z_2 = 2 + i$, find
(i) z^3;

(ii) z^4;

(iii) $(z_1 z_2)^2$;

(iv) z_1^{-2}.

Solution

(i) $z^3 = z^2 z = (1 + i)^2(1 + i) = (1 + 2i + i^2)(1 + i)$
$$= (1 + 2i - 1)(1 + i)$$

$$= 2i(1 + i)$$
$$= 2i + 2i^2 = -2 + 2i.$$

(ii) $z^4 = (z^2)^2 = [(1 + i)^2]^2 = [2i]^2 = 4i^2 = -4.$

(iii) $(z_1 z_2)^2 = [(1 - 2i)(2 + i)]^2 = [2 + i - 4i - 2i^2]^2$

$$= [2 - 3i + 2]^2$$
$$= (4 - 3i)^2$$
$$= 16 - 24i + 9i^2$$
$$= 16 - 24i - 9$$
$$= 7 - 24i.$$

Equivalently, we have

$$(z_1 z_2)^2 = z_1^2 z_2^2 = (1 - 2i)^2 (z + i)^2$$
$$= (1 - 4i + 4i^2)(4 + 4i + i^2)$$
$$= (-3 - 4i)(3 + 4i)$$
$$= (-9 - 12i - 12i - 16i^2)$$
$$= -9 - 24i - 16(-1)$$
$$= 7 - 24i.$$

(iv) $z_1^{-2} = \dfrac{1}{(1 - 2i)^2} = \dfrac{1}{1 - 4i + 4i^2}$

$$= \frac{1}{1 - 4i - 4}$$

$$= \frac{-1}{3 + 4i}$$

$$= \frac{-(3 - 4i)}{(3 + 4i)(3 - 4i)}$$

$$= \frac{-3 + 4i}{3^2 + 4^2}$$

$$= \frac{(-3 + 4i)}{25}.$$ ▲

PROBLEMS 10

1. Find (a) i^3; (b) i^4; (c) i^5; (d) i^6; (e) $(i)^{-2}$; (f) $(i)^{-4}$; and (g) $(i)^{-5}$.

2. Find (a) $\sqrt{-9}$; (b) $\sqrt{-25}$; (c) $\sqrt{-49}$; (d) $\sqrt{-\pi^2}$.

Find the complex numbers in problems 3 to 10 when $z_1 = 3 + i$, $z_2 = 1 - 2i$, $z_3 = 4i$ and $z_4 = -1 + 3i$.

3.   (a) $z_1 + z_2$; (b) $z_1 - z_2$; (c) $z_2 + z_3$; (d) $z_1 - z_4$.

4.   (a) $z_1 z_2$; (b) $z_1 z_3$; (c) $z_2 z_4$.

5.   (a) $(2z_1 + 1)(z_2 - 1)$; (b) $(z_4 + 4)(1 - 3z_3)$; (c) $(2z_1 + 1)(2z_2 - 3i)$.

6.   (a) z_1/z_2; (b) z_2/z_1; (c) z_2/z_3.

7.   (a) z_3/z_4; (b) $z_2/(i + 3z_2)$; (c) $\dfrac{z_4 + 2}{z_1 - 2i}$.

8.   (a) $z_1 z_2 z_3$; (b) $z_2^2 z_4$; (c) $z_1 z_3 z_4$.

9.   (a) $z_1^2 z_4^2$; (b) $z_2^2 z_3^{-2}$; (c) z_3^{-3}.

10. (a) $z_2^2(z_1 + z_3)$; (b) $z_4(z_2^2 + z_4^2)$.

11. Find a, b if

$$2a - (1 + 2i)(a - bi) = 1 + 2i.$$

12. Find a, b if

$$- 2a + (3 - i)(a + 2bi) = 2 + i.$$

13. Find a, b if

$$\frac{a + 2bi}{3 + 2i} = 1 + 2i.$$

14. Find a, b if

$$\frac{a - bi}{1 + 2i} = 1 - 2i.$$

In the following problems find by inspection a real root of the given cubic equation and then, with the aid of the quadratic formula, find the other two roots.

15. $x^3 - 1 = 0$.

16. $x^3 - 2x^2 + 5x - 10 = 0$.

17. $2x^3 + 3x^2 + 6x + 5 = 0$.

18. $x^3 - x^2 + 8x - 8 = 0$.

Geometry of complex numbers   **11**

The complex number

$$z = a + ib$$

can be represented graphically either as a **point**, or as a **directed line (vector)**, in what is called the **complex plane** (also the z-**plane** or an **Argand diagram**). In this representation rectangular Cartesian axes are used with the real axis (x-axis) horizontal and the imaginary axis (y-axis) vertical. The complex number $z = a + ib$ is then represented either as the point with coordinates (a, b), or as the directed line from the origin to the point (a, b) with the direction indicated by an arrow on the line pointing away from the origin.

Thus $z = 4 + 2i$ can be represented in the complex plane either as the point P in Fig. 36(a), or as the directed line OP in Fig. 36(b).

It follows from the law for addition of complex numbers that if $z_1 = a + ib$ and $z_2 = c + id$, then

$$z_1 + z_2 = (a + c) + i(b + d).$$

Geometrically, this is equivalent to the following construction. Draw the directed line representing z_1 from the origin, and then draw from the tip of this line (the end towards which the arrow is directed) the line corresponding to z_2. The **sum** $z_1 + z_2$ then corresponds to the line drawn from the origin to the tip of the line representing z_2.

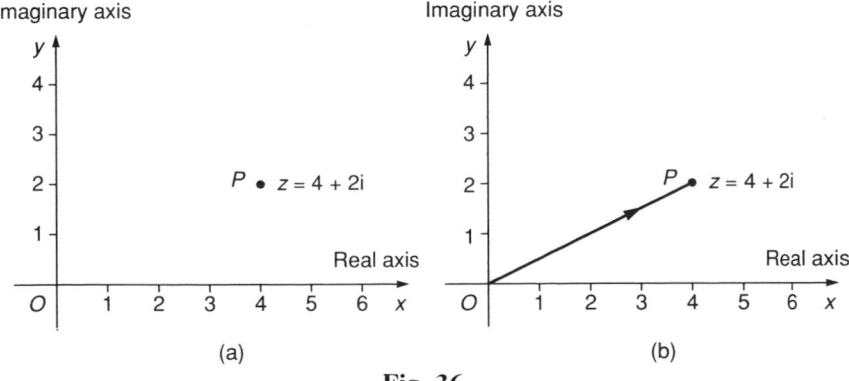

Fig. 36

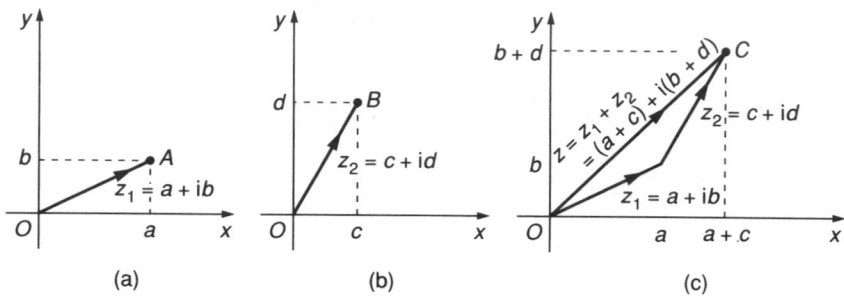

Fig. 37

The geometrical representation of the sum $z_1 + z_2$, with $z_1 = a + ib$ and $z_2 = c + id$ is shown in Fig. 37. The diagrams in Fig. 37(a) and (b) represent, respectively, $z_1 = a + ib$ (the line OA) and $z_2 = c + id$ (the line OB), while Fig. 37(c) represents the sum $z_1 + z_2 = (a + c) + i(b + d)$ (the line OC). This geometrical rule for addition is called the **triangle law** for addition.

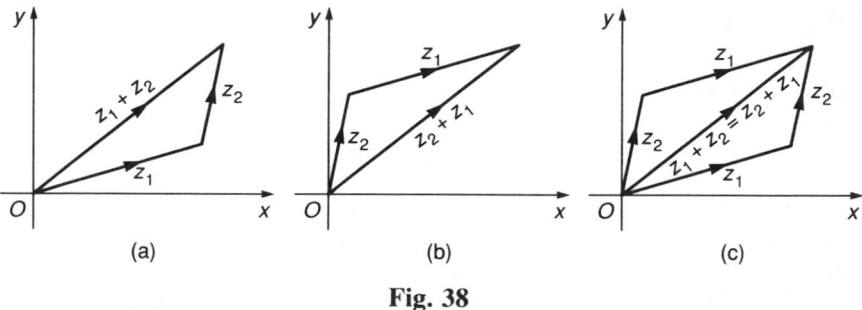

Fig. 38

As addition is a commutative operation $z_1 + z_2 = z_2 + z_1$, so the sum may be evaluated in either of the ways shown in Fig. 38(a) and (b). This leads to the **parallelogram law** for addition shown in Fig. 38(c). In this the complex numbers z_1 and z_2 are represented as shown (the arrows 'follow through') and the parallelogram is completed. The sum $z_1 + z_2$ is then represented by the diagonal of the parallelogram drawn as shown, with the direction along the line away from the origin. The triangle law and parallelogram law for addition are equivalent.

The **difference** $z_1 - z_2$ is formed in similar fashion by writing

$$z_1 - z_2 = z_1 + (-z_2)$$

and adding to z_1 the complex number $-z_2$. This is illustrated in Fig. 39.

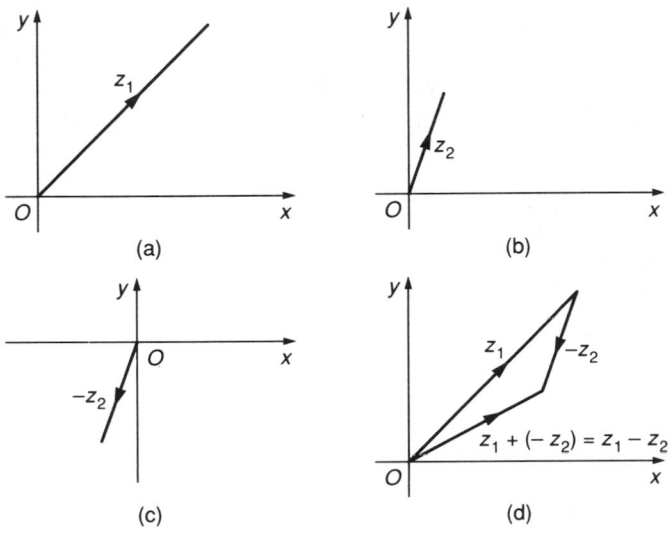

Fig. 39

Example 11.1

Given $z_1 = 2 + i$, $z_2 = 3 + 3i$
(i)   form $z_1 + z_2$, $z_1 - z_2$ and plot them as points in the complex plane;
(ii)   represent $z_1 + z_2$ and $z_1 - z_2$ geometrically and verify that the ends of the directed lines corresponding to these complex numbers coincide with the points in (i).

Solution
(i) $z_1 + z_2 = (2 + i) + (3 + 3i) = 5 + 4i$

$z_1 - z_2 = (2 + i) - (3 + 3i) = -1 - 2i.$

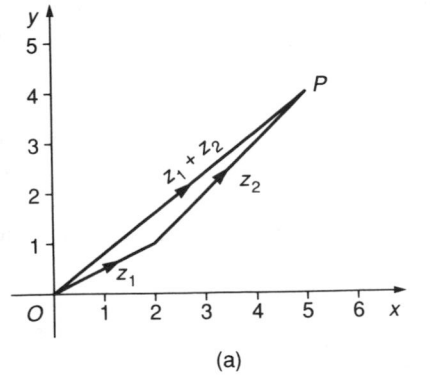

(a)

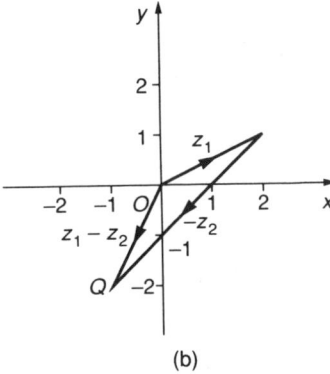

(b)

Fig. 40

(ii)   The sum $z_1 + z_2$ constructed by means of the triangle law is shown in Fig. 40(a). The end of the directed line OP lies at the point $(5, 4)$ in agreement with the result that $z_1 + z_2 = 5 + 4i$. The difference $z_1 - z_2$ constructed by means of the triangle law by adding z_1 and $- z_2$ is shown in Fig. 40(b). The end of the directed line OQ lies at the point $(- 1, - 2)$ in agreement with the result $z_1 - z_2 = - 1 - 2i$.   ▲

The graphical interpretation of the complex conjugate $\bar{z} = a - ib$ of the complex number $z = a + ib$ is reflection of the point (a, b) or of the directed line from the origin to (a, b) in the real axis, as shown in Fig. 41.

The **modulus** of the complex number $z = a + ib$ is denoted by writing $|z|$, and it is defined as

$$|z| = (a^2 + b^2)^{1/2}.$$

When expressed in terms of z and $\bar{z}$,

$$|z|^2 = z\bar{z}.$$

It is seen from Fig. 41 that

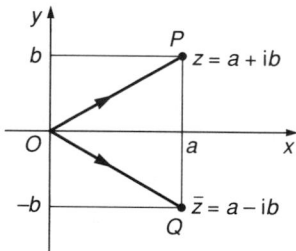

Fig. 41

$$|z| = OP.$$

Example 11.2

Show $|z| = |\bar{z}|$ for all z, and find $|z|$ given that
(i) $z = 2 + 3i$;
(ii) $z = - 3$;
(iii) $z = 5i$;

Solution
If $z = a + ib$ then $|z| = (a^2 + b^2)^{1/2}$, and $\bar{z} = a - ib$ so $|\bar{z}| = (a^2 + (- b)^2)^{1/2} = (a^2 + b^2)^{1/2}$, and thus $|z| = |\bar{z}|$ for all z.

(i) $|z| = (2^2 + 3^2)^{1/2} = \sqrt{13}$, $|\bar{z}| = (2^2 + (- 3)^2)^{1/2} = \sqrt{13}$.
(ii) $|z| = \sqrt{(- 3)^2} = 3$, $|\bar{z}| = \sqrt{(- 3)^2} = 3$.
(iii) $|z| = \sqrt{5^2} = 5$, $|\bar{z}| = \sqrt{(- 5)^2} = 5$.   ▲

Properties of $|z|$

1 $|z^n| = |z|^n.$

2 $|z|^m|z|^n = |z|^{m+n}.$

3 $|z^{-n}| = 1/|z|^n.$

4 $|z\bar{z}| = |z|^2 = |\bar{z}|^2.$

5 $|z_1/z_2| = |z_1|/|z_2|.$

6 $|z_1 + z_2| \leq |z_1| + |z_2|$ (triangle inequality).

7 $||z_1| - |z_2|| \leq |z_1 - z_2|.$

Example 11.3

Prove property 6 (the triangle inequality) and property 7 of the modulus function for complex numbers, and interpret the triangle inequality in geometrical terms.

Solution

$$|z_1 + z_2|^2 = (z_1 + z_2)(\bar{z}_1 + \bar{z}_2) = z_1\bar{z}_1 + z_1\bar{z}_2 + \bar{z}_1 z_2 + z_2\bar{z}_2.$$

However, $z_1\bar{z}_1 = |z_1|^2$, $z_2\bar{z}_2 = |z_2|^2$ and

$$z_1\bar{z}_2 + \bar{z}_1 z_2 = 2\ Re(z_1\bar{z}_2) \leqslant 2|z_1\bar{z}_2| = 2|z_1||z_2|,$$

so

$$|z_1 + z_2|^2 \leqslant |z_1|^2 + 2|z_1||z_2| + |z_2|^2 = (|z_1| + |z_2|)^2.$$

Property 6 now follows by taking the square root. Property 7 follows in similar fashion by writing

$$|z_1 - z_2|^2 = (z_1 - z_2)(\bar{z}_1 - \bar{z}_2).$$

Thus the required results are established, and it only remains for us to provide a geometrical interpretation of the first result. As $|z|$ is the length of the directed line representing z, inspection of Fig. 42 shows that $|z_1 + z_2| \leq |z_1| + |z_2|$ merely asserts that the length of side AC of the triangle ABC cannot exceed the sum of the lengths of sides AB and BC. Equality is possible only

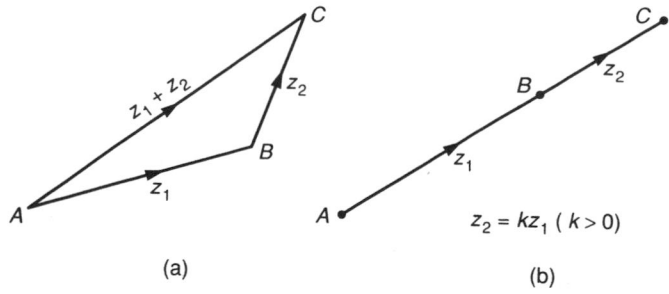

(a)   (b)

Fig. 42

when A, B and C are colinear, for then $z_2 = kz_1$ ($k > 0$ real). This is a familiar result of Euclidean geometry, and it is because of it that this inequality is called the **triangle inequality**. ▲

Example 11.4

Verify the inequalities

(i) $\quad \left|z_1 + z_2\right| \leqslant \left|z_1\right| + \left|z_2\right|$;

(ii) $\quad \left||z_1| - |z_2|\right| \leqslant \left|z_1 - z_2\right|$,

when $z_1 = 1 + i$ and $z_2 = 2 - 3i$.

Solution

$$\left|z_1\right| = \sqrt{2}, \ \left|z_2\right| = \sqrt{13}, \ \left|z_1 + z_2\right| = \left|3 + 2i\right| = \sqrt{13}, \ \left|z_1 - z_2\right| = \left|-1 + 4i\right| = \sqrt{17}.$$

(i) $\quad \left|z_1 + z_2\right| = \sqrt{13} < \left|z_1\right| + \left|z_1\right| = \sqrt{2} + \sqrt{13}.$

(ii) $\quad \left||z_1| - |z_2|\right| = \left|\sqrt{2} - \sqrt{13}\right| = \sqrt{13} - \sqrt{2} < \left|z_1 - z_2\right| = \sqrt{17}.$ ▲

PROBLEMS 11

In problems 1 to 6 use the given complex numbers z_1 and z_2 to find $z_1 + z_2$ and $z_1 - z_2$ and then verify the results graphically by means of the triangle law.

1. $z_1 = 3 + i, \quad z_2 = 2 + 2i.$

2. $z_1 = 4 - 3i, \quad z_2 = -1 - 2i.$

3. $z_1 = 2 - i, \quad z_2 = 2 + i.$

4. $z_1 = -1 - 2i, \quad z_2 = 2 - 3i.$

5. $z_1 = 3 + i, \quad z_2 = 4i.$

6. $z_1 = -3, \quad z_2 = 3i.$

7. Find $|z|$ given (a) $z = 4 + 2i$; (b) $z = -2 - i$; (c) $z = 1 + i$.

8. Find $|\bar{z}|$ given (a) $z = 3 - i$; (b) $z = 2 + i$; (c) $z = -1 - 2i$.

9. Verify the inequalities

$$\left|z_1 + z_2\right| \leqslant \left|z_1\right| + \left|z_2\right|$$

and

$$\left||z_1| - |z_2|\right| \leqslant \left|z_1 - z_2\right|$$

when

(a) $z_1 = 3 + 4i, \quad z_2 = 1 - i$;

(b) $z_1 = 2 + 4i, \quad z_2 = 1 + 2i$;

(c) $z_1 = 6 + 4i, \quad z_2 = -3 - 2i.$

Modulus–argument form of a complex number 12

An alternative and important representation of a complex number involves the use of polar coordinates. If a complex number z is regarded as a point P in the complex plane, it can be identified uniquely by specifying the radial distance r from the origin to P, together with the polar angle θ measured anticlockwise from the positive real axis to the line OP. The distance r is simply the modulus of z, while the angle θ is called the **argument** of z, and it is written arg z. The specification of r and θ is called the **modulus–argument** form of a complex number. The modulus–argument representation of z is shown in Fig. 43.

Clearly, although for a given point P the radial distance r is unique, the argument θ is determined only up to a multiple of 2π. This is because when $r = |z|$ is given, the same point P will be identified by specifying any of the angles arg $z = \theta \pm 2n\pi$, with $n = 0, 1, 2, ...,$. It is necessary to remove this ambiguity, so by convention the value of θ is chosen so that it lies in the interval $-\pi < \theta \leqslant \pi$. This value of θ is called the **principal value** of the argument. All other values of the argument merely differ from the principal value by a multiple of 2π.

Inspection of Fig. 43 shows that if P is the point (r, θ) in polar coordinates and (x, y) in Cartesian coordinates, then when r and θ are given, x and y follow from the results

$$x = r \cos \theta, \quad y = r \sin \theta.$$

Conversely, to express a complex number given in the form $z = x + iy$ in modulus–argument form we use the fact that

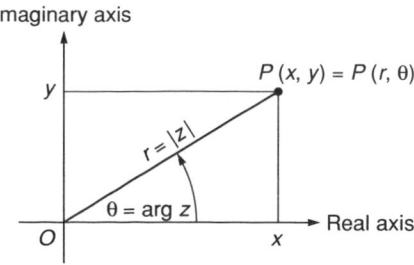

Fig. 43

$$r = |z| = (x^2 + y^2)^{1/2},$$

and θ is such that

$$\cos \theta = \frac{x}{r} = \frac{x}{(x^2 + y^2)^{1/2}} \quad \text{and} \quad \sin \theta = \frac{y}{r} = \frac{y}{(x^2 + y^2)^{1/2}}.$$

Thus if

1   $x > 0$, $y > 0$, θ lies in the first quadrant;
2   $x < 0$, $y > 0$, θ lies in the second quadrant;
3   $x < 0$, $y < 0$, θ lies in the third quadrant;
4   $x > 0$, $y < 0$, θ lies in the fourth quadrant.

Recalling that $\theta = \arg z$ must be selected so that $-\pi < \theta \leqslant \pi$, this leads to the following rule for determining θ.

Rule to determine $\theta = \arg z$ such that $-\pi < \theta \leqslant \pi$
If

1   $x > 0$, $y > 0$, then $\theta = \arg z = \arctan y/x$;
2   $x < 0$, $y > 0$, then $\theta = \arg z = \pi - \arctan |y/x|$;
3   $x < 0$, $y < 0$, then $\theta = \arg z = \arctan y/x - \pi$;
4   $x > 0$, $y < 0$, then $\theta = \arg z = -\arctan |y/x|$.

Example 12.1

(i)   Find the Cartesian form of the complex number z for which

$$|z| = 3 \quad \text{and} \quad \arg z = \pi/6.$$

(ii)   Find the modulus–argument form of

$$z = -5 - 5\sqrt{3}i.$$

Solution
(i)   Here $r = 3$ and $\theta = \arg z = \pi/6$, so

$$x = 3 \cos \pi/6 = 3\sqrt{3}/2$$

and

$$y = 3 \sin \pi/6 = 3/2.$$

(ii)   As $z = -5 - 5\sqrt{3}i$ we have $x = -5$, $y = -5\sqrt{3}$, so

$$r = [(-5)^2 + (-5\sqrt{3})^2]^{1/2} = 10,$$

and from 3 above

$$\theta = \arg z = \arctan \sqrt{3} - \pi = -2.0944 = -2\pi/3. \qquad \blacktriangle$$

In modulus–argument form a complex number z may be written

$$z = r(\cos \theta + i \sin \theta)$$

with

$$\text{Re}\{z\} = r \cos \theta, \quad \text{Im}\{z\} = r \sin \theta.$$

Then it follows by appeal to elementary trigonometric identities that if

$$z_1 = r_1(\cos \theta_1 + i \sin \theta_1) \quad \text{and} \quad z_2 = r(\cos \theta_2 + i \sin \theta_2),$$

$$z_1 z_2 = r_1 r_2(\cos(\theta_1 + \theta_2) + i \sin(\theta_1 + \theta_2))$$

and

$$\frac{z_1}{z_2} = \frac{r_1}{r_2}(\cos(\theta_1 - \theta_2) + i \sin(\theta_1 - \theta_2)).$$

Thus

$$\left| z_1 z_2 \right| = r_1 r_2 \quad \text{and} \quad \arg(z_1 z_2) = \theta_1 + \theta_2$$

and

$$\left| z_1/z_2 \right| = r_1/r_2 \quad \text{and} \quad \arg(z_1/z_2) = \theta_1 - \theta_2.$$

In general, if $z_1 = r_1(\cos \theta_1 + i \sin \theta_1)$, $z_2 = r_2(\cos \theta_2 + i \sin \theta_2)$, ..., $z_n = r_n(\cos \theta_n + i \sin \theta_n)$,

$$z_1 z_2 \ldots z_n = r_1 r_2 \ldots r_n [\cos(\theta_1 + \theta_2 + \ldots + \theta_n) + i \sin(\theta_1 + \theta_2 + \ldots + \theta_n)],$$

with

$$\left| z_1 z_2 \ldots z_n \right| = r_1 r_2 \ldots r_n$$

and

$$\arg(z_1 + z_2 + \ldots + z_n) = \theta_1 + \theta_2 + \ldots + \theta_n.$$

In particular, if $z_1 = z_2 = \ldots = z_n = z = r(\cos \theta + i \sin \theta)$, the above result reduces to

$$z^n = [r(\cos \theta + i \sin \theta)]^n = r^n(\cos n\theta + i \sin n\theta).$$

When $r = 1$ this result becomes

$$(\cos \theta + i \sin \theta)^n = \cos n\theta + i \sin n\theta,$$

and in this form it is known as **de Moivre's theorem**.

Example 12.2

Given $z_1 = 2\left[\cos \dfrac{\pi}{4} + i \sin \dfrac{\pi}{4}\right]$ and $z_2 = 3\left[\cos \dfrac{\pi}{3} + i \sin \dfrac{\pi}{3}\right]$ find

(i) $z_1 z_2$;   and

(ii) z_1/z_2.

Solution

$$z_1 z_2 = 2 \times 3 \left[\cos\left(\frac{\pi}{4} + \frac{\pi}{3}\right) + i \sin\left(\frac{\pi}{4} + \frac{\pi}{3}\right) \right]$$

$$= 6 \left[\cos\frac{7\pi}{12} + i \sin\frac{7\pi}{12} \right].$$

$$z_1/z_2 = \frac{2}{3} \left[\cos\left(\frac{\pi}{4} - \frac{\pi}{3}\right) + i \sin\left(\frac{\pi}{4} - \frac{\pi}{3}\right) \right]$$

$$= \frac{2}{3} \left[\cos\left(-\frac{\pi}{12}\right) + i \sin\left(-\frac{\pi}{12}\right) \right]$$

$$= \frac{2}{3} \left[\cos\frac{\pi}{12} - i \sin\frac{\pi}{12} \right]. \qquad \blacktriangle$$

Example 12.3

Find

(i) $(1 + i)^{25}$; and

(ii) $(2\sqrt{3} - 2i)^{30}$.

Solution

(i) Setting $z = 1 + i$ we see that

$$r = |z| = \sqrt{2},$$

and from rule 1 above for determining arg z

$$\theta = \arg z = \arctan 1 = \pi/4.$$

Thus

$$z^{25} = \left[\sqrt{2}\left(\cos\frac{\pi}{4} + i \sin\frac{\pi}{4} \right) \right]^{25}$$

$$= (\sqrt{2})^{25} \left[\cos\frac{25\pi}{4} + i \sin\frac{25\pi}{4} \right]$$

$$= 2^{25/2} \left[\cos\frac{\pi}{4} + i \sin\frac{\pi}{4} \right]$$

$$= 2^{25/2} \left[\frac{1}{\sqrt{2}} + \frac{i}{\sqrt{2}} \right]$$

$$= 2^{12}(1 + i).$$

(ii) Setting $z = 2\sqrt{3} - 2i$ we see that

$$r = |z| = [(2\sqrt{3})^2 + (-2)^2]^{1/2} = 4,$$

and from rule 4 above for determining arg z

$$\theta = \arg z = -\arctan\left|\frac{-2}{2\sqrt{3}}\right| = -\arctan\frac{1}{\sqrt{3}} = -\pi/6.$$

Thus

$$z^{30} = \left\{4\left[\cos\left(\frac{-\pi}{6}\right) + i\sin\left(\frac{-\pi}{6}\right)\right]\right\}^{30} = 4^{30}\left[\cos(-5\pi) + i\sin(-5\pi)\right]$$

$$= 4^{30}\left[\cos 5\pi - \sin 5\pi\right] = 4^{30}\cos\pi = -4^{30}.$$ ▲

Section 49 develops the Maclaurin series for e^θ, $\sin\theta$ and $\cos\theta$. Replacing θ by $i\theta$ in the series for e^θ, grouping real and imaginary terms and comparing the series involved with those for $\cos\theta$ and $\sin\theta$, respectively, gives the **Euler formula**

$$e^{i\theta} = \cos\theta + i\sin\theta.$$

This has many uses and, for example, since $(e^{i\theta})^n = e^{in\theta}$, an application of the Euler formula yields **de Moivre's theorem**

$$(\cos\theta + i\sin\theta)^n = \cos n\theta + i\sin n\theta.$$

Also, as $e^{i\theta_1}\cdot e^{i\theta_2} = e^{i(\theta_1 + \theta_2)}$, applying the Euler formula gives

$$(\cos\theta_1 + i\sin\theta_1)(\cos\theta_2 + i\sin\theta_2) = \cos(\theta_1 + \theta_2) + i\sin(\theta_1 + \theta_2).$$

Equating real and imaginary parts then gives rise to the trigonometric identities for $\sin(\theta_1 + \theta_2)$ and $\cos(\theta_1 + \theta_2)$ listed on page 810. Other trigonometric identities follow in similar fashion.

PROBLEMS 12

In problems 1 to 6 use the stated modulus–argument form of z to express it in the form $z = x + iy$.

1. $|z| = 3$, $\arg z = 3\pi/4$.

2. $|z| = \sqrt{5}$, $\arg z = -3\pi/4$.

3. $|z| = 4$, $\arg z = 2\pi/3$.

4. $|z| = 2$, $\arg z = -\pi/4$.

5. $|z| = 7$, $\arg z = 5\pi/6$.

6. $|z| = 6$, $\arg z = \pi/6$.

In problems 7 to 12 determine the modulus–argument form of the given complex number.

7. $z = 2 + 2i$.   10. $z = -3 + 3i$.

8. $z = 11i$.   11. $z = 3 - 2i$.

9. $z = -3\sqrt{3} - 3i$.   12. $z = -4$.

13. Given

$$z_1 = 3\left[\cos\frac{\pi}{4} + i\sin\frac{\pi}{4}\right]$$

and

$$z_2 = 2\left[\cos\frac{\pi}{3} + i\sin\frac{\pi}{3}\right],$$

find (a) $z_1 z_2$ and   (b) z_1/z_2.

14. Given

$$z_1 = 4\left[\cos\frac{\pi}{6} - i\sin\frac{\pi}{6}\right]$$

and

$$z_2 = 3\left[\cos\frac{\pi}{3} + i\sin\frac{\pi}{3}\right],$$

find (a) $z_1 z_2$ and   (b) z_1/z_2.

15. Given

$$z_1 = 4\left[\cos\frac{\pi}{3} + i\sin\frac{\pi}{3}\right]$$

and

$$z_2 = 5\left[\cos\frac{\pi}{4} - i\sin\frac{\pi}{4}\right],$$

find (a) $z_1 z_2$ and   (b) z_1/z_2.

16. Find $(1 + i)^{30}$.

17. Find $\left[\dfrac{1+i}{\sqrt{3}-i}\right]^5$.

18. Find $\left[\dfrac{1+i\sqrt{3}}{1-i}\right]^{20}$.

19. Show that

$$\left[\frac{1 + i\tan\theta}{1 - i\tan\theta}\right]^n = \frac{1 + i\tan n\theta}{1 - i\tan n\theta}.$$

20. Find $\left|z^n\right|$ and arg z^n when $z = \dfrac{1 + i\tan\theta}{1 - i\tan\theta}$.

Roots of complex numbers

The modulus–argument representation of complex numbers allows the solution of an equation of the form

$$w^n = z,$$

where z is a complex number and n is an integer. The n different solutions w to this equation are the nth **roots** of z, denoted by $\sqrt[n]{z}$ or, equivalently, by $z^{1/n}$.

Writing $z = r(\cos\theta + i\sin\theta)$ and $w = \rho(\cos\varphi + i\sin\varphi)$ the equation $w^n = z$ is seen to be equivalent to

$$\rho^n(\cos n\varphi + i\sin n\varphi) = r(\cos\theta + i\sin\theta).$$

Equality of two complex numbers z_1 and z_2 in modulus–argument form means that $|z_1| = |z_2|$ but that arg z_1 and arg z_2 may differ by a multiple of 2π, say $2k\pi$ with $k = 0, \pm 1, \pm 2, \dots$. Thus the above equation derived from $w^n = z$ is seen to imply that

$$\rho = r^{1/n} \quad \text{and} \quad \varphi = \frac{\theta + 2k\pi}{n},$$

with $k = 0, 1, 2, \dots, n-1$. Making $k > n-1$ merely repeats the same n roots.

Rule for finding the roots of $w^n = z$
The n roots $w_0, w_1, \dots, w_{n-1}$ of

$$w^n = z,$$

where $z = r(\cos\theta + i\sin\theta)$ and $w = \rho(\cos\varphi + i\sin\varphi)$ are given by

$$w_k = r^{1/n}\left[\cos\left(\frac{\theta + 2k\pi}{n}\right) + i\sin\left(\frac{\theta + 2k\pi}{n}\right)\right],$$

with $k = 0, 1, 2, \dots, n-1$.

Example 13.1

Find $\sqrt[8]{1}$.

Solution

$1 = \cos 0 + i \sin 0$, so setting $z = 1$ we see that $r = |z| = 1$ and $\theta = \arg z = 0$. Thus the **eight roots of unity** are

$$w_k = \cos \frac{2k\pi}{8} + \sin \frac{2k\pi}{8}$$

$$= \cos \frac{k\pi}{4} + i \sin \frac{k\pi}{4} \quad \text{with} \quad k = 0, 1, 2, \ldots, 7.$$

Thus locations of these points around the unit circle $|z| = 1$ (the circle of radius 1 centred on the origin) are shown in Fig. 44, from which it is seen that they are equally spaced around the circle with their arguments differing only by a multiple of $\pi/4$.

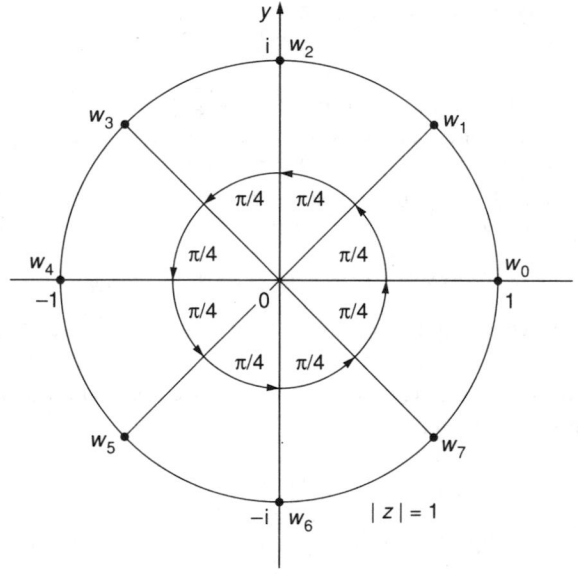

Fig. 44

It is easily seen that:

$w_0 = 1,$

$w_1 = (1 + i)/\sqrt{2},$

$w_2 = i,$

$w_3 = (-1 + i)/\sqrt{2},$

$w_4 = -1,$

$w_5 = (-1 - i)/\sqrt{2},$

$w_6 = -i,$

$w_7 = (1 - i)/\sqrt{2}$

Example 13.2

Find $^5\sqrt{(\sqrt{3} - i)}$.

Solution
We have $\sqrt{3} - i = 2[\cos(-\pi/6) + i\sin(-\pi/6)]$, so setting $z = \sqrt{3} - i$ we see that $r = |z| = 2$ and $\theta = \arg z = -\pi/6$. Thus the five roots are seen to be given by

$$w_k = 2^{1/5}\left[\cos\left(\frac{(12k-1)\pi}{30}\right) + i\sin\left(\frac{(12k-1)\pi}{30}\right)\right],$$

with $k = 0, 1, 2, 3, 4$.
  Consequently the required roots are

$$w_k = 2^{1/5}\left[\cos\left(\frac{11k\pi}{30}\right) + i\sin\left(\frac{11k\pi}{30}\right)\right],$$

with $k = 0, 1, 2, 3, 4$.
  The five roots are seen to lie on the circle $|z| = 2^{1/5}$ with their arguments only differing by a multiple of $11\pi/30$.   ▲

Example 13.1

Find $i^{2/3}$.

Solution
If we find the three cube roots of i, that is, if we solve the equation

$$w^3 = i$$

for the numbers w_0, w_1 and w_2, the three values of $i^{2/3}$ will be w_0^2, w_1^2 and w_2^2. This follows by setting $w = i^{1/3}$, because then

$$w^3 = i,$$

so that

$$w^2 = i^{2/3}.$$

Setting $z = i = [\cos\pi/2 + i\sin\pi/2]$ it follows that $r = |z| = 1$ and $\theta = \arg z = \pi/2$, and so the three cube roots of i are

$$w_k = \cos\left(\frac{\pi/2 + 2k\pi}{3}\right) + i\sin\left(\frac{\pi/2 + 2k\pi}{3}\right),$$

with $k = 0, 1, 2$.
Hence

$$w_0 = \cos\frac{\pi}{6} + i\sin\frac{\pi}{6} = \frac{1}{2}(\sqrt{3} + i),$$

$$w_1 = \cos \frac{5\pi}{6} + i \sin \frac{5\pi}{6} = \frac{1}{2}(-\sqrt{3} + i),$$

$$w_2 = \cos \frac{9\pi}{6} + i \sin \frac{9\pi}{6} = -i,$$

and so the three roots of $i^{2/3}$ are

$$w_0^2 = \frac{1}{2}(1 + i\sqrt{3}),$$

$$w_1^2 = \frac{1}{2}(1 - i\sqrt{3}),$$

$$w_2^2 = -1. \qquad \blacktriangle$$

Example 13.4

Let $w \neq 1$ be any one of the n roots of $w^n = 1$ (the nth roots of unity). Prove that for any positive integer $n > 1$

$$1 + w + w^2 + \ldots + w^{n-1} = 0.$$

Solution
Set

$$S = 1 + w + w^2 + \ldots + w^{n-1}$$

and multiply by w to obtain

$$wS = w + w^2 + w^3 + \ldots + w^n.$$

Substracting this result from the expression for S gives $S(1 - w) = 1 - w^n$, or

$$S = \frac{1 - w^n}{1 - w}.$$

However, $w^n = 1$, so as $w \neq 1$ we see that $S = 0$ and the result is proved. $\qquad \blacktriangle$

We remark for future use that when working with either real or complex numbers the expression $\sqrt[n]{a^m}$ is defined as $a^{m/n}$. Thus $\sqrt[3]{5^2} = 5^{2/3}$, $\sqrt[4]{9^3} = 9^{3/4}$ and $\sqrt[5]{[(1 + i)^4]} = (1 + i)^{4/5}$.

PROBLEMS 13

Find the roots of the following complex numbers.

1. $\sqrt[4]{1}$.
2. $(\sqrt{3} - i)^{1/6}$.
3. $(2 + i)^{1/3}$.
4. $(2 + 5i)^{1/4}$.

5. $\sqrt[3]{(3-i)}$.

6. $\sqrt[4]{-4}$.

7. $\left[\dfrac{1+i}{1-i}\right]^{1/6}$.

8. $1^{1/n}$.

14   Limits

The development of the calculus is based on the concept of a limit of a function. In what follows, instead of using the rigorous definition of a limit, it will suffice for our purposes to use the following intuitive definition.

The function $f(x)$ will be said to have the **limit** L as x tends to the value c if, when x is arbitrarily close to either side of c, $f(x)$ is arbitrarily close to L. The statement 'x tends to c' is written $x \rightarrow c$, and when the limit of $f(x)$ exists as $x \rightarrow c$ this will be shown by writing

$$\lim_{x \rightarrow c} f(x) = L.$$

When a limit exists it is **unique**, but the mere existence of the limit L of $f(x)$ as $x \rightarrow c$ does not necessarily imply that $f(c) = L$ or, indeed, that $f(c)$ is even defined.

The essential ideas underlying the limit of a function are illustrated by considering the function

$$f(x) = \frac{x^3 - x^2 - x - 2}{x - 2}.$$

The function $f(x)$ is defined for all x with the exception of the single point $x = 2$, at which point both numerator and denominator of $f(x)$ vanish. When this occurs $f(x)$ is not defined, and at such a point $f(x)$ is said to be an **indeterminate form**. Roughly speaking, $f(x)$ is an indeterminate form of this type if when $x = c$ the function $f(x)$ reduces to '$0 \div 0$'. Factorizing the numerator of $f(x)$ leads to the result

$$x^3 - x^2 - x - 2 = (x^2 + x + 1)(x - 2),$$

so

$$f(x) = \frac{(x^2 + x + 1)(x - 2)}{x - 2} = x^2 + x + 1,$$

for $x \neq 2$, but it must be remembered that $f(x)$ is not defined at $x = 2$. The graph of $f(x)$ is shown in Fig. 45, where the small circle at the point corresponding to $x = 2$ indicates that this point is missing from the graph.

Where the graph is unbroken, as, for example, at the typical point P corresponding to $x = -1$, it is seen that as x increases to the value -1, or decreases to it, so $f(x)$ approaches the actual functional value at P, which in this case is 1. Thus

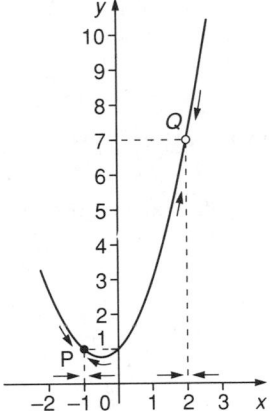

Fig. 45

$$\lim_{x \to -1} \frac{x^3 - x^2 - x - 2}{x - 2} = 1,$$

and it is also true here that $f(-1) = 1$. The equality of the limit and the functional value at the limit is true at any point on the graph of $f(x)$ through which the line of the graph passes and is unbroken, but not at a point like Q corresponding to $x = 2$ where a point is missing. At Q, as x increases to the value 2, or decreases to it, so $f(x)$ approaches arbitrarily closely to the value 7, but does not attain the value. Thus in this case

$$\lim_{x \to 2} \frac{x^3 - x^2 - x - 2}{x - 2} = 7,$$

but $f(2) \neq 7$ because $f(2)$ is not defined.

Elementary properties of limits

1 $\lim_{x \to c} [k f(x)] = k \lim_{x \to c} f(x) \quad (k = \text{const.}).$

2 $\lim_{x \to c} [f(x) \pm g(x)] = \lim_{x \to c} f(x) \pm \lim_{x \to c} g(x).$

3 $\lim_{x \to c} [f(x) \, g(x)] = \left[\lim_{x \to c} f(x) \right] \left[\lim_{x \to c} g(x) \right].$

4 $\lim_{x \to c} \left[\dfrac{f(x)}{g(x)} \right] = \left[\lim_{x \to c} f(x) \right] \bigg/ \left[\lim_{x \to c} g(x) \right]$ if $\lim_{x \to c} g(x) \neq 0.$

5 $\lim_{x \to c} f(g(x)) = f \left[\lim_{x \to c} g(x) \right].$

6 $\lim\limits_{x \to c} [f(x)]^n = \left[\lim\limits_{x \to c} f(x) \right]^n$.

TECHNIQUES FOR EVALUATING LIMITS

The following examples illustrate some of the most important ways of evaluating limits.

Example 14.1 (direct evaluation)

Find

$$\lim_{x \to 2} \left[\frac{x^2 + 5x + 3}{2x^3 - x + 4} \right].$$

Solution
This is not an indeterminate form, because setting $f(x) = x^2 + 5x + 3$, $g(x) = 2x^3 - x + 4$, the numerator and denominator do not vanish when $x = 2$. Thus, by property 4 above,

$$\lim_{x \to 2} \left[\frac{x^2 + 5x + 3}{2x^3 - x + 4} \right] = \frac{\lim\limits_{x \to 2} (x^2 + 5x + 3)}{\lim\limits_{x \to 2} (2x^3 - x + 4)} = \frac{17}{18}. \qquad \blacktriangle$$

Example 14.2 (finding a limit by factorization)

Find

$$\lim_{x \to 1} \left[\frac{2x^2 + x - 3}{x^2 + x - 2} \right].$$

Solution
This example is similar to the one used to introduce limits. It is an indeterminate form and factorization of the expression shows that

$$\lim_{x \to 2} \left[\frac{2x^2 + x - 3}{x^2 + x - 2} \right] = \lim_{x \to 1} \left[\frac{(x - 1)(2x + 3)}{(x - 1)(x + 2)} \right]$$

$$= \lim_{x \to 1} \left[\frac{2x + 3}{x + 2} \right] = \frac{5}{3}. \qquad \blacktriangle$$

Example 14.3 (a limit as $x \to \infty$)

Find

(i) $\lim\limits_{x \to \infty} \left[\frac{2x^3 + x^2 - 2x + 4}{3x^3 - x^2 + 1} \right];$

(ii) $\lim\limits_{x \to \infty} \left[\dfrac{x^4 - x^2 + 3x + 1}{4x^3 + x^2 + 3} \right]$;

(iii) $\lim\limits_{x \to \infty} \left[\dfrac{x^2 + 7x - 6}{x^3 + 4x^2 + 3x - 1} \right]$.

Solution

There are examples of indeterminate forms in which the limiting form of $f(x)$ looks like '$\infty \div \infty$'.

(i) Divide numerator and denominator by the highest power of x in the denominator, namely x^3, and then proceed to the limit using the fact that if n is a positive integer $1/x^n \to 0$ as $x \to \infty$ to obtain

$$\lim\limits_{x \to \infty} \left[\frac{2 + 1/x - 2/x^2 + 4/x^3}{3 - 1/x + 1/x^3} \right] = \frac{2}{3}.$$

(ii) Proceeding as in (i) gives

$$\lim\limits_{x \to \infty} \left[\frac{x^4 - x^2 + 3x + 1}{4x^3 + x^2 + 3} \right] = \lim\limits_{x \to \infty} \left[\frac{x - 1/x + 3/x^2 + 1/x^3}{4 + 1/x + 3/x^3} \right] = \infty.$$

(iii) Proceeding as in (i) gives

$$\lim\limits_{x \to \infty} \left[\frac{x^2 + 7x - 6}{x^3 + 4x^2 + 3x - 1} \right] = \lim\limits_{x \to \infty} \left[\frac{1/x + 7/x^2 - 6/x^3}{1 + 4/x + 3/x^2 - 1/x^3} \right] = 0. \qquad \blacktriangle$$

Example 14.4 (using the binomial theorem)

Find

$$\lim\limits_{x \to 0} \left[\frac{\sqrt{(1 + x)} - 1}{\sqrt{(1 - 2x)} - 1} \right].$$

Solution

This is an indeterminate form, and to evaluate it we expand $\sqrt{(1 + x)}$ and $\sqrt{(1 - 2x)}$ by the binomial theorem, using only the first few power of x, and then proceed to the limit. We have

$$\sqrt{(1 + x)} = (1 + x)^{1/2} = 1 + \frac{x}{2} - \frac{x^2}{8} + \frac{x^3}{16} - \dots .$$

$$\sqrt{(1 - 2x)} = (1 - 2x)^{1/2} = 1 - x - \frac{x^2}{2} - \frac{x^3}{2} - \dots .$$

Thus

$$\frac{\sqrt{(1 + x)} - 1}{\sqrt{(1 - 2x)} - 1} = \frac{[1 + x/2 - x^2/8 + x^3/16 - \dots] - 1}{[1 - x - x^2/2 - x^3/2 - \dots] - 1},$$

$$= \frac{x/2 - x^2/8 + x^3/16 - \dots}{-[x + x^2/2 + x^3/2 + \dots]}$$

$$= \frac{1/2 - x/8 + x^2/16 - \dots}{-[1 + x/2 + x^2/2 + \dots]},$$

and so

$$\lim_{x \to 0} \left[\frac{\sqrt{(1+x)} - 1}{\sqrt{(1-2x)} - 1} \right] = \lim_{x \to 0} \left[\frac{1/2 - x/8 + x^2/16 - \dots}{-[1 + x/2 + x^2/2 + \dots]} \right] = -\frac{1}{2}. \qquad \blacktriangle$$

Example 14.5 (combining limits)

Find

$$\lim_{x \to 0} \left\{ \left[\frac{(1 + 2x)^{1/3} - 1}{3x} \right] \left[\frac{\sqrt{(1+x)} - 1}{\sqrt{(1-2x)} - 1} \right] \right\}.$$

Solution
This involves the product of two indeterminate forms, so we use property 3 in the above list. Setting

$$f(x) = \frac{(1 + 2x)^{1/3} - 1}{3x}$$

and

$$g(x) = \frac{\sqrt{(1+x)} - 1}{\sqrt{(1-2x)} - 1},$$

we use the fact that

$$\lim_{x \to 0} [f(x)\, g(x)] = \left[\lim_{x \to 0} f(x) \right] \left[\lim_{x \to 0} g(x) \right].$$

Now

$$(1 + 2x)^{1/3} = 1 + \frac{2x}{3} - \frac{4x^2}{9} + \frac{40x^3}{81} - \dots,$$

so

$$\frac{(1 + 2x)^{1/3} - 1}{3x} = \frac{2x/3 - 4x^2/9 + 40x^3/81 + \dots}{3x}$$

$$= \frac{2}{9} - \frac{4x}{27} + \frac{40x^2}{243} - \dots,$$

and thus

$$\lim_{x \to 0} f(x) = \lim_{x \to 0} \left[\frac{7}{9} - \frac{4x}{27} + \frac{40x^2}{243} - \dots \right] = \frac{2}{9}.$$

It was shown in Example 14.4 that

$$\lim_{x \to 0} g(x) = -\frac{1}{2},$$

and so

$$\lim_{x \to 0} \left\{ \left[\frac{(1 + 2x)^{1/3} - 1}{3x} \right] \left[\frac{\sqrt{(1 + x)} - 1}{\sqrt{(1 - 2x)} - 1} \right] \right\} = \left[\lim_{x \to 0} f(x) \right] \left[\lim_{x \to 0} g(x) \right]$$

$$= \left[\frac{2}{9} \right] \left(-\frac{1}{2} \right) = -\frac{1}{9}. \qquad \blacktriangle$$

The following are important and useful trigonometric limits:

1 $\lim\limits_{x \to 0} \left[\dfrac{\sin kx}{x} \right] = k;$

2 $\lim\limits_{x \to 0} \left[\dfrac{\tan kx}{x} \right] = k;$

3 $\lim\limits_{x \to 0} \left[\dfrac{1 - \cos kx}{x} \right] = 0;$

4 $\lim\limits_{x \to 0} \left[\dfrac{1 - \cos kx}{x^2} \right] = \dfrac{k^2}{2}.$

Example 14.6

Prove limits 1 and 2, namely that

$$\lim_{x \to 0} \left[\frac{\sin kx}{x} \right] = k \quad \text{and} \quad \lim_{x \to 0} \left[\frac{\tan kx}{x} \right] = k.$$

Solution
Inspection of Fig. 46 shows that

area of triangle $OAC <$ area of sector $OAC <$ area of triangle OAB.

In terms of OA which is of unit length and the angle x, the above inequalities become

$$\frac{1}{2} \sin x < \frac{1}{2} x < \frac{1}{2} \tan x.$$

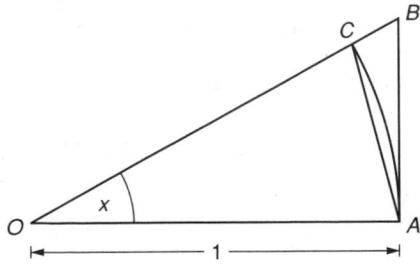

Fig. 46

When x is small, $\sin x$ is positive, so taking reciprocals and multiplying by $\frac{1}{2} \sin x$ gives, after reversing the inequality because of 9 on page 3,

$$\cos x < \frac{\sin x}{x} < 1.$$

Taking the limit of this inequality as $x \to 0$ gives

$$\lim_{x \to 0} \cos x < \lim_{x \to 0} \left[\frac{\sin x}{x} \right] < 1,$$

but $\lim_{x \to 0} \cos x = 1$, and hence

$$\lim_{x \to 0} \left[\frac{\sin x}{x} \right] = 1.$$

Replacing x by kx in the above result gives

$$\lim_{kx \to 0} \left[\frac{\sin kx}{kx} \right] = 1,$$

but $kx \to 0$ as $x \to 0$, so this is equivalent to

$$\lim_{x \to 0} \left[\frac{\sin kx}{kx} \right] = 1,$$

and hence to

$$\lim_{x \to 0} \left[\frac{\sin kx}{x} \right] = k.$$

The proof of limit 2 follows in similar fashion.   ▲

Example 14.7

Find

$$\lim_{x \to 0} \left[\frac{\tan 4x}{\sin 5x} \right].$$

Solution

$$\frac{\tan 4x}{\sin 5x} = \frac{\sin 4x}{\cos 4x} \cdot \frac{1}{\sin 5x} = \frac{1}{\cos 4x} \left[\frac{\sin 4x}{x} \right] \cdot \left[\frac{x}{\sin 5x} \right].$$

Thus, appealing to property 3 we see that

$$\lim_{x \to 0} \left[\frac{\tan 4x}{\sin 5x} \right] = \lim_{x \to 0} \left[\frac{1}{\cos 4x} \right] \cdot \lim_{x \to 0} \left[\frac{\sin 4x}{x} \right] \cdot \lim_{x \to 0} \left[\frac{x}{\sin 5x} \right].$$

We have

$$\lim_{x \to 0} \left[\frac{1}{\cos 4x} \right] = 1,$$

and from Example 14.6

$$\lim_{x \to 0} \left[\frac{\sin 4x}{x} \right] = 4$$

and

$$\lim_{x \to 0} \left[\frac{x}{\sin 5x} \right] = \frac{1}{5},$$

and so

$$\lim_{x \to 0} \left[\frac{\tan 4x}{\sin 5x} \right] = 1 \times 4 \times \frac{1}{5} = \frac{4}{5}.$$

▲

PROBLEMS 14

Find the following limits.

1. $\lim\limits_{x \to 1} \left[\dfrac{3x^2 + 9x - 1}{2x^3 + x^2 + 4} \right].$

2. $\lim\limits_{x \to -1} \left[\dfrac{x^2 + 2x + 1}{3x^2 + 4x + 2} \right].$

3. $\lim\limits_{x \to 2} \left[\dfrac{x^2 + 9x - 6}{2x^2 - 3x - 2} \right].$

4. $\lim\limits_{x \to \infty} \left[\dfrac{4x^3 + 9x^2 - 3}{3x^3 + 4x^2 + 4} \right].$

5. $\lim\limits_{x \to \infty} \left[\dfrac{5 - 7x^2 - 21x^3}{7x^3 + 2x + 4} \right].$

6. $\lim\limits_{h \to 0} \left[\dfrac{(x + h)^3 - x^3}{h} \right].$

7. $\lim\limits_{h \to 0} \left[\dfrac{(3 + h)^2 - 9}{h} \right].$

8. $\lim\limits_{x \to 0} \left[\dfrac{x}{\sqrt{(1 + x)} - 1} \right].$

9. $\lim\limits_{x \to -2} \left[\dfrac{x^3 + 4x^2 + 4x}{x^2 - x - 6} \right].$

10. $\lim\limits_{x \to 4} \left[\dfrac{\sqrt{(2x+1)} - 3}{\sqrt{(x-2)} - \sqrt{2}} \right]$.

11. $\lim\limits_{x \to 0} \left[\dfrac{\sqrt{(x^2 + 4)} - 2}{\sqrt{(x^2 + 9)} - 3} \right]$.

12. $\lim\limits_{x \to 0} \left[\dfrac{\sin^2 (x/4)}{x^2} \right]$.

13. $\lim\limits_{x \to 0} \left[\dfrac{\sin 5x}{\tan 7x} \right]$.

14. $\lim\limits_{x \to 4} \left[\dfrac{x^4 - 64x}{(x-1)\tan 3(x-4)} \right]$.

15. $\lim\limits_{x \to 0} \left[\dfrac{\sin mx}{\sin nx} \right]$.

16. $\lim\limits_{x \to \infty} \left[\dfrac{\sqrt{(x^2 + 14)} + x}{\sqrt{(x^2 - 2)} + x} \right]$.

17. $\lim\limits_{x \to -\infty} \left[\dfrac{\sqrt{(x^2 + 14)} + x}{\sqrt{(x^2 - 2)} + x} \right]$.

18. $\lim\limits_{x \to 1} \left[\dfrac{x-1}{\sin \pi x} \right]$.

19. $\lim\limits_{x \to 0} \left[\dfrac{x - \sin 2x}{x - \sin 5x} \right]$.

20. $\lim\limits_{x \to 0} \left[\dfrac{\sin x}{\sin 6x - \sin 7x} \right]$.

21. $\lim\limits_{x \to 0} \left[\dfrac{\cos 3x - \cos 7x}{x^2} \right]$.

22.   By writing $1 - \cos kx = 2\sin^2 \tfrac{1}{2} kx$, so that

$$\frac{1 - \cos kx}{x} = 2\left[\frac{\sin \frac{1}{2} kx}{x} \right] \sin \tfrac{1}{2} kx \quad \text{and} \quad \frac{1 - \cos kx}{x^2} = 2\left[\frac{\sin \frac{1}{2} kx}{x} \right]^2,$$

show that

$$\lim\limits_{x \to 0} \left[\frac{1 - \cos kx}{x} \right] = 0 \quad \text{and} \quad \lim\limits_{x \to 0} \left[\frac{1 - \cos kx}{x^2} \right] = \frac{k^2}{2}.$$

One-sided limits: continuity

15

It can happen that although a function does not have a limit as $x \to c$ in the sense of Section 14, it does have a limit in a more restricted sense when x approaches c from one side or the other. Such limits are called **one-sided limits**, and although a one-sided limit may exist when x approaches c from one direction, there may or may not be another one-sided limit when it approaches c from the other direction.

To work with one-sided limits we need to modify the notation introduced in Section 14. If x approaches c from the **left**, that is if x **increases** to the value c, we will write $x \to c -$. Correspondingly, if x approaches c from the **right**, that is if x **decreases** to the value c, we will write $x \to c +$.

We can now define limits from the left and right. The function $f(x)$ will be said to have a **limit from the left** L_1 if when x is arbitrarily close to the left of c, $f(x)$ is arbitrailry close to L_1. Analogously, the function $f(x)$ will be said to have a **limit from the right** L_2 if when x is arbitrarily close to the right of c, $f(x)$ is arbitrarily close to L_2.

Thus we write

$$\lim_{x \to c -} f(x) = L_1 \quad \text{and} \quad \lim_{x \to c +} f(x) = L_2.$$

The function $f(x)$ may, or may not, be defined at a one-sided limit.

Figure 47 illustrates a function $f(x)$ defined for $a \leqslant x < c$ and $c < x \leqslant b$

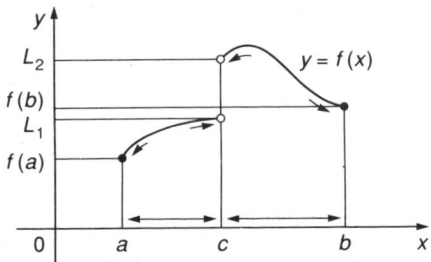

Fig. 47

which has different limits from the left and right at $x = c$, only a limit from the right at $x = a$ and only a limit from the left at b. We see from the graph that

$$\lim_{x \to a+} f(x) = f(a) \quad \text{and} \quad \lim_{x \to b-} f(x) = f(b),$$

because the values of $f(x)$ corresponding to $x = a$ and $x = b$ lie on the curve, whereas

$$\lim_{x \to c-} f(x) = L_1 \quad \text{and} \quad \lim_{x \to c+} f(x) = L_2.$$

with $L_1 \neq L_2$. The function $f(x)$ shown in the diagram is not defined at $x = c$.

Example 15.1 (a function with different one-sided limits)

Show that $f(x) = x/|x|$ has two different one-sided limits as $x \to 0$.

Solution
The graph of $f(x) = x/|x|$ is shown in Fig. 48, from which we see that

$$\lim_{x \to 0-} \frac{x}{|x|} = -1 \quad \text{and} \quad \lim_{x \to 0+} \frac{x}{|x|} = 1.$$

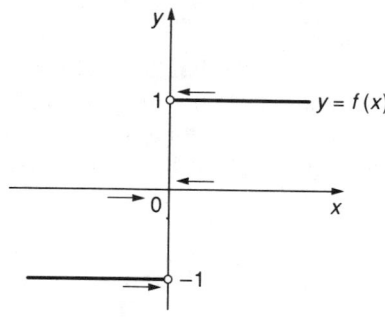

Fig. 48

Example 15.2 (a function with only a single one-sided limit)

Examine the limiting behaviour of

$$f(x) = 1 + \sqrt{(5 - x)}$$

as $x \to 5$.

Solution
The function $f(x) = 1 + \sqrt{(5 - x)}$ is only defined (in terms of real variables) if $5 - x \geq 0$. Thus a limit can exist as $x \to 5 -$, but it certainly cannot exist as $x \to 5+$ because then $5 - x < 0$. The function is illustrated in Fig. 49, from which it is seen that

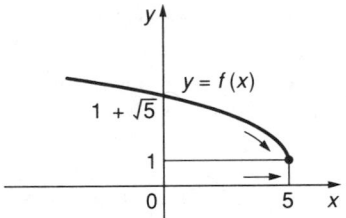

Fig. 49

$$\lim_{x \to 5-} [1 + \sqrt{(5-x)}] = 1.$$ ▲

Example 15.3

Given

$$f(x) = \frac{3}{4^{1/x} + 7},$$

find

(i) $\lim_{x \to 0-} f(x)$; and

(ii) $\lim_{x \to 0+} f(x)$.

Solution

(i) If x is small and negative, $1/x$ is large and negative, so $\lim_{x \to 0-} 4^{1/x} = 0$, and thus

$$\lim_{x \to 0-} \left[\frac{3}{4^{1/x} + 7}\right] = \frac{3}{7}.$$

(ii) If x is small and positive, $1/x$ is large and positive, so $\lim_{x \to 0+} 4^{1/x} = \infty$, and thus

$$\lim_{x \to 0+} \left[\frac{3}{4^{1/x} + 7}\right] = 0.$$ ▲

The concept of limits from the left and right lead directly to the definition of another fundamental idea called continuity. A function $f(x)$ will be said to be **continuous** at $x = c$ if

1 $\lim_{x \to c-} f(x) = \lim_{x \to c+} f(x) = L$; and

2 $f(c) = L$.

Thus a function is continuous at $x = c$ (and also in its immediate neighbourhood) if the limits of $f(x)$ from both the left and right at $x = c$ exist and are equal to L and, moreover, $f(c)$ is defined and is such that $f(c) = L$. Intuitively, this means that in the immediate neighbourhood of $x = c$, the curve representing the graph of $y = f(x)$ is an unbroken line passing through the point (c, L) in the (x, y)-plane. In general, if $f(x)$ is continuous for $a \leqslant x \leqslant b$, its graph is an unbroken curve starting at the point $(a, f(a))$ and ending at the point $(b, f(b))$.

When it happens that

$$\lim_{x \to c-} f(x) = L_1 \quad \text{and} \quad \lim_{x \to c+} f(x) = L_2,$$

but $L_1 \neq L_2$, the function $f(x)$ is said to be **discontinuous** at $x = c$. Such discontinuities are often called **jump discontinuities**. The function shown in Fig. 47 is discontinuous at $x = c$.

A weak form of discontinuity arises when

$$\lim_{x \to c-} f(x) = \lim_{x \to c+} f(x) = L,$$

but $f(x)$ is not defined at $x = c$. Thus the graph of such a function has a single point missing at $x = c$ as, for example, at $x = 2$ in Fig. 45. In these circumstances, if we define $f(x)$ by setting $f(c) = L$ the function becomes continuous at (and in the neighbourhood of) $x = c$. A discontunuity of this type is called a **removable discontinuity**.

Example 15.4

Show that

$$f(x) = \frac{\sin x}{x}$$

is a continuous function with a single removable discontinuity at the origin.

Solution
The function $f(x) = (\sin x)/x$ is the quotient of two continuous functions and it is defined for all x other than at $x = 0$ at which point it becomes an indeterminate form. Thus its graph will be an unbroken curve except at $x = 0$. Appealing to Example 14.6 we see that

$$\lim_{x \to 0-} \left[\frac{\sin x}{x} \right] = \lim_{x \to 0+} \left[\frac{\sin x}{x} \right] = 1.$$

The equality of the limits from the left and right follows because $(\sin x)/x$ is an **even** function.

Consequently $f(x) = (\sin x)/x$ has a removable discontinuity at $x = 0$, and if we define $f(0) = 1$ the function becomes continuous for all x. A graph of $y = (\sin x)/x$ is shown in Fig. 50.

Thus the function

$$f(x) = \begin{cases} \dfrac{\sin x}{x}, & \text{for } x \neq 0 \\ 1, & \text{for } x = 0 \end{cases}$$

is continuous for all x.   ▲

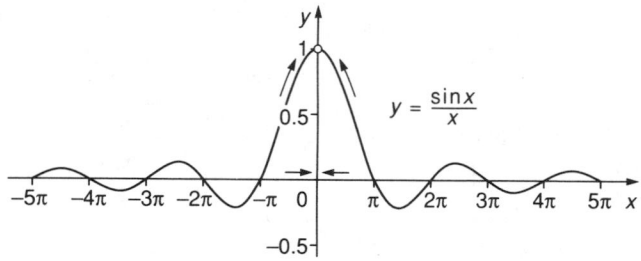

Fig. 50

Example 15.5

Examine the contunity of $f(x) = 1/x$

(i)   in the open interval $0 < x < k$; and

(ii)   in the closed interval $0 \leqslant x \leqslant k$.

Solution

(i) $f(x)$ is finite in the open interval $0 < x < k$ because the interval does not contain the value $x = 0$. The graph is represented by an unbroken curve, so the function is continuous for any k.

(ii)   As the closed interval $0 \leqslant x \leqslant k$ contains the value $x = 0$ the function becomes infinite at the origin and thus is not continuous for any choice of k.   ▲

Consequences of continuity

Let $f(x)$ and $g(x)$ be continuous for $a \leqslant x \leqslant b$, then:

1    $kf(x)$ is continuous for $a \leqslant x \leqslant b$ $(k = \text{const.})$;

2    $f(x) = \pm g(x)$ is continuous for $a \leqslant x \leqslant b$;

3    $f(x) g(x)$ is continuous for $a \leqslant x \leqslant b$;

4    $f(x)/g(x)$ is continuous for $a \leqslant x \leqslant b$, provided $g(x) \neq 0$;

5   If $a < c < b$, then the composite function $f \circ g(x) = f(g(x))$ is continuous at $x = c$.

One of the important consequences of continutity is the following theorem which applies to any function which is continuous on a closed interval.

Intermediate value theorem

If $f(x)$ is continuous on the closed interval $a \leqslant x \leqslant b$, and k is any number between $f(a)$ and $f(b)$, then the graph of $y = f(x)$ will pass at least once through the value k.

The meaning of this theorem is illustrated graphically in Fig. 51. It is seen from the diagram that as the graph of $y = f(x)$ is an unbroken line (the function

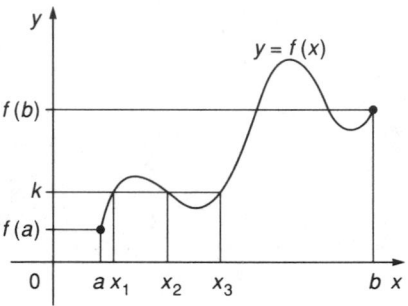

Fig. 51

is continuous), starting at $(a, f(a))$ and ending at $(b, f(b))$, the line representing the graph must pass at least once through any number k which lies between $f(a)$ and $f(b)$. In Fig. 51 the graph of $y = f(x)$ actually crosses the line $y = k$ three times, corresponding to $x = x_1$, $x = x_2$ and $x = x_3$.

Example 15.6 (an application of the intermediate value theorem)

Show the equation

$$\sin x = \frac{1}{2} x$$

has a root in the interval $\pi/2 \leqslant x \leqslant \pi$.

Solution
Set

$$f(x) = \sin x - \frac{1}{2} x,$$

then as $\sin x$ and $\frac{1}{2} x$ are continuous functions for $\pi/2 \leqslant x \leqslant \pi$, $f(x)$ is a continuous function for $-\pi/2 \leqslant x \leqslant \pi$, and so the intermediate value theorem applies. A simple calculation shows that

$$f(\pi/2) = 0.215$$

and

$$f(\pi) = -1.571,$$

so by the intermediate value theorem there must be at least one value of x, say $x = c$ (a root of $f(x)$), strictly between $\pi/2$ and π for which $f(c) = 0$, and the result is proved.

Figure 52 shows a graph of $y = \sin x - \frac{1}{2} x$, from which it can be seen that, approximately, $c = 1.9$ (the point where the graph crosses the x-axis). For purposes of comparison, the graphs of $y = \sin x$ and $y = \frac{1}{2} x$ are also shown and, of course, the value of x at the point P at which they intersect corresponds to the required root c. ▲

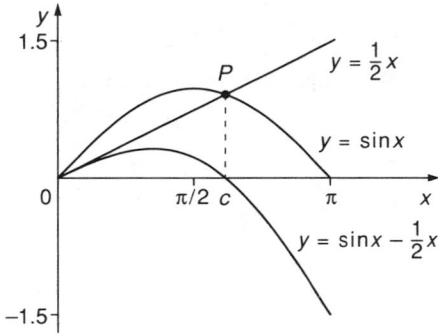

Fig. 52

PROBLEMS 15

In problems 1 to 10 find the one-sided limits when they exist, and determine whether the function $f(x)$ involved has a removable discontinuity.

1. (a) $\lim\limits_{x \to 3-} \left[\dfrac{x-3}{x^2-9}\right]$; (b) $\lim\limits_{x \to 3+} \left[\dfrac{x-3}{x^2-9}\right]$.

2. (a) $\lim\limits_{x \to 1-} \sqrt{(1-x)}$; (b) $\lim\limits_{x \to 1+} \sqrt{(1-x)}$.

3. (a) $\lim\limits_{x \to 2-} |x^2-4|^{1/2}$; (b) $\lim\limits_{x \to 2+} |x^2-4|^{1/2}$.

4. (a) $\lim\limits_{x \to 0-} \left[\dfrac{3^{1/x}}{3^{1/x}+4}\right]$; (b) $\lim\limits_{x \to 0+} \left[\dfrac{3^{1/x}}{3^{1/x}+4}\right]$.

5. (a) $\lim\limits_{x \to 0-} \left[\dfrac{\sin 3x}{|x|}\right]$; (b) $\lim\limits_{x \to 0+} \left[\dfrac{\sin 3x}{|x|}\right]$.

6. (a) $\lim\limits_{x \to 0-} \left[\dfrac{2^{1/x}+3\times 4^{1/x}}{4^{1/x}+9}\right]$; (b) $\lim\limits_{x \to 0+} \left[\dfrac{2^{1/x}+3\times 4^{1/x}}{4^{1/x}+9}\right]$.

7. (a) $\lim\limits_{x \to 0-} \left[\dfrac{5^{1/x}}{3^{1/x}+5}\right]$; (b) $\lim\limits_{x \to 0+} \left[\dfrac{5^{1/x}}{3^{1/x}+5}\right]$.

8. (a) $\lim\limits_{x \to 4-} \left[\dfrac{\sqrt{(2x+1)}-3}{\sqrt{(x-2)}-\sqrt{2}}\right]$; (b) $\lim\limits_{x \to 4+} \left[\dfrac{\sqrt{(2x+1)}-3}{\sqrt{(x-2)}-\sqrt{2}}\right]$.

9. (a) $\lim\limits_{x \to 0-} \left[\dfrac{\tan |5x|}{\sin 3x}\right]$; (b) $\lim\limits_{x \to 0+} \left[\dfrac{\tan |5x|}{\sin 3x}\right]$.

10.   (a) $\displaystyle \lim_{x \to 0-} \left[\frac{x + |x|}{\sin x} \right]$; (b) $\displaystyle \lim_{x \to 0+} \left[\frac{x + |x|}{\sin x} \right]$

In problems 11 to 20 determine where, if at all, the given function is discontinuous.

11. $f(x) = |x|$,   for $-3 \leqslant x \leqslant 4$.

12. $f(x) = 1/(x - 3)$,   for $-1 \leqslant x \leqslant 2$.

13. $f(x) = \begin{cases} 1 + x, & \text{for } 0 \leqslant x \leqslant 2 \\ 2 + 3x, & \text{for } x > 2. \end{cases}$

14. $f(x) = x^n$ for $n \leqslant x < n$ and $n = 0, 1, 2, \dots$.

15. $f(x) = \tan x$,   for $-\pi/4 \leqslant x \leqslant \pi/4$.

16. $f(x) = \dfrac{x^2}{x^2 - 4}$.

17. $f(x) = \dfrac{|x + 5|}{x + 5}$.

18. $f(g(x))$ when $f(x) = \dfrac{3}{x + 2}$ and $g(x) = x^2 + 6$.

19. $f(g(x))$ when $f(x) = 3/x$ and $g(x) = \sin 2x$.

20. $f(g(x))$ when $f(x) = \sin(2x + 1)$ and $g(x) = \dfrac{1}{2} \cos 3x$.

Derivatives   16

When the limit exists, the derivative of the function $f(x)$ at $x = a$, denoted by $f'(a)$, is defined as

$$f'(a) = \lim_{h \to 0} \left[\frac{f(a+h) - f(a)}{h} \right].$$

The symbol $'$ used here is called a 'prime', and the expression $f'(a)$ is read 'f prime a'. It follows from this definition that $f'(a)$ is a **number** determined as the limit of an indeterminate form as $x \to a$. If the number a in this definition is replaced by the variable x, giving

$$f'(x) = \lim_{h \to 0} \left[\frac{f(x+h) - f(x)}{h} \right],$$

the expression $f'(x)$ becomes a **function** of x, and it is called the **first order derivative** of $f(x)$ with respect to x. Equivalent notations for the first order derivative of $f(x)$ with respect to x are

$$f'(x), \quad \frac{d}{dx}[f(x)] \quad \text{and, if} \quad y = f(x), \quad \frac{dy}{dx}.$$

The operation of determining the derivative of a function is called **differentiation**, and a function for which a derivative exists is said to be **differentiable**. Inspection of Fig. 53 shows that

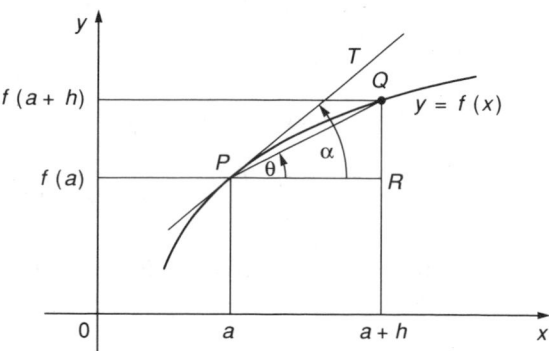

Fig. 53

$$f'(a) = \lim_{h \to 0} \left[\frac{f(a+h) - f(a)}{h} \right] = \lim_{h \to 0} \left[\frac{QR}{PR} \right]$$

$$= \lim_{h \to 0} [\tan \theta].$$

However, as $h \to 0$, so $Q \to P$, and the secant line (chord) PQ approaches the tangent line PT to the graph of $y = f(x)$ at $x = a$. If the tangent line PT is inclined at an angle α to the x-axis, it then follows that $\theta \to \alpha$ as $h \to 0$, and so

$$f'(a) = \tan \alpha.$$

Thus the **geometrical interpretation** of the derivative of $f(x)$ at any point $x = x_0$ is that it is the tangent of the angle between the tangent line PT to the graph $y = f(x)$ at x_0 and the x-axis, with the angle α measured as shown in Fig. 53.

It follows directly from the above definition that

$$\frac{dy}{dx} = 1 \bigg/ \left[\frac{dx}{dy} \right].$$

Example 16.1

Show that

(i) $\dfrac{d}{dx} [k] = 0;$ and

(ii) $\dfrac{d}{dx} [kf(x)] = kf(x),$ ($k = $ const.),

Solution
(i)   Setting $f(x) = k = $ const., it follows that

$$f(x+h) = k$$

and so

$$f(x+h) - f(x) = k - k \equiv 0.$$

Thus from the definition of a derivative:

$$\frac{d}{dx} [k] = \lim_{h \to 0} \left[\frac{f(x+h) - f(x)}{h} \right] = \lim_{h \to 0} \left[\frac{0}{h} \right] \equiv 0.$$

(ii)   We must differentiate the function $kf(x)$, with $k = $ const. From the definition of a derivative:

$$\frac{d}{dx} [kf(x)] = \lim_{h \to 0} \left[\frac{kf(x+h) - kf(x)}{h} \right] = k \lim_{h \to 0} \left[\frac{f(x+h) - f(x)}{h} \right] = kf'(x). \quad \blacktriangle$$

Example 16.2

If $y = x^n$,   find $\dfrac{dy}{dx}$ and $\dfrac{dx}{dy}$.

Solution
From the definition of a derivative:

$$\frac{dy}{dx} = \frac{d}{dx}[x^n] = \lim_{h \to 0} \left[\frac{(x+h)^n - x^n}{h} \right].$$

However, expanding $(x + h)^n$ by the binomial theorem, and retaining only the first few powers of h because we are only interested in the case when $h \to 0$, gives

$$\frac{d}{dx}[x^n] = \lim_{h \to 0} \left[\frac{\left[x^n + nx^{n-1}h + \dfrac{n(n-1)(n-2)}{2!} x^{n-2}h^2 + \ldots \right] - x^n}{h} \right]$$

$$= \lim_{h \to 0} \left[nx^{n-1} + \frac{n(n-1)(n-2)}{2!} x^{n-2}h + \ldots \right]$$

$$= nx^{n-1},$$

and so

$$\frac{dy}{dx} = \frac{d}{dx}[x^n] = nx^{n-1}.$$

As $dx/dy = 1/(dy/dx)$ it follows that

$$\frac{dx}{dy} = \frac{1}{nx^{n-1}}.$$

Example 16.3

Find

$$\frac{d}{dx}\left[\frac{1}{1+x} \right]. \qquad\qquad \blacktriangle$$

Solution

$$\frac{d}{dx}\left[\frac{1}{1+x} \right] = \lim_{h \to 0} \left[\frac{1/[1 + (x + h)] - 1/(1+x)}{h} \right]$$

$$= \lim_{h \to 0} \left[\frac{-1}{(1+x+h)(1+x)} \right] = \frac{-1}{(1+x)^2} \qquad \blacktriangle$$

Example 16.4

Show that

(i) $\dfrac{\mathrm{d}}{\mathrm{d}x}[\sin\ kx]=k\ \cos\ kx;$

(ii) $\dfrac{\mathrm{d}}{\mathrm{d}x}[\cos\ kx]=-k\ \sin\ kx$ (k = const.).

Solution

(i) $\dfrac{\mathrm{d}}{\mathrm{d}x}[\sin\ kx]=\lim_{h\to 0}\left[\dfrac{\sin\ k(x+h)-\sin\ kx}{h}\right]$

$\qquad\qquad=\lim_{h\to 0}\left[\dfrac{\sin\ kx\ \cos\ kh+\cos\ kx\ \sin\ kh-\sin\ kx}{h}\right]$

$\qquad\qquad=\lim_{h\to 0}\left[\left(\dfrac{\cos\ kh-1}{h}\right)\sin\ kx+\cos\ kx\left(\dfrac{\sin\ kh}{h}\right)\right]$

However, from Section 14 we have

$$\lim_{h\to 0}\left[\dfrac{\cos\ kh-1}{h}\right]=0\ \ \text{and}\ \ \lim_{h\to 0}\left[\dfrac{\sin\ kh}{h}\right]=k,$$

so

$$\dfrac{\mathrm{d}}{\mathrm{d}x}[\sin\ kx]=k\ \cos\ kx.$$

(ii) $\dfrac{\mathrm{d}}{\mathrm{d}x}[\cos\ kx]=\lim_{h\to 0}\left[\dfrac{\cos\ k(x+h)-\cos\ kx}{h}\right]$

$\qquad\qquad=\lim_{h\to 0}\left[\dfrac{\cos\ kx\ \cos\ kh-\sin\ kx\ \sin\ kh-\cos\ kx}{h}\right]$

$\qquad\qquad=\lim_{h\to 0}\left[\left(\dfrac{\cos\ kh-1}{h}\right)\cos\ kx-\sin\ kx\left(\dfrac{\sin\ kh}{h}\right)\right],$

so using the limiting values of the bracketed expressions already quoted in (i) gives

$$\dfrac{\mathrm{d}}{\mathrm{d}x}[\cos\ kx]=-k\ \sin\ kx.$$ ▲

Example 16.5 (a function which is not differentiable at a point)

Show that $f(x)=|x|$ is differentiable everywhere except at $x=0$.

Solution
If $x>0$, then $f(x)=x$ and it follows from Example 16.2 with $n=1$ that

$$\dfrac{\mathrm{d}}{\mathrm{d}x}[|x|]=1,\quad\text{for}\quad x>0.$$

If $x<0$, then $f(x)=-x$ and it follows from Example 16.1(ii) with $k=-1$ and Example 16.2 with $n=1$ that

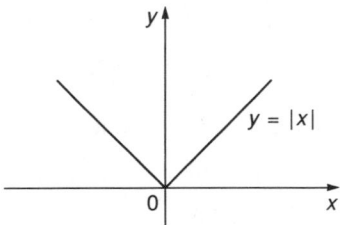

Fig. 54

$$\frac{\mathrm{d}}{\mathrm{d}x}[|x|] = -1, \quad \text{for} \quad x < 0.$$

However, the graph of $y = |x|$ has no tangent at the point $x = 0$, as may be seen from Fig. 54, so from the geometrical interpretation of a derivative it follows that $f(x) = |x|$ is not differentiable at the origin. Thus from the definition of $|x|$ we see that

$$\frac{\mathrm{d}}{\mathrm{d}x}[|x|] = \frac{x}{|x|}, \quad \text{for} \quad x \neq 0. \qquad \blacktriangle$$

Table 2 lists the derivatives of some commonly occurring elementary functions.

Table 2 A short table of derivatives

$f(x)$	$f'(x)$
$k = \text{const.}$	0
x^α	$\alpha x^{\alpha - 1}$
$\sin x$	$\cos x$
$\cos x$	$-\sin x$
$\tan x$	$\sec^2 x$
$\sec x$	$\sec x \tan x$
$\operatorname{cosec} x$	$-\operatorname{cosec} x \cot x$
$\cot x$	$-\operatorname{cosec}^2 x$

The basic rules for differentiating functions formed as simple combinations of differentiable functions are listed below.

Fundamental rules for differentiation
Let $f(x)$ and $g(x)$ be differentiable functions, then:

1 $\dfrac{\mathrm{d}}{\mathrm{d}x}[kf(x)] = kf'(x), \; k = \text{const.}$;

2 $\dfrac{\mathrm{d}}{\mathrm{d}x}[f(x) \pm g(x)] = f'(x) \pm g'(x)$ (differentiation of a sum or difference);

3 $\dfrac{\mathrm{d}}{\mathrm{d}x}[f(x)\, g(x)] = g(x)f'(x) + f(x)g'(x)$ (differentiation of a product);

4 $\dfrac{d}{dx}\left[\dfrac{f(x)}{g(x)}\right] = \dfrac{f'(x)\ g(x) - f(x)\ g'(x)}{[g(x)]^2}$, $(g(x) \ne 0)$ (differentiation of a quotient);

5 If $y = f(u)$ and $u = g(x)$, then $y = f(g(x))$ and

$$\frac{dy}{dx} = \frac{df}{du}\frac{du}{dx} \quad \text{(chain rule)}.$$

If a function of a function of a function is involved, and $y = f\,[g[h(x)]]$, then by setting $u = g(v)$ and $v = h(x)$ the chain rule generalizes to

$$\frac{dy}{dx} = \frac{df}{du}\frac{du}{dv}\frac{dv}{dx}.$$

Example 16.6

(i)   Find $\dfrac{d[f(x)]}{dx}$ given that $f(x) = x^3 + 4\cos x$.

(ii) Find $\dfrac{d}{dx}\,[x^3 \sin x]$,

(iii) Find $\dfrac{d}{dx}\left[\dfrac{x^4}{1+x}\right]$.

(iv) Prove that

$$\frac{d}{dx}\,[\tan x] = \sec^2 x.$$

Solution

(i)   From rule 2 above we have

$$\frac{d}{dx}\,[x^3 + 4\ \cos\ x] = \frac{d}{dx}\,[x^3] + \frac{d}{dx}\,[4\cos x],$$

and applying rule 1 to the second term on the right-hand side this becomes

$$\frac{d}{dx}\,[x^3 + 4\ \cos\ x] = \frac{d}{dx}\,[x^3] + 4\frac{d}{dx}\,[\cos\ x].$$

From the table of derivatives this is seen to reduce to

$$\frac{d}{dx}\,[x^3 + 4\ \cos\ x] = 3x^2 - 4\ \sin\ x.$$

(ii) Applying rule 3 with $f(x) = x^3$ and $g(x) = \sin\ x$ gives

$$\frac{d}{dx}\,[x^3\ \sin\ x] = \frac{d}{dx}\,[x^3]\ \sin\ x + x^3\ \frac{d}{dx}\,[\sin\ x]$$

$$= 3x^2 \sin x + x^3 \cos x.$$

(iii) This may be evaluated in either of the following two different ways;

(a) as the derivative of the quotient $\dfrac{x^4}{1+x}$, or

(b) as the derivative of the product $x^4 \left[\dfrac{1}{1+x} \right]$.

In method (a) we use rule 4 with $f(x) = x^4$ and $g(x) = 1 + x^2$, so that

$$\frac{d}{dx}\left[\frac{x^4}{1+x}\right] = \frac{\dfrac{d}{dx}[x^4](1+x) - x^4\dfrac{d}{dx}[1+x]}{(1+x)^2}$$

$$= \frac{4x^3(1+x) - x^4\cdot 1}{(1+x^2)}$$

$$= \frac{4x^3 + 3x^4}{(1+x)^2}.$$

In method (b) we use rule 3 with $f(x) = x^4$ and $g(x) = \dfrac{1}{1+x}$. Then

$$\frac{d}{dx}\left[\frac{x^4}{1+x}\right] = \frac{d}{dx}[x^4]\left[\frac{1}{1+x}\right] + x^4\frac{d}{dx}\left[\frac{1}{1+x}\right],$$

but from Example 16.3

$$\frac{d}{dx}\left[\frac{1}{1+x}\right] = \frac{-1}{(1+x)^2},$$

and so

$$\frac{d}{dx}\left[\frac{x^4}{1+x}\right] = \frac{4x^3}{1+x} - \frac{x^4}{(1+x)^2}$$

$$= \frac{4x^3 + 3x^4}{(1+x)^2}.$$

(iv) As $\tan x = \sin x / \cos x$, we have

$$\frac{d}{dx}[\tan x] = \frac{d}{dx}\left[\frac{\sin x}{\cos x}\right],$$

so setting $f(x) = \sin x$, $g(x) = \cos x$ in rule 4 gives

$$\frac{d}{dx}[\tan x] = \frac{\dfrac{d}{dx}[\sin x]\cos x - \sin x\dfrac{d}{dx}[\cos x]}{\cos^2 x}$$

$$= \frac{\cos^2 x + \sin^2 x}{\cos^2 x} = \frac{1}{\cos^2 x} = \sec^2 x,$$

where use has been made of the trigonometric identity

$$\sin^2 x + \cos^2 x = 1.$$

▲

Example 16.7

Find

(i) $\dfrac{d}{dx}[\sin(3x^2 + 2x - 1)]$;

(ii) $\dfrac{d}{dx}[\sqrt{(1 + x^2)}]$;

(iii) $\dfrac{d}{dx}\left[\dfrac{1}{\sqrt{(1 + 4x + x^3)}}\right]$;

(iv) $\dfrac{d}{dx}\{\sin[1 + \cos(x^2 + 3)]\}$.

Solution

These examples involve the use of the chain rule, since they involve differentiation of a function of a function.

(i)   Set $u = 3x^2 + 2x - 1$ and $f(u) = \sin u$, then from rule 4

$$\frac{d}{dx}[\sin(3x^2 + 2x - 1)] = \frac{d}{du}[\sin u] \cdot \frac{du}{dx}$$

$$= \frac{d}{du}[\sin u]\,\frac{d}{dx}[3x^2 + 2x - 1]$$

$$= \cos u \cdot (6x + 2),$$

but $u = 3x^2 + 2x - 1$, so

$$\frac{d}{dx}[\sin(3x^2 + 2x - 1)] = (6x + 2)\cos(3x^2 + 2x - 1).$$

(ii)   Set $u = x^2 + 1$ and $f(u) = u^{1/2}$, then from rule 4

$$\frac{d}{dx}[(x^2 + 1)^{1/2}] = \frac{d}{du}[u^{1/2}] \cdot \frac{du}{dx}$$

$$= \frac{d}{du}[u^{1/2}] \cdot \frac{d}{dx}[x^2 + 1]$$

$$= \frac{1}{2}u^{-1/2} \cdot 2x,$$

but as $u = x^2 + 1$ this reduces to

$$\frac{d}{dx}[(x^2 + 1)^{1/2}] = \frac{x}{(x^2 + 1)^{1/2}}.$$

(iii) Set $u = 1 + 4x + x^3$ and $f(u) = u^{-1/2}$, then from rule 4

$$\frac{d}{dx}\left[\frac{1}{\sqrt{(1 + 4x + x^3)}}\right] = \frac{d}{du}[u^{-1/2}] \cdot \frac{du}{dx}$$

$$= \frac{d}{du}[u^{-1/2}] \cdot \frac{d}{dx}[1 + 4x + x^3]$$

$$= -\frac{1}{2}u^{-3/2} \cdot (4 + 3x^2),$$

but as $u = 1 + 4x + x^3$ this becomes

$$\frac{d}{dx}\left[\frac{1}{(1 + 4x + x^3)^{1/2}}\right] = \frac{-(4 + 3x^2)}{2(1 + 4x + x^3)^{3/2}}.$$

(iv) Setting $v = x^2 + 3$ and $u = 1 + \cos v$, so that $f(x) = \sin u$, we have

$$\frac{df}{dx} = \frac{df}{du}\frac{du}{dv}\frac{dv}{dx} = \cos u(-\sin v) \cdot 2x$$

$$= -2x \cos[1 + \cos(x^2 + 3)] \sin(x^2 + 3). \qquad \blacktriangle$$

Higher order derivatives of $f(x)$ are defined by successive application of the operation of differentiation with respect to x. Thus the second order derivative of $f(x)$ with respect to x, written d^2f/dx^2, is defined as

$$\frac{d^2f}{dx^2} = \frac{d}{dx}\left[\frac{df}{dx}\right].$$

Analogously, the nth order derivative of $f(x)$ with respect to x, written d^nf/dx^n, is defined as

$$\frac{d^nf}{dx^n} = \frac{d}{dx}\left[\frac{d^{n-1}f}{dx^{n-1}}\right].$$

Example 16.8

Find the first four derivatives of
(i) $f(x) = \sin x$; and
(ii) $f(x) = \cos x$.

Solution
(i) By repeated use of the results

$$\frac{d}{dx}[\sin x] = \cos x \quad \text{and} \quad \frac{d}{dx}[\cos x] = -\sin x$$

we see that

$$\frac{df}{dx} = \frac{d}{dx}[\sin x] = \cos x, \qquad \frac{d^3 f}{dx^3} = \frac{d}{dx}[-\sin x] = -\cos x,$$

$$\frac{d^2 f}{dx^2} = \frac{d}{dx}[\cos x] = -\sin x, \qquad \frac{d^4 f}{dx^4} = \frac{d}{dx}[-\cos x] = \sin x.$$

(ii) $\dfrac{df}{dx} = \dfrac{d}{dx}[\cos x] = -\sin x, \qquad \dfrac{d^3 f}{dx^3} = \dfrac{d}{dx}[-\cos x] = \sin x,$

$$\frac{d^2 f}{dx^2} = \frac{d}{dx}[-\sin x] = -\cos x, \qquad \frac{d^4 f}{dx^4} = \frac{d}{dx}[\sin x] = \cos x$$

▲

Example 16.9

Find

$$\frac{df}{dx} \quad \text{and} \quad \frac{d^2 f}{dx^2} \text{ given that } f(x) = x^2 \sin 3x.$$

Solution
Setting $f(x) = x^2$, $g(x) = \sin 3x$, it follows from rule 3 that

$$\frac{d}{dx}[x^2 \sin 3x] = \frac{d}{dx}[x^2]\sin 3x + x^2 \frac{d}{dx}[\sin 3x]$$

$$= 2x \sin 3x + x^2 \frac{d}{dx}[\sin 3x]$$

However, appeal to rule 5 with $u = 3x$ and $f(u) = \sin u$ shows that

$$\frac{d}{dx}[\sin 3x] = 3 \cos 3x,$$

so

$$\frac{df}{dx} = \frac{d}{dx}[x^2 \sin 3x] = 2x \sin 3x + 3x^2 \cos 3x.$$

To find $d^2 f/dx^2$ we must now differentiate this last result with respect to x.
Proceeding in similar fashion we find that

$$\frac{d^2 f}{dx^2} = \frac{d}{dx}\left[\frac{df}{dx}\right] = \frac{d}{dx}[2x \sin 3x + 3x^2 \cos 3x]$$

$$= \frac{d}{dx}[2x \sin 3x] + \frac{d}{dx}[3x^2 \cos 3x]$$

$$= \frac{d}{dx}[2x]\sin 3x + 2x \frac{d}{dx}[\sin 3x] + \frac{d}{dx}[3x^2]\cos 3x$$

$$+ 3x^2 \frac{d}{dx}[\cos 3x]$$

$$= 2 \sin 3x + 6x \cos 3x + 6x \cos 3x - 9x^2 \sin 3x$$

$$= 2 \sin 3x + 12x \cos 3x - 9x^2 \sin 3x.$$ ▲

A useful alternative condensed notation for derivatives is

$$f^{(n)}(x) = \frac{d^n f}{dx^n}, \quad \text{with} \quad n = 1, 2, 3, \dots ,$$

so that, for example,

$$f^{(1)}(x) = \frac{df}{dx} = f'(x), \; f^{(2)}(x) = \frac{d^2 f}{dx^2} \quad \text{and} \quad f^{(3)}(x) = \frac{d^3 f}{dx^3}.$$

Equivalently, if we set $y = f(x)$, we have

$$\frac{d^n y}{dx^n} = f^{(n)}(x).$$

This notation is often used when the nth derivative of $f(x)$ needs to be specified for some specific value of x, say at $x = x_0$ for then by $f^{(n)}(x_0)$ we mean

$$f^{(n)}(x_0) = \left[\frac{d^n f}{dx^n} \right]_{x = x_0}$$

Example 16.10

Find $f^{(1)}(2)$ and $f^{(2)}(3)$ given

(i) $f(x) = 3x^2 - \dfrac{2}{x}$; and

(ii) $f(x) = x \sin \pi x.$

Solution

(i) $f^{(1)}(x) = \dfrac{df}{dx} = \dfrac{d}{dx} [3x^2] - \dfrac{d}{dx} \left[\dfrac{2}{x} \right]$

$$= 6x + \frac{2}{x^2}$$

and

$$f^{(2)}(x) = \frac{d}{dx} \left[6x + \frac{2}{x^2} \right] = \frac{d}{dx} [6x] + \frac{d}{dx} \left[\frac{2}{x^2} \right]$$

$$= 6 - \frac{4}{x^3}.$$

Thus

$$f^{(1)}(2) = 6 \times 2 + \frac{2}{2^2} = \frac{25}{2}$$

and

$$f^{(2)}(3) = 6 - \frac{4}{3^3} = \frac{158}{27}.$$

(ii) $f^{(1)}(x) = \dfrac{d}{dx}[x \sin \pi x] = \dfrac{d}{dx}[x] \sin \pi x + x \dfrac{d}{dx}[\sin \pi x]$

$$= \sin \pi x + \pi x \cos \pi x,$$

and

$$f^{(2)}(x) = \frac{d}{dx}[\sin \pi x + \pi x \cos \pi x]$$

$$= \frac{d}{dx}[\sin \pi x] + \frac{d}{dx}[\pi x \cos \pi x]$$

$$= \pi \cos \pi x + \pi \left\{ \frac{d}{dx}[x] \cos \pi x + x \frac{d}{dx}[\cos \pi x] \right\}$$

$$= \pi \cos \pi x + \pi \cos \pi x - \pi x \sin \pi x$$

$$= \pi(2 \cos \pi x - \pi x \sin \pi x).$$

Thus

$$f^{(1)}(2) = \sin 2\pi + 2\pi \cos 2\pi = 2\pi,$$

and

$$f^{(2)}(3) = \pi(2 \cos 3\pi - 3\pi \sin 3\pi) = -2\pi.$$

PROBLEMS 16

In problems 1 to 12 find df/dx and $f^{(1)}(x_0)$ for the given value of x_0.

1. $f(x) = 3 \cos x + 7 \sin x;$ $x_0 = \pi/4.$

2. $f(x) = x^4 - 3x^2 + x - 3;$ $x_0 = 1.$

3. $f(x) = x^{2/3} + 2x + 1;$ $x_0 = 2.$

4. $f(x) = \dfrac{x}{x^2 + 1};$ $x_0 = -1.$

5. $f(x) = x\sqrt{(1 + x)};$ $x_0 = 0.$

6. $f(x) = x\sqrt{(1 + x^2)};$ $x_0 = 0.$

7. $f(x) = \dfrac{2x + 3}{x^2 - 5x + 5};$ $x_0 = 1.$

8. $f(x) = \dfrac{2}{2x - 1} - \dfrac{1}{x};$ $x_0 = -1.$

9. $f(x) = x^3 \sin 2x; \quad x = \pi.$

10. $f(x) = \dfrac{\sin x + \cos x}{\sin x - \cos x}; \quad x = 0.$

11. $f(x) = \dfrac{1 + \sqrt{x}}{1 - \sqrt{x}}; \quad x = 2.$

12. $f(x) = \dfrac{\sqrt{x}}{2 + x^{2/3}}; \quad x = 1.$

13. Find the equation of the tangent to the curve

$$y = x^3 + 4x^2 - 3$$

at $x = 3$.

14. Find the equation of the tangent to the curve

$$y = \sqrt{x} + \sqrt[3]{x} + \sqrt[4]{x}$$

at $x = 1$.

15. Find the tangent line to the curve

$$y = 5x \cos x$$

at $x = \pi/2$.

16. Find the two points on the curve

$$y = 2x^3 + x^2 + 1$$

at which the tangent lines to the curve each have gradient 4.

17. Find the equation of the line normal (perpendicular) to the curve

$$y = 1 + \sin 2\pi x + 3 \cos \pi x$$

at the point P corresponding to $x = 1/2$.

18. Find the equation of the line normal to the curve

$$y = 3x^2 - 2x - 3$$

at the point P corresponding to $x = 1$.

In problems 19 to 30 find df/dx.

19. $f(x) = \tan 5x$.

20. $f(x) = \cot x^2$.

21. $f(x) = \sec(1 + x^2)^{1/2}$.

22. $f(x) = \dfrac{\sin 3x}{\cos 2x}$.

23. $f(x) = \tan^2 3x$.

24. $f(x) = \dfrac{\cos 2x}{1 + x^2}$.

25. $f(x) = \sin(\cos 3x)$.

26. $f(x) = \dfrac{1 + \cos 5x}{(x^2 - 1)^{3/2}}$.

27. $f(x) = 3 \cos 2x \sin^3(5x + 1)$.

28. $f(x) = \sqrt{[3 - \sin^2(2x + 1)]}$.

29. $f(x) = [4 + \cos(x^2 + 2)]^{3/2}$.

30. $f(x) = [3 + (1 + \sin 2x)^2]^{1/2}$.

In problems 31 to 38 find the first three derivatives of $f(x)$.

31. $f(x) = \dfrac{1}{x^2 - 9}$.

32. $f(x) = \sin 4x$.

33. $f(x) = x \sin x$.

34. $f(x) = (x + 4)^{1/2}$.

35. $f(x) = x \cos 3x$.

36. $f(x) = (1 + x^3)^4$.

37. $f(x) = \sin x \cos 2x$.

38. $f(x) = \dfrac{\sin x}{1 + x}$.

Leibniz's formula 17

The result we now describe provides a generalization of the derivative of a product. Let $\Phi(x) = f(x)g(x)$, where $f(x)$ and $g(x)$ are functions which may both be differentiated n times. Applying the rule for the differentiation of a product to $\Phi(x)$ gives

$$\frac{d\Phi}{dx} = \frac{d[fg]}{dx} = f\frac{dg}{dx} + g\frac{df}{dx}.$$

A further differentiation gives

$$\frac{d^2\Phi}{dx^2} = \frac{d^2[fg]}{dx^2} = f\frac{d^2g}{dx^2} + 2\frac{df}{dx}\frac{dg}{dx} + g\frac{d^2f}{dx^2},$$

and one more differentiation gives

$$\frac{d^3[fg]}{dx^3} = f\frac{d^3g}{dx^3} + 3\frac{df}{dx}\frac{d^2g}{dx^2} + 3\frac{d^2f}{dx^2}\frac{dg}{dx} + g\frac{d^3f}{dx^2}.$$

Continuing in this manner it is not difficult to show (by induction) that, in general,

$$\frac{d^n[fg]}{dx^n} = f\frac{d^ng}{dx^n} + n\frac{df}{dx}\frac{d^{n-1}g}{dx^{n-1}} + \frac{n(n-1)}{2!}\frac{d^2f}{dx^2}\frac{d^{n-2}g}{dx^{n-2}}$$

$$+ \frac{n(n-1)(n-2)}{3!}\frac{d^3f}{dx^3}\frac{d^{n-3}g}{dx^{n-3}} + \ldots + n\frac{d^{n-1}f}{dx^{n-1}}\frac{dg}{dx} + g\frac{d^nf}{dx^n}.$$

This result is called **Leibniz's formula**, and the coefficients n, $n(n-1)/2\,!$, $n(n-1)(n-2)/3\,!$ are seen to be the **binomial coefficients** $\binom{n}{k}$. On account of this, Leibniz's formula may be written more concisely as

$$\frac{d^n}{dx^n}[f(x)\,g(x)] = \sum_{k=0}^{n}\binom{n}{k} f^{(k)}(x)\,g^{(n-k)}(x),$$

with the convention that $f^{(0)} = f(x)$ and $g^{(0)} = g(x)$.

In general the nth derivative $d^n[f(x)\,g(x)]/dx^n$ will contain $n+1$ terms, but if $f(x)$ (or $g(x)$) is a polynomial of degree m, $f^{(n)}(x) = 0$ (or $g^{(n)}(x) = 0$) for $n > m$ and then $d^n[f(x)\,g(x)]/dx^n$ will only contain $m+1$ terms when $n > m$.

This result is particularly convenient if, say, $f(x)$ is a polynomial of degree m and a simple expression can be found for $d^n g/dx^n$.

This happens, for example, when $g(x)$ involves either a sine or cosine function, for then $d^n[\sin x]/dx^n$ and $d^n[\cos x]/dx^n$ take on simple forms. To see how this happens, notice that if we consider

$$\sin\left(x + \frac{n\pi}{2}\right), \quad \text{for} \quad n = 0, 1, 2 \dots$$

and compare the results for successive values of n with the results of Example 16.8(i), we have:

$$(n = 1) \quad \sin\left(x + \frac{n\pi}{2}\right) = \cos x = \frac{d}{dx}[\sin x]$$

$$(n = 2) \quad \sin(x + \pi) = -\sin x = \frac{d^2}{dx^2}[\sin x]$$

$$(n = 3) \quad \sin\left(x + \frac{3\pi}{2}\right) = -\cos x = \frac{d^3}{dx^3}[\sin x]$$

$$(n = 4) \quad \sin(x + 2\pi) = \sin x = \frac{d^4}{dx^4}[\sin x]$$

Further differentiation of $\sin x$ will simply repeat the above pattern of results, so we see that

$$\frac{d^n}{dx^n}[\sin x] = \sin\left(x + \frac{n\pi}{2}\right), \quad \text{for} \quad n = 0, 1, 2, 3, \dots ,$$

where we define

$$\frac{d^0}{dx^0}[\sin x] = \sin x \text{ (the \textbf{undifferentiated} function).}$$

A similar argument may be applied to $d^n[\cos x]/dx^n$, and so we arrive at the following useful results:

$$\frac{d^n}{dx^n}[\sin x] = \sin\left(x + \frac{n\pi}{2}\right), \quad \text{for} \quad n = 1, 2, \dots ,$$

and

$$\frac{d^n}{dx^n}[\cos x] = \cos\left(x + \frac{n\pi}{2}\right), \quad \text{for} \quad n = 1, 2, \dots ,$$

Example 17.1

Find

$$\frac{d^n}{dx^n}[x^2 \sin x],$$

and use the result to find the derivative when $n = 5$ and $n = 10$.

Solution

Set $f(x) = x^2$ and $g(x) = \sin x$ in Leibniz's formula. Then $f(x) = x^2, \dfrac{d}{dx}[f(x)]$

$= 2x, \dfrac{d^2}{dx^2}[f(x)] = 2$ and $\dfrac{d^n}{dx^n}[f(x)] = 0$ for $n > 2$, while $d^n[\sin x]/dx^n$

$= \sin\left(x + \dfrac{n\pi}{2}\right)$. Substitution into Leibniz's formula gives

$$\dfrac{d^n}{dx^n}[x^2 \sin x] = x^2 \sin\left(x + \dfrac{n\pi}{2}\right) + n(2x)\sin\left(x + \left[\dfrac{n-1}{2}\right]\pi\right)$$

$$+ \dfrac{n(n-1)}{2!}(2)\sin\left(x + \left[\dfrac{n-2}{2}\right]\pi\right)$$

$$\dfrac{d^n}{dx^n}[x^2 \sin x] = x^2 \sin\left(x + \dfrac{n\pi}{2}\right) + 2nx\sin\left(x + \left[\dfrac{n-1}{2}\right]\pi\right)$$

$$+ n(n-1)\sin\left(x + \left[\dfrac{n-2}{2}\right]\pi\right),$$

for $n \geqslant 2$.

Thus setting $n = 5$ and simplifying the result we find that

$$\dfrac{d^5}{dx^5}[x^2 \sin x] = (x^2 - 20)\cos x + 10x \sin x,$$

while setting $n = 10$ and simplifying the result gives

$$\dfrac{d^{10}}{dx^{10}}[x^2 \sin x] = 20x \cos x + (90 - x^2)\sin x.$$

▲

Example 17.2

Find an equation relating the three successive derivatives $d^n g/dx^n$, $d^{n-1}g/dx^{n-1}$ and $d^{n-2}g/dx^{n-2}$ of

$$g(x) = \dfrac{1}{1 + x^2},$$

and use it to find $d^3 g/dx^3$.

Solution

We have $1 = (1 + x^2)g(x)$,
so identifying this with $\Phi(x) = f(x)g(x)$ in Leibniz's formula, we see that
$\Phi(x) = 1$ and $f(x) = 1 + x^2$.

Now

$$f(x) = 1 + x^2, \quad \dfrac{d}{dx}[f(x)] = 2x, \quad \dfrac{d^2}{dx^2}[f(x)] = 2, \quad \text{and} \quad \dfrac{d^n}{dx^n}[f(x)] = 0$$

for $n > 2$. Thus substituting into Leibniz's formula and using the fact that

$$\frac{d^n \Phi}{dx^n} = \frac{d^n [1]}{dx^n} = 0,$$

gives

$$0 = (1 + x^2) \frac{d^n}{dx^n} [g(x)] + n(2x) \frac{d^{n-1}}{dx^{n-1}} [g(x)] + \frac{n(n-1)}{2!} (2) \frac{d^{n-2}}{dx^{n-2}} [g(x)]$$

for $n \geqslant 2$, and hence

$$(1 + x^2) \frac{d^n g}{dx^n} + 2nx \frac{d^{n-1} g}{dx^{n-1}} + n(n-1) \frac{d^{n-2} g}{dx^{n-2}} = 0,$$

for $n \geqslant 2$.

This is called a **recursion relation** or **algorithm** for derivatives, since it relates higher order derivatives to lower order ones. Knowing $g(x)$, if we find dg/dx and set $n = 2$ in the above recursion relation we can find d^2g/dx^2, then setting $n = 3$ and using dg/dx and d^2g/dx^2 we can find d^3g/dx^3, and so on. Thus each derivative $d^n g/dx^n$ is defined recursively in terms of the two successively lower order derivatives.

In this case

$$g(x) = \frac{1}{1 + x^2} \quad \text{and} \quad \frac{dg}{dx} = \frac{-2x}{(1 + x^2)^2}$$

so using the recursion relation with $n = 2$ gives

$$(1 + x^2) \frac{d^2 g}{dx^2} + 4x \left[\frac{-2x}{(1 + x^2)^2} \right] + 2(2 - 1) \frac{1}{1 + x^2} = 0$$

and so

$$\frac{d^2 g}{dx^2} = \frac{2(3x^2 - 1)}{(1 + x^2)^3}.$$

Similarly, setting $n = 3$ in the recursion relation gives

$$(1 + x^2) \frac{d^3 g}{dx^3} + 6x \frac{2(3x^2 - 1)}{(1 + x^2)^3} + 3(3 - 1) \left[\frac{-2x}{(1 + x^2)^2} \right] = 0,$$

and so

$$\frac{d^3 g}{dx^3} = \frac{-24x(x^2 - 1)}{(1 + x^2)^4}. \qquad \blacktriangle$$

PROBLEMS 17

1. Show

$$\frac{d^n}{dx^n} [\sin kx] = k^n \sin \left(kx + \frac{n\pi}{2} \right),$$

for $n = 1, 2, \ldots$.

2. Show

$$\frac{d^n}{dx^n}[\cos kx] = k^n \cos\left(kx + \frac{n\pi}{2}\right),$$

for $n = 1, 2, \ldots$.

3. Use the result of problem 1 to determine

$$\frac{d^n}{dx^n}[x^2 \sin kx].$$

4. Use the result of problem 2 to determine

$$\frac{d^n}{dx^n}[x^2 \cos kx].$$

5. Find a recursion relation connecting the two successive derivatives $d^n g/dx^n$ and $d^{n-1}g/dx^{n-1}$ given that

$$g(x) = \frac{1}{1 + kx},$$

and use it to deduce that

$$\frac{d^n}{dx^n}\left[\frac{1}{1+kx}\right] = \frac{(-1)^n k^n n!}{(1+kx)^{n+1}},$$

for $n = 1, 2, \ldots$.

6. Find a recursion relation connecting $d^n g/dx^n$, $d^{n-1}g/dx^{n-1}$ and $d^{n-1}g/d^{n-2}$, given that

$$g(x) = \frac{1}{1 - 2x^2}.$$

Use the result to find

$$\frac{d^3}{dx^3}\left[\frac{1}{1 - 2x^2}\right].$$

18 Differentials

If $y = f(x)$, the notation dy/dx signifies the **derivative** of $f(x)$ with respect to x so that

$$\frac{dy}{dx} = f'(x).$$

Although suggestive, the notation does not mean that $f'(x)$ is the quotient of two finite quantities dy and dx. However, it is often helpful to treat dy/dx as though this were the case, and to do this we introduce small finite numbers dx and dy called differentials. This is accomplished by considering a differentiable function $y = f(x)$ defined for some $a < x < b$, taking a fixed point x_0 in this interval, defining the **differential of** x, written dx, to be any small non-zero number, and the differential of y corresponding to $x = x_0$, written dy, to be given by

$$dy = f'(x_0)dx.$$

The geometrical meaning of differentials can be seen by examination of Fig. 55. The tangent line PT to the curve at P (the point $(x_0, f(x_0))$) has gradient $\tan \alpha = f'(x_0)$, so the ratio $dy : dx$ of the differentials dx and dy at P equals the gradient of the curve at P. If a small **non-zero** change in x from x_0 is denoted by Δx, we can set $dx = \Delta x$, and then the approximate change in $f(x)$ due to the

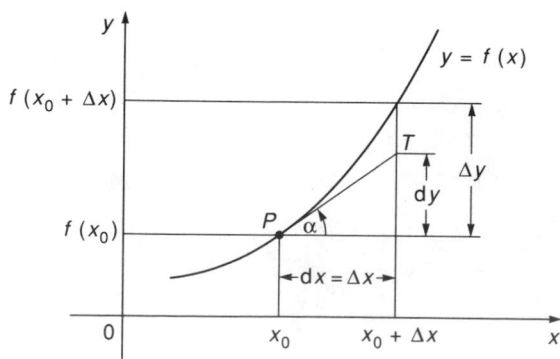

Fig. 55

change Δx in x may be taken to be dy. The exact change Δy will differ from dy, as seen in Fig. 55, but when the differential dx is small, the differential dy will be a good approximation to the exact change Δy.

This is called the **tangent line approximation** to the graph of $y = f(x)$ at $x = x_0$. We see from this that

$$\lim_{\Delta x \to 0} \left[\frac{\Delta y}{dy} \right] = 1,$$

with $dy = f'(x_0)dx$ and $\Delta y = f(x_0 + \Delta x) - f(x_0)$.

If the point x_0 is allowed to vary, so the suffix zero is omitted, we obtain the expression

$$dy = f'(x)dx$$

relating dy to dx as a **function** of x.

Example 18.1

Find the differential dy for the function $y = f(x)$ given that

(i) $f(x) = 3x^2 - 4x + 3$;

(ii) $f(x) = x \sin 2x$; and

(iii) $f(x) = (1 + x^2)^{1/2}$.

Solution

(i)   Here $y = f(x) = 3x^2 - 4x + 3$, so

$$f'(x) = 6x - 4,$$

and thus

$$dy = (6x - 4)dx.$$

(ii)   Here $y = f(x) = x \sin 2x$, so

$$f'(x) = \sin 2x + 2x \cos 2x,$$

and thus

$$dy = (\sin 2x + 2x \cos 2x)dx.$$

(iii) Here $y = (1 + x^2)^{1/2}$, so

$$f'(x) = \frac{x}{(1 + x^2)^{1/2}},$$

and thus

$$dy = \frac{x}{(1 + x^2)^{1/2}} dx.$$ ▲

Differentials can be used to estimate the effect on y of small changes in the variable x, given that $y = f(x)$.

Example 18.2

(i)   In a certain piece of test equipment the pressure p is given in terms of the radius r of a tube by the expression

$$p = 25k(15 - r^2)^{3/2},$$

with $k = $ const. Find the approximate percentage change in p in terms of a small change dr in r.

(ii)   Use the result to estimate the percentage change when $r = 2$ and the radius is changed to $r = 1.95$.

Solution

(i)   A routine calculation shows

$$\frac{dp}{dr} = -75kr(15 - r^2)^{1/2},$$

so

$$dp = -75kr(15 - r^2)^{1/2} \, dr.$$

The approximate fractional change is dp/p, so

$$\frac{dp}{p} = \frac{-75 \, kr(15 - r^2)^{1/2}}{25k(15 - r^2)^{3/2}} \, dr,$$

$$= -\left[\frac{3r}{15 - r^2} \right] dr.$$

Thus the approximate percentage change in dp/p when r is changed by dr is given by

$$\text{approximate \% change in } p = -\left[\frac{300 \, r}{15 - r^2} \right] dr.$$

(ii)   Here $r = 2$ and as r changes from $r = 2$ to $r = 1.95$, it follows that d$r = -0.05$. Hence

$$\text{approximate \% change in } p = -\left[\frac{300 \, r}{15 - r^2} \right](-0.05) = 2.73\%.$$

The exact percentage change is

$$100 \left[\frac{p(1.95) - p(2)}{p(2)} \right] = 2.705 \, 77. \qquad \blacktriangle$$

The differential notation extends in the following obvious manner to combinations of functions.

Constant multiple of u:

$$d[ku] = kdu \ (k = \text{const.}).$$

Sum or difference:

$$d[u \pm v] = du \pm dv.$$

Product

$$d[uv] = u\,dv + v\,du.$$

Quotient:

$$d[u/v] = \frac{v\,du - u\,dv}{v^2} \quad (v \neq 0).$$

Example 18.3

Find the differentials in the four cases listed above given that $u = \cos(2x + 1)$ and $v = x^3$.

Solution

$$d[k \cos(2x + 1)] = -\, 2k \sin(2x + 1)dx,$$

$$d[\cos(2x + 1) \pm x^3] = [-\, 2 \sin(2x + 1) \pm 3x^2]dx,$$

$$d[x^3 \cos(2x + 1)] = [3x^2 \cos(2x + 1) - 2x^3 \sin(2x + 1)]dx,$$

$$d\left[\frac{\cos(2x + 1)}{x^3}\right] = -\left[\frac{3 \cos(2x + 1) + 2x \sin(2x + 1)}{x^4}\right]dx, \ x \neq 0. \qquad \blacktriangle$$

PROBLEMS 18

In problems 1 to 14 find the differential dy when $y = f(x)$ and $f(x)$ has the given form.

1. $f(x) = x^{3/2}.$
2. $f(x) = \sin(4x - 1).$
3. $f(x) = (1 + x^2)^{5/2}.$
4. $f(x) = x \cos(5x - 3).$
5. $f(x) = x^2(1 - x^2)^{1/2}.$
6. $f(x) = x \cos(3x^2 - 6).$
7. $f(x) = x^3/\sin 4x.$
8. $f(x) = \tan x/\tan 3x.$
9. $f(x) = \sin x \tan 4x.$
10. $f(x) = 5x^2 + 3 + x \sin x.$
11. $f(x) = x \sin x \cos 2x.$
12. $f(x) = \dfrac{x + 7}{x - 9}.$

13. $f(x) = x^{1/2} + \dfrac{1}{x^{1/4}}$.

14. $f(x) = x \sec x$.

15. The period of oscillation T of a pendulum of length l is given by

$$T = 2\pi \sqrt{\dfrac{l}{g}},$$

where g is a constant (acceleration due to gravity). Find the approximate percentage change in T if (a) the length of the pendulum is increased by 3% and (b) it is reduced by 5%.

16. The mass M of a cube of metal of side l is given by

$$M = \rho l^3,$$

where ρ is the density of the metal. Find the approximate percentage change in M if (a) the length is decreased by 2% and (b) it is increased by 3%.

17. The drag F on a body moving with speed v through air is given by

$$F = k_1 v^{3/2} + k_2 v^2,$$

where k_1 and k_2 are constants. Find the approximate fractional change in F when v is increased by 4%.

Differentiation of inverse trigonometric functions   19

Let us consider the inverse sine function

$$y = \arcsin \frac{x}{a} \quad \text{for} \quad -1 \leqslant x/a \leqslant 1 \qquad \text{and} \qquad -\pi/2 \leqslant y \leqslant \pi/2.$$

The graph is shown in Fig. 56.
  The statements

$$y = \arcsin \frac{x}{a}$$

and

$$x = a \sin y$$

are equivalent, so differentiating the last expression with respect to y (regarding x as the dependent variable) gives

$$\frac{\mathrm{d}x}{\mathrm{d}y} = a \cos y.$$

However, $\mathrm{d}x/\mathrm{d}y = 1/(\mathrm{d}y/\mathrm{d}x)$, so

$$\frac{\mathrm{d}y}{\mathrm{d}x} = \frac{1}{a \cos y} = \frac{1}{\pm a \sqrt{(1 - \sin^2 y)}} = \frac{\pm 1}{a[1 - [x/a]^2]^{1/2}} = \frac{\pm 1}{(a^2 - x^2)^{1/2}}.$$

The choice of sign introduced by the square root operation is determined by inspection of Fig. 56 which shows that $\mathrm{d}y/\mathrm{d}x$ is **positive**, so

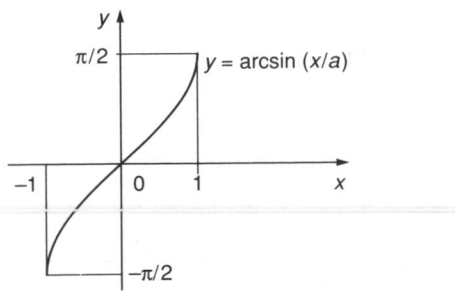

Fig. 56

$$\frac{dy}{dx} = \frac{d}{dx}\left[\arcsin\frac{x}{a}\right] = \frac{1}{(a^2 - x^2)^{1/2}}, \quad \text{for } -1 \leqslant x/a \leqslant 1 \quad \text{and} \quad -\pi/2 \leqslant y \leqslant \pi/2.$$

Similar arguments may be used to determine the derivatives of the other inverse trignomtric functions, and they lead to the results listed below.

SUMMARY OF DERIVATIVES OF INVERSE TRIGONOMETRIC FUNCTIONS

$$\frac{d}{dx}\left[\arcsin\frac{x}{a}\right] = \frac{1}{(a^2 - x^2)^{1/2}}, \quad |x/a| \leqslant 1, \quad -\pi/2 \leqslant \arcsin\frac{x}{a} \leqslant \pi/2,$$

$$\frac{d}{dx}\left[\arctan\frac{x}{a}\right] = \frac{a}{a^2 + x^2}, \quad |x| < \infty, \quad -\pi/2 < \arctan\frac{x}{a} < \pi/2,$$

$$\frac{d}{dx}\left[\operatorname{arcsec}\frac{x}{a}\right] = \frac{a}{|x|\,(x^2 - a^2)^{1/2}}, \quad |x/a| \geqslant 1, \quad 0 \leqslant \operatorname{arcsec}\frac{x}{a} \leqslant \pi \ (\neq \pi/2).$$

The three derivatives which follow are comparatively unimportant, because they only differ from those above by a change of sign.

$$\frac{d}{dx}\left[\arccos\frac{x}{a}\right] = \frac{-1}{(a^2 - x^2)^{1/2}}, \quad |x/a| \leqslant 1, \quad 0 \leqslant \arccos\frac{x}{a} \leqslant \pi,$$

$$\frac{d}{dx}\left[\operatorname{arccot}\frac{x}{a}\right] = \frac{-a}{(a^2 + x^2)^{1/2}}, \quad |x| < \infty, \quad 0 < \operatorname{arccot}\frac{x}{a} < \pi,$$

$$\frac{d}{dx}\left[\operatorname{arccosec}\frac{x}{a}\right] = \frac{-a}{|x|\,(x^2 - a^2)^{1/2}}, \quad |x/a| \geqslant 1, \quad 0 \leqslant \operatorname{arccosec}\frac{x}{a} \leqslant \pi/2 \ (\neq 0).$$

The reason for the occurance of the factor $|x|$ in the denominator of the derivative of arcsec x/a can be understood by inspection of the graph of $y = \operatorname{arcsec} x/a$ in Fig. 57, which is seen to have a positive gradient, for x/a positive and such that $x/a \geqslant 1$ and also for x/a negative and such that $x/a \leqslant -1$. The occurance of $|x|$ in the derivative of arccosec x/a is for a similar reason, though in this case it is because the gradient of arccosec x/a is everywhere negative.

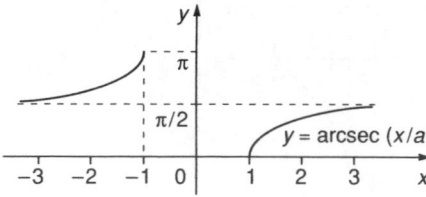

Fig. 57

A more general form of the three most important derivatives of inverse trignometric functions follows by use of the chain rule and leads to the following results.

DERIVATIVES OF INVERSE TRIGONOMETRIC FUUNCTIONS OF A FUNCTION

Let $u = u(x)$ be a differentiable function of x. Then

$$\frac{d}{dx}[\arcsin u] = \frac{1}{(1-u^2)^{1/2}}\frac{du}{dx}, \quad |u| \leqslant 1, \; \pi/2 \leqslant \arcsin u \leqslant \pi/2,$$

$$\frac{d}{dx}[\arctan u] = \frac{1}{1+u^2}\frac{du}{dx}, \quad |u| < \infty, \; -\pi/2 < \arctan u < \pi/2,$$

$$\frac{d}{dx}[\text{arcsec } u] = \frac{1}{|u|\,(u^2-1)^{1/2}}\frac{du}{dx}, \quad |u| \geqslant 1, \; 0 \leqslant \text{arcsec } u \leqslant \pi \,(\neq \pi/2).$$

Example 19.1

Find

(i) $\dfrac{d}{dx}[\arcsin 3x]$;

(ii) $\dfrac{d}{dx}\left[\arctan \dfrac{x}{4}\right]$;

(iii) $\dfrac{d}{dx}[\text{arcsec } 2x]$.

Solution
(i)   Identifying the function with

$$\frac{d}{dx}\left[\arcsin \frac{x}{a}\right]$$

shows we must set $a = 1/3$, and so

$$\frac{d}{dx}[\arcsin 3x] = \frac{3}{(1-9x^2)^{1/2}}, \quad \text{for } -1/3 \leqslant x \leqslant 1/3.$$

(ii)   Identifying the function with

$$\frac{d}{dx}\left[\arctan \frac{x}{a}\right]$$

shows we must set $a = 4$, and so

$$\frac{d}{dx}\left[\arctan \frac{x}{4}\right] = \frac{4}{x^2+16}, \quad \text{for } -\infty < x < \infty.$$

(iii) Identifying the function with

$$\frac{d}{dx}[\text{arcsec } 2x]$$

shows we must set $a = 1/2$, and so

$$\frac{d}{dx}[\text{arcsec } 2x] = \frac{1}{|x|\,(4x^2-1)^{1/2}}, \quad \text{for} \quad -1/2 \leqslant x \leqslant 1/2.$$

▲

Example 19.2

Find df/dx given that

(i) $f(x) = (1 + 3x^2)\arcsin\dfrac{x}{4}$;

(ii) $f(x) = (1 + x^2)\arctan x$;

(iii) $f(x) = \text{arcsec}\,(x^2 - 3)$;

(iv) $f(x) = \arcsin\left[\dfrac{\sqrt{(4-x^2)}}{2}\right]$.

Solution

(i) $\dfrac{df}{dx} = 6x\arcsin\dfrac{x}{4} + (1 + 3x^2)\dfrac{d}{dx}\left[\arcsin\dfrac{x}{4}\right]$

$$= 6x\arcsin\frac{x}{4} + \frac{3x^2+1}{(16-x^2)^{1/2}}.$$

(ii) $\dfrac{df}{dx} = 2x\arctan x + (1 + x^2)\dfrac{d}{dx}[\arctan x]$

$$= 2x\arctan x + 1.$$

(iii) Set $u = x^2 - 3$. Then from the chain rule

$$\frac{df}{dx} = \frac{d}{du}[\text{arcsec } u]\frac{du}{dx}$$

$$= \left[\frac{1}{|u|\,(u^2-1)^{1/2}}\right](2x)$$

$$= \frac{2x}{|x^2-3|\,(x^4-6x^2+8)^{1/2}}.$$

(iv) Set $u = \dfrac{1}{2}\sqrt{(4-x^2)}$. Then from the chain rule

$$\frac{df}{dx} = \frac{d}{du}[\arcsin u]\frac{du}{dx}$$

$$= \frac{1}{(1-u^2)^{1/2}}\left[\frac{-x}{2(4-x^2)^{1/2}}\right]$$

$$= \frac{2}{x}\left[\frac{-x}{2(4-x^2)^{1/2}}\right] = \frac{-1}{(4-x^2)^{1/2}} \qquad \blacktriangle$$

PROBLEMS 19

Differentiate the following functions.

1. $f(x) = \arctan 4x$.
2. $f(x) = x \arcsin 3x$.
3. $f(x) = (1 - x^2)\arcsin x$.
4. $f(x) = 3x^2 \operatorname{arcsec} 3x$.
5. $f(x) = \arcsin (x - 3)$.
6. $f(x) = \arctan \sqrt{x}$.
7. $f(x) = \arcsin\left[\frac{\sqrt{(81 - x^2)}}{9}\right]$.
8. $f(x) = \operatorname{arcsec} \sqrt{(1 + x^2)}$.
9. $f(x) = x \arctan (1 + x^2)$.
10. $f(x) = \arcsin\left[\frac{1}{1 + x^2}\right]$.
11. $f(x) = (1 + x) \arctan (\sqrt{x}/2)$.
12. $f(x) = x^3 \arcsin \sqrt{x}$.

20   Implicit differentiation

If an equation relating the independent variable x and the dependent variable y can be solved for y in the form

$$y = f(x),$$

with $f(x)$ a function of x, the equation is said to be solvable **explicitly** for y. However, the complexity of many equations is such that an explicit solution for y is impossible to obtain, yet given x, y can be found by numerical means. When this occurs the equation is said to define y **implicitly** in terms of x. Thus, for example, the equation

$$xy - x^2 \sin x + 1 = 0$$

can be solved explicitly for y in the form

$$y = x \sin x - \frac{1}{x},$$

but the equation

$$y = x \sin y + 3x^2 + 1$$

merely determines y implicitly in terms of x.

When y is only known implicitly in terms of x it may still be necessary to determine dy/dx. This may be accomplished by regarding y as a function of x (as it is) and differentiating the implicit equation with respect to x. A further differentiation will, of course, determine d^2y/dx^2 in terms of x, y and dy/dx. It is important to recognize that when y is only known implicitly, its derivatives are also likely to be determined implicitly, and so will involve both x and y. Thus the values of x and y to be used in a derivative, say dy/dx, are not arbitrary, but must satisfy the original undifferentiated implicit equation.

Example 20.1

Given that

$$y - x \sin y - 3x^2 - 1 = 0,$$

find

(i) dy/dx in terms of x and y;

(ii) dy/dx when $x = 0$, $y = 1$;

(iii) d^2y/dx^2 when $x = 0$, $y = 1$.

Solution

(i)   Differentiation of the equation with respect to x, regarding y as a function of x and the term $x \sin y$ as a product of x and a function of a function of x gives

$$\frac{dy}{dx} - \sin y - x\frac{d}{dx}[\sin y] - 6x = 0,$$

but

$$\frac{d}{dx}[\sin y] = \cos y\frac{dy}{dx},$$

and thus

$$\frac{dy}{dx} - \sin y - x\cos y\frac{dy}{dx} - 6x = 0,$$

or

$$\frac{dy}{dx}[1 - x\cos y] = \sin y + 6x,$$

and so

$$\frac{dy}{dx} = \frac{\sin y + 6x}{1 - x\cos y}.$$

(ii)   Substituting $x = 0$, $y = 1$ into the original equation verifies that it is, indeed, a solution, and so it is appropriate to seek the numerical value of the derivative dy/dx at $x = 0$, $y = 1$. Using the result in (i) gives

$$\left[\frac{dy}{dx}\right]_{(0,\,1)} = \left[\frac{\sin y + 6x}{1 - x\cos y}\right]_{(0,\,1)} = \sin 1 = 0.8415.$$

(Remember that the argument in $\sin 1$ is in radians).

(iii) To determine d^2y/dx^2 it is simplest to return to the result in (i):

$$\frac{dy}{dx}[1 - x\cos y] = \sin y + 6x,$$

and to differentiate this with respect to x. The result is

$$\frac{d^2y}{dx^2}[1 - x\cos y] + \frac{dy}{dx}\left[-\cos y - x\frac{d}{dx}[\cos y]\right] = \frac{d}{dx}[\sin y] + 6.$$

However,

$$\frac{d}{dx}[\cos y] = -\sin y\frac{dy}{dx} \quad \text{and} \quad \frac{d}{dx}[\sin y] = \cos y\frac{dy}{dx},$$

and so

$$\frac{d^2y}{dx^2}[1 - x\cos y] - \cos y\frac{dy}{dx} + x\sin y\left[\frac{dy}{dx}\right]^2 = \cos y\frac{dy}{dx} + 6,$$

or

$$\frac{d^2y}{dx^2}[1 - x \cos y] = 2 \cos y \frac{dy}{dx} - x \sin y \left[\frac{dy}{dx}\right]^2 + 6.$$

Substituting $x = 0$, $y = 1$ and $(dy/dx)_{(0, 1)} = \sin 1$ gives

$$\left[\frac{d^2y}{dx^2}\right]_{(0, 1)} = 2(\cos 1)(\sin 1) + 6 = 6.9093$$

▲

PROBLEMS 20

In problems 1 to 4 find dy/dx as a function of x and y, and also its value at the given point $x = x_0$, $y = y_0$.

1. $x^2 + 3xy + y^2 - x - 4 = 0$; $x_0 = 1$, $y_0 = 1$.

2. $x^2 + x^2y^2 + y^3 - 13 = 0$; $x_0 = 1$, $y = 2$.

3. $x^2 + y^2 + xy - 17 = 0$; $x_0 = 4$, $y_0 = 3$.

4. $x^2y^3 - x^2 + 3y - 3 = 0$; $x_0 = 3$, $y_0 = 1$.

In problems 5 and 6 find the values of dy/dx and d^2y/dx^2 at the given point $x = x_0$, $y = y_0$.

5. $3x^2 + y^2 + 3xy - 3 = 0$; $x_0 = 1$, $y_0 = 0$.

6. $\sin(x + y) + 3xy - \dfrac{3\pi^2}{4} = 0$; $x_0 = \dfrac{\pi}{2}$, $y_0 = \dfrac{\pi}{2}$.

Parametrically defined curves and parametric differentiation

A more general description of a curve than the one provided by the explicit representation $y = f(x)$ occurs when points on a curve in the (x, y)-plane are defined by setting $x = X(t)$ and $y = Y(t)$, for $a \leqslant t \leqslant b$, with $X(t)$ and $Y(t)$ given functions of t.

This is called a **parametric representation** of a curve, with t as the **parameter**. To see that this does indeed define a curve, notice that for any value of t in $a \leqslant t \leqslant b$ there corresponds a single point $(X(t), Y(t))$ in the (x, y)-plane. As t traverses the interval from a to b, so the points $(X(t), Y(t))$ generate a curve in the (x, y)-plane.

In general, it is usually impossible to eliminate t between $x = X(t)$ and $y = Y(t)$ in order to obtain an explicit equation for the curve in the form $y = f(x)$. It should, however, be clearly understood that a parametrically defined curve does not necessarily define a function $y = f(x)$, because it may describe a curve for which more than one y corresponds to a given value of x (a one–many mapping), and such a curve may even intersect itself and form loops. We will see that, provided $X(t)$ and $Y(t)$ are differentiable functions, a parametrically specified curve is unambiguously defined. It also has a uniquely defined tangent at each point, provided the point is identified by its associated value of t.

An enlightening and easy way to construct a parametrically defined curve is by first drawing the graphs of x and y as functions of t. The curve in the (x, y)-plane is then constructed by taking a set of points $t_1 < t_2 < \ldots < t_n$ in the interval $a \leqslant t \leqslant b$, for each t_i plotting the point $(X(t_i), Y(t_i))$ using the graphs $x = X(t)$, $y = Y(t)$ and finally joining up the points to arrive at the required curve.

Example 21.1 (a non-self-intersecting one–many mapping)

Draw the curve described parametrically by $x = X(t)$ and $y = Y(t)$, with

$$X(t) = t^3 - 3t \quad \text{and} \quad Y(t) = 1 + 2t + \sin t,$$

for $-3 \leqslant t \leqslant 3$.

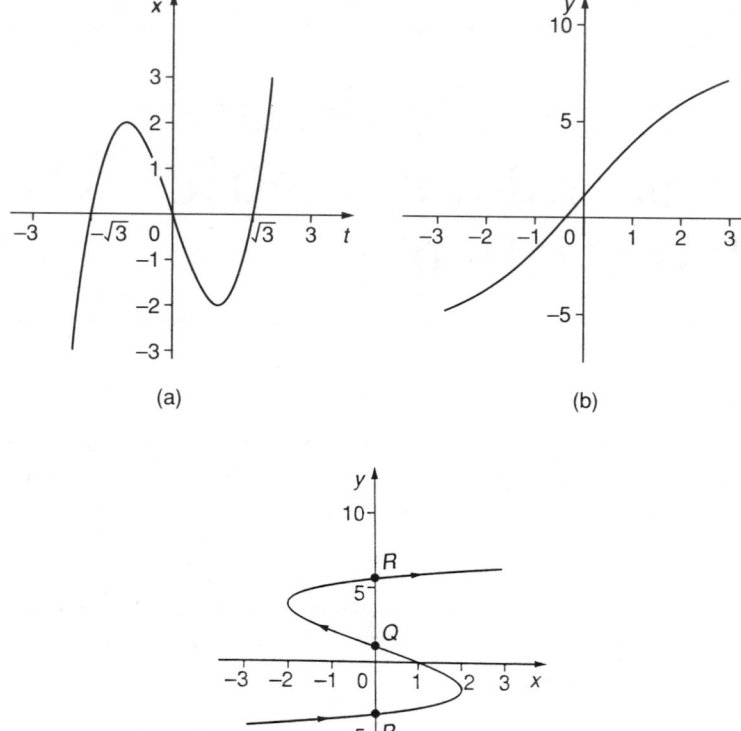

(a)

(b)

(c)

Fig. 58

Solution

The graphs of $x = X(t)$ and $y = Y(t)$ corresponding to the given functions are shown in Fig. 58(a) and (b), and the graph of the parametrically defined curve in the (x, y)-plane which is constructed from them is shown in Fig. 58(c). The arrows on the graph show the direction in which t increases, with point P corresponding to $t = -\sqrt{3}$, Q to $t = 0$ and R to $t = \sqrt{3}$. It is clear that the curve in the (x, y)-plane is a one–many mapping, because to any single value of x in the interval $-2 < x < 2$ there correspond three values of y. However, P, Q and R correspond to different values of t, and so in terms of the parameter t they are uniquely defined, as are all points on the curve.   ▲

Example 21.2 (a self-intersecting one–many mapping)

Draw the curve represented parametrically by $x = X(t)$ and $y = Y(t)$, with

$$X(t) = t^2 \quad \text{and} \quad Y(t) = t^3 - 2t$$

for $-4 \leqslant t \leqslant 4$.

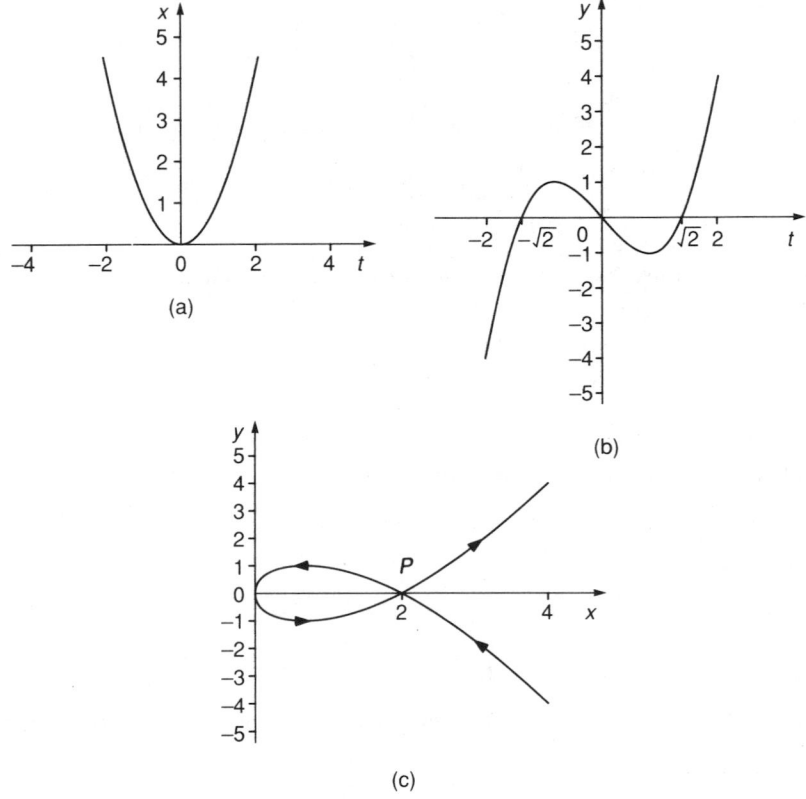

Fig. 59

Solution

The graphs of $x = X(t)$ and $y = Y(t)$ are shown in Fig. 59(a) and (b), and the parametrically defined curve in the (x, y)-plane constructed from these graphs is shown in Fig. 59(c) which exhibits a loop. Thus this curve is another example of a one–many mapping, because to any single value of x in $x > 0$, there correspond two values of y. The parameter t increases in the sense shown by the arrows, and the first time P is reached corresponds to $t = -\sqrt{2}$ and the second time to $t = \sqrt{2}$. Thus the part of the curve with negative gradient through P corresponds to $t = -\sqrt{2}$ and the part with positive gradient through P to $t = \sqrt{2}$. The curve has two different tangents at P, but each corresponds to a different value of t.   ▲

Let $X(t)$ and $Y(t)$ be differentiable functions. To find the gradient of any point on the curve corresponding to a specific value of t we use the fact that, by definition,

$$\frac{dy}{dx} = \lim_{h \to 0} \left(\frac{Y(t + h) - Y(t)}{X(t + h) - X(t)} \right)$$

$$= \lim_{h \to 0} \left(\frac{Y(t - h) - Y(t)}{h} \cdot \frac{h}{X(t - h) - X(t)} \right)$$

$$= \lim_{h \to 0} \left(\frac{Y(t - h) - Y(t)}{h} \right) \lim_{h \to 0} \left(\frac{h}{X(t - h) - X(t)} \right)$$

$$= \frac{dY}{dt} \cdot \frac{dt}{dX} = \frac{dY}{dt} \bigg/ \frac{dX}{dt}$$

so that dy/dx is itself a function of t, as would be expected.

Writing

$$\frac{dy}{dx} = \frac{dt}{dX} \frac{dY}{dt},$$

and omitting y and Y, converts the result from a statement about the relationship between derivatives to one about operations of differentiation; namely

$$\frac{d}{dx} = \frac{dt}{dX} \frac{d}{dt},$$

or

$$\frac{d}{dx} \equiv \frac{1}{[dX/dt]} \frac{d}{dt}.$$

This result allows higher order derivatives with respect to x to be determined, because

$$\frac{d^2y}{dx^2} = \frac{d}{dx}\left[\frac{dy}{dx}\right],$$

but as dy/dx is a function of t it cannot be differentiated with respect to x. However, using the above result we have

$$\frac{d^2y}{dx^2} = \frac{d}{dx}\left[\frac{dy}{dx}\right] = \frac{1}{[dX/dt]} \frac{d}{dt}\left[\frac{dy}{dx}\right],$$

and so d^2y/dx^2 can be found.

A further differentiation gives

$$\frac{d^3y}{dx^3} = \frac{d}{dx}\left[\frac{d^2y}{dx^2}\right] = \frac{1}{[dX/dt]} \frac{d}{dt}\left[\frac{d^2y}{dx^2}\right],$$

and still higher order derivatives may be found by repetition of the same form of argument.

Example 21.3

Find dy/dx as a function of t when $X(t)$ and $Y(t)$ are the functions given in Example 21.1. Use the result to find the gradient of the curve at the points $P(t = -\sqrt{3})$, $Q(t = 0)$ and $R(t = \sqrt{3})$ in Fig, 58(c).

Solution

$$\frac{dX}{dt} = 3t^2 - 3 \quad \text{and} \quad \frac{dY}{dt} = 2 + \cos t,$$

so

$$\frac{dy}{dx} = \frac{1}{[dX/dt]}\left[\frac{dY}{dt}\right] = \frac{2 + \cos t}{3t^2 - 3}.$$

Thus, as can be seen, dy/dx is itself also determined in terms of *t*.
   Point *P* corresponds to $t = -\sqrt{3}$, so

$$\left[\frac{dy}{dx}\right]_P = \frac{2 + \cos(-\sqrt{3})}{3(-\sqrt{3})^2 - 3} = \frac{2 + \cos\sqrt{3}}{6}.$$

Setting $t = -\sqrt{3}$ in $X(t)$ and $Y(t)$ shows *P* is located at $(0, \ 1 - 2\sqrt{3} - \sin\sqrt{3})$.
   Point *Q* corresponds to $t = 0$, so

$$\left[\frac{dy}{dx}\right]_Q = \frac{3}{-3} = -1.$$

Setting $t = 0$ in $X(t)$ and $Y(t)$ shows that *Q* is located at $(0, 1)$.
   Point *R* corresponds to $t = \sqrt{3}$, so

$$\left[\frac{dy}{dx}\right]_R = \frac{2 + \cos(\sqrt{3})}{3(\sqrt{3})^2 - 3} = \frac{2 + \cos\sqrt{3}}{6}.$$

Setting $t = \sqrt{3}$ in $X(t)$ and $Y(t)$ shows that *Q* is located at $(0, \ 1 + 2\sqrt{3} + \sin\sqrt{3})$.   ▲

Example 21.4

Find dy/dx and d^2y/dx^2 as functions of *t* when $X(t)$ and $Y(t)$ are the functions given in Example 21.2. Use the result to find the gradients of the two tangent lines to the curve at *P* corresponding to $t = \pm\sqrt{2}$, and find the values of d^2y/dx^2 at *P*.

Solution

$$\frac{dX}{dt} = 2t \quad \text{and} \quad \frac{dY}{dt} = 3t^2 - 2,$$

so

$$\frac{dy}{dx} = \frac{1}{[dX/dt]}\left[\frac{dY}{dt}\right] = \frac{3t^2 - 2}{2t}$$

$$= \frac{3}{2}t - \frac{1}{t}.$$

Thus

$$\left[\frac{dy}{dx}\right]_{P(t=\sqrt{2})} = \frac{3}{2}\sqrt{2} - \frac{1}{\sqrt{2}} = \sqrt{2},$$

and

$$\left[\frac{dy}{dx}\right]_{P(t=\sqrt{2})} = \frac{3}{2}(-\sqrt{2}) - \left[\frac{1}{-\sqrt{2}}\right] = -\sqrt{2}.$$

$$\frac{d^2y}{dx^2} = \frac{1}{[dX/dt]}\frac{d}{dt}\left[\frac{dy}{dx}\right]$$

$$= \frac{1}{2t}\frac{d}{dt}\left[\frac{3}{2}t - \frac{1}{t}\right] = \frac{3t^2 + 2}{4t^3}.$$

If we now substitute the values $t = \pm\sqrt{2}$ we obtain

$$\left[\frac{d^2y}{dx^2}\right]_{P(t=-\sqrt{2})} = \frac{3(-\sqrt{2})^2 + 2}{4(-\sqrt{2})^3} = \frac{-\sqrt{2}}{2},$$

and

$$\left[\frac{d^2y}{dx^2}\right]_{P(t=\sqrt{2})} = \frac{3(\sqrt{2})^2 + 2}{4(\sqrt{2})^3} = \frac{\sqrt{2}}{2}.$$

This example illustrates how a parametric description of a curve with a loop (a self-intersecting curve) allows the two different gradients of the tangent lines at the point of intersection (and elsewhere) to be determined. It also emphasizes yet again the necessity to relate the operations of differentiation with respect to x and t through the result

$$\frac{d}{dx} \equiv \frac{1}{[dX/dt]}\frac{d}{dt},$$

because dy/dx is a function of t and not x. ▲

PROBLEMS 21

In problems 1 to 10 find dy/dx.

1. $x = \sin^2 t,\ y = \cos^2 t$ for $0 < t < \pi/2$.

2. $x = a\cos t,\ y = b\sin t$ for $0 < t < \pi$.

3. $x = t^2 + 6t + 5,\ y = \dfrac{t^3 - 54}{t}$ for $-\infty < t < 0$.

4. $x = a(t - \sin t),\ y = a(1 - \cos t)$ for $-\infty < t < \infty$.

5. $x = 2t + 3t^2$, $y = t^2 + 2t^3$ for $-\infty < t < \infty$.

6. $x = \sqrt{(1 + t^2)}$, $y = \dfrac{t - 1}{\sqrt{(1 + t^2)}}$ for $-\infty < t < \infty$.

7. $x \doteq a \cos^2 t$, $y = b \sin^2 t$ for $0 < t < \pi/2$.

8. $x = a \cos^3 t$, $y = b \sin^3 t$ for $0 < t < \pi/2$.

9. $x = \dfrac{3t}{1 + t^3}$, $y = \dfrac{3t^2}{1 + t^3}$ for $-\infty < t < \infty$.

10. $x = a(\cos t + t \sin t)$, $y = a(\sin t - t \cos t)$ for $0 < t < \pi$.

In problems 11 to 14 find dy/dx and d^2y/dx^2 when $t = t_0$.

11. $x = 5 + \sin t$, $y = 3 - \cos t$; $t_0 = \pi/4$.

12. $x = -2 + 3t - t^3$, $y = t + 2t^2 + t^3$; $t_0 = -2$.

13. $x = a(t - \sin t)$, $y = a(1 - \cos t)$; $t_0 = \pi/3$.

14. $x = \dfrac{2t - t^2}{t - 1}$, $y = \dfrac{t^2}{t - 1}$; $t_0 = -2$.

In problems 15 to 16 find d^3y/dx^3.

15. $x = a \cos t$, $y = a \sin t$.

16. $x = a \cos^3 t$, $y = a \sin^3 t$.

22 The Exponential function

The **Euler constant** e and the associated **exponential function** e^x can be defined in several different ways. The approach adopted here is a geometrical one, and it is motivated by consideration of the derivative of the function

$$y = a^x \quad (a > 1)$$

and the behaviour of the tangent line to the graph of this function when $x = 0$. To be specific, we take as the defining property of the Euler constant e, that value of a which makes the tangent line to the graph at $x = 0$ have gradient 1. Thus we define e to be the value of a for which

$$\left[\frac{d}{dx} [a^x] \right]_{x=0} = 1.$$

The function

$$y = e^x$$

is then called the **exponential function**.

The behaviour of $y = a^x$ for different positive values of a is shown in Fig. 60. It is seen from this that the gradient of the tangent line to the graph at $x = 0$ increases as a increases, starting from 0 when $a = 1$ and becoming arbitrarily large as $a \to \infty$.

By definition, for any choice of a, we have

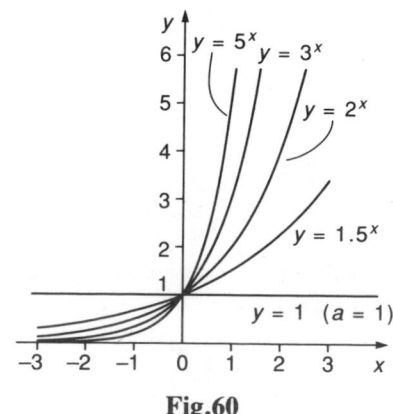

Fig.60

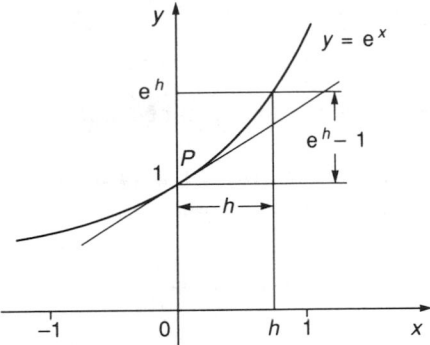

Fig. 61

$$\left[\frac{d}{dx}[a^x]\right]_{x=0} = \lim_{h \to 0}\left(\frac{a^h - 1}{h}\right).$$

Setting $a = e$ and requiring the gradient of the tangent line to the curve at P in Fig. 61 to be 1 we have

$$\lim_{h \to 0}\left(\frac{e^h - 1}{h}\right) = 1.$$

Writing $h = 1/n$, so that $h \to 0$ corresponds to $n \to \infty$, causes the above limit to become

$$\lim_{n \to \infty}\left(\frac{e^{1/n} - 1}{1/n}\right) = 1.$$

Arguing intuitively, but with the concept of a limit in mind, we recognize that this last result means that for n greater than some suitably large number N,

$$\frac{e^{1/n} - 1}{1/n} \approx 1,$$

where the symbol $\approx$ is to be read 'is approximately equal to', and thus

$$e^{1/n} \approx 1 + \frac{1}{n},$$

or

$$e \approx \left(1 + \frac{1}{n}\right)^n.$$

Proceeding to the limit this result becomes exact and we arrive at the following definition of the Euler constant e as the limit

$$e = \lim_{n \to \infty}\left(1 + \frac{1}{n}\right)^n.$$

The numerical value of e determined not from the above limit, but from a series to be derived later, is

$$e = 2.718\,281\,828\,459\ldots .$$

It can be shown that e is an irrational number so its decimal representation is non-recurring.

If in the above argument we had set $h = k/n$, with $k = \text{const.}$, the same reasoning would have led to the more general result

$$e^k = \lim_{n \to \infty} \left(1 + \frac{k}{n}\right)^n.$$

At this point it is useful to recall the following general properties of exponents, and hence of the exponential function e^x in particular.

GENERAL PROPERTIES OF EXPONENTS

For any $a > 0, b > 0$ and for any real numbers x and y:

1 $a^0 = 1$;

2 $a^x a^y = a^{x+y}$;

3 $\dfrac{a^x}{a^y} = a^{x-y}$;

4 $(a^x)^y = a^{xy}$;

5 $a^{-x} = \dfrac{1}{a^x}$;

6 $(ab)^x = a^x b^x$;

7 $\left(\dfrac{a}{b}\right)^x = \dfrac{a^x}{b^x}$.

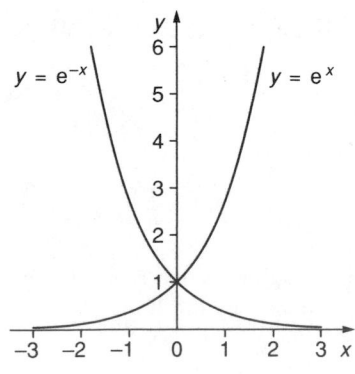

Fig. 62

For reference purposes, graphs of $y = e^x$ and $y = e^{-x}$ are shown in Fig. 62, from which it can be seen that each graph is the reflection of the other in the y-axis. This fact is, of course, a consequence of property 5 listed above.

We now determine the derivative of the exponential function

$$\frac{d}{dx}[e^x]$$

when $x = x_0$, for any arbitrary value of x_0. By definition,

$$\left[\frac{d}{dx}[e^x]\right]_{x=x_0} = \lim_{h \to 0}\left[\frac{e^{x_0+h} - e^{x_0}}{h}\right]$$

$$= e^{x_0}\lim_{h \to 0}\left[\frac{e^h - 1}{h}\right]$$

$$= e^{x_0}.$$

As x_0 was arbitrary the subscript zero may be omitted, causing this to become the fundamental general result

$$\frac{d}{dx}[e^x] = e^x.$$

The derivative of $e^{f(x)}$ follows by applying the chain rule, for setting $u = f(x)$ we have

$$\frac{d}{dx}\left[e^{f(x)}\right] = \frac{d}{du}[e^u]\frac{du}{dx}$$

$$= e^{f(x)}f'(x),$$

where $f'(x)$ denotes the derivative of $f(x)$. Thus we have shown that

$$\frac{d}{dx}\left[e^{f(x)}\right] = f'(x)\,e^{f(x)}.$$

In particular, when $f(x) = kx$, it follows directly that

$$\frac{d}{dx}[e^{kx}] = k\,e^{kx}.$$

We remark that an alternative notation for $e^{f(x)}$ which is often used is $\exp[f(x)]$, so that

$$\exp[f(x)] = e^{f(x)}.$$

Example 22.1

Find

(i) $\displaystyle \lim_{n \to \infty}\left(1 - \frac{1}{3n}\right)^n$;

(ii) $\displaystyle \lim_{n \to \infty} \left(1 + \frac{1}{n+k}\right)^n$;

(iii) $\displaystyle \lim_{n \to \infty} \left(\frac{4^n + 2}{4^n}\right)^{4^n}$.

Solution

(i)   Comparison with

$$\lim_{n \to \infty} \left(1 + \frac{k}{n}\right)^n = e^k$$

shows $k = -1/3$, so

$$\lim_{n \to \infty} \left(1 - \frac{1}{3n}\right) = e^{-1/3}.$$

(ii) $\displaystyle \lim_{n \to \infty} \left(1 + \frac{1}{n+k}\right)^n = \lim_{n \to \infty} \left(1 + \frac{1}{n+k}\right)^{-k} \left(1 + \frac{1}{n+k}\right)^{n+k}$

$\displaystyle \qquad = \lim_{n \to \infty} \left(1 + \frac{1}{n+k}\right)^{-k} \lim_{n \to \infty} \left(1 + \frac{1}{n+k}\right)^{n+k}$

Now

$$\lim_{n \to \infty} \left(1 + \frac{1}{n+k}\right)^{-k} = 1,$$

and setting $m = n + k$ we see that

$$\lim_{n \to \infty} \left(1 + \frac{1}{n+k}\right)^{n+k} = \lim_{m \to \infty} \left(1 + \frac{1}{m}\right)^m = e,$$

and thus

$$\lim_{n \to \infty} \left(1 + \frac{1}{n+k}\right)^n = e.$$

(iii)   Set $m = 4^n$, then as $n \to \infty$ so also does m and we have

$$\lim_{n \to \infty} \left(\frac{4^n + 2}{4^n}\right)^{4^n} = \lim_{m \to \infty} \left(1 + \frac{2}{m}\right)^m = e^2. \qquad \blacktriangle$$

Example 22.2

Find the first and second derivatives of

(i) e^{3x};

(ii) $e^{\sin x}$;

(iii) $\exp\left[\dfrac{x}{1+x^2}\right]$.

Solution

(i)   If we identify e^{3x} with e^{kx} by setting $k = 3$, and then use the result already established that

$$\frac{d}{dx}[e^{kx}] = k\,e^{kx},$$

it follows that

$$\frac{d}{dx}[e^{3x}] = 3e^{3x}.$$

To obtain the second derivative we start from the fact that

$$\frac{d^2}{dx^2}[e^{3x}] = \frac{d}{dx}\left[\frac{d}{dx}[e^{3x}]\right] = \frac{d}{dx}[3e^{3x}] = 3\frac{d}{dx}[e^{3x}].$$

Thus substituting the derivative of e^{3x} shows that

$$\frac{d^2}{dx^2}[e^{3x}] = 3(3e^{3x}) = 9e^{3x}.$$

Alternatively, setting $u = 3x$ and using the chain rule gives

$$\frac{d}{dx}[e^{3x}] = \frac{d}{du}[e^u] = \frac{du}{dx} = e^u \cdot 3 = 3e^{3x}.$$

The second derivative follows in similar fashion.

(ii)   If we identify $e^{\sin x}$ with $e^{f(x)}$ by setting $f(x) = \sin x$, and then use the result established above that

$$\frac{d}{dx}\left[e^{f(x)}\right] = f'(x)\,e^{f(x)},$$

we have

$$\frac{d}{dx}[e^{\sin x}] = e^{\sin x}\frac{d}{dx}[\sin x] = e^{\sin x}\cos x,$$

and so

$$\frac{d}{dx}[e^{\sin x}] = \cos x\, e^{\sin x}.$$

To find the second derivative we differentiate this product, and as a result obtain

$$\frac{d}{dx}[e^{\sin x}] = \frac{d}{dx}[\cos x]\, e^{\sin x} + \cos x \frac{d}{dx}[e^{\sin x}]$$

$$= -\sin x\, e^{\sin x} + \cos^2 x\, e^{\sin x},$$

and so

$$\frac{d}{dx}[e^{\sin x}] = (\cos^2 x - \sin x)e^{\sin x}.$$

Alternatively, setting $u = \sin x$ and using the chain rule gives

$$\frac{d}{dx}[e^{\sin x}] = \frac{d}{du}[e^u]\frac{du}{dx} = e^u \cos x = \cos x\, e^{\sin x}.$$

The second derivative follows in similar fashion after a further differentiation.

(iii)   The result in this case may either be obtained as in (ii) above by setting $f(x) = x/(1 + x^2)$ and using the result that

$$\frac{d}{dx}\{\exp f(x)]\} = f'(x)\exp[f(x)],$$

followed by a further differentiation to find the second derivative, or the chain rule may be used. We only give the details for the last method. Setting $u = x/(1 + x^2)$ and using the chain rule gives

$$\frac{d}{dx}\left[\exp\left(\frac{x}{1+x^2}\right)\right] = \frac{d}{du}[e^u]\frac{du}{dx} = e^u\frac{d}{dx}\left[\frac{x}{1+x^2}\right]$$

$$= e^u\left[\frac{1-x^2}{(1+x^2)^2}\right],$$

and so

$$\frac{d}{dx}\left[\exp\left(\frac{x}{1+x^2}\right)\right] = \frac{1-x^2}{(1+x^2)^2}\exp\left(\frac{x}{1+x^2}\right).$$

A further differentiation gives

$$\frac{d^2}{dx^2}\left[\exp\left(\frac{x}{1+x^2}\right)\right] = \frac{d}{dx}\left[\frac{d}{dx}\left[\exp\left(\frac{x}{1+x^2}\right)\right]\right]$$

$$= \frac{d}{dx}\left[\left(\frac{1-x^2}{(1+x^2)^2}\right)\exp\left(\frac{x}{1+x^2}\right)\right]$$

$$= \exp\left(\frac{x}{1+x^2}\right)\frac{d}{dx}\left[\frac{1-x^2}{(1+x^2)^2}\right] + \frac{1-x^2}{(1+x^2)^2}\frac{d}{dx}\left[\exp\left(\frac{x}{1+x^2}\right)\right]$$

$$= \left(\frac{2x^5 + x^4 - 4x^3 - 2x^2 - 6x + 1}{(1+x^2)^4}\right)\exp\left(\frac{x}{1+x^2}\right).$$

▲

PROBLEMS 22

In problems 1 to 6 find the required limit.

1. $\lim\limits_{n \to \infty} \left(1 - \dfrac{1}{4n}\right)^n$.

2. $\lim\limits_{n \to \infty} \left(1 + \dfrac{2}{5n}\right)^n$.

3. $\lim\limits_{n \to \infty} \left(3^n + \dfrac{4}{3^{n+1}}\right)^{3^n}$.

4. $\lim\limits_{n \to \infty} \left(5^n - \dfrac{1}{5^{n+1}}\right)^{5^n}$.

5. $\lim\limits_{n \to \infty} \left(1 + \dfrac{2x}{n}\right)^n$.

6. $\lim\limits_{n \to \infty} \left(2^n - \dfrac{\cos x}{2^{n+2}}\right)^{2^n}$.

In problems 7 to 14 find dy/dx and d^2y/dx^2.

7. $y = e^{\cos x}$.

8. $y = e^{x^3}$.

9. $y = e^{1/x}$.

10. $y = e^x \cdot e^{x^2}$.

11. $y = \dfrac{1}{2}\left(e^{kx} + e^{-kx}\right)$.

12 $y = \dfrac{1}{2}\left(e^{kx} - e^{-kx}\right)$.

13. $y = \exp\left(\sqrt{x}\right)$.

14. $y = \exp\left(1 - x^2\right)$.

In problems 15 and 16 find dy/dx by implicit differentiation.

15. $x^2 e^y + 3x - y^2 + 2 = 0$.

16. $x e^{y^2} + 5xy + x^2 + y + 1 = 0$.

23   The logarithmic function

Let $a > 0$ with $a \neq 1$ be any real number. Then if
$$x = a^y,$$
we say y is the **logarithm** of x to the **base** a, and write
$$y = \log_a x.$$
Thus the statements
$$x = a^y \quad \text{and} \quad y = \log_a x$$
are equivalent, and so each expression is the **inverse** of the other. When used for multiplication or division in numerical calculations, the base of the logarithmic function is usually taken to be 10. By convention, when logarithms to the base 10 are used, the suffix 10 is usually omitted and it is understood that $\log x$ means $\log_{10} x$. However, in the calculus, logarithms to the base e are always used, and to indicate this we write
$$\ln x,$$
with the understanding that
$$\ln x = \log_e x.$$
Logarithms to the base e are called **natural logarithms**.

The following elementary properties of logarithms to any base will be assumed to be familiar, and so will not be discussed.

Basic properties of the logarithmic function
For any base $a > 0$ such that $a \neq 1$, and any two real numbers $x > 0, y > 0$, we have:

1   $\log_a a = 1$;

2   $\log_a (xy) = \log_a x + \log_a y$;

3   $\log_a [x/y] = \log_a x - \log_a y$;

4   $\log_a (x^y) = y \log_a x$;

5   $\log_a x = \ln x / \ln a$;

6   $\log_a x = \log_b x / \log_b a$ for any $b > 0$ such that $b \neq 1$.

Working now with natural logarithms, we recall from Section 9 that the graph of the natural logarithmic function $y = \ln x$

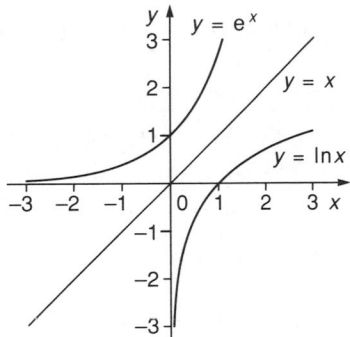

Fig. 63

may be deduced graphically from the graph of

$$y = e^x$$

by reflection in the line $y = x$. The result is shown in Fig. 63, from where it can be seen that:

1   the domain of $f(x) = \ln x$ is $(0, \infty)$, and its range is $(-\infty, \infty)$;

2   the function $f(x) = \ln x$ is continuous and one–one;

3   the y-axis is an asymptote and

$$\lim_{x \to 0+} \ln x = -\infty, \quad \text{while} \quad \lim_{x \to \infty} \ln x = \infty.$$

Example 23.1

Use the properties of the natural logarithmic function and its inverse, the exponential function, to simplify expressions **(i)** to **(vi)** and solve **(vii)** for x:

(i) $\log_2 3$;

(ii) $\ln e^{5x}$;

(iii) $e^{\ln 2x}$;

(iv) $e^{2\ln 4x}$;

(v) $\ln e^{x^2} - \ln e^{3x}$;

(vi) $\ln 10^x$;

(vii) $\ln(x^2 - 9) = 2$.

Solution

(i)   As $\log_a x = \ln x / \ln a$, by setting $a = 2$ and $x = 3$ we have

$$\log_2 3 = \ln 3 / \ln 2 = 1.098\,61 / 0.693\,147 = 1.584\,96.$$

(ii)   The natural logarithmic function is the inverse of the exponential function, so

$$\ln e^{5x} = 5x.$$

(iii)   The exponential function is the inverse of the natural logarithmic function, so

$$e^{\ln 2x} = 2x.$$

(iv)   Using property 4 of the logarithmic function (which is true for $a = e$) we have $2 \ln 4x = \ln(4x)^2 = \ln(16x^2)$, so arguing as in **(ii)** shows that

$$e^{2\ln 4x} = 16x^2.$$

(v)   Using property 3 of the logarithmic function we have

$$\ln e^{x^2} - \ln e^{3x} = \ln \left(\frac{e^{x^2}}{e^{3x}} \right)$$
$$= \ln [\exp(x^2 - 3x)]$$
$$= x^2 - 3x.$$

(vi)   Using property 4 of the logarithmic function with $a = e$ gives

$$\ln 10^x = x\ln 10.$$

(vii)   Taking the exponential of both sides of the equation

$$\ln(x^2 - 9) = 2$$

gives

$$\exp[\ln(x^2 - 9)] = e^2,$$

and thus

$$x^2 - 9 = e^2.$$

Hence

$$x^2 = 9 + e^2,$$

and so the solution is not unique since it is seen to be given by

$$x = \pm (9 + e^2)^{1/2}. \qquad \blacktriangle$$

The derivative of the natural logarithmic function follows from the fact that the results $y = \ln x$ and $x = e^y$ are equivalent, since each is the inverse of the other. Differentiation of

$$x = e^y$$

with respect to y gives

$$\frac{dx}{dy} = e^y,$$

but

$$\frac{dx}{dy} = 1 \Big/ \left[\frac{dy}{dx} \right],$$

so that

$$\frac{dy}{dx} = \frac{1}{e^y} = \frac{1}{x}.$$

Thus we have proved that

$$\frac{d}{dx}[\ln x] = \frac{1}{x}.$$

A more general result follows by using the chain rule to differentiate $\ln f(x)$ by setting $u = f(x)$ to obtain

$$\frac{d}{dx}[\ln f(x)] = \frac{d}{du}[\ln u]\frac{du}{dx} = \frac{1}{u}\frac{du}{dx} = \frac{f'(x)}{f(x)}.$$

Thus, provided $f(x) > 0$, the function $f(x)$ exists, and when $f(x)$ is differentiable we have shown that

$$\frac{d}{dx}[\ln f(x)] = \frac{f'(x)}{f(x)}.$$

Example 23.2

Find

(i) $\quad \dfrac{d}{dx}[\ln(3x)];$

(ii) $\quad \dfrac{d}{dx}[e^x \ln x];$

(iii) $\quad \dfrac{d}{dx}[\ln(4 + x^2 + 2\sin x)].$

Solution

(i) Setting $u = 3x$ and using the chain rule gives

$$\frac{d}{dx}[\ln(3x)] = \frac{d}{du}[\ln u]\frac{du}{dx} = \frac{1}{u}\frac{du}{dx} = \frac{3}{3x} = \frac{1}{x}.$$

Alternatively, as $\ln(3x) = \ln 3 + \ln x$, we have

$$\frac{d}{dx}[\ln(3x)] = \frac{d}{du}[\ln 3] + \frac{du}{dx}[\ln x] = 0 + \frac{1}{x} = \frac{1}{x}.$$

(ii) $\dfrac{d}{dx}[e^x \ln x] = \dfrac{d}{dx}[e^x]\ln x + e^x\dfrac{d}{dx}[\ln x]$

$$= e^x \ln x + \frac{e^x}{x} = e^x\left(\ln x + \frac{1}{x}\right).$$

(iii) Setting $u = 4 + x^2 + 2\sin x$ and using the chain rule gives

$$\frac{d}{dx}[\ln(4 + x^2 + 2\sin x)] = \frac{d[\ln u]}{du}\frac{du}{dx}$$

$$= \frac{1}{u}\frac{du}{dx}$$

$$= \frac{2(x + \cos x)}{4 + x^2 + 2\sin x}.$$

▲

The process of using the properties of the natural logarithmic function to simplify the task of differentiating a function which does not involve natural logarithms is called **logarithmic differentiation**. This process involves first taking the natural logarithm of both sides of an equation, using the properties of logarithms to simplify the result, differentiating the simplified result, substituting for y and solving for dy/dx.

Example 23.3

Use logarithmic differentiation to obtain the derivative of

$$y = \frac{(x+1)^3}{(x^2+4)^{3/2}} .$$

Solution
Taking natural logarithms gives

$$\ln y = \ln\left[\frac{(x+1)^3}{(x^3+2)^{3/2}}\right] \quad \text{(taking logarithms)},$$

$$= \ln(x+1)^3 - \ln(x^2+4)^{3/2}$$

$$= 3 \ln(x+1) - \frac{3}{2} \ln(x^2+4) \quad \text{(simplifying).}$$

Differentiating with respect to x and using the chain rule with $u = x+1$ in the first term on the right and $v = x^2+4$ in the second gives

$$\frac{d}{dy}[\ln y]\frac{dy}{dx} = 3 \frac{d}{du}[\ln u]\frac{du}{dx} - \frac{3}{2}\frac{d}{dy}[\ln v]\frac{dv}{dx} \quad \text{(differentiating)}$$

and so

$$\frac{1}{y}\frac{dy}{dx} = \frac{3}{x+1} - \frac{3}{2}\left(\frac{2x}{x^2+4}\right)$$

$$= \frac{3}{x+1} - \frac{3x}{x^2+4} .$$

Thus

$$\frac{dy}{dx} = 3y\left(\frac{1}{x+1} - \frac{x}{x^2+4}\right),$$

and so substituting for y we find that

$$\frac{dy}{dx} = \frac{3(x+1)^3}{(x^2+4)^{3/2}}\left(\frac{1}{x+1} - \frac{x}{x^2+4}\right) \quad \text{simplifying and solving}$$

for dy/dx gives

$$\frac{dy}{dx} = \frac{3(x+1)^2 (4-x)}{(x^2+4)^{5/2}} .$$

▲

Example 23.4

Use logarithmic differentiation to relate the differentials dx and dy, given that $y = x^x$.

Solution
Taking the natural logarithm of each side of the given expression we have

$$\ln y = \ln x^x = x \ln x.$$

Differentiation with respect to x gives

$$\frac{d}{dx} [\ln y] = \frac{d}{dx} [x \ln x],$$

or, applying the chain rule to the left-hand side,

$$\frac{d}{dy} [\ln y] \frac{dy}{dx} = \frac{d}{dx} [x] \ln x + \frac{d}{dx} [\ln x],$$

and so

$$\frac{1}{y} \frac{dy}{dx} = \ln x + x \left(\frac{1}{x} \right)$$

$$= \ln x + 1.$$

Multiplying by y then shows that

$$\frac{dy}{dx} = (1 + \ln x)x^x,$$

and so in terms of differentials

$$dy = (1 + \ln x)x^x \, dx. \qquad \blacktriangle$$

The natural logarithmic function is only defined for positive arguments, so sometimes it is necessary to differentiate $\ln |f(x)|$. Let us show that the result can be obtained by ignoring the absolute value sign and formally differentiating $\ln f(x)$ without regard to the sign of $f(x)$.

Set $u = f(x)$ and consider $d[\ln u]/dx$. Then if $f(x) > 0$, $|u| = u$ and so

$$\frac{d}{dx} [\ln |f(x)|] = \frac{d}{du} [\ln u] \frac{du}{dx} = \frac{f'(x)}{f(x)}.$$

Now suppose $f(x) < 0$, so that $|u| = -u$. Then

$$\frac{d}{dx} [\ln |f(x)|] = \frac{d}{du} [\ln |u|] \frac{d|u|}{dx}$$

$$= \frac{1}{|u|} \frac{d|u|}{dx}$$

$$= \left(\frac{1}{-u} \right) \left(\frac{\mathrm{d}(-u)}{\mathrm{d}x} \right)$$

$$= \frac{u'}{u} = \frac{f'(x)}{f(x)}.$$

Example 23.5

Find

$$\frac{\mathrm{d}}{\mathrm{d}x} \left[\ln |x - 3 \sin^3 x| \right].$$

Solution
Setting $f(x) = x - 3 \sin^3 x$, and using the last result, gives

$$\frac{\mathrm{d}}{\mathrm{d}x} \left[\ln |x - 3 \sin^3 x| \right] = \frac{\mathrm{d}}{\mathrm{d}x} \left[\ln |f(x)| \right]$$

$$= \frac{f'(x)}{f(x)} = \frac{1 - 9 \sin^2 x \cos x}{x - 3 \sin^3 x}. \qquad \blacktriangle$$

PROBLEMS 23

Use the properties of the natural logarithmic function and its inverse, the exponential function, to simplify the expressions in problems 1 to 8.

1. $\log_7 4$.
2. $\ln e^{(1 + 4x)^2}$.
3. $\exp[\frac{1}{2} \ln x^3]$.
4. $e^{3 \ln 3x^2}$.
5. $\ln e^{\sin x} + \ln e^x$.
6. $\ln e^{x^2} - \ln e^{x^2/2}$.
7. $\ln e^{\sin x} - \ln e^{\cos x} + \ln e^x$.
8. $e^{2 \ln \sin x} + e^{2 \ln \cos x}$.

In problems 9 to 10 solve for x.

9. $2 \ln(x^2 - 1) = 3$.
10. $\ln[(x + 4)^2] = \ln[(x + 1)^2]$.

Differentiate the functions in problems 11 to 20 once with respect to x.

11. $\ln(x + 1)$.
12. $\ln(5x)$.
13. $e^{2x} \ln(3x)$.

14. $\ln(2 + \cos^2 x + e^x)$.

15. $\ln(4x^2 + \sin x)$.

16. $\ln(\cos x)$.

17. $\ln(\tan 2x)$.

18. $\ln(\sec x)$.

19. $\sin 2x \ln(\cos 2x)$.

20. $e^{x^2} \ln(x^2 + 1)$.

Use logarithmic differentiation to determine the derivatives of function in problems 21 to 26.

21. $(x + 2)^2/(x^2 + 3)^{5/2}$.

22. $(x - 3)^3/(x^2 + 1)^{3/2}$.

23. $(e^x + 2)/(e^x + 3)$.

24. $(x + 1)^{1/2}/(x^2 + 3)^{3/2}$.

25. x^{x^x}.

26. $x e^{\sin x}$.

Differentiate the functions in problems 27 to 38 once with respect to x.

27. $\ln |x^2 - 2 \cos^2 x|$.

28. $\ln |e^x - e^{-x}|$.

29. $\ln |x^2 - 2 \sin^2 x + 1|$.

30. $\ln |e^{-x} \ln x|$.

31. $\ln |e^{-x} \ln x - x|$.

32. $\ln |x - \ln x|$.

33. $\ln \dfrac{x}{\sqrt{(1 - x^2)}}$.

34. $\ln |1 + \sec x|$.

35. $3 \ln [\sqrt{(x + 3)} + \sqrt{x}] - \sqrt{(x^2 + 3x)}$.

36. $\ln[e^{2x} + \sqrt{(e^{4x} + 1)}]$.

37. $\ln \sqrt{\left(\dfrac{e^{4x}}{e^{4x} + 1}\right)}$.

38. $\ln \cos x - \dfrac{1}{2} \cos^2 x$.

39. Find dy/dx given that $x = \ln \sin(t/2)$ and $y = \ln \sin t$, for $0 < t < \pi$.

40. Find dy/dx given that $x = \ln(1 + e^t)$ and $y = \ln(1 + e^{-t})$, for $-\infty < t < \infty$.

24 Hyperbolic functions

The **hyperbolic sine, cosine** and **tangent functions**, written sinh x, cosh x and tanh x, are defined in terms of the exponential function as follows:

$$\sinh x = \frac{e^x - e^{-x}}{2} \quad \textbf{(hyperbolic sine } \text{function)},$$

$$\cosh x = \frac{e^x + e^{-x}}{2} \quad \textbf{(hyperbolic cosine } \text{function)},$$

$$\tanh x = \frac{\sinh x}{\cosh x} \quad \textbf{(hyperbolic tangent } \text{function)}.$$

By analogy with trigonometric functions the **hyperbolic cosecant, secant** and **cotangent functions** written cosech x, sech x and coth x, are defined as

$$\operatorname{cosech} x = \frac{1}{\sinh x} \quad (x \neq 0) \quad \textbf{(hyperbolic cosecant } \text{function)},$$

$$\operatorname{sech} x = \frac{1}{\cosh x} \quad \textbf{(hyperbolic secant } \text{function)},$$

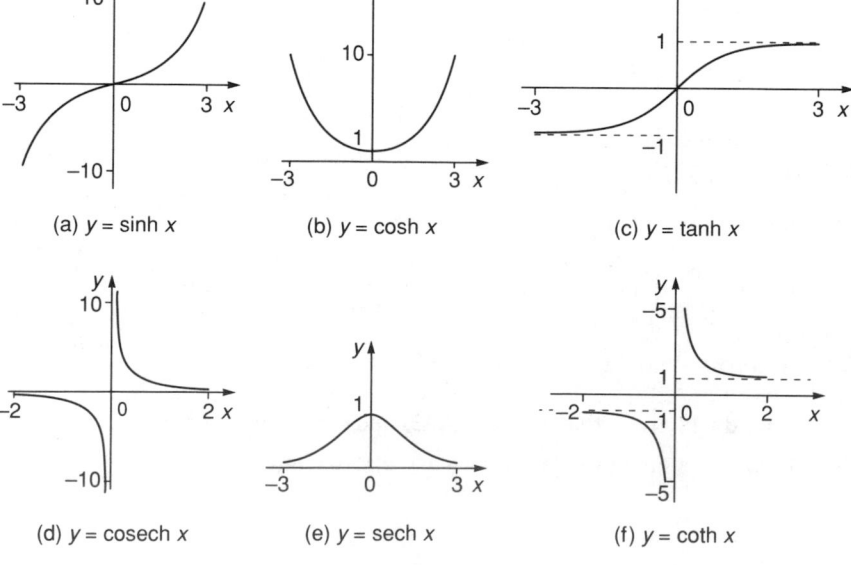

(a) $y = \sinh x$ (b) $y = \cosh x$ (c) $y = \tanh x$

(d) $y = \operatorname{cosech} x$ (e) $y = \operatorname{sech} x$ (f) $y = \coth x$

Fig. 64

$$\coth x = \frac{1}{\tanh x} \quad (x \neq 0) \quad \textbf{(hyperbolic cotangent } \text{function).}$$

Their graphs, which are not periodic, are shown in Fig. 64. It can be seen from the definitions, and also from the graphs, that $\sinh x$, $\tanh x$, $\operatorname{cosech} x$ and $\coth x$ are **odd** functions, while $\cosh x$ and $\operatorname{sech} x$ are **even** functions.

A number of useful identities exist relating hyperbolic functions. The key identities are listed in Table 3, and each can be verified by direct appeal to the definitions of the hyperbolic functions involved. The similarities and dissimilarities between trigonometric and the corresponding hyperbolic identities should be noticed.

Table 3   Hyperbolic identities and the corresponding trigonometric identities

Hyperbolic identities	Trigonometric identities
1. $\cosh^2 x - \sinh^2 x = 1$	$\sin^2 x + \cos^2 x = 1$
2. $\tanh^2 x + \operatorname{sech}^2 x = 1$	$\sec^2 x = 1 + \tan^2 x$
3. $\coth^2 x - \operatorname{cosech}^2 x = 1$	$\operatorname{cosec}^2 x = 1 + \cot^2 x$
4. $\sinh(x + y) = \sinh x \cosh y + \cosh x \sinh y$	$\sin(x + y) = \sin x \cos y + \cos x \sin y$
5. $\sinh(x - y) = \sinh x \cosh y - \cosh x \sinh y$	$\sin(x - y) = \sin x \cos y - \cos x \sin y$
6. $\cosh(x + y) = \cosh x \cosh y + \sinh x \sinh y$	$\cos(x + y) = \cos x \cos y - \sin x \sin y$
7. $\cosh(x - y) = \cosh x \cosh y - \sinh x \sinh y$	$\cos(x - y) = \cos x \cos y + \sin x \sin y$
8. $\sinh 2x = 2 \sinh x \cosh x$	$\sin 2x = 2 \sin x \cos x$
9. $\cosh 2x = \cosh^2 x + \sinh^2 x$	$\cos 2x = \cos^2 x - \sin^2 x$
$\quad = 1 + 2 \sinh^2 x$	$= 1 - 2 \sin^2 x$
$\quad = 2 \cosh^2 x - 1$	$= 2 \cos^2 x - 1$

We only prove hyperbolic identities 1 and 4. To prove the first identity we substitute the definitions of $\cosh x$ and $\sinh x$ into the left-hand side of the identity, to obtain

$$\cosh x - \sinh x = \left(\frac{e^x + e^{-x}}{2}\right)^2 - \left(\frac{e^x + e^{-x}}{2}\right)^2$$

$$= \frac{e^{2x} + 2 + e^{-2x}}{4} - \frac{e^{2x} - 2 + e^{-2x}}{4} = 1,$$

and the result is verified.

To establish the second identity we substitute the definitions of $\sinh x$ and $\cosh x$ into the right-hand side to obtain

$$\sinh x \cosh y + \cosh x \sinh y = \left(\frac{e^x - e^{-x}}{2}\right)\left(\frac{e^y + e^{-y}}{2}\right) + \left(\frac{e^x + e^{-x}}{2}\right)\left(\frac{e^y - e^{-y}}{2}\right)$$

$$= \frac{e^{x+y} - e^{-(x+y)}}{2} = \sinh (x + y),$$

and the result is verified. We could have substituted the exponential form for $\sinh(x + y)$ on the left-hand side instead, but the subsequent manipulation to rearrange the result into the form on the right would have been harder.

The derivatives of hyperbolic functions follow by differentiating their definitions and using the results

$$\frac{d}{dx}[e^x] = e^x \quad \text{and} \quad \frac{d}{dx}[e^{-x}] = -e^{-x}.$$

Thus

$$\frac{d}{dx}[\sinh x] = \frac{d}{dx}\left[\frac{e^x - e^{-x}}{2}\right] = \frac{e^x + e^{-x}}{2} = \cosh x,$$

and

$$\frac{d}{dx}[\cosh x] = \frac{d}{dx}\left[\frac{e^x + e^{-x}}{2}\right] = \frac{e^x - e^{-x}}{2} = \sinh x.$$

Derivatives of hyperbolic functions

1 $\dfrac{d}{dx}[\sinh x] = \cosh x;$

2 $\dfrac{d}{dx}[\cosh x] = \sinh x;$

3 $\dfrac{d}{dx}[\tanh x] = \operatorname{sech}^2 x;$

4 $\dfrac{d}{dx}[\coth x] = -\operatorname{cosech}^2 x;$

5 $\dfrac{d}{dx}[\operatorname{sech} x] = -\operatorname{sech} x \tanh x;$

6 $\dfrac{d}{dx}[\operatorname{cosech} x] = -\operatorname{cosech} x \coth x.$

Example 24.1

Differentiate the following functions:
(i) $\cosh 3x;$
(ii) $\tanh(3x^2 + 5x + 1);$
(iii) $x \sinh(x^2 - 3);$
(iv) $\operatorname{sech}(x^2 + 1)^{1/2}.$

Solution
(i)   Setting $u = 3x$ and using the chain rule gives

$$\frac{d}{dx}[\cosh 3x] = \frac{d}{du}[\cosh u]\frac{du}{dx} = \sinh u \cdot 3,$$

so

$$\frac{d}{dx}[\cosh 3x] = 3\sinh 3x.$$

(ii)   Setting $u = 3x^2 + 5x + 1$ and using the chain rule gives

$$\frac{d}{dx}[\tanh(3x^2 + 5x + 1)] = \frac{d}{du}[\tanh u]\frac{du}{dx} = \operatorname{sech}^2 u(6x + 5),$$

so

$$\frac{d}{dx}[\tanh(3x^2 + 5x + 1)] = (6x + 5)\operatorname{sech}^2(3x^2 + 5x + 1).$$

(iii)   Differentiating the product gives

$$\frac{d}{du}[x\sinh(x^2 - 3)] = \frac{d}{dx}[x]\sinh(x^2 - 3) + x\frac{d}{dx}[\sinh(x^2 - 2)].$$

Setting $u = x^2 - 3$ in the last term and using the chain rule, this becomes

$$\frac{d}{dx}[x\sinh(x^2 - 3)] = \sinh(x^2 - 3) + x\frac{d}{du}[\sinh u]\frac{du}{dx}$$

$$= \sinh(x^2 - 3) + x\cosh u(2x)$$

and so

$$\frac{d}{dx}[x\sinh(x^2 - 3)] = \sinh(x^2 - 3) + 2x^2\cosh(x^2 - 3).$$

(iv)   Setting $u = (x^2 + 1)^{1/2}$ and using the chain rule gives

$$\frac{d}{dx}[\operatorname{sech}(x^2 + 1)^{1/2}] = \frac{d}{du}[\operatorname{sech} u]\frac{du}{dx} = -\operatorname{sech} u\tanh u\frac{du}{dx}$$

and so

$$\frac{d}{dx}[\operatorname{sech}(x^2 + 1)^{1/2}] = -\frac{x}{(x^2 + 1)^{1/2}}\operatorname{sech}(x^2 + 1)^{1/2}\tanh(x^2 + 1)^{1/2}. \qquad \blacktriangle$$

PROBLEMS 24

Verify the identities in problems 1 to 4.

1. $\tanh^2 x + \operatorname{sech}^2 x = 1.$

2. $\coth^2 x - \operatorname{cosech}^2 x = 1.$

3. $\cosh(x - y) = \cosh x\cosh y - \sinh x\sinh y.$

4. $\cosh 2x = \cosh^2 x + \sinh^2 x.$

$$= 1 + 2\sinh^2 x$$

$$= 2\cosh^2 x - 1$$

5.   Prove

$$\frac{d}{dx}[\tanh x] = \operatorname{sech}^2 x.$$

6. Prove

$$\frac{d}{dx}[\coth x] = -\operatorname{cosech}^2 x.$$

7. Prove

$$\frac{d}{dx}[\operatorname{sech} x] = -\operatorname{sech} x \tanh x.$$

8. Prove

$$\frac{d}{dx}[\operatorname{cosech} x] = -\operatorname{cosech} x \coth x.$$

Differentiate the functions in problems 9 to 16.

9. $\sinh(2x + 1)$.

10. $\cosh(3x^2 + x - 1)$.

11. $x \tanh \sqrt{x}$.

12. $\operatorname{sech}(e^x + x + 1)$.

13. $\coth(2x^2 + 3)^{1/2}$.

14. $\operatorname{cosech}(e^x + x^2 + 3x)$.

15. $\sqrt{(x^2 + 1)} \sinh \sqrt{(x^2 + 1)}$.

16. $(x + \ln x) \operatorname{sech}(3x + 1)$.

17. Given that $x = \tanh t$ and $y = \cosh t$, for $-\infty < t < \infty$, show that

$$\frac{dy}{dx} = \frac{1}{2} \sinh 2t \cosh t.$$

Eliminate t between x and y and obtain the explicit equation of the curve.

18. Given that $x = t \cosh t - \sinh t$ and $y = t \sinh t - \cosh t$, for $-\infty < t < \infty$, show that

$$\frac{d^2 y}{dx^2} = \frac{-1}{t \sinh^3 t}.$$

19. Given that $x = a \cosh t$ and $y = a \sinh t$, for $-\infty < t < \infty$ show that

$$\frac{d^3 y}{dx^3} = \frac{3 \cosh t}{a^2 \sinh^5 t}.$$

Inverse hyperbolic functions   25

The **inverse hyperbolic functions** may be found geometrically by reflecting the hyperbolic functions of Fig. 64 in the line $y = x$. As the hyperbolic sine, cosecant, tangent and cotangent functions are one–one they will have unique inverses. These are denoted, respectively, by arsinh x, arcosech x, artanh x and arcoth x or, alternatively, by $\sinh^{-1} x$, $\operatorname{cosech}^{-1} x$, $\tanh^{-1} x$ and $\coth^{-1} x$.

The graphs of the hyperbolic cosine and secant functions are not one–one, but they can be made so if their domains are restricted to $x > 0$. The corresponding inverse functions are then denoted by arcosh x and arsech x or, alternatively, by $\cosh^{-1} x$ and $\operatorname{sech}^{-1} x$. The graphs of the inverse hyperbolic functions are shown in Fig. 65.

The following pairs of functions are thus inverses:

1 $y = \operatorname{arsinh} x$ and $x = \sinh y$;

2 $y = \operatorname{arcosh} x$ and $x = \cosh y$;

3 $y = \operatorname{artanh} x$ and $x = \tanh y$;

4 $y = \operatorname{arcosech} x$ and $x = \operatorname{cosech} y$;

5 $y = \operatorname{arsech} x$ and $x = \operatorname{sech} y$;

6 $y = \operatorname{arcoth} x$ and $x = \coth y$.

It is possible to express the inverse hyperbolic functions in terms of natural logarithms. To see how this is accomplished consider, for example,

$$y = \operatorname{arsinh} x$$

which is equivalent to $x = \sinh y$. Thus

$$x = \frac{e^y - e^{-y}}{2},$$

and so after multiplication by e^y and rearranging terms we find that

$$e^{2y} - 2xe^y - 1 = 0.$$

Setting $u = e^y$ the equation becomes

$$u^2 - 2xu - 1 = 0,$$

which is seen to be a quadratic in u. Applying the quadratic formula shows that

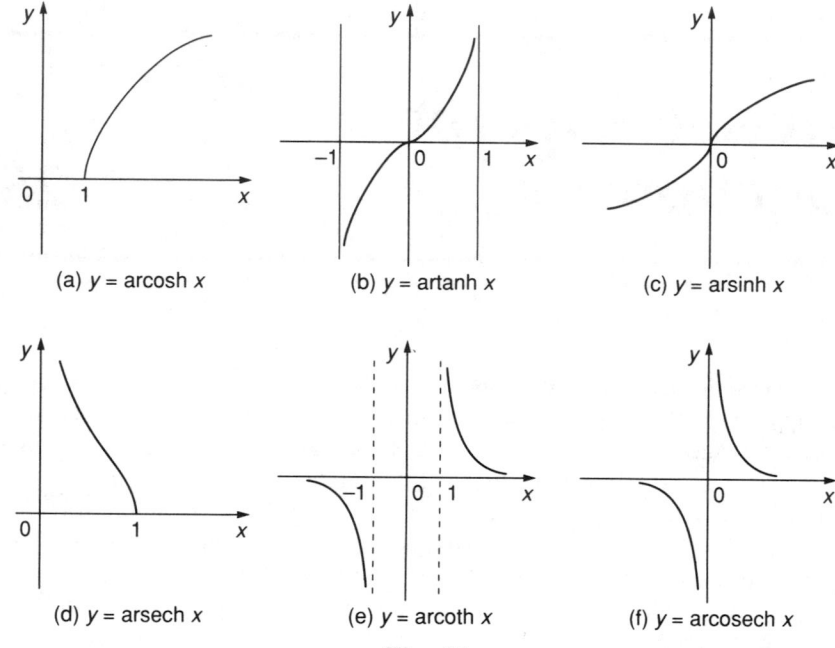

(a) $y = \text{arcosh } x$ (b) $y = \text{artanh } x$ (c) $y = \text{arsinh } x$

(d) $y = \text{arsech } x$ (e) $y = \text{arcoth } x$ (f) $y = \text{arcosech } x$

Fig. 65

$$u = e^y = x \pm \sqrt{(x^2 + 1)}.$$

However, as $e^y > 0$, the positive square root must be taken, so

$$e^y = x + \sqrt{(x^2 + 1)}.$$

Finally, taking natural logarithms gives

$$y = \ln [x + \sqrt{(x^2 + 1)}],$$

and thus

$$\text{arsinh } x = \ln [x + \sqrt{(x^2 + 1)}], \quad \text{for } -\infty < x < \infty.$$

Similar arguments give rise to the following list.

Inverse hyperbolic function defined in terms of natural logarithms

1 $\text{arsinh } x = \ln [x + \sqrt{(x^2 + 1)}], \quad \text{for } -\infty < x < \infty;$

2 $\text{arcosh } x = \ln[x + \sqrt{(x^2 - 1)}], \quad \text{for } 1 \leqslant x < \infty;$

3 $\text{artanh } x = \dfrac{1}{2} \ln [(1 + x)/(1 - x)], \quad \text{for } -1 < x < 1;$

4 $\text{arcosech } x = \ln \left[\dfrac{1 + \sqrt{(x^2 + 1)}}{|x|} \right], \quad \text{for } -\infty < x < \infty \quad \text{and} \quad x \neq 0;$

5 $\text{arsech } x = \ln \left[\dfrac{1 + \sqrt{(1 - x^2)}}{|x|} \right], \quad \text{for } 0 < x \leqslant 1;$

6 $\operatorname{arcoth} x = \dfrac{1}{2} \ln\left[\dfrac{x+1}{x-1}\right]$,   for $-\infty < x < \infty$ and $x \neq 0$.

Routine differentiation of these results gives rise to the following derivatives.

Derivatives of inverse hyperbolic functions

1 $d/dx\, [\operatorname{arsinh} x] = 1/\sqrt{(x^2 + 1)}$;

2 $d/dx\, [\operatorname{arcosh} x] = 1/\sqrt{(x^2 - 1)}$; $[x > 1]$

3 $d/dx\, [\operatorname{artanh} x] = 1/(1 - x^2)$; $[x^2 < 1]$

4 $d/dx\, [\operatorname{arcosech} x] = 1/[|x|\,\sqrt{(x^2 + 1)}]$; $[x \neq 0]$

5 $d/dx\, [\operatorname{arsech} x] = -1/[x\sqrt{(1 - x^2)}]$; $[0 < x < 1]$

6 $d/dx\, [\operatorname{arcoth} x] = 1/(1 - x^2)$; $[x^2 > 1]$

We prove only the first result, since the rest follow in similar fashion. Differentiating the definition of arsinh x gives

$$\frac{d}{dx}[\operatorname{arsinh} x] = \frac{d}{dx}[\ln(x + \sqrt{(x^2 - 1)})]$$

$$= \left(\frac{1}{x + \sqrt{(x^2 + 1)}}\right)\left(1 + \frac{x}{\sqrt{(x^2 + 1)}}\right)$$

$$= \left(\frac{1}{x + \sqrt{(x^2 + 1)}}\right)\left(\frac{\sqrt{(x^2 + 1)} + x}{\sqrt{(x^2 + 1)}}\right) = \frac{1}{\sqrt{(x^2 + 1)}}.$$

Example 25.1

Differentiate

(i) $\operatorname{arsinh}(4x + 1)$;

(ii) $\operatorname{artanh} \sqrt{(1 - 2x^2)}$;

(iii) $\operatorname{arsech}\left(\dfrac{1}{2 + x^2}\right)$.

Solution

(i)   Setting $u = 4x + 1$ and using the chain rule gives

$$\frac{d}{dx}[\operatorname{arsinh}(4x + 1)] = \frac{d}{du}[\operatorname{arsinh} u]\frac{d}{du}$$

$$= \frac{1}{\sqrt{(u^2 + 1)}} \cdot 4$$

and so

$$\frac{d}{dx}[\operatorname{arsinh}(4x + 1)] = \frac{2\sqrt{2}}{\sqrt{(8x^2 + 4x + 1)}}.$$

(iii)   Setting $u = (1 - 2x^2)^{1/2}$ and using the chain rule gives

$$\frac{d}{dx}[\text{artanh}\,\sqrt{(1 - 2x^2)}] = \frac{d}{du}[\text{artanh}\,u]\frac{du}{dx}$$

$$= \frac{1}{1 - u^2}\left(\frac{-2x}{\sqrt{(1 - 2x^2)}}\right)$$

and so

$$\frac{d}{dx}[\text{artanh}\sqrt{(1 - 2x^2)}] = \frac{-1}{x\sqrt{(1 - 2x^2)}}.$$

(iii)   Setting $u = (2 + x^2)^{-1}$ and using the chain rule gives

$$\frac{d}{dx}\left[\text{arsech}\left(\frac{1}{2 + x^2}\right)\right] = \frac{d}{du}[\text{arsech}\,u]\frac{du}{dx}$$

$$= \left(\frac{-2}{u\sqrt{(1 - u^2)}}\right)\left(\frac{-2x}{(2 + x^2)^2}\right)$$

$$= \frac{2x}{\sqrt{(1 + x^2)}\sqrt{(3 + x^2)}}. \qquad ▲$$

Example 25.2

Find dy/dx, given that

$$x = \text{arsinh}\,t \quad \text{and} \quad y = \text{arsech}\,t.$$

Solution

$$\frac{dx}{dt} = \frac{1}{\sqrt{(1 + x^2)}} \quad \text{and} \quad \frac{dy}{dt} = \frac{-1}{x\sqrt{(1 - x^2)}},$$

so

$$\frac{dy}{dx} = \frac{dy}{dt}\bigg/\frac{dx}{dt} = \left(\frac{-1}{x\sqrt{(1 - x^2)}}\right)\sqrt{(1 + x^2)}$$

$$= -\frac{1}{x}\left(\frac{1 + x^2}{1 - x^2}\right)^{1/2} \qquad ▲$$

Example 25.3

Find dy/dx by implicit differentiation, given that
$$1 + x^2 + 3xy + \text{artanh}\,y = 0.$$

Solution
Differentiating with respect to x gives

$$2x + 3y + 3x\frac{dy}{dx} + \frac{dy}{dx}\frac{d}{dy}[\text{artanh}\,y] = 0,$$

and so

$$2x + 3y + 3x\frac{dy}{dx} + \frac{dy}{dx} \cdot \frac{1}{1-y^2} = 0.$$

Solving for dy/dx gives

$$\frac{dy}{dx} = \frac{(y^2-1)(2x+3y)}{(3x-3xy^2+1)}.$$ ▲

PROBLEMS 25

1. Prove that
$$\operatorname{arcosh} x = \ln[x + \sqrt{(x^2-1)}], \quad \text{for} \quad 1 \leqslant x < \infty.$$

2. Prove that
$$\operatorname{artanh} x = \frac{1}{2}\ln\left[\frac{1+x}{1-x}\right], \quad \text{for} \quad -1 < x < 1.$$

In problems 3 to 7 derive the stated results by differentiation of the definitions of the inverse hyperbolic functions in terms of natural logarithms.

3. $\dfrac{d}{dx}[\operatorname{arcosh} x] = \dfrac{1}{\sqrt{(x^2-1)}}.$

4. $\dfrac{d}{dx}[\operatorname{artanh} x] = \dfrac{1}{1-x^2}.$

5. $\dfrac{d}{dx}[\operatorname{arcosech} x] = \dfrac{-1}{|x|\sqrt{(1+x^2)}}.$

6. $\dfrac{d}{dx}[\operatorname{arsech} x] = \dfrac{-1}{x\sqrt{(1-x^2)}}.$

7. $\dfrac{d}{dx}[\operatorname{arcoth} x] = \dfrac{1}{1-x^2}.$

Differentiate the functions in problems 8 to 15 once with respect to x.

8. $\operatorname{arsinh}(3x+5).$

9. $\operatorname{artanh}(\sin x).$

10. $\operatorname{arsech}\left(\dfrac{1}{3-x^2}\right).$

11. $\operatorname{artanh}[\tanh(\sin^2 x)].$

12. $\operatorname{arsinh}(2\sin x).$

13. $\operatorname{arcosh}[\cosh(x^2+1)].$

14. $\operatorname{artanh}\left(\dfrac{x^2-4}{x^2+4}\right).$

15. Use implicit differentiation to find dy/dx, given that
$$3 + 2x^2 + x\operatorname{artanh}\left(\frac{3-y^2}{y^2+4}\right) = 0.$$

26 Properties and applications of differentiability

DIFFERENTIABILITY IMPLIES CONTINUITY

An examination of the definition of differentiability shows that for the derivative $f'(x)$ of a function $f(x)$ to exist at a point $x = x_0$, it is necessary that $f(x_0)$ is defined and such that

$$\lim_{x \to x_0} f(x) = f(x_0).$$

This establishes the important result that **differentiability at a point implies continuity at that point.**

The converse is untrue, because continuity at $x = x_0$ does not imply differentiability at that point. A function which is continuous at a point may, or may not, be differentiable there. This is easily seen by considering the function

$$f(x) = |x|, \quad \text{for} \quad -\infty < x < \infty.$$

This function, which is shown in Fig. 66, is continuous for all x and differentiable for $x < 0$ with $f'(x) = -1$, and for $x > 0$ with $f'(x) = 1$, but $f'(x)$ is not defined at the origin, despite the fact that $f(x)$ is continuous there.

EXTREMA AND STATIONARY POINTS

A function $f(x)$ is said to have an **absolute maximum** at $x = c$ if

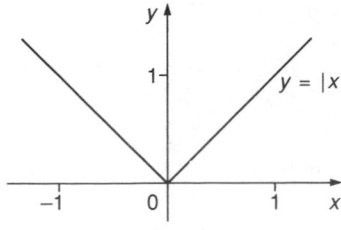

Fig. 66

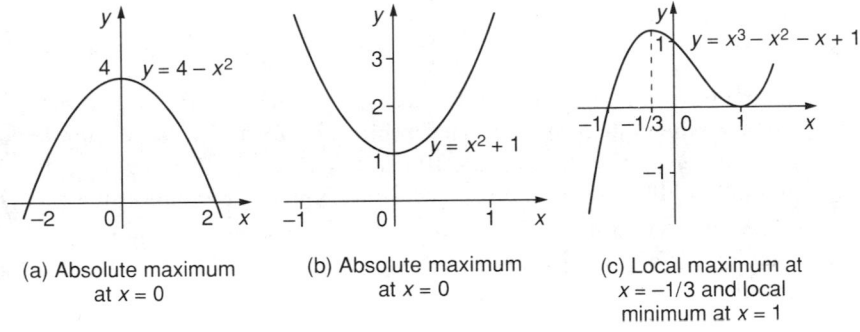

(a) Absolute maximum
at $x = 0$

(b) Absolute maximum
at $x = 0$

(c) Local maximum at
$x = -1/3$ and local
minimum at $x = 1$

Fig. 67

$$f(c) - f(x) \geqslant 0 \quad \text{for all} \quad x,$$

and an **absolute minimum** at $x = c$ if

$$f(c) - f(x) \leqslant 0 \quad \text{for all} \quad x.$$

A function $f(x)$ will be said to have a **local**, or **relative**, **maximum** or **minimum** at $x = c$ if the above conditions are only satisfied locally in some finite interval containing $x = c$. Examples of these situations are illustrated in Fig. 67.

These definitions of maxima and minima, collectively called **extrema**, apply to continuous functions irrespective of whether or not they are differentiable at every point in their domain of definition. For example, the definitions apply to the function

$$f(x) = x(x + 1)^{2/3}$$

illustrated in Fig. 68 which is continuous everywhere, but not differentiable at the single point $x = -1$. The function has a local maximum at $x = -1$ despite its non-differentiability at that point, and a local minimum in the interval $-1 < x < 0$ at which point it is differentiable.

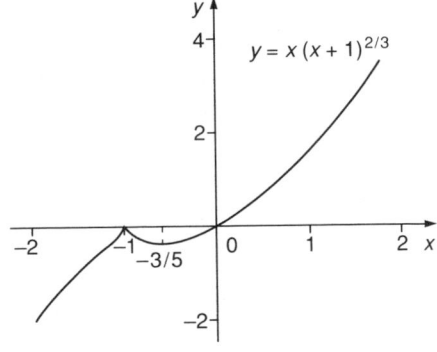

Fig. 68

If $f(x)$ is differentiable, its **stationary points** are defined to be those values of x for which

$$f'(x) = 0.$$

These are points at which the tangent line to the graph of $y = f(x)$ is **horizontal**. This is clearly the case at maxima and minima at which $f(x)$ is differentiable as, for example, in the three cases illustrated in Fig. 67 and at the local minimum in Fig. 68. However, it is not the case when an extreme value occurs at a point where $f(x)$ is not differentiable, as at $x = -1$ in Fig. 68.

Thus the extrema of a differentiable function $f(x)$ can be located by solving the equation

$$f'(x) = 0$$

or, equivalently, if we write $y = f(x)$, by finding the values of x such that

$$\frac{dy}{dx} = 0.$$

Not every stationary point is necessarily a maximum or minimum, because the function may change **monotonically** across a stationary point (i.e. either continue to **increase** or to **decrease** across it). For obvious reasons, stationary points corresponding to maxima or minima are often called **turning points**.

Example 26.1

Find the stationary points of the following functions and sketch them:

(i) $f(x) = x^3 - x^2 - x + 1$;

(ii) $f(x) = x^3 + 1$.

Solution

(i)   Differentiation gives

$$f'(x) = 3x^2 - 2x - 1,$$

so solving $f'(x) = 0$ to determine the stationary points leads to the equation

$$3x^2 - 2x - 1 = 0,$$

with the solutions

$$x = -1/3 \quad \text{and} \quad x = 1.$$

There are thus two stationary points and the graph of this function has already been given in Fig. 67(c). The stationary point at $x = -1/3$ is seen to be a local maximum, and the one at $x = 1$ is a local minimum.

(ii)   Differentiation gives

$$f'(x) = 3x^2,$$

so solving $f'(x) = 0$ leads to the equation

$$3x^2 = 0,$$

with the solution

$$x = 0$$

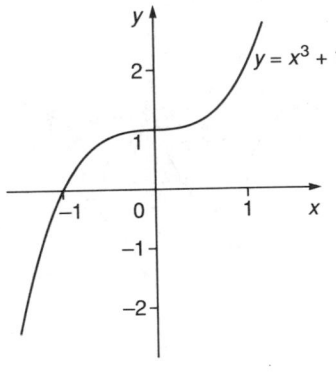

Fig. 69

Thus this function has only one stationary point and it occurs when $x = 0$. The graph of this function is given in Fig. 69, from which it is seen that this stationary point is neither a maximum nor a minimum as the function increases monotonically across $x = 0$.   ▲

The sign of the derivative $f'(x)$ to the immediate left and right of a stationary point can be used to identify its nature. Inspection of Fig. 70 shows how this can be accomplished. We see that $f'(x) > 0$ to the immediate left of a maximum such as P or R, irrespective of the differentiability property of $f(x)$ at these points, while to the immediate right of a maximum $f'(x) < 0$. Conversely, we see that $f'(x) < 0$ to the immediate left of a minimum like Q or S, irrespective of the differentiability property of $f(x)$ at these points, while to the immediate right of a minimum $f'(x) > 0$.

A stationary point across which $f(x)$ changes monotonically (increases or decreases steadily) is characterized by the fact that $f'(x)$ is the same sign to the immediate left and right of such a point. In Fig. 70 the point T at $x = x_4$ is a stationary point across which $f(x)$ increases monotonically, as is also the point $x = 0$ in Fig. 69. Such stationary points are called **points of inflection**. More generally, a *point of inflection* is a stationary point of $f'(x)$, so it occurs when $f''(x) = 0$.

Table 4   Identification of the nature of stationary points using the sign of $f'(x)$

Type of stationary point	Condition
Local maximum of $f(x)$ at $x = c$.	$f'(x) > 0$ to the immediate left of $x = c$ and $f'(x) < 0$ to the immediate right.
Local minimum of $f(x)$ at $x = c$.	$f'(x) < 0$ to the immediate left of x and $f'(x) > 0$ to the immediate right.
Stationary point at $x = c$ with $f(x)$ changing monotonically across $x = c$. (point of inflection)	$f'(x)$ has the same sign to the immediate left and right of $x = c$. Monotonic increasing if $f'(x) > 0$ and monotonic decreasing if $f'(x) < 0$.

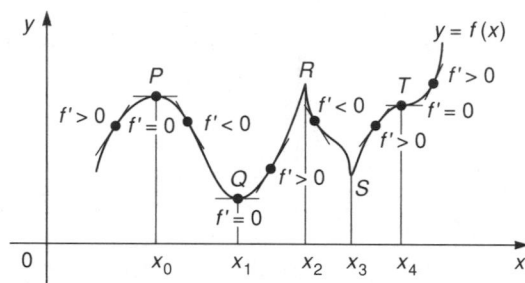

Fig. 70

Example 26.2

Identify by means of the criteria in Table 4 the nature of the stationary points found in examples considered in Figs. 67 to 69.

Solution
In Fig. 67(a) we have $f(x) = 4 - x^2$, so $f'(x) = -2x$, and hence the only stationary point occurs when $x = 0$. To the left of the origin $f'(x) > 0$ and to the right $f'(x) < 0$, so $x = 0$ corresponds to a maximum. Inspection of the nature of the function shows this to be an absolute maximum.

In Fig. 67(b) we have $f(x) = x^2 + 1$, so $f'(x) = 2x$, and hence the only stationary point occurs when $x = 0$. To the left of the origin $f'(x) < 0$ and to the right $f'(x) > 0$, so $x = 0$ corresponds to a minimum. Inspection of the nature of the function shows this to be an absolute minimum.

The stationary points of the function $f(x) = x^3 - x^2 - x + 1$ shown in Fig. 67(c) were found in Example 26.1 and shown to be $x = -1/3$ and $x = 1$. As in this case

$$f'(x) = 3x^2 - 2x - 1$$

it can be shown by routine numerical computation (or algebraically) that $f'(x) > 0$ to the left of $x = -1/3$ and $f'(x) < 0$ to the immediate right so this must be a local maximum. Similarly, $f'(x) < 0$ to the immediate left of $x = 1$ and $f'(x) > 0$ to the right so this must be a local minimum.

To show algebraically, for example, that $x = 1$ is a local minimum, we set $x = 1 + h$ where h is small. Then points to the left of $x = 1$ correspond to $h < 0$ and those to the right to $h > 1$. Setting $x = 1 + h$ we find that

$$f'(x) = 3x^2 - 2x - 1$$

becomes

$$f'(1 + h) = 3(1 + h)^2 - 2(1 + h) - 1$$

or

$$f'(1 + h) = 3h^2 + 4h.$$

When h is small and negative, so x is to the immediate left of $x = 1$, h^2 may be neglected showing $f'(1 + h)$ carries the sign of h and so is negative. Thus

$f'(x)$ is negative to the immediate left of $x = 1$. If $h > 0$, corresponding to a point x to the immediate right of $x = 1$ it follows that $f'(x) > 0$. The identification of the nature of the stationary point located at $x = 1$ then follows as before.

The function

$$f(x) = x(x + 1)^{2/3}$$

is shown in Fig. 68. Differentiation gives

$$f'(x) = \frac{5(x + 3/5)}{3(x + 1)^{1/3}}$$

so $f'(x) = 0$ when $x = -3/5$ and $f(x)$ is not differentiable when $x = -1$.

The only stationary point occurs when $x = -3/5$, and a simple calculation shows $f'(x) < 0$ to the immediate left of $x = -3/5$ and $f'(x) > 0$ to the immediate right, so $x = -3/5$ is a local minimum.

The only other point to be examined is $x = -1$ where $f(x)$ is not differentiable. A simple calculation shows $f'(x)$ is positive to the left of $x = -1$ and negative to the immediate right, so $x = -1$ is a local maximum.

The function $f(x) = x^3 + 1$ shown in Fig. 69 has its only stationary point located at the origin. Thus as

$$f'(x) = 3x^2,$$

we see that $f'(x) > 0$ to both the left and right of the origin, so the stationary point at $x = 0$ is seen to be a point of inflection ($f''(x) = 0$ at $x = 0$).   ▲

When $f(x)$ is twice differentiable, the sign of $f''(x)$ at a stationary point can be used to identify its nature. To see how this comes about, consider the definition of a second derivative at a point x_0, namely

$$f''(x_0) = \lim_{x \to x_0} \left[\frac{f'(x) - f'(x_0)}{x - x_0} \right] = L, \quad \text{say.}$$

Now let x_0 be a stationary point, and suppose that $L < 0$. Then it follows that $f'(x_0) = 0$, and thus

$$f''(x) = \lim_{x \to x_0} \left[\frac{f'(x)}{x - x_0} \right] = L < 0.$$

If x lies to the left of x_0, then $x - x_0 < 0$ and since $L < 0$ it follows that $f'(x) > 0$. Conversely, if x lies to the right of x_0, then $x - x_0 > 0$ and as $L < 0$ it follows that $f'(x) < 0$. We deduce from the signs of $f'(x)$ to the left and right of x_0 that a (local) maximum of $f(x)$ must occur at $x = x_0$ if $f'(x_0) = 0$ and $f''(x_0) < 0$.

Correspondingly, if $L > 0$, the same form of argument shows that a (local) minimum of $f(x)$ must occur at $x = x_0$ if $f'(x_0) = 0$ and $f''(x_0) > 0$. We have arrived at the second derivative test for maxima and minima.

Second derivative test for maxima and minima

Let $f(x)$ be twice differentiable with a stationary point at $x = x_0$ at which $f''(x_0) \neq 0$. Then x_0 is a (local) maximum if $f''(x_0) < 0$ and a (local) minimum if $f''(x_0) > 0$.

To see how this test works, let us apply it to Example 26.1(i) in which

$$f(x) = x^3 - x^2 - x + 1.$$

It was shown that stationary points occurred at $x = -1/3$ and $x = 1$. Now

$$f'(x) = 3x^2 - 2x - 1$$

and

$$f''(x) = 6x - 2,$$

so that $f''(-1/3) = -4$ and $f''(1) = 4$. Thus from the second derivative test, as $f''(-1/3) < 0$, $x = -1/3$ must be a maximum, whereas since $f''(1) > 0$, $x = 1$ must be a minimum.

A similar form of argument may be applied to the function

$$f(x) = x(x + 1)^{2/3}$$

shown in Fig. 68, but only at $x = -3/5$ since $f''(x)$ is not defined at $x = -1$.

ROLLE'S THEOREM

A simple but important result on which many others depend is **Rolle's theorem** which may be stated as follows.

Rolle's theorem

Let the function $f(x)$ be continuous in the (closed) interval $a \leqslant x \leqslant b$ and differentiable in the (open) interval $a < x < b$ and such that $f(a) = f(b)$. Then there is at least one number X strictly between a and b such that

$$f'(X) = 0.$$

The geometrical meaning of this theorem is simple, because it gives the conditions under which the tangent line to the graph of $y = f(x)$ shown in Fig. 71 is parallel to the x-axis at a point (there may be more than one) strictly between a and b.

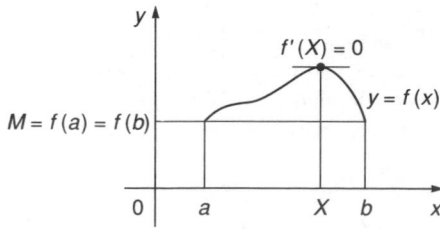

Fig. 71

To prove this result analytically we proceed as follows. Suppose $f(a) = f(b) = M$. Then if $f(x) \equiv M$ the result is obviously true for all X such that $a < X < b$.

Now suppose that $f(X) > M$, so that the function must have a **maximum** at some point $x = X$ strictly between a and b. As the function is differentiable it then follows that $f'(X) = 0$. A similar argument applies if $f(X) < M$, so the result is proved.

Example 26.3

(i)   Show that Rolle's theorem applies to the function

$$f(x) = \sin x \sin 3x \quad \text{for} \quad 0 \leqslant x \leqslant 2\pi,$$

and determine at how many points $f'(x) = 0$ in this interval.

(ii)   Explain why Rolle's theorem does not apply to the function

$$f(x) = \begin{cases} \tan^2 x & \text{for } 0 \leqslant x \leqslant \pi/4 \\ 1 - \tan\left(x - \dfrac{\pi}{4}\right) & \text{for } \pi/4 \leqslant x \leqslant \pi/2. \end{cases}$$

Solution

(i)   The function

$$f(x) = \sin x \sin 3x$$

is both continuous and differentiable on the interval $0 \leqslant x \leqslant 2\pi$, and $f(0) = f(2\pi) = 0$, so Rolle's theorem applies. The points at which $f'(x) = 0$ may be obtained analytically by solving the equation $f'(x) = 0$, but they are most easily determined graphically by inspection of Fig. 72(a). It may be seen from this figure that $f'(x) = 0$ at the seven points P, Q, R, S, T, U and V.

(ii)   Rolle's theorem does not apply to this function because although $f(x)$ is continuous, with $f(0) = f(\pi/2) = 0$, and differentiable on $0 < x < \pi/4$ and $\pi/4 < x < \pi/2$, it is not differentiable at $x = \pi/4$, as may be seen from Fig. 71(b). ▲

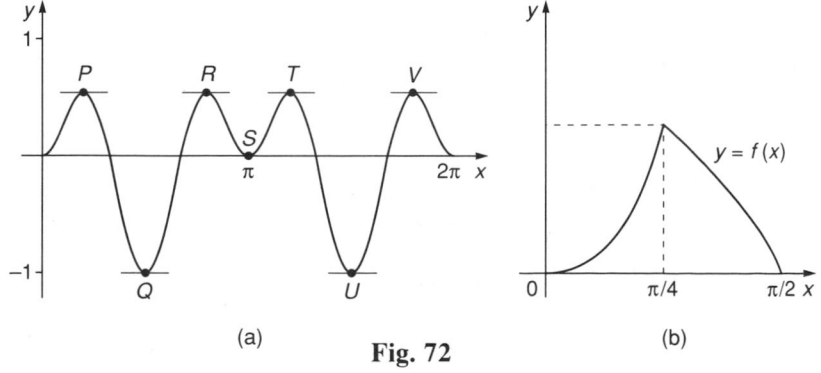

(a)   Fig. 72   (b)

MEAN VALUE THEOREM

One of the main uses for Rolle's theorem is to be found in the proof of other theorems. An important example of such a use is to be found in the proof to the mean value theorem which may be regarded as an extension of Rolle's theorem.

Mean value theorem
Let $f(x)$ be continuous on the (closed) interval $a \leqslant x \leqslant b$ and differentiable on the (open) interval $a < x < b$. Then there is a number X strictly between a and b such that

$$f'(X) = \frac{f(b) - f(a)}{b - a}.$$

The geometrical meaning of this theorem can be seen by examination of Fig. 73. The theorem gives the conditions under which the tangent line T to the graph of $y = f(x)$ at a point X strictly between a and b is **parallel** to the chord AB.

The proof is accomplished by constructing a special function $F(x)$ involving $f(x)$ in such a way that $F(x)$ satisfies Rolle's theorem for $a \leqslant x \leqslant b$.
Define

$$F(x) = f(x) - \left[\frac{f(b) - f(a)}{b - a} \right](x - a) - f(a).$$

Then as $f(x)$ and $x - a$ are both continuous on $a \leqslant x \leqslant b$ and differentiable on $a < x < b$ it follows that $F(x)$ has these same properties. Furthermore, $F(a) = F(b) = 0$, so $F(x)$ satisfies the conditions of Rolle's theorem. Thus there exists a point $x = X$ strictly between a and b, such that $F'(X) = 0$. However,

$$F'(x) = f'(x) - \left(\frac{f(b) - f(a)}{b - a} \right),$$

so if $F'(X) = 0$, we have the result

$$f'(X) = \frac{f(b) - f(a)}{b - a}, \quad \text{for} \quad a < X < b,$$

and the theorem is proved.

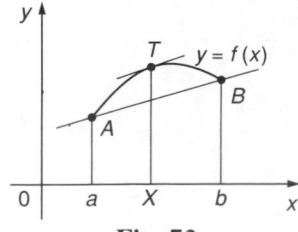

Fig. 73

EVALUATION OF INDETERMINATE FORMS: L'HÔPITAL'S RULE

The mean value theorem may be used to simplify the task of determining limits involving **indeterminate forms**.

Suppose $f(x)$ and $g(x)$ are differentiable in an interval containing the point $x = c$ and that $f(c) = g(c) = 0$, so

$$\lim_{x \to c} \frac{f(x)}{g(x)}$$

is an indeterminate form. We now replace $f(x)$ and $g(x)$ using the mean value theorem as follows. Setting $a = c$ and $b = x$ we obtain

$$f(x) = f(c) + (x - c) f'(X), \quad \text{with} \quad c < X < x$$

and

$$g(x) = g(c) + (x - c) (\tilde{X}), \quad \text{with} \quad c < \tilde{X} < x$$

(X and $\tilde{X}$ are not necessarily the same). Since, by hypothesis, $f(c) = g(c) = 0$, it then follows that

$$\frac{f(x)}{g(x)} = \frac{f'(X)}{g'(\tilde{X})}.$$

Now as $x \to c$ it follows that $X \to c$ and $\tilde{X} \to c$, so we conclude that

$$\lim_{x \to c} \left[\frac{f(x)}{g(x)} \right] = \lim_{x \to c} \left[\frac{f'(x)}{g'(x)} \right],$$

provided the limit on the right-hand side is not itself an indeterminate form.

This method of evaluating indeterminate forms is called **L'Hôpital's rule**. If it happens that the limit on the right-hand side is also an indeterminate form a further application of the rule then shows that if $f(c) = g(c) = 0$ and $f'(c) = g'(c) = 0$ but $f''(x)/g''(x)$ is not an indeterminate form, then

$$\lim_{x \to c} \left[\frac{f(x)}{g(x)} \right] = \lim_{x \to c} \left[\frac{f''(x)}{g''(x)} \right].$$

The rule may be extended in an obvious manner to arrive at the following generalization.

Generalized L'Hôpital's rule
Let $f(x)$ and $g(x)$ be such that $f(c) = g(c) = 0$ and the first $n - 1$ derivatives of $f(x)$ and $g(x)$ all vanish when $x = c$, so that $f^{(1)}(c) = g^{(1)}(c) = f^{(2)}(c) = g^{(2)}(c) = \ldots = f^{(n-1)}(c) = g^{(n-1)}(c) = 0$, but the nth order derivatives $f^{(n)}(x) = d^n f/dx^n$ and $g^{(n)}(x) = d^n g/dx^n$ do not both vanish when $x = c$. Then

$$\lim_{x \to c} \left[\frac{f(x)}{g(x)} \right] = \lim_{x \to c} \left[\frac{f^{(n)}(x)}{g^{(n)}(x)} \right].$$

It is important to notice that the repeated differentiation of the numerator and denominator in the generalized L'Hôpital's rule only continues until the *first* occasion on which the limit on the right-hand side ceases to be an indeterminate form. Any further differentiation is incorrect and will lead to the wrong result. This is because L'Hôpital's rule may only be applied to an indeterminate form.

Example 26.4

Evaluate

$$\lim_{x \to 1} \left[\frac{x^3 + 2x^2 - x - 2}{x^2 - 1} \right],$$

and show the consequence of applying L'Hôpital's rule to a limit which is not an indeterminate form.

Solution
The limit is an indeterminate form, so setting $f(x) = x^3 + 2x^2 - x - 2$ and $g(x) = x^2 - 1$ and differentiating gives

$$g'(x) = 3x^2 + 4x - 1 \quad \text{and} \quad g'(x) = 2x.$$

These derivatives do not both vanish as $x \to 1$, so from L'Hôpital's rule

$$\lim_{x \to 1} \left[\frac{f(x)}{g(x)} \right] = \lim_{x \to 1} \left[\frac{f'(x)}{g'(x)} \right] = \lim_{x \to 1} \left[\frac{3x^2 + 4x - 1}{2x} \right] = \frac{6}{2} = 3.$$

If, mistakenly, L'Hôpital's rule is applied once again to this last limit (it is not an indeterminate form), the result would be

$$\lim_{x \to 1} \left[\frac{3x^2 + 4x - 1}{2x} \right] = \lim_{x \to 1} \left[\frac{6x + 4}{2} \right] = 5,$$

which is incorrect.   ▲

Example 26.5

Evaluate

$$\lim_{x \to 0} \left[\frac{\sqrt{(1 + 4x)} - 1}{3x} \right].$$

Solution
This is an indeterminate form so we start by setting

$$f(x) = \sqrt{(1 + 4x)} - 1 \quad \text{and} \quad g(x) = 3x,$$

and differentiating to obtain

$$f'(x) = \frac{2}{(1 + 4x)^{1/2}} \quad \text{and} \quad g'(x) = 3.$$

As these are not both zero when $x = 0$ (the value of x at which the limit is required) we may use the simple form of L'Hôpital's rule to obtain

$$\lim_{x \to 0} \left[\frac{\sqrt{(1 + 4x)} - 1}{3x} \right] = \lim_{x \to 0} \left[\frac{f'(x)}{g'(x)} \right] = \frac{2}{3}.$$
▲

Example 26.6

Evaluate

$$\lim_{x \to 3} \left[\frac{2^x - 8}{\sin \pi x} \right].$$

Solution
Setting $f(x) = 2^x - 8$ and $g(x) = \sin \pi x$ and differentiating gives

$$f'(x) = 2^x \ln 2$$

and

$$g'(x) = \pi \cos \pi x.$$

The limit is required as $x \to 3$ and as $f'(3)$ and $g'(3)$ do not vanish we may use the simple form of L'Hôpital's rule to obtain

$$\lim_{x \to 3} \left[\frac{2^x - 8}{\sin \pi x} \right] = \lim_{x \to 3} \left[\frac{f'(x)}{g'(x)} \right] = -\frac{8 \ln 2}{\pi}.$$

This limit could not have been evaluated by using one of the elementary methods described in Section 14.
▲

Example 26.7

Evaluate

$$\lim_{x \to 0} \left[\frac{x \sin x - x^2}{2 \cos x - 2 + x^2} \right].$$

Solution
This is an indeterminate form, so we start by setting

$$f(x) = x \sin x - x^2$$

and

$$g(x) = 2 \cos x - 2 + x^2.$$

Repeated differentiation of $f(x)$ and $g(x)$ shows that the first three derivatives of each function vanish at $x = 0$, because

$$f'(x) = \sin x + x \cos x - 2x, \quad \text{so} \quad f'(0) = 0;$$
$$g'(x) = -2 \sin x + 2x, \quad \text{so} \quad g'(0) = 0;$$
$$f^{(2)}(x) = 2 \cos x - x \sin x - 2, \quad \text{so} \quad f^{(2)}(0) = 0;$$
$$g^{(2)}(x) = -2 \cos x + 2, \quad \text{so} \quad g^{(2)}(0) = 0;$$

$$f^{(3)}(x) = -3\sin x - x\cos x, \quad \text{so} \quad f^{(3)}(0) = 0;$$

$$g^{(3)}(x) = 2\sin x, \quad \text{so} \quad g^{(3)}(0) = 0.$$

However, a further differentiation shows that

$$f^{(4)}(x) = -4\cos x + x\sin x, \quad \text{so} \quad f^{(4)}(0) = -4,$$

and

$$g^{(4)}(x) = 2\cos x, \quad \text{so} \quad g^{(4)}(0) = 2.$$

Thus as these derivatives are not both zero we may use the generalized form of L'Hôpital's rule (corresponding to $n=4$) to deduce that

$$\lim_{x \to 0} \left[\frac{x\sin x - x^2}{2\cos x - 2 + x^2} \right] = \lim_{x \to 0} \left[\frac{f^{(4)}(x)}{g^{(4)}(x)} \right] = -2.$$

As in Example 26.6, this limit could not have been evaluated by using one of the elementary methods described in Section 14.   ▲

It should be remarked that L'Hôpital's rule does not always lead to the evaluation of an indeterminate form because, on occasions, $\lim_{x \to c} [f'(x)/g'(x)]$ is more complicated than the original expression $\lim_{x \to c} [f(x)/g(x)]$. This happens, for example, with

$$\lim_{x \to +\infty} [xe^{-x}] = \lim_{x \to +\infty} \left[\frac{e^{-x}}{(1/x)} \right].$$

An application of L'Hôpital's rule gives

$$\lim_{x \to +\infty} [xe^{-x}] = \lim_{x \to +\infty} \left[\frac{-e^{-x}}{(-1/x^2)} \right] = \lim_{x \to \infty} [x^2 e^{-x}],$$

and although the result is not incorrect, it is a limit which is more complicated than the original one.

L'Hôpital's rule may also be applied to indeterminate forms of the type '$\infty \div \infty$' when it takes the following form.

L'Hôpital's rule applied to an indeterminate form of the type '$\infty \div \infty$'
Let $f(x)$ and $g(x)$ be such that as $x \to c$, so $f(x) \to \pm\infty$ and $g(x) \to \pm\infty$. Then if

$$\lim_{x \to c} \left[\frac{f'(x)}{g'(x)} \right] = L,$$

it follows that

$$\lim_{x \to c} \left[\frac{f(x)}{g(x)} \right] = \lim_{x \to c} \left[\frac{f'(x)}{g'(x)} \right] = L.$$

Example 26.8

Evaluate

$$\lim_{x \to \infty} [xe^{-x}].$$

Solution
Writing the limit as

$$\lim_{x \to \infty} [xe^{-x}] = \lim_{x \to \infty} \left[\frac{x}{e^x} \right],$$

it is seen to be of the form '$\infty \div \infty$'.
Setting $f(x) = x$ and $g(x) = e^x$ and differentiating gives

$$f'(x) = 1$$

and

$$g'(x) = e^x,$$

so an application of L'Hôpital's rule gives

$$\lim_{x \to \infty} [xe^{-x}] = \lim_{x \to \infty} \left[\frac{x}{e^x} \right] = 0$$

▲

It is often possible to use L'Hôpital's rule to evaluate indeterminate forms of the type '$0 \cdot \infty$' and '$\infty - \infty$'. Indeed, the limit in Example 26.8 was of the form '$0 \cdot \infty$' when written in its original form

$$\lim_{x \to +\infty} [xe^{-x}].$$

Indeterminate forms of the type '$0 \cdot \infty$' arise when the limit concerned has the form $\lim_{x \to c} [f(x) g(x)]$, where as $x \to c$ so $f(x) \to 0$ and $g(x) \to \pm\infty$. This may be transformed into a limit of the form '$0 \div 0$' by writing it as

$$\lim_{x \to c} [f(x) g(x)] = \lim_{x \to c} \left[\frac{f(x)}{1/g(x)} \right],$$

or to one of the form '$\infty \div \infty$' by writing it as

$$\lim_{x \to c} [f(x) g(x)] = \lim_{x \to c} \left[\frac{g(x)}{1/f(x)} \right],$$

to both of which L'Hôpital's rule may be applied, as in Example 26.8. Indeterminate forms of the type '$\infty \div \infty$' can be transformed either into the form '$0 \div 0$' or '$\infty \div \infty$' by algebraic manipulation, as shown in the last example.

Example 26.9

Evaluate

$$\lim_{x \to 0} \left(\frac{1}{\sin^2 x} - \frac{1}{x^2} \right).$$

Solution
This limit is of the form '$\infty - \infty$'. Combining terms gives

$$\lim_{x \to 0} \left(\frac{x^2 - \sin^2 x}{x^2 \sin^2 x} \right),$$

which is now in the form '0 ÷ 0' to which L'Hôpital's rule may be applied. To avoid making repeated applications of L'Hôpital's rule we will make use of simple trigonometric identities and the fact that in Section 14 we showed that $\lim_{x\to 0} (\sin x/x) = 1$. This means that for small x, $\sin x$ may be approximated by x. The approximation becomes exact in the limit as $x \to 0$. Thus for small x (the only situation which concerns us):

$$\lim_{x \to 0} \left(\frac{1}{\sin^2 x} - \frac{1}{x^2} \right) = \lim_{x \to 0} \left(\frac{x^2 - \sin^2 x}{x^4} \right).$$

Applying L'Hôpital's rule gives

$$\lim_{x \to 0} \left(\frac{1}{\sin^2 x} - \frac{1}{x^2} \right) = \lim_{x \to 0} \left(\frac{2x - 2\sin x \cos x}{4x^3} \right),$$

so as $\sin 2x = 2\sin x \cos x$ we have

$$\lim_{x \to 0} \left(\frac{1}{\sin^2 x} - \frac{1}{x^2} \right) = \lim_{x \to 0} \left(\frac{2x - 2\sin 2x}{4x^3} \right).$$

A further application of L'Hôpital's rule gives

$$\lim_{x \to 0} \left(\frac{1}{\sin^2 x} - \frac{1}{x^2} \right) = \lim_{x \to 0} \left(\frac{2 - 2\cos 2x}{12x^2} \right) = \lim_{x \to 0} \left(\frac{1 - \cos 2x}{6x^2} \right).$$

However, $1 - \cos 2x = 2\sin^2 x$, so

$$\lim_{x \to 0} \left(\frac{1}{\sin^2 x} - \frac{1}{x^2} \right) = \lim_{x \to 0} \frac{1}{3} \left(\frac{\sin x}{x} \right)^2 = \frac{1}{3},$$

where we have used the fact that $(\sin x/x)^2 = (\sin x/x)(\sin x/x)$, and $\lim_{x \to 0} (\sin x/x) = 1$.   ▲

PROBLEMS 26

In problems 1 to 16 locate and identify the stationary points and find the equations of any asymptotes that exist.

1. $f(x) = x^3 - 3x^2$.

2. $f(x) = 6x^2 - x^4$.

3. $f(x) = \dfrac{x^2 - 2x + 2}{x - 1}$.

4. $f(x) = \dfrac{x^4 + 3}{x}$.

5. $f(x) = \dfrac{8}{x^2 - 4}$.

6. $f(x) = \dfrac{4x - 12}{(x - 2)^2}$.

7. $f(x) = x(x + 3)^{1/2}$.

8. $f(x) = (x^3 - 3x)^{1/2}$.

9. $f(x) = xe^{-x}$.

10. $f(x) = \dfrac{1}{2} x^2 \ln\left(\dfrac{x}{a}\right)$ $(a > 0)$.

11. $f(x) = \sin x + \cos x$.

12. $f(x) = \dfrac{x^3}{4(2 - x)^2}$.

13. $f(x) = 2x + 3x^{2/3}$.

14. $f(x) = (x^2 - 1)^{2/3}$.

15. $f(x) = \dfrac{4}{(x^2 + 8)^{1/2}}$.

16. $f(x) = x(x^2 - 4)^{-2/3}$.

Evaluate the indeterminate forms in problems 17 to 40.

17. $\displaystyle\lim_{x \to 2}\left[\dfrac{x - 2}{x^2 - 3x + 2}\right]$.

18. $\displaystyle\lim_{x \to 3}\left[\dfrac{x^2 - 9}{x - 3}\right]$.

19. $\displaystyle\lim_{x \to 0}\left[\dfrac{x}{\sqrt{(1 + 3x)} - 1}\right]$.

20. $\displaystyle\lim_{x \to \pi/4}\left[\dfrac{\sin x - \cos x}{\cos 2x}\right]$.

21. $\displaystyle\lim_{x \to \pi}\left[\dfrac{\tan x}{\sin 2x}\right]$.

22. $\displaystyle\lim_{x \to 1}\left[\dfrac{x^{1/3} - 1}{x^{1/2} - 1}\right]$.

23. $\displaystyle\lim_{x \to 0}\left[\dfrac{\sqrt{(1 + x)} - \sqrt{(1 - x)}}{x}\right]$.

24. $\displaystyle\lim_{x \to \pi/4}\left[\dfrac{1 + \sin 2x}{1 - \cos 4x}\right]$.

25. $\displaystyle\lim_{x \to 0}\left[\dfrac{\sin 3x}{\sqrt{2} - \sqrt{(x + 2)}}\right]$.

26. $\lim\limits_{x \to \pi} \left[\dfrac{\sqrt{(1 + \tan x)} - \sqrt{(1 - \tan x)}}{\sin 2x} \right].$

27. $\lim\limits_{x \to 0+} \left[\dfrac{\ln x}{\cot x} \right].$

28. $\lim\limits_{x \to +\infty} \left[\dfrac{\ln x}{x^k} \right], \quad (k > 0).$

29. $\lim\limits_{x \to 1/2} \left[\dfrac{\arcsin(1 - 2x)}{4x^2 - 1} \right].$

30. $\lim\limits_{x \to 0} \left[\dfrac{2x \sin x}{\sec x - 1} \right].$

31. $\lim\limits_{x \to +\infty} \left[x^n\, e^{-x} \right].$

32. $\lim\limits_{x \to +\infty} \left[\dfrac{\ln(2x)}{x} \right].$

33. $\lim\limits_{x \to \pi/2} \left[\dfrac{\tan x}{\tan 3x} \right].$

34. $\lim\limits_{x \to 0-} \left[x \ln x \right].$

35. $\lim\limits_{x \to \pi} (\pi - x) \tan \dfrac{x}{2}.$

36. $\lim\limits_{x \to 0+} \left[\dfrac{\ln(kx)}{\cot x} \right], \quad (k > 0).$

37. $\lim\limits_{x \to 1} \left[\dfrac{1}{x - 1} - \dfrac{2}{x^2 - 1} \right].$

38. $\lim\limits_{x \to +\infty} \left[\sqrt{(x^2 + x + 1)} - \sqrt{(x^2 - x)} \right].$

39. $\lim\limits_{x \to 0} \left[\dfrac{1}{\sin^2 x} - \dfrac{1}{4 \sin^2 x/2} \right].$

40. $\lim\limits_{x \to 1} \left[\dfrac{1}{x - 1} - \dfrac{1}{\ln x} \right].$

Functions of two variables

27

A rule which assigns a unique number z to each point (x, y) in part or all of the (x, y)-plane is said to define a **function** of the two variables x and y. The variables x and y are called **independent variables** and z is called the **dependent variable**. It is usual to show this relationship by writing

$$z = f(x, y),$$

where $f(x, y)$ is the rule relating x and y to the (dependent) variable z.

The region in the (x, y)-plane for which z is defined is called the **domain of definition** of the function $f(x, y)$. Unless stated otherwise, the domain of definition of a function $f(x, y)$ of the two independent variables x and y is taken to be all the points (x, y) for which $f(x, y)$ is defined. For example, the function

$$z = x^2 + y^2$$

is defined for all points in the (x, y)-plane, so, unless otherwise stated, its domain of definition is the entire plane. However, if the function concerned is

$$z = \sqrt{(1 - x^2 - y^2)}$$

where the positive square root is taken, z is only defined for all points such that $x^2 + y^2 \leq 1$, and so its largest possible domain of definition is the interior and boundary of a circle of radius 1 centred on the origin.

It is often convenient to define a domain of definition of a function by means of inequalities as shown by the example which now follows.

Example 27.1

A function has for its domain of definition a region in the (x, y)-plane satisfying the following inequalities

$$x^2 + y^2 > 1, \quad y > x, \quad x \leq 2.$$

Construct a diagram in which the region is shown as a shaded area, and on which boundaries belonging to the region are represented by a solid line, and ones which are excluded from the region are represented by a dashed line.

Solution
The inequality

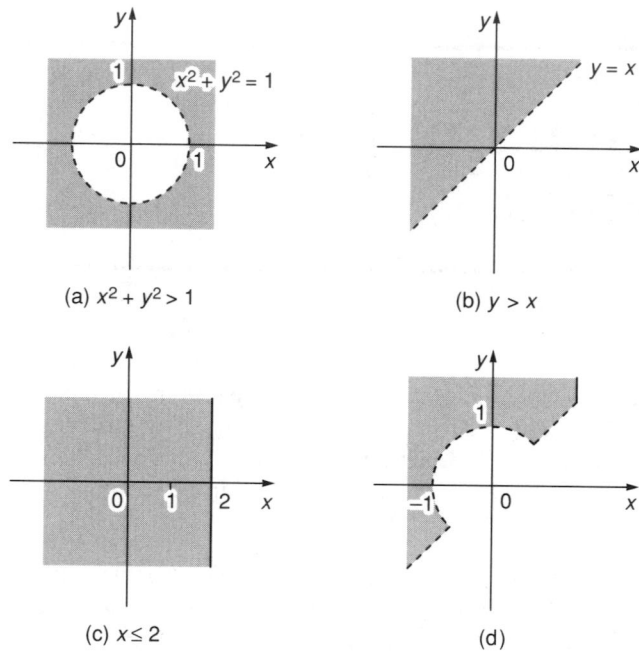

(a) $x^2 + y^2 > 1$

(b) $y > x$

(c) $x \leq 2$

(d)

Fig. 74

$$x^2 + y^2 > 1$$

describes all points lying strictly **outside** a circle of radius 1 centred on the origin. This follows because replacing the sign > by an equality gives $x^2 + y^2 = 1$, which is the equation of a circle of radius 1 centred on the origin. Thus the condition $x^2 + y^2 > 1$ defines points strictly outside this circle. We remark here that had the inequality been $x^2 + y^2 < 1$ then the points would have been **inside** the circle. The region in the (x, y)-plane satisfying this inequality is shown in Fig. 74(a). The circle $x^2 + y^2 = 1$ is shown as a dashed line because points on its boundary do not belong to the shaded region.

A similar argument shows that $y > x$ describes all the points strictly above the line $y = x$ as shown in Fig. 74(b). The line $y = x$ is again shown as a dashed line because its points do not belong to the shaded region. The inequality $x \leq 2$ describes the points to the left of and on the line $x = 2$. These points are shown as the shaded region in Fig. 74(c), to which belong the points on the line $x = 2$ which, accordingly, is shown as a solid line. The points in the plane satisfying all these inequalities are obtained by superimposing the three regions. The required region together with its boundaries obtained in this manner is shown in Fig. 74(d). ▲

If rectangular Cartesian axes $O(x, y, z)$ are adopted, the points

$$z = f(x, y)$$

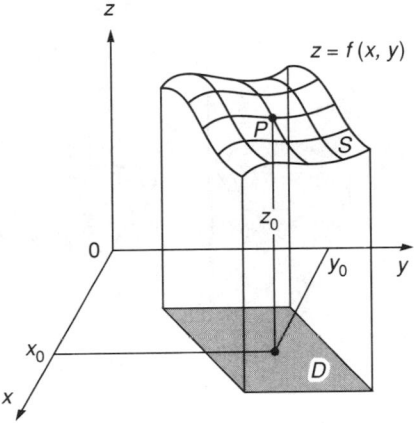

$z = f(x, y)$

Fig. 75

describe a **surface** S above the domain of definition D of $f(x, y)$ in the (x, y)-plane. This interpretation is illustrated by Fig. 75.

The surface S can be visualized in two different ways, one of which uses a **cutting plane** technique, and the other **contour lines**.

CUTTING PLANE TECHNIQUE

In this method the curves of intersection of $z = f(x, y)$ and first the planes $x = $ constant and then the planes $y = $ constant are constructed. These are called **cutting planes** because if the surface $z = f(x, y)$ is considered as a thin sheet, these planes 'cut' it to form plane curves. An examination of the shape of these curves for different values of $x = $ constant and $y = $ constant then enables the shape of the surface to be visualized.

For example, if

$$z = 2x^2 + y^2,$$

the curves of intersection with the plane $x = a$ (the plane parallel to the y and z-axes passing through $x = a$ on the x-axis) is

$$z = 2a^2 + y^2,$$

which is a parabola. Varying the value of a simply moves the parabola up or down relative to the (x, y)-plane.

Similarly, the curve of intersection with the plane $y = b$ (the plane parallel to the x and z-axes passing through the point $y = b$ on the y-axis) is

$$z = 2x^2 + b^2$$

which is another parabola. Here also, changing the value of b merely moves the parabola up or down relative to the (x, y)-plane.

The surface

$$z = 2x^2 + y^2,$$

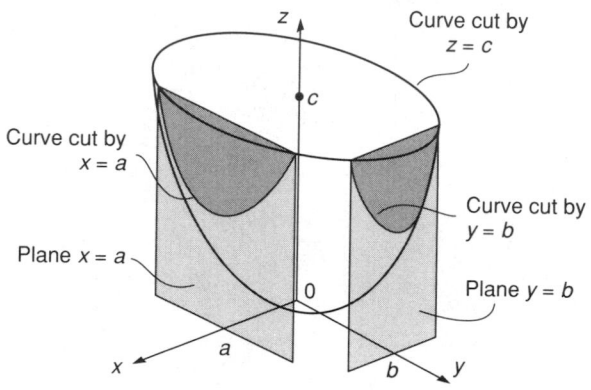

Fig. 76

which is a **paraboloid**, can be visualized by sketching the curves produced by these cutting planes, as shown in Fig. 76.

CONTOUR LINE METHOD

This method enables the visualization of a surface by making use of the familiar concept of the **contour lines** (also called **level curves**) on maps; namely, the lines joining points on the surface

$$z = f(x, y)$$

which all lie at a constant 'height' z above the (x, y)-plane. To represent contour lines in a two-dimensional manner, the curves of constant z are projected on to the (x, y)-plane, each being associated with a (different) constant

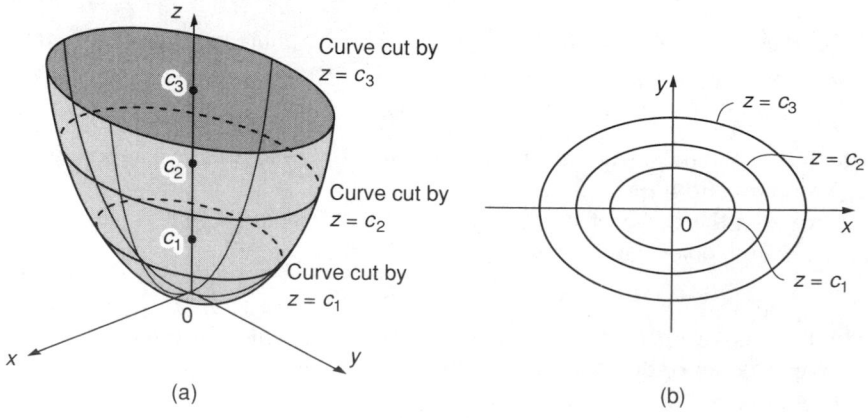

(a)   (b)

Fig. 77

value of z. The equation of the curve in the (x, y)-plane determining all points for which $z = c$ is thus given by cutting the surface with the cutting plane $z = c$ to obtain

$$c = f(x, y).$$

For example, if

$$z = 2x^2 + y^2,$$

the contour lines are determined by the equation

$$c = 2x^2 + y^2,$$

which describes a family of ellipses. This approach is illustrated in Fig. 77(a). The curves in Fig. 77(b) are obtained by projecting the elliptical curves in Fig. 77(a) on to the (x, y)-plane.

PROBLEMS 27

Sketch the regions satisfying the inequalities in problems 1 to 4.

1. $x^2 + y^2 \geqslant 4$, $y \leqslant 2$, $x > -3$.
2. $x^2/4 + y^2/9 < 1$, $y < 1$, $x > -1$.
3. $y \geqslant 1/x$, $x \geqslant 2$, $y < x$.
4. $(x - 1)^2 + (y - 1)^2 > 1$, $x \geqslant 0$, $y \geqslant 0$.

In problems 5 to 10 determine the largest possible domains of definition for the stated functions.

5. $f(x, y) = \ln(1 - x^2 - 2y^2)$.
6. $f(x, y) = (x + y) e^{-(x^2 + y^2)}$.
7. $f(x, y) = \operatorname{artanh}\left(\dfrac{x^2 + 6}{x^2 + y^2 + 4}\right)$.
8. $f(x, y) = (x + y) \ln(\sinh xy)$.
9. $f(x, y) = \dfrac{4x^2 + y^2 + 9}{\sqrt{(x^2 + y^2 - 1)}}$.
10. $f(x, y) = [(x - 1)^2 + (y - 1)^2 - 4]^{1/2} \ln(1 - x^2 - y^2)$.
11. Find the equation of the contour lines for the **hyperbolic paraboloid** function

$$z = \frac{x^2}{4} - \frac{y^2}{16},$$

and verify by inspection that they lie on the saddle-shaped surface shown in Fig. 78. This is called a hyperbolic paraboloid because cutting planes in one direction produce hyperbolas while in another direction they produce parabolas.

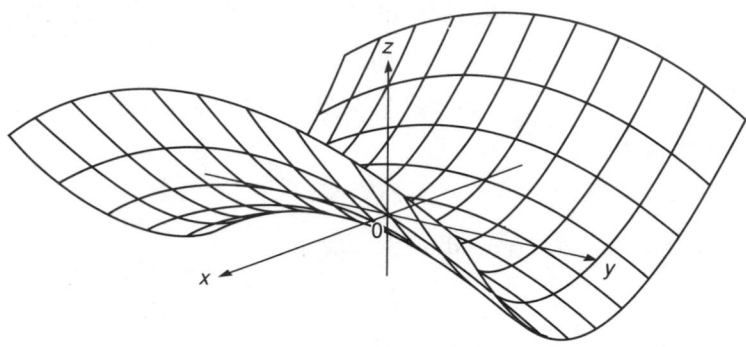

Fig. 78

12.   Find the equation of the contour lines for the function

$$z = x^2 + 2xy + y^2$$

and verify by inspection that they lie on the u-shaped surface shown in Fig. 79.

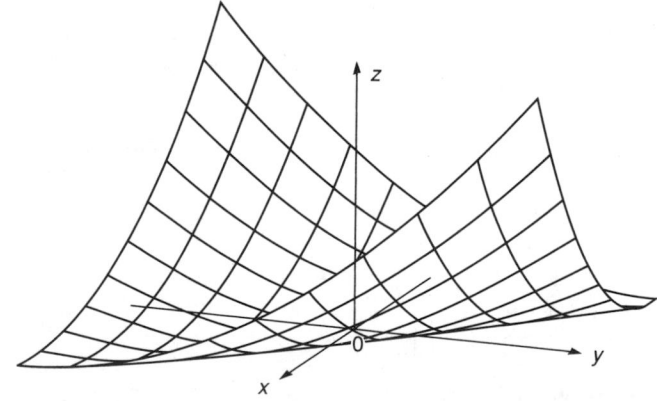

Fig. 79

Limits and continuity of functions of two real variables

28

Let a function $f(x, y)$ of the two real variables x and y have domain of definition D in which there lies the point Q at (x_0, y_0), and let L be a real number. In addition, let γ be any **path** (curve in the (x, y)-plane) joining an arbitrary point P in D to the point Q at (x_0, y_0). We shall say a point (x, y) on γ **approaches arbitrarily closely** to the point (x_0, y_0), written either $x \to x_0$, $y \to y_0$ or $(x, y) \to (x_0, y_0)$, if the distance from (x, y) to (x_0, y_0) becomes arbitrarily small.

The function $f(x, y)$ will be said to have the **limit** L as $(x, y) \to (x_0, y_0)$, written

$$\lim_{(x, y) \to (x_0, y_0)} f(x, y) = L,$$

if $f(x, y)$ becomes arbitrarily close to L as (x, y) becomes arbitrarily close to (x_0, y_0) and, furthermore, the result is true for **every** path joining P to Q. Here, by requiring $f(x, y)$ to be arbitrarily close to the number L we mean that the number

$$|f(x, y) - L|$$

becomes arbitrarily small, say less than some small number $\varepsilon > 0$, so

$$|f(x, y) - L| < \varepsilon.$$

Correspondingly, the distance from (x, y) to (x_0, y_0) is by Pythagoras' theorem (see Section 3):

$$[(x - x_0)^2 + (y - y_0)^2]^{1/2},$$

so for (x, y) to be arbitrarily close to (x_0, y_0) we mean that this distance is less than some small number $\delta > 0$, so

$$[(x - x_0)^2 + (y - y_0)^2]^{1/2} < \delta.$$

Thus the mathematical definition of the limit L of $f(x, y)$ as $(x, y) \to (x_0, y_0)$ is as follows:

$$\lim_{(x, y) \to (x_0, y_0)} f(x, y) = L$$

if for any $\varepsilon > 0$ there corresponds a $\delta > 0$ such that

$$|f(x, y) - L| < \varepsilon \quad \text{when} \quad [(x - x_0)^2 + (y - y_0)^2]^{1/2} < \delta.$$

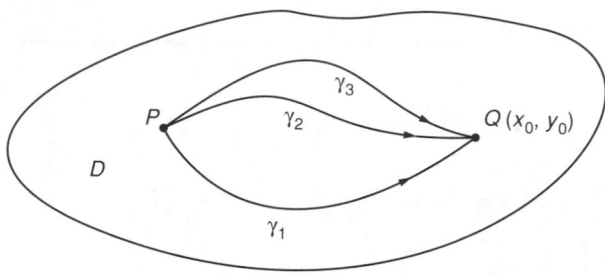

Fig. 80

To see that the point Q located at (x_0, y_0) may be approached along infinitely many different paths, it is only necessary to consider Fig. 80 which shows three possible paths γ_1, γ_2 and γ_3 in D joining P to Q. Geometrically, the existence of a limit L of the function $f(x, y)$ as $(x, y) \to (x_0, y_0)$ implies that in the **neighbourhood** of the point (x_0, y_0) the surface S represented by the graph of

$$z = f(x, y)$$

is **unbroken**. This follows because in whatever manner $(x, y) \to (x_0, y_0)$, if the limit exists $f(x, y)$ must always **approach** the value L. Notice the important fact that the value of $f(x, y)$ at (x_0, y_0) does not enter into the definition of the limit. Thus $f(x, y)$ need not even be defined at (x_0, y_0) for the limit as $(x, y) \to (x_0, y_0)$ to exist. Indeed, in many important cases $f(x, y)$ becomes an indeterminate form at a point at which a limit is to be evaluated.

This property is illustrated in Fig. 81, in which a limit of $z = f(x, y)$ is seen to exist as both Q located at (x_0, y_0) and R at (x_1, y_1) are approached by (x, y). The respective values of these limits are L_0 and L_1. However, $f(x, y)$ is not even defined at (x_0, y_0), whereas it is at (x_1, y_1) at which point $f(x_1, y_1) = L_1$. The small circle in the surface S above Q indicates that in this case $f(x, y)$ is not defined at Q. The arrows in the (x, y)-plane indicate, respectively, different

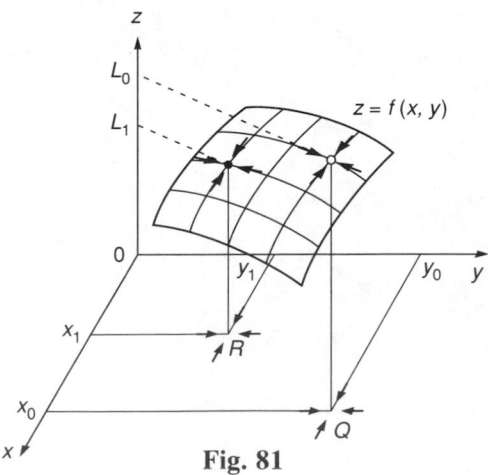

Fig. 81

paths of approach to Q and R, while the arrows on the surface S indicate the corresponding manner of approach to the limiting values L_0 and L_1 on S.

Example 28.1

Evaluate the limits

(i) $\displaystyle \lim_{(x,\,y)\,\to\,(\pi/2,\,1)} \left[\frac{\sin xy}{x^2 + y^2 + 1} \right]$;   and

(ii) $\displaystyle \lim_{(x,\,y)\,\to\,(0,\,0)} \left[\frac{\sin xy}{x^2 + y^2 + 1} \right]$.

Solution

(i)   The function $\sin xy$ is a continuous function of its arguments x and y, so (see Section 15):

$$\lim_{(x,\,y)\,\to\,(\pi/2,\,1)} (\sin xy) = \sin \frac{\pi}{2} = 1$$

and, similarly,

$$\lim_{(x,\,y)\,\to\,(\pi/2,\,1)} (x^2 + y^2 + 1) = \frac{\pi^2}{4} + 2 = (\pi^2 + 8)/4,$$

and so

$$\lim_{(x,\,y)\,\to\,(\pi/2,\,1)} \left[\frac{\sin xy}{x^2 + y^2 + 1} \right] = \frac{4}{\pi^2 + 8}.$$

(ii)   Arguing as in (i),

$$\lim_{(x,\,y)\,\to\,(0,\,0)} (\sin xy) = 0$$

and, similarly,

$$\lim_{(x,\,y)\,\to\,(0,\,0)} (x^2 + y^2 + 1) = 1,$$

and so

$$\lim_{(x,\,y)\,\to\,(0,\,0)} \left[\frac{\sin xy}{x^2 + y^2 + 1} \right] = \frac{0}{1} = 0.$$ ▲

On occasions a limit does not exist at a particular point, and this is illustrated by the following example.

Example 28.2

Show that

$$f(x, y) = \frac{2x^2 - 3y^2}{x^2 + y^2}$$

has a limit everywhere except at the point $(0, 0)$.

Solution

Consider any point (a, b) where not both a and b are zero. Then as both numerator and denominator are continuous functions of their arguments (see Section 15), it follows that

$$\lim_{(x, y) \to (a, b)} (2x^2 - 3y^2) = 2a^2 - 3b^2$$

and

$$\lim_{(x, y) \to (a, b)} (x^2 + y^2) = a^2 + b^2 \neq 0.$$

Thus we see that

$$\lim_{(x, y) \to (a, b)} \left[\frac{3x^2 - 3y^2}{x^2 + y^2} \right] = \frac{2a^2 - 3b^2}{a^2 + b^2},$$

so the limit is defined for all $(x, y) \neq (0, 0)$.

It follows from the above argument that the function becomes an indeterminate form of the type '$0 \div 0$' at the origin.

To discover whether or not a limit exists at the origin we determine the value approached by $f(x, y)$ for different directions of approach of (x, y) to $(0, 0)$. Setting $y = kx$, and allowing $x \to 0$, the point $(x, y) \to (0, 0)$ along a straight line through the origin with gradient k, and we have

$$\lim_{(x, kx) \to (0, 0)} \left[\frac{2x^2 - 3y^2}{x^2 + y^2} \right] = \lim_{x \to 0} \left[\frac{2x^2 - 3k^2 x^2}{x^2 + k^2 x^2} \right]$$

$$= \lim_{x \to 0} \left[\frac{2 - 3k^2}{1 + k^2} \right] = \frac{2 - 3k^2}{1 + k^2}.$$

This value depends on k, and so is not independent of the direction of approach of (x, y) to $(0, 0)$. Thus the function does not have a limit at the origin, though it does have one at every other point in the (x, y)-plane.   ▲

Closely associated with the notion of a limit of a function $f(x, y)$ of two independent variables is the concept of continuity. A function $f(x, y)$ is said to be **continuous** at (x_0, y_0) if
1 $f(x, y)$ has a limit L as $(x, y) \to (x, y_0)$;   and
2 $f(x_0, y_0) = L$.

In geometrical terms this means that $f(x, y)$ is continuous at (x_0, y_0) if the surface S represented by the graph of

$$z = f(x, y)$$

is unbroken at the point corresponding to (x_0, y_0). This is because when $f(x, y)$ is continuous at (x, y_0)

$$\lim_{(x, y) \to (x_0, y_0)} f(x, y) = L \quad \text{and} \quad f(x_0, y_0) = L.$$

A function which is not continuous at a point (x_0, y_0) is said to be **discontinuous**. These ideas are illustrated graphically in Fig. 81, in which $f(x, y)$ is seen to be continuous at R, but discontinuous at Q because, in this case,

$f(x, y)$ is not even defined at Q. Similarly, it is easily seen that the function in Example 28.1 is continuous everywhere, whereas the function in Example 28.2 is discontinuous at the single point $(0, 0)$, and continuous at all others in the (x, y)-plane.

The related notions of a limit and continuity extend in an obvious manner to functions of n real variables

$$z = f(x_1, x_2, ..., x_n),$$

in which z is the dependent variable and $x_1, x_2, ..., x_n$ are n independent variables. Here, $f(x_1, x_2, ..., x_n)$ is a rule which associates with any 'point' $(x_1, x_2, ..., x_n)$ a unique real number z. The n-dimensional space in which lie all the points $(x_1, x_2, ..., x_n)$ for which z is defined is again called the **domain of definition** of the function.

Simple examples of functions of more than two real variables are

$$z = u^2 + v^2 + w^2$$

(when three independent variables are involved they are not always taken to be x_1, x_2 and x_3), and

$$\varphi = (x^2 + y^2 + z^2)^{-1/2}$$

(the dependent variable is not always taken to be z), and the independent variables are often the Cartesian coordinates (x, y, z) of a point in ordinary three-dimensional space.

Note that the consequences of the continuity of a function of a single real variable listed as properties 1 to 5 in Section 15 apply also to functions of several real variables.

Example 28.3

Determine where the function

$$f(x, y, z) = \frac{1}{\sinh xyz}$$

is continuous.

Solution
The denominator $\sinh xyz$ is non-vanishing provided $xyz \neq 0$, which occurs when $x = 0, y = 0$ or $z = 0$. Thus $f(x, y, z)$ is uniquely defined for any point (x, y, z) away from the x, y and z-axes. Consequently the function $f(x, y, z)$ is continuous at all points away from the x, y and z-axes. However, as $\sinh xyz$ vanishes on each axis the function is discontinuous at each point on each of these axes.   ▲

PROBLEMS 28

Find the following limits when they exist.

1. $\lim\limits_{(x, y) \to (1, 2)} (2x + 3y + 1)$.

2. $\lim\limits_{(x, y) \to (0,0)} [(x^2 + 2y^2 + 3) \sin xy]$.

3. $\lim\limits_{(x, y) \to (0,0)} \left[\dfrac{x + y + 1}{x - y + 3} \right]$.

4. $\lim\limits_{(x, y) \to (1,3)} \left[\dfrac{x^2 + 2xy - 4}{x^3 + 2y^2 + 3} \right]$.

5. $\lim\limits_{(x, y) \to (0,1)} \left[\dfrac{x \sin(x + 2y)}{x^2 + y^2} \right]$.

6. $\lim\limits_{(x, y) \to (0,0)} \left[\dfrac{xy^2}{2x^2 + 3y^2} \right]$.

7. $\lim\limits_{(x, y) \to (0,0)} \left[\dfrac{x^2}{x^2 - 4y^2} \right]$.

8. $\lim\limits_{(x, y) \to (0,0)} \left[\dfrac{\sin xy}{x^2 + y^2} \right]$.

In the following problems determine where, if at all, the functions are discontinuous.

9. $f(x, y) = \dfrac{x^2 + y^2 + 1}{x^2 + y^2 - 1}$.

10. $f(x, y) = \exp(2xy + 1)$.

11. $f(x, y) = \dfrac{8x^2 + y^2 + 4}{x^2 - y}$.

12. $f(x, y) = \ln[x \sin(x^2 + y^2)]$.

Partial differentiation

29

To extend the concept of a derivative to a function of more than one independent variable in a manner consistent with an ordinary derivative, the idea of a cutting plane is utilized. Let us consider the case of a function $f(x, y)$ of the two independent variables x and y which is defined in a neighbourhood of the point (x_0, y_0). Cutting the surface

$$z = f(x, y)$$

by the plane $y = y_0$ gives a curve of intersection in the plane $y = y_0$ with the equation

$$z = f(x, y_0).$$

The gradient of this curve at the point (x_0, y_0) is defined to be the first order **partial derivative** of $f(x, y)$ with respect to x at (x_0, y_0). To distinguish this partial derivative from an ordinary derivative with respect to x it is denoted by writing $(\partial f/\partial x)_{(x_0, y_0)}$. Thus, from the definition of an ordinary derivative, as $z = f(x, y_0)$ is only a function of x it follows that

$$\left(\frac{\partial f}{\partial x}\right)_{(x_0, y_0)} = \lim_{h \to 0} \left[\frac{f(x_0 + h, y_0) - f(x_0, y_0)}{h}\right],$$

provided this limit exists.

Similarly, by cutting $z = f(x, y)$ by the plane $x = x_0$, a curve of intersection

$$z = (x_0, y)$$

is produced. The gradient of this curve at the point (x_0, y_0) is defined to be the first order partial derivative of $f(x, y)$ with respect to y at (x_0, y_0). This partial derivative is written $(\partial f/\partial y)_{(x_0, y_0)}$ and it follows that

$$\left(\frac{\partial f}{\partial y}\right)_{(x_0, y_0)} = \lim_{k \to 0} \left[\frac{f(x_0, y_0 + k) - f(x_0, y_0)}{k}\right],$$

provided the limit exists. As these two gradients are evaluated at (x_0, y_0) it follows that they are numbers.

The geometrical meaning of these partial derivatives can be understood by inspection of Fig. 82. It can be seen from this that the partial derivative

$$\left(\frac{\partial f}{\partial x}\right)_{(x_0, y_0)}$$

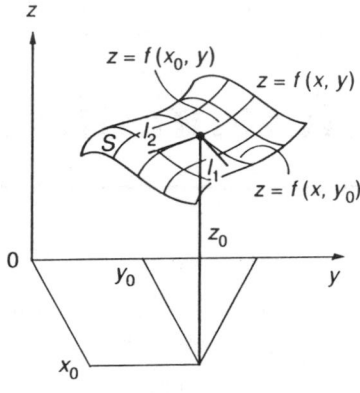

Fig. 82

is the gradient of the tangent line l_1 to

$$z = f(x, y_0)$$

at $x = x_0$, while the partial derivative

$$\left(\frac{\partial f}{\partial y}\right)_{(x_0, y_0)}$$

is the gradient of the tangent line l_2 to

$$z = f(x_0, y)$$

at $y = y_0$.

Removing the suffixes from x_0 and y_0 and allowing x and y to become variables, it follows that $\partial f/\partial x$ and $\partial f/\partial y$ become **functions**, which are defined as the limits

$$\frac{\partial f}{\partial x} = \lim_{h \to 0} \left[\frac{f(x + h, y) - f(x, y)}{h}\right]$$

and

$$\frac{\partial f}{\partial y} = \lim_{k \to 0} \left[\frac{f(x, y + k) - f(x, y)}{k}\right].$$

Thus, unlike a function of one variable, the function $f(x, y)$ has **two** first order partial derivatives; one is the partial derivative $\partial f/\partial x$ with respect to x, and the other is the partial derivative $\partial f/\partial y$ with respect to y.

On occasions it will be convenient to use a more concise notation for these partial derivatives which makes use of suffixes to denote partial differentiation. Thus we will write f_x in place of $\partial f/\partial x$ and f_y in place of $\partial f/\partial y$, so that

$$f_x = \frac{\partial f}{\partial x} \quad \text{and} \quad f_y = \frac{\partial f}{\partial y}.$$

It follows directly from the definition of partial differentiation that the rules for partial differentiation are the same as those for ordinary differentiation summarized in Section 16, save only that when determining $\partial f/\partial x$ the variable y is regarded as a constant, whereas when determining $\partial f/\partial y$ the variable x is regarded as a constant.

Example 29.1

Find the first order partial derivatives of
(i) $f(x, y) = x^3 y^2 + 3x^2 y + x + 5$;
(ii) $f(r, \theta) = r^2(\cos \theta + 2\sin \theta)$.

Solution
(i)   To determine $\partial f/\partial x$ we differentiate $f(x, y)$ with respect to x regarding y · as a constant, and as a result obtain

$$\frac{\partial f}{\partial x} = \frac{\partial}{\partial x} [x^3] y^2 + 3 \frac{\partial}{\partial x} [x^2] y + \frac{\partial}{\partial x} [x] + \frac{\partial}{\partial x} [5].$$

However, when partial differentiation with respect to x acts on a function of x it behaves like an ordinary derivative with respect to x so that

$$\frac{\partial f}{\partial x} = 3x^2 y^2 + 6xy + 1.$$

To determine $\partial f/\partial y$ we differentiate $f(x, y)$ with respect to y, regarding x as a constant, and as a result obtain

$$\frac{\partial f}{\partial y} = x^3 \frac{\partial}{\partial y} [y^2] + 3x^2 \frac{\partial}{\partial y} [y] + \frac{\partial}{\partial y} [x] + \frac{\partial}{\partial y} [5]$$

$$= 2x^3 y + 3x^2.$$

This follows because x behaves as a constant when differentiated partially with respect to y so $\partial[x]/\partial y = 0$, and 5 is an absolute constant, so $\partial[5]/\partial y = 0$.

(ii) Here the independent variables are r and θ, so partial differentiation with respect to r means regarding θ as a constant, while partial differentiation with respect to θ means regarding r as a constant. Thus

$$\frac{\partial f}{\partial r} = \frac{\partial}{\partial r} [r^2] (\cos \theta + 2\sin \theta)$$

$$= 2r(\cos \theta + 2\sin \theta)$$

and

$$\frac{\partial f}{\partial \theta} = r^2 \frac{\partial}{\partial \theta} [\cos \theta + 2\sin \theta]$$

$$= -r^2 \sin \theta + 2r^2 \cos \theta. \qquad \blacktriangle$$

Example 29.2

Find the first order partial derivatives of

$$f(x, y) = x^2 \cosh(2x + 3y)$$

and determine their values at the point $(2, -1)$.

Solution

To determine $\dfrac{\partial f}{\partial x}$ we differentiate $f(x, y)$ with respect to x regarding y as a constant, and as a result obtain

$$\frac{\partial f}{\partial x} = \frac{\partial}{\partial x} [x^2] \cosh(2x + 3y) + x^2 \frac{\partial}{\partial x} [\cosh(2x + 3y)].$$

Performing the indicated differentiation in the first term, setting $u = 2x + 3y$ in the second term and using the chain rule gives

$$\frac{\partial f}{\partial x} = 2x \cosh(2x + 3y) + x^2 \frac{d}{du} [\cosh u] \frac{\partial u}{\partial x}$$

$$= 2x \cosh(2x + 3y) + x^2 \sinh u (2),$$

and thus the partial derivative $\partial f/\partial x$ as a function of x and y becomes

$$\frac{\partial f}{\partial x} = 2x \cosh(2x + 3y) + 2x^2 \sinh(2x + 3y).$$

Substituting $x = 2, y = -1$ it now follows that

$$\left(\frac{\partial f}{\partial x} \right)_{(2, -1)} = 4 \cosh 1 + 8 \sinh 1.$$

To determine $\partial f/\partial y$ we differentiate $f(x, y)$ with respect to y, regarding x as a constant, and as a result obtain

$$\frac{\partial f}{\partial y} = x^2 \frac{\partial}{\partial y} [\cosh(2x + 3y)].$$

Setting $u = 2x + 3y$ and using the chain rule gives

$$\frac{\partial f}{\partial y} = x^2 \frac{d}{du} [\cosh u] \frac{\partial u}{\partial y}$$

$$= x^2 \sinh u (3),$$

and thus the partial derivative $\partial f/\partial y$ as a function of x and y becomes

$$\frac{\partial f}{\partial y} = 3x^2 \sinh(2x + 3y).$$

Substituting $x = 2, y = -1$ then shows that

$$\left(\frac{\partial f}{\partial y} \right)_{(2, -1)} = 12 \sinh 1 \qquad \blacktriangle$$

Example 29.3

Find the first order partial derivatives of

(i) $f(x, y) = \dfrac{x}{y}$;

(ii) $f(x, y) = \exp(x^2 - y^2)$;

(iii) $f(x, y) = \ln(1/(x + 2y))$;

(iv) $f(x, y) = \arctan(y/x)$.

Solution

(i) $\dfrac{\partial f}{\partial x} = \dfrac{1}{y} \dfrac{\partial}{\partial x} [x] = \dfrac{1}{y}$,   so $\dfrac{\partial f}{\partial x} = \dfrac{1}{y}$;

$\dfrac{\partial f}{\partial x} = x \dfrac{\partial f}{\partial x}\left[\dfrac{1}{y}\right] = \dfrac{x}{y^2}$,   so $\dfrac{\partial f}{\partial x} = \dfrac{x}{y^2}$.

(ii)   Set $u = x^2 - y^2$ and use the chain rule to obtain

$$\frac{\partial f}{\partial x} = \frac{d}{du} [e^u] \frac{\partial u}{\partial x} = e^u(2x), \quad \text{so} \quad \frac{\partial f}{\partial x} = 2x \exp(x^2 - y^2);$$

$$\frac{\partial f}{\partial y} = \frac{d}{du} [e^u] \frac{\partial u}{\partial y} = e^u(2y), \quad \text{so} \quad \frac{\partial f}{\partial y} = 2y \exp(x^2 - y^2).$$

(iii) Set $u = 1/(x + 2y)$ and use the chain rule to obtain

$$\frac{\partial f}{\partial x} = \frac{d}{du} [\ln u] \frac{\partial u}{\partial x} = \frac{1}{u} \left[\frac{-1}{(x + 2y)^2} \right],$$

so

$$\frac{\partial f}{\partial x} = \frac{-1}{(x + 2y)},$$

while

$$\frac{\partial f}{\partial y} = \frac{d}{du} [\ln u] \frac{\partial u}{\partial y} = \frac{1}{u} \left[\frac{-2}{(x + 2y)^2} \right],$$

so

$$\frac{\partial f}{\partial y} = \frac{-2}{(x + 2y)}.$$

These results could have been obtined more simply had we used the fact that

$$f(x, y) = \ln\left(\frac{1}{x + 2y}\right) = \ln 1 - \ln(x + 2y) = -\ln(x + 2y),$$

for setting $u = x + 2y$ it follows that

$$\frac{\partial f}{\partial y} = -\frac{d}{du} [\ln u] \frac{\partial u}{\partial y} = \frac{-1}{x + 2y},$$

while

$$\frac{\partial f}{\partial x} = \frac{d}{du} [\ln u] \frac{\partial u}{\partial y} = \frac{-2}{x+2y} .$$

(iv)   Set $u = y/x$ and use the chain rule to obtain

$$\frac{\partial f}{\partial x} = \frac{d}{du} [\arctan u] \frac{\partial u}{\partial x} = \frac{1}{1+u^2} \left(-\frac{y}{x^2} \right) .$$

Substituting for u then shows that

$$\frac{\partial f}{\partial x} = \frac{-y}{x^2+y^2} .$$

Similarly,

$$\frac{\partial f}{\partial y} = \frac{d}{du} [\arctan u] \frac{\partial u}{\partial y} = \frac{1}{1+u^2} \left(\frac{1}{x} \right) ,$$

so substituting for a we arrive at the result

$$\frac{\partial f}{\partial y} = \frac{x}{x^2+y^2} .$$ ▲

In general $\partial f/\partial x$ and $\partial f/\partial y$ are functions of x and y, so they also may be differentiated partially with respect to x and y to arrive at second order partial derivatives. Proceeding in this way we arrive at the four partial derivatives:

$$\frac{\partial}{\partial x} \left(\frac{\partial f}{\partial x} \right), \ \frac{\partial}{\partial x} \left(\frac{\partial f}{\partial y} \right), \ \frac{\partial}{\partial y} \left(\frac{\partial f}{\partial x} \right) \ \text{and} \ \frac{\partial}{\partial y} \left(\frac{\partial f}{\partial y} \right).$$

There are two different notations for these four partial derivatives, the first being

$$\frac{\partial^2 f}{\partial x^2}, \ \frac{\partial^2 f}{\partial x \partial y}, \ \frac{\partial^2 f}{\partial y \partial x} \ \text{and} \ \frac{\partial^2 f}{\partial y^2},$$

respectively. Notice that in this notation the order in which differentiations with respect to x and y are to be performed is to be read from right to left. The second, more concise, notation represents the same four partial derivatives in the form

$$f_{xx}, \ f_{xy}, \ f_{yx} \ \text{and} \ f_{yy},$$

respectively.
  The derivatives

$$\frac{\partial}{\partial x} \left(\frac{\partial f}{\partial y} \right) = \frac{\partial^2 f}{\partial x \partial y} = f_{xy}$$

and

$$\frac{\partial}{\partial y} \left(\frac{\partial f}{\partial x} \right) = \frac{\partial^2 f}{\partial y \partial x} = f_{yx}$$

are called **mixed second order partial derivatives**.

There would appear to be four second order partial derivatives associated with a general function $f(x, y)$. However, in most cases of practical importance the mixed partial derivatives are equal, thus reducing the number of different second order partial derivatives of $f(x, y)$ to three, usually taken to be

$$\frac{\partial^2 f}{\partial x^2}, \frac{\partial^2 f}{\partial x \partial y} \quad \text{and} \quad \frac{\partial^2 f}{\partial y^2}.$$

The conditions for this to occur are set out in the following theorem which will not be proved, but which follows almost directly from the definitions of continuity and differentiability.

Theorem of equality of mixed derivatives
If $f(x, y)$ is such that $\partial f/\partial x$, $\partial f/\partial y$ and $\partial^2 f/\partial x \partial y$ exist and are continuous, then $\partial^2 f/\partial y \partial x$ exists and

$$\frac{\partial^2 f}{\partial x \partial y} = \frac{\partial^2 f}{\partial y \partial x}.$$

Example 29.4

Find all four second order partial derivatives of

$$f(x, y) = \ln(x^2 + y),$$

and verify that the conditions of the above theorem apply.

Solution
Setting $u = x^2 + y$ and using the chain rule gives

$$\frac{\partial f}{\partial x} = \frac{d}{du}[\ln u]\frac{\partial u}{\partial x} = \frac{2x}{x^2 + y}$$

and

$$\frac{\partial f}{\partial y} = \frac{d}{du}[\ln u]\frac{\partial u}{\partial y} = \frac{1}{x^2 + y}.$$

It then follows that

$$\frac{\partial^2 f}{\partial x^2} = \frac{\partial}{\partial x}\left[\frac{2x}{x^2 + y}\right]$$

$$= \frac{\partial}{\partial x}[2x]\left(\frac{1}{x^2 + y}\right) + 2x\frac{\partial}{\partial x}\left[\frac{1}{x^2 + y}\right]$$

$$= \frac{2}{x^2 + y} + 2x\left[\frac{-2x}{(x^2 + y)^2}\right]$$

$$= \frac{2(y - x^2)}{(x^2 + y^2)^2}.$$

Now, by definition:

$$\frac{\partial^2 f}{\partial y \partial x} = \frac{\partial}{\partial y}\left[\frac{\partial f}{\partial x}\right]$$

$$= \frac{\partial}{\partial y}\left[\frac{2x}{x^2 + y}\right]$$

$$= 2x\frac{\partial}{\partial y}\left[\frac{1}{x^2 + y}\right]$$

$$= 2x\left[\frac{-1}{(x^2 + y)^2}\right]$$

$$= \frac{-2x}{(x^2 + y)^2}.$$

As $\partial f/\partial x$, $\partial f/\partial y$ and $\partial^2 f/\partial y \partial x$ all exist and are continuous, it follows that the theorem on mixed derivatives applies, so that $\partial^2 f/\partial x \partial y$ also exists and is given by

$$\frac{\partial^2 f}{\partial x \partial y} = \frac{-2x}{(x^2 + y)^2}.$$

This can be confirmed by direct differentiation because by definition

$$\frac{\partial^2 f}{\partial x \partial y} = \frac{\partial}{\partial x}\left[\frac{\partial f}{\partial y}\right] = \frac{\partial}{\partial x}\left[\frac{1}{x^2 + y}\right]$$

$$= \frac{-2x}{(x^2 + y)^2}.$$

Finally, by definition,

$$\frac{\partial^2 f}{\partial y^2} = \frac{\partial}{\partial y}\left[\frac{\partial f}{\partial y}\right] = \frac{\partial}{\partial y}\left[\frac{1}{x^2 + y}\right]$$

$$= \frac{-1}{(x^2 + y)^2}.$$

▲

Example 29.5

Show that if

$$w = \arctan\left(\frac{2y}{x}\right),$$

then

$$4\frac{\partial^2 w}{\partial x^2} + \frac{\partial^2 w}{\partial y^2} = 0.$$

Solution
Proceeding in the same manner as in Example 29.3(iv) it is easily established that

$$\frac{\partial w}{\partial x} = \frac{-2y}{x^2 + 4y^2} \quad \text{and} \quad \frac{\partial w}{\partial y} = \frac{2x}{x^2 + 4y^2} .$$

Further differentiation then shows that

$$\frac{\partial^2 w}{\partial x^2} = \frac{4xy}{(x^2 + 4y^2)^2} \quad \text{while} \quad \frac{\partial^2 w}{\partial y^2} = \frac{-16xy}{(x^2 + 4y^2)^2} ,$$

and thus

$$4\frac{\partial^2 w}{\partial x^2} + \frac{\partial^2 w}{\partial y^2} = 0.$$

▲

Still higher order partial derivatives may be obtained in similar fashion. Thus third order partial derivatives may be associated with $f(x, y)$ in an obvious manner by writing

$$\frac{\partial}{\partial x}\left(\frac{\partial^2 f}{\partial x^2}\right) = \frac{\partial^3 f}{\partial x^3}$$

$$\frac{\partial}{\partial y}\left(\frac{\partial^2 f}{\partial x^2}\right) = \frac{\partial^3 f}{\partial y \partial x^2} = \frac{\partial^2}{\partial x^2}\left(\frac{\partial f}{\partial y}\right)$$

.
.
.

$$\frac{\partial}{\partial y}\left(\frac{\partial^2 f}{\partial y^2}\right) = \frac{\partial^3 f}{\partial y^3} .$$

These are evaluated by carrying out the differentiations indicated on the left.

Example 29.6

Find $\partial^3 f/\partial y^2 \partial x$ and $\partial^3 f/\partial y^3$ given that

$$f(x, y) = \ln(x^2 + y).$$

Solution
The second order partial derivative $\partial^2 f/\partial y^2$ was found in Example 29.4, so by definition

$$\frac{\partial^3 f}{\partial y^2 \partial x} = \frac{\partial^3 f}{\partial x \partial y^2} = \frac{\partial}{\partial x}\left(\frac{\partial^2 f}{\partial y^2}\right) = \frac{\partial}{\partial x}\left[\frac{-1}{(x^2 + y)^2}\right] = \frac{4x}{(x^2 + y)^3} ,$$

and

$$\frac{\partial^3 f}{\partial y^3} = \frac{\partial}{\partial y}\left(\frac{\partial^2 f}{\partial y^2}\right) = \frac{\partial}{\partial y}\left[\frac{-1}{(x^2 + y)^2}\right] = \frac{2}{(x^2 + y)^3} .$$

▲

The operation of partial differentiation extends immediately to functions of more than two independent variables. Thus if a function $f(x, y, z)$ of the three independent variables x, y and z is involved, to obtain the first order partial derivative $\partial f/\partial x$, differentiation with respect to x is carried out regarding both y and z as constants. Higher order partial derivatives are obtained as before, so that, for example,

$$\frac{\partial^2 f}{\partial x^2} = \frac{\partial}{\partial x}\left(\frac{\partial f}{\partial x}\right) = f_{xx},$$

$$\frac{\partial^2 f}{\partial y \partial x} = \frac{\partial}{\partial y}\left(\frac{\partial f}{\partial x}\right) = f_{yx},$$

$$\frac{\partial^2 f}{\partial z \partial x} = \frac{\partial}{\partial z}\left(\frac{\partial f}{\partial x}\right) = f_{zx}.$$

Example 29.7

Find the first order partial derivatives of

$$f(x, y, z) = x^2 yz^3 + 2xy + yz^2 + 4,$$

and the second order mixed derivative $\partial^2 f/\partial x \partial z$.

Solution
To find $\partial f/\partial x$ we differentiate $f(x, y, z)$ with respect to x, regarding y and z as constants, and as a result obtain

$$\frac{\partial f}{\partial x} = \frac{\partial}{\partial x}[x^2]yz^3 + 2\frac{\partial}{\partial x}[x]y + \frac{\partial}{\partial x}[yz^2] + \frac{\partial}{\partial x}[4]$$

$$= 2xyz^3 + 2y.$$

Proceeding in similar fashion we find that

$$\frac{\partial f}{\partial y} = x^2\frac{\partial}{\partial y}[y]z^3 + 2x\frac{\partial}{\partial y}[y] + \frac{\partial}{\partial y}[y]z^2 + \frac{\partial}{\partial y}[4]$$

$$= x^2 z^3 + 2x + z^2.$$

and

$$\frac{\partial f}{\partial z} = x^2 y\frac{\partial}{\partial x}[z^3] + \frac{\partial}{\partial z}[xy] + y\frac{\partial}{\partial z}[z^2] + \frac{\partial}{\partial z}[4]$$

$$= 3x^2 yz^2 + 2yz.$$

Finally, by definition,

$$\frac{\partial^2 f}{\partial z \partial x} = \frac{\partial}{\partial z}\left[\frac{\partial f}{\partial x}\right]$$

$$= \frac{\partial}{\partial z}[2xyz^3 + 2y]$$

$$= 2xy \frac{\partial}{\partial z} [z^3] + 2 \frac{\partial}{\partial z} [y]$$

$$= 6xyz^2.$$

▲

PROBLEMS 29

In problems 1 to 9 find the first order partial derivatives.

1. $f(x, y) = x^3 + 3x^2y^2 - y^3 + 4$.

2. $f(x, y) = \ln(x^2 + y^2)$.

3. $f(x, y) = \dfrac{xy}{x - y}$.

4. $f(x, y) = \arctan \dfrac{x}{y}$.

5. $f(x, y) = \cos(3x - 4y)$.

6. $f(x, t) = \dfrac{2x - t}{x + 2t}$.

7. $f(r, \theta) = \arcsin(\theta/\sqrt{r})$.

8. $f(x, g) = \ln \sin(x - 2y)$.

9. $f(x, y) = \dfrac{x}{3y - 2x}$.

10. Show that if $w = \ln(\sqrt{x} + \sqrt{y})$, then

$$x \frac{\partial w}{\partial x} + y \frac{\partial w}{\partial y} = \frac{1}{2}.$$

11. Show that if $u = e^{x/y^2}$, then

$$2x \frac{\partial u}{\partial x} + y \frac{\partial u}{\partial y} = 0.$$

12. Show that if $u = \sqrt{x} \sin(y/x)$, then

$$x \frac{\partial u}{\partial x} + y \frac{\partial u}{\partial y} = \frac{1}{2} u.$$

13. Find $\partial^2 w/\partial x^2$, $\partial^2 w/\partial x \partial y$ and $\partial^2 w/\partial y^2$, given that

$$w = x^2 y^3 + 2xy + y^2.$$

14. Find $\partial^2 u/\partial x \partial y$, given that

$$u = (2xy + y^2)^{1/2}.$$

15. Find $\partial^2 u/\partial x \partial y$, given that

$$u = \arctan \left(\frac{x + y}{1 - xy} \right).$$

16. Show that $\partial^2 f/\partial x \partial y = \partial^2 f/\partial y \partial x$, given that

$$f(x, y) = \arcsin\left(\frac{x-y}{x}\right)^{1/2}.$$

17. Show that if

$$u(x, t) = A \sin(c\lambda t + \omega) \sin \lambda x,$$

then

$$\frac{\partial^2 u}{\partial t^2} = c^2 \frac{\partial^2 u}{\partial x^2}.$$

18. Show that if $u = (x^2 + y^2 + z^2)^{1/2}$, then

$$\left(\frac{\partial u}{\partial x}\right)^2 + \left(\frac{\partial u}{\partial y}\right)^2 + \left(\frac{\partial u}{\partial z}\right)^2 = 1.$$

19. Find $\partial^3 f/\partial x \partial y^2$, given that

$$f(x, y) = \sin(xy).$$

20. Show that if

$$u(x, t) = \exp(x - at) + \exp[3(x + at)],$$

then

$$\frac{\partial^2 u}{\partial t^2} = a^2 \frac{\partial^2 u}{\partial x^2}.$$

The total differential 30

If $f(x, y)$ is a differentiable function of the two independent variables x and y, and we set

$$z = f(x, y),$$

then

$$dz = \frac{\partial f}{\partial x}\, dx + \frac{\partial f}{\partial y}\, dy$$

is called the **total differential** of $f(x, y)$. To understand its meaning, let us consider a fixed point (x_0, y_0) in the (x, y)-plane and start by holding y constant at the value $y = y_0$, so $f(x, y_0)$ is then a function only of x. If we now change x from x_0 to $x_0 + dx$, where dx is a differential change in x, it follows that

$$\{dz\}_x = \left(\frac{\partial f}{\partial x}\right)_{(x_0, y_0)} dx$$

is the corresponding differential change in z, produced by this change in x. Similarly, if we hold x constant at $x = x_0$ and change y from $y_0 + dy$, where dy is a differential change in y, it follows that

$$\{dz\}_y = \left(\frac{\partial f}{\partial y}\right)_{(x_0, y_0)} dy$$

is the corresponding differential change in z produced by this change in y.

Thus by allowing both x and y to change from x_0 and y_0 by the respective differentials dx and dy, the corresponding **total differential** change dz is given by $dz = \{dz\}_x + \{dz\}_y$, so

$$dz = \left(\frac{\partial f}{\partial x}\right)_{(x_0, y_0)} dx + \left(\frac{\partial f}{\partial y}\right)_{(x_0, y_0)} dy.$$

The choice of the point (x_0, y_0) was arbitrary, so freeing the point (x_0, y_0) we arrive at the general expression for the total differential:

$$dz = \frac{\partial f}{\partial x}\, dx + \frac{\partial f}{\partial y}\, dy.$$

Example 30.1

Given $z = f(x, y)$, with

$$f(x, y) = 3x^2 \sin y + y \cos y + y \cosh 2x,$$

find the total differential dz.

Solution
Partial differentiation shows that

$$\frac{\partial f}{\partial x} = 6x \sin y + 2y \sinh 2x$$

and

$$\frac{\partial f}{\partial y} = 3x^2 \cos y + \cos y - y \sin y + \cosh 2x,$$

and thus

$$dz = (6x \sin y + 2y \sinh 2x)dx + [(3x^2 + 1)\cos y - y \sin y + \cosh 2x]dy. \quad \blacktriangle$$

The geometrical meaning of the total differential follows directly from the cutting plane interpretation of the partial derivatives of $f(x, y)$ at the point (x_0, y_0). These show that the total differential change

$$dz = \left(\frac{\partial f}{\partial x}\right)_{(x_0, y_0)} dx + \left(\frac{\partial f}{\partial y}\right)_{(x_0, y_0)} dy,$$

from the value $z_0 = f(x_0, y_0)$, is the change in z produced by using a tangent plane approximation to the surface $z = f(x, y)$ at (x_0, y_0) and changing x_0 to $x_0 + dx$ and y_0 to $y_0 + dy$, and so moving to the point $(x_0 + dx, y_0 + dy)$ on the plane. This interpretation is shown in Fig. 83, in which the tangent plane to $z = f(x_0, y_0)$ at (x_0, y_0) is shown in Fig. 83(a), and the way in which dx and

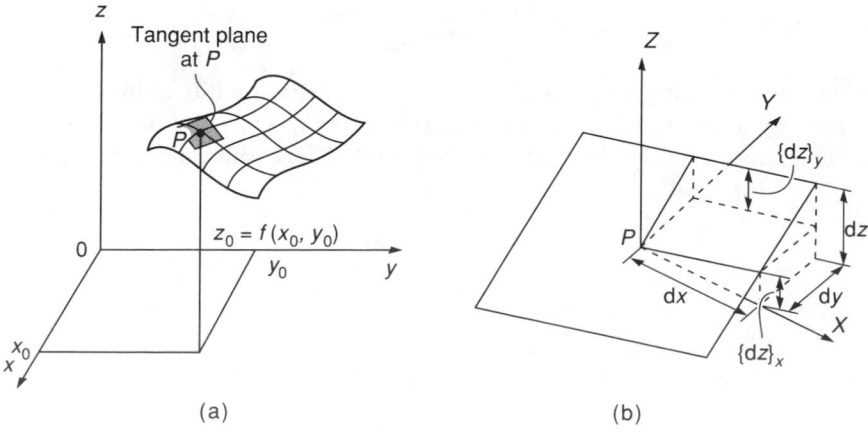

(a)   (b)

Fig. 83

dy contribute to dz is shown in Fig. 83(b), in which PX, PY and PZ are parallel to the x, y and z-axes, respectively.

It is seen from Fig. 83 that when dx and dy are finite, the total differential dz is the approximate change in z when x and y are changed by the small amounts dx and dy, respectively. This result extends in an obvious manner to the case in which n independent variables $x_1, x_2, ..., x_n$ are involved and

$$z = f(x_1, x_2, ..., x_n).$$

In this case, similar reasoning shows that the total differential

$$dz = \frac{\partial f}{\partial x_1} dx_1 + \frac{\partial f}{\partial x_2} dx_2 + ... + \frac{\partial f}{\partial x_n} dx_n.$$

The next example illustrates how the total differential may sometimes be used to find the approximate percentage change in z when small changes are made in dx_1, dx_2, ..., dx_n.

Example 30.2

The drag F on a sphere of volume V moving slowly with speed u in a fluid of viscosity η is given by

$$F = K V^{1/3} \eta u,$$

where K is a numerical constant. Find the approximate percentage change in F produced by small changes dV, dη and du in the volume, viscosity and speed.

Solution
The drag F depends on the three independent variables V, η and u, so it follows that

$$dF = \left(\frac{\partial F}{\partial V}\right) dV + \left(\frac{\partial F}{\partial \eta}\right) d\eta + \left(\frac{\partial F}{\partial u}\right) du.$$

Now

$$\frac{\partial F}{\partial V} = \frac{1}{3} KV^{-2/3} \eta u, \quad \frac{\partial F}{\partial \eta} = KV^{1/3} u, \quad \frac{\partial F}{\partial u} = KV^{1/3} \eta,$$

so

$$dF = \frac{1}{3} KV^{-2/3} \eta u\, dV + KV^{1/3} u\, d\eta + KV^{1/3} \eta\, du.$$

Dividing this result by F gives the approximate fractional change in F due to the changes dV, dη and du in V, η and u, respectively, so multiplying the result by 100 gives the approximate percentage change in F. Thus

$$\text{approximate percentage change in } F = \frac{100\, dF}{F}$$

and hence

approximate percentage change in $F = 100\left(\dfrac{1}{3V} dV + \dfrac{1}{\eta} d\eta + \dfrac{1}{u} du\right)$. ▲

APPLICATION TO IMPLICIT DIFFERENTIATION OF $f(x, y) =$ CONSTANT

If in the expression

$$z = f(x, y)$$

z is kept constant while allowing x and y to vary (we say the **constraint** $z =$ constant is imposed) it follows that y is then a function of x. However, unless the form of $f(x, y)$ is expecially simple, y is usually defined **implicitly** in terms of x.

Applying the total differential to

$$\text{constant} = z = f(x, y)$$

then gives

$$0 = \frac{\partial f}{\partial x} dx + \frac{\partial f}{\partial y} dy,$$

because if $z =$ constant, $dz = 0$. Hence dividing by dx, rearranging terms and recalling that the quotient $dy \div dx$ of the differentials is precisely the derivative dy/dx, shows that

$$\frac{dy}{dx} = -\left(\frac{\partial f}{\partial x}\right) \Big/ \left(\frac{\partial f}{\partial y}\right).$$

This, then, is a way to perform implicit differentiation in terms of partial differentiation. The result will, of course, be the same as the result obtained using the approach discussed in Section 20.

Example 30.3

Given that

$$x \sin y + 2x^2 y - \cosh y + 1 = 0,$$

find dy/dx.

Solution
To apply the approach described above we first set

$$f(x, y) = x \sin y + 2 x^2 y - \cosh y + 1,$$

and then write

$$z = f(x, y)$$

and constrain z to be constant at $z = 0$.

Then it follows at once that the required derivative

$$\frac{dy}{dx} = -\left(\frac{\partial f}{\partial x}\right)\bigg/\left(\frac{\partial f}{\partial y}\right).$$

but

$$\frac{\partial f}{\partial x} = \sin y + 4xy$$

and

$$\frac{\partial f}{\partial x} = x\cos y + 2x^2 - \sinh y,$$

so

$$\frac{dy}{dx} = -\left(\frac{\sin y + 4xy}{x\cos y + 2x^2 - \sinh y}\right).$$

If, instead of using partial differentiation, we had proceeded as in Section 20 and differentiated $f(x, y) = 0$ directly with respect to x we would have obtained the result

$$\sin y + x\cos y\,\frac{dy}{dx} + 4xy + 2x^2\,\frac{dy}{dx} - \sinh y\,\frac{dy}{dx} = 0.$$

Solving for dy/dx then gives rise to the result found above, so the two methods are seen to be equivalent.   ▲

DETERMINING $\partial f/\partial x$ AND $\partial z/\partial y$ GIVEN $f(x, y, z) = 0$

It may happen that x, y and z are related implicitly by the expression

$$f(x, y, z) = 0,$$

yet it is still necessary to find $\partial z/\partial x$ and $\partial z/\partial y$. This may be accomplished as follows. If we define w such that

$$w = f(x, y, z),$$

then taking the total differential we have

$$dw = \frac{\partial f}{\partial x}\,dx + \frac{\partial f}{\partial y}\,dy + \frac{\partial f}{\partial z}\,dz.$$

However, as $f(x, y, z) = 0$ it follows that w is constrained such that $w = 0$ and so $dw = 0$, giving

$$0 = \frac{\partial f}{\partial x}\,dx + \frac{\partial f}{\partial y}\,dy + \frac{\partial f}{\partial z}\,dz.$$

Now suppose it had been possible to solve for z explicitly, and that

$$z = h(x, y).$$

Then taking the total differential we have

$$dz = \frac{\partial h}{\partial x} dx + \frac{\partial h}{\partial y} dy.$$

Substituting this expression for dz in the above result gives

$$0 = \frac{\partial f}{\partial x} dx + \frac{\partial f}{\partial y} dy + \frac{\partial f}{\partial z}\left(\frac{\partial h}{\partial x} dx + \frac{\partial h}{\partial y} dy\right),$$

and so

$$0 = \left(\frac{\partial f}{\partial x} + \frac{\partial f}{\partial z}\frac{\partial h}{\partial x}\right) dx + \left(\frac{\partial f}{\partial y} + \frac{\partial f}{\partial z}\frac{\partial h}{\partial y}\right) dy.$$

However, since $f(x, y, z) = 0$, we know the dependent variable z is a function of the two independent variables x and y, so the differentials dx and dy must be arbitrary. Hence it follows that for the above result to be true we must have

$$\frac{\partial f}{\partial x} + \frac{\partial f}{\partial z}\frac{\partial h}{\partial x} = 0 \quad \text{and} \quad \frac{\partial f}{\partial y} + \frac{\partial f}{\partial z}\frac{\partial h}{\partial y} = 0.$$

However, as $z = h(x, y)$ this result may be rewritten as

$$\frac{\partial f}{\partial x} + \frac{\partial f}{\partial z}\frac{\partial z}{\partial x} = 0 \quad \text{and} \quad \frac{\partial f}{\partial y} + \frac{\partial f}{\partial z}\frac{\partial z}{\partial y} = 0,$$

and so the required partial derivatives are

$$\frac{\partial z}{\partial x} = -\left(\frac{\partial f}{\partial x}\right) \bigg/ \left(\frac{\partial f}{\partial z}\right)$$

and

$$\frac{\partial z}{\partial y} = -\left(\frac{\partial f}{\partial y}\right) \bigg/ \left(\frac{\partial f}{\partial z}\right).$$

Example 30.4

Find $\partial z/\partial x$ and $\partial z/\partial y$, given that

$$xyz^2 + \sinh(x - 2y + 3z) = 0.$$

Solution
To apply the above result we first make the identification

$$f(x, y, z) = xyz^2 + \sinh(x - 2y + 3z).$$

Then

$$\frac{\partial f}{\partial x} = yz^2 + \cosh(x - 2y + 3z),$$

$$\frac{\partial f}{\partial y} = xz^2 - 2\cosh(x - 2y + 3z)$$

and

$$\frac{\partial f}{\partial z} = 2xyz + 3\cosh(x - 2y + 3z).$$

Thus substituting into the above result gives

$$\frac{\partial z}{\partial x} = -\left[\frac{yz^2 + \cosh(x - 2y + 3z)}{2xyz + 3\cosh(x - 2y + 3z)}\right]$$

and

$$\frac{\partial z}{\partial y} = -\left[\frac{xz^2 - 2\cosh(x - 2y + 3z)}{2xyz + 3\cosh(x - 2y + 3z)}\right]. \qquad \blacktriangle$$

PROBLEMS 30

In problems 1 to 6 find the total differential.

1. $f(x, y) = x^2 + 3xy^2 - y^3 + 4.$

2. $f(x, y) = \sin(xy) + x^2 - 3y + 1.$

3. $f(x, y) = \sinh x \cosh(xy) + x^2 + y^2.$

4. $f(x, y) = \ln(x^2 + y^2) + xy - 4.$

5. $f(r, \theta, \varphi) = r^2 \sin\theta + r\cos\varphi + \sin\theta \sin\varphi + 1.$

6. $f(u, v, w) = u^2 \sin v + v^2 \sin u + uvw^2.$

7. If

$$f(u, v, w) = \frac{u^2 v^{1/2}}{w^{1/2}},$$

find the approximate percentage change in $f(u, v, w)$ when u, v and w are changed by the small amounts du, dv and dw, respectively.

8. If

$$f(x, y) = (x/y)^{1/2},$$

find the approximate percentage change in $f(x, y)$ when x and y are changed by the small amounts dx and dy.

9. Find dy/dx, given that

$$3x^2y - 2xy^2 + x^2 + y^2 + 1 = 0.$$

10. Find dy/dx, given that

$$\cosh(x + 2y + 1) - x^2 + 2y^2 - 3 = 0.$$

11. Find $\partial z/\partial x$ and $\partial z/\partial y$, given that

$$x + 2yz^2 + \cos(x + 2y - z) = 0.$$

12. Find $\partial z/\partial x$ and $\partial z/\partial y$, given that

$$z \ln(x^2 + 2y^2 + 1) - 2xyz^2 + 3x = 0.$$

31   The chain rule

The **chain rule** for the function

$$w = f(x,\ y)$$

of the two independent variables x and y is a direct extension of the chain rule in the calculus of one real variable. It is most easily derived from the expression for the total derivative

$$dw = \frac{\partial f}{\partial x}\,dx + \frac{\partial f}{\partial y}\,dy.$$

Let us suppose that x and y depend only on a single real variable t with

$$x = X(t) \qquad \text{and} \qquad y = Y(t),$$

where $X(t)$ and $Y(t)$ are differentiable functions of t. Then in terms of differentials

$$dx = X'(t)\,dt \qquad \text{and} \qquad dy = Y'(t)\,dt,$$

so substituting into the expression for dw gives

$$dw = \frac{\partial f}{\partial x}\,X'(t)\,dt + \frac{\partial f}{\partial y}\,Y'(t)\,dt.$$

Dividing by dt and using the fact that the quotient of the differentials dw and dt is, by virtue of the definition of differentials, the derivative dw/dt, we arrive at the result

$$\frac{dw}{dt} = \frac{\partial f}{\partial x}\,X'(t) + \frac{\partial f}{\partial y}\,Y'(t).$$

However,

$$X'(t) = \frac{dx}{dt} \qquad \text{and} \qquad Y'(t) = \frac{dy}{dt},$$

so we find that

$$\frac{dw}{dt} = \frac{\partial f}{\partial x}\frac{dx}{dt} + \frac{\partial f}{\partial y}\frac{dy}{dt}.$$

This result is called the **chain rule** for the function $w = f(x, y)$, and it shows that the function $f(X(t), Y(t))$ is a differentiable function with respect to t. The chain rule also shows how the derivative dw/dt may be determined without the need to differentiate $w = f(X(t), Y(t))$ directly with respect to t. For obvious reasons, the derivative dw/dt computed from $w = f(X(t), Y(t))$ when both x and y are functions of t is called the **total derivative**.

This result extends to the case of a differentiable function

$$w = f(x_1, x_2, ..., x_n)$$

of the n independent variables $x_1, x_2, ..., x_n$ in an obvious manner. Suppose $x_1, x_2 ..., x_n$ are all differentiable functions of the single variable t with

$$x_1 = X_1(t), \quad x_2 = X_2(t), \quad ..., \quad x_n = X_n(t),$$

Then the chain rule for the function $w = f(x_1, x_2, ..., x_n)$ takes the form

$$\frac{dw}{dt} = \frac{\partial f}{\partial x_1}\frac{dx_1}{dt} + \frac{\partial f}{\partial x_2}\frac{dx_2}{dt} + ... + \frac{\partial f}{\partial x_n}\frac{dx_n}{dt},$$

and it shows how the derivative dw/dt may be determined without the need to differentiate

$$w = f(X_1(t), X_2(t), ..., X_n(t))$$

directly with respect to t.

Example 31.1

Given that

$$w = \ln(x^2 + 2y^2 + 1),$$

where

$$x = \sin t \quad \text{and} \quad y = e^{-t},$$

find dw/dt and hence determine its value when $t = 0$.

Solution
Setting $w = f(x, y)$, with

$$f(x, y) = \ln(x^2 + 2y^2 + 1),$$

it follows that

$$\frac{\partial f}{\partial x} = \frac{2x}{x^2 + 2y^2 + 1} \quad \text{and} \quad \frac{\partial f}{\partial y} = \frac{4y}{x^2 + 2y^2 + 1}.$$

Differentiating the expressions for x and y with respect to t gives

$$\frac{dx}{dt} = \cos t \quad \text{and} \quad \frac{dy}{dt} = -e^{-t},$$

so applying the chain rule and substituting for x and y in terms of t we arrive at the result

$$\frac{dw}{dt} = \frac{\partial f}{\partial x}\frac{dx}{dt} + \frac{\partial f}{\partial y}\frac{dy}{dt} = \frac{2\sin t \cos t}{\sin^2 t + 2e^{-2t} + 1} - \frac{4e^{-2t}}{\sin^2 t + 2e^{-2t} + 1}.$$

After using the trigonometric identity $\sin 2t = 2 \sin t \cos t$ this reduces to

$$\frac{dw}{dt} = \frac{\sin 2t - 4e^{-2t}}{\sin^2 t + 2e^{-2t} + 1}.$$

Thus setting $t = 0$ in this last result to determine dw/dt at $t = 0$, that is at the point $(0, 1)$ in the (x, y)–plane, gives

$$\left(\frac{dw}{dt}\right)_{(t=0)} = -\frac{4}{3}. \qquad \blacktriangle$$

Example 31.2

Given that

$$w = \exp(x_1^2 + x_1 x_2 + x_2 x_3),$$

with

$$x_1 = \frac{1}{t}, \qquad x_2 = 1 - \frac{2}{t} \qquad \text{and} \qquad x_3 = 1 - \frac{1}{t},$$

find dw/dt.

Solution
Setting $w = f(x_1, x_2, x_3)$, with

$$f(x_1, x_2, x_3) = \exp(x_1^2 + x_1 x_2 + x_2 x_3),$$

differentiation followed by substituting for x_1, x_2 and x_3 in terms of t gives

$$\frac{\partial f}{\partial x_1} = (2x_1 + x_2) \exp(x_1^2 + x_1 x_2 + x_2 x_3) = \exp\left(1 - \frac{2}{t} + \frac{1}{t^2}\right),$$

$$\frac{\partial f}{\partial x_2} = (x_1 + x_3) \exp(x_1^2 + x_1 x_2 + x_2 x_3) = \exp\left(1 - \frac{2}{t} + \frac{1}{t^2}\right),$$

$$\frac{\partial f}{\partial x_3} = x_2 \exp(x_1^2 + x_1 x_2 + x_2 x_3) = \left(1 - \frac{2}{t}\right) \exp\left(1 - \frac{2}{t} + \frac{1}{t^2}\right).$$

Differentiation of x_1, x_2 and x_3 with respect to t gives

$$\frac{dx_1}{dt} = -\frac{1}{t^2}, \qquad \frac{dx_2}{dt} = \frac{2}{t^2}, \qquad \frac{dx_3}{dt} = \frac{1}{t^2},$$

so substituting these and the previous results into the chain rule gives

$$\frac{dw}{dt} = \frac{\partial f}{\partial x_1}\frac{dx_1}{dt} + \frac{\partial f}{\partial x_2}\frac{dx_2}{dt} + \frac{\partial f}{\partial x_3}\frac{dx_3}{dt} = \frac{2}{t^2}\left(1 - \frac{1}{t}\right)\exp\left(1 - \frac{2}{t} + \frac{1}{t^2}\right). \qquad \blacktriangle$$

A useful application of the chain rule is to the determination of dw/dx when $w = f(x, y)$, and the variables x and y are related **implicitly** by an equation of the form $g(x, y) = 0$. In such a case it is impossible to substitute for y in terms of x in $w = f(x, y)$ and then to find dw/dx by direct differentiation. To resolve this problem we proceed as follows. Setting $t = x$ and $y = y(x)$ in the chain rule for $w = f(x, y)$ gives

$$\frac{dw}{dx} = \frac{\partial f}{\partial x}\frac{d[x]}{dx} + \frac{\partial f}{\partial y}\frac{dy}{dx},$$

which reduces to

$$\frac{dw}{dx} = \frac{\partial f}{\partial x} + \frac{\partial f}{\partial y}\frac{dy}{dx}.$$

It now remains for us to determine dy/dx, but it follows from Section 30 that

$$\frac{\partial g}{\partial x} + \frac{\partial g}{\partial y}\frac{dy}{dx} = 0,$$

so

$$\frac{dy}{dx} = -\left(\frac{\partial g}{\partial x}\right)\Big/\left(\frac{\partial g}{\partial y}\right),$$

and thus

$$\frac{dw}{dx} = \frac{\partial f}{\partial x} - \left(\frac{\partial f}{\partial y}\right)\left(\frac{\partial g}{\partial x}\right)\Big/\left(\frac{\partial g}{\partial y}\right).$$

Example 31.3

Given that

$$w = x^2 + 4xy + 1,$$

and

$$x + \sin(x + 3y) = 0,$$

find dw/dx.

Solution
Setting $w = f(x, y)$, with

$$f(x, y) = x^2 + 4xy + 1,$$

it follows that

$$\frac{\partial f}{\partial x} = 2x + 4y \quad \text{and} \quad \frac{\partial f}{\partial y} = 4x.$$

Making the identification

$$g(x, y) = x + \sin(x + 3y),$$

we have

$$\frac{\partial g}{\partial x} = 1 + \cos(x + 3y) \quad \text{and} \quad \frac{\partial g}{\partial y} = 3\cos(x + 3y).$$

Finally, substituting the above results into the expression

$$\frac{dw}{dz} = \frac{\partial f}{\partial x} - \left(\frac{\partial f}{\partial y}\right)\left(\frac{\partial g}{\partial x}\right) \bigg/ \left(\frac{\partial g}{\partial y}\right),$$

gives

$$\frac{dw}{dz} = 2x + 4y - \frac{4x[1 + \cos(x + 3y)]}{3\cos(x + 3y)}.$$

Notice that the implicit relationship between x and y means that dw/dz is also determined implicity. The values of x and y in the expression for dw/dz are not independent, but must satisfy $g(x, y) = 0$.   ▲

PROBLEMS 31

1. Use the chain rule to find dw/dt given that
$$w = \exp(2x - 3y),$$
where $x = t^2$ and $y = 1/t$.
   Check the result by direct substitution followed by differentiation with respect to t.

2. Use the chain rule to find dw/dt given that
$$w = \sinh[3xy + 1],$$
where
$$x = \frac{1}{1 + t} \quad \text{and} \quad y = \frac{1}{1 - t}.$$
   Check the result by direct substitution followed by differentiation with respect to t.

3. Use the chain rule to find dw/dt given that
$$w = x^3 + 2y^2 - 4z^2,$$
where $x = t$, $y = \sin t$ and $z = \tan t$.
   Check the result by direct substitution followed by differentiation with respect to t.

4. Use the chain rule to find dw/dt given that
$$w = \frac{x}{y + 2z},$$
where $x = 1/t$, $y = 2t$ and $z = 2/t^2$.
   Check the result by direct substitution followed by differentiation with respect to t.

5. Find dw/dx given that
$$w = \sin x + \sinh(x^2 + y),$$

and

$$\cosh(x - y) - x^3 = 0.$$

6. Find dw/dx given that

$$w = \ln(xy + 4),$$

and

$$xy + \ln(x^2 + y) = 0.$$

Change of variable in partial differentiation

32

Many applications of the calculus of several variables lead to equations involving partial derivatives with respect to a specific system of coordinates which is usually determined by the nature of the application. For various reasons, it often becomes necessary to change to a different system of coordinates, so it is important to know how the partial derivatives involved transform. It is the purpose of this section to examine this problem and to establish the rules by which such transformations may be accomplished.

For simplicity, and because it is the most important case, we only give a detailed account of the way in which derivatives of functions of two independent variables transform. The extension to n independent variables is straightforward, so we will only present the result.

Let $w = f(x, y)$ be a differentiable function of the two independent variables x and y and suppose that x and y are themselves differentiable functions of two new independent variables u and v, so

$$x = X(u, v) \qquad \text{and} \qquad y = Y(u, v).$$

If these expressions are substituted into $f(x, y)$ the function takes on a new form $F(u, v)$, say. Thus under this change of variable $w = f(x, y)$ becomes $w = F(u, v)$, and we see from this that the total differential dw can be expressed in the two different but equivalent forms:

$$dw = \frac{\partial f}{\partial x} dx + \frac{\partial f}{\partial y} dy \tag{A}$$

and

$$dw = \frac{\partial F}{\partial u} du + \frac{\partial f}{\partial v} dv. \tag{B}$$

Now the differentials dx and dy can be related to the differentials du and dv by differentiation of the expressions for x and y:

$$dx = \frac{\partial X}{\partial u} du + \frac{\partial X}{\partial v} dv$$

and

$$dy = \frac{\partial Y}{\partial u} du + \frac{\partial Y}{\partial v} dv$$

or, as $x = X(u, v)$ and $y = Y(u, v)$,

$$dx = \frac{\partial x}{\partial u} du + \frac{\partial x}{\partial v} dv$$

and

$$dy = \frac{\partial y}{\partial u} du + \frac{\partial y}{\partial v} dv.$$

Substituting these results into (A) and rearranging terms gives

$$dw = \left(\frac{\partial f}{\partial x} \frac{\partial x}{\partial u} + \frac{\partial f}{\partial y} \frac{\partial y}{\partial u} \right) du + \left(\frac{\partial f}{\partial x} \frac{\partial x}{\partial v} + \frac{\partial f}{\partial y} \frac{\partial y}{\partial v} \right) dv.$$

As this result expresses dw in terms of du and dv it is simply an alternative form of (B). Thus comparing the coefficients of du and dv we arrive at the following result.

Rule for changing variables in partial derivatives of $f(x, y)$ from x and y to $x = X(u, v)$, $y = Y(u, v)$ when $f(x, y)$ becomes $F(u, v)$

$$\frac{\partial F}{\partial u} = \frac{\partial f}{\partial x} \frac{\partial x}{\partial u} + \frac{\partial f}{\partial y} \frac{\partial y}{\partial u}$$

$$\frac{\partial F}{\partial v} = \frac{\partial f}{\partial x} \frac{\partial x}{\partial v} + \frac{\partial f}{\partial y} \frac{\partial y}{\partial v}.$$

When, later, we come to consider how to determine higher order partial derivatives, it will be necessary to relate partial differentiation **operations** rather than **derivatives**. In anticipation of this need we first rewrite the above results as follows:

$$\frac{\partial F}{\partial u} = \frac{\partial x}{\partial u} \frac{\partial f}{\partial x} + \frac{\partial y}{\partial u} \frac{\partial f}{\partial y}$$

$$\frac{\partial F}{\partial v} = \frac{\partial x}{\partial v} \frac{\partial f}{\partial x} + \frac{\partial y}{\partial v} \frac{\partial f}{\partial y}.$$

Omitting the functions F and f from these results converts them from relationships between derivatives to the following relationships between partial differentiation operations:

$$\frac{\partial}{\partial u} \equiv \frac{\partial x}{\partial u} \frac{\partial}{\partial x} + \frac{\partial y}{\partial u} \frac{\partial}{\partial y}$$

$$\frac{\partial}{\partial v} \equiv \frac{\partial x}{\partial v} \frac{\partial}{\partial x} + \frac{\partial y}{\partial v} \frac{\partial}{\partial y}.$$

The rule for change of variables extends to functions of n independent variables in an obvious manner. Let

$$w = f(x_1, x_2, ..., x_n)$$

be a differentiable function of the n independent variables $x_1, x_2, ..., x_n$ and let $u_1, u_2, ..., u_n$ be n new independent variables such that

$$x_1 = X_1(u_1, u_2, ..., u_n)$$
$$x_2 = X_2(u_1, u_2, ..., u_n)$$
$$\vdots$$
$$x_n = X_n(u_1, u_2, ..., u_n),$$

where $X_1, X_2, ..., X_n$ are differentiable functions of their arguments. Then if $w = f(x_1, x_2, ..., X_n)$ becomes the function $w = F(u_1, u_2, ..., u_n)$ under this change of variable, the rule for changing variables becomes

$$\frac{\partial F}{\partial u_1} = \frac{\partial f}{\partial x_1}\frac{\partial x_1}{\partial u_1} + \frac{\partial f}{\partial x_2}\frac{\partial x_2}{\partial u_1} + ... + \frac{\partial f}{\partial x_n}\frac{\partial x_n}{\partial u_1}$$

$$\frac{\partial F}{\partial u_2} = \frac{\partial f}{\partial x_1}\frac{\partial x_1}{\partial u_2} + \frac{\partial f}{\partial x_2}\frac{\partial x_2}{\partial u_2} + ... + \frac{\partial f}{\partial x_n}\frac{\partial x_n}{\partial u_2}$$

$$\vdots$$

$$\frac{\partial F}{\partial u_n} = \frac{\partial f}{\partial x_1}\frac{\partial x_1}{\partial u_n} + \frac{\partial f}{\partial x_2}\frac{\partial x_2}{\partial u_n} + ... + \frac{\partial f}{\partial x_n}\frac{\partial x_n}{\partial u_n}.$$

The connection between partial differentiation operations for functions of two independent variables may be extended in an obvious manner to give

$$\frac{\partial}{\partial u_1} \equiv \frac{\partial x_1}{\partial u_1}\frac{\partial}{\partial x_1} + \frac{\partial x_2}{\partial u_1}\frac{\partial}{\partial x_2} + ... + \frac{\partial x_n}{\partial u_1}\frac{\partial}{\partial x_n}$$

$$\frac{\partial}{\partial u_2} \equiv \frac{\partial x_1}{\partial u_2}\frac{\partial}{\partial x_1} + \frac{\partial x_2}{\partial u_2}\frac{\partial}{\partial x_2} + ... + \frac{\partial x_n}{\partial u_2}\frac{\partial}{\partial x_n}$$

$$\vdots$$

$$\frac{\partial}{\partial u_n} \equiv \frac{\partial x_1}{\partial u_n}\frac{\partial}{\partial x_1} + \frac{\partial x_2}{\partial u_n}\frac{\partial}{\partial x_2} + ... + \frac{\partial x_n}{\partial u_n}\frac{\partial}{\partial x_n}.$$

An important and frequently used change of variable involves the transformation from the Cartesian coordinates (x, y) to the cylindrical polar coordinates (r, θ), in which (see Section 4)

$$x = r \cos \theta \quad \text{and} \quad y = r \sin \theta.$$

The first example shows how partial derivatives with respect to r and θ are related to partial derivatives with respect to x and y.

Example 32.1

The differentiable function $f(x, y)$ becomes the function $F(r, \theta)$ under the change of variable

$$x = r \cos \theta, \quad y = r \sin \theta.$$

Find $\partial F/\partial r$ and $\partial F/\partial \theta$ in terms of partial derivatives of f with respect to x and y.

Solution
Partial differentiation with respect to r means regarding θ as a constant, while partial differentiation with respect to θ means regarding r as a constant, so

$$\frac{\partial x}{\partial r} = \cos\theta, \qquad \frac{\partial x}{\partial \theta} = -r\sin\theta$$

$$\frac{\partial y}{\partial r} = \sin\theta, \qquad \frac{\partial y}{\partial \theta} = r\cos\theta.$$

Thus the rule for change of variable becomes (here we have r, θ in place of u, v)

$$\frac{\partial F}{\partial r} = \frac{\partial f}{\partial x}\frac{\partial x}{\partial r} + \frac{\partial f}{\partial y}\frac{\partial y}{\partial r} = \cos\theta\frac{\partial f}{\partial x} + \sin\theta\frac{\partial f}{\partial y}$$

and

$$\frac{\partial F}{\partial \theta} = \frac{\partial f}{\partial x}\frac{\partial x}{\partial \theta} + \frac{\partial f}{\partial y}\frac{\partial y}{\partial \theta} = \frac{\partial f}{\partial x}(-r\sin\theta) + \frac{\partial f}{\partial y}r\cos\theta$$

$$= -r\sin\theta\frac{\partial f}{\partial x} + r\cos\theta\frac{\partial f}{\partial y}.$$

The change of coordinates has thus given rise to the results

$$\frac{\partial F}{\partial r} = \cos\theta\frac{\partial f}{\partial x} + \sin\theta\frac{\partial f}{\partial y}$$

and

$$\frac{\partial F}{\partial \theta} = -r\sin\theta\frac{\partial f}{\partial x} + r\cos\theta\frac{\partial f}{\partial y} \qquad \blacktriangle$$

Example 32.2

The twice differentiable function $f(x, y)$ becomes the function $F(u, v)$ under the change of variable:

$$x = u^2 + v^2, \qquad y = uv.$$

Find $\partial F/\partial u$, $\partial F/\partial v$, $\partial^2 F/\partial u^2$ and $\partial^2 F/\partial v\partial u$ in terms of u, v and partial derivatives of f with respect to x and y.

Solution
Partial differentiation of x and y with respect to u and v shows that

$$\frac{\partial x}{\partial u} = 2u, \qquad \frac{\partial x}{\partial v} = 2v,$$

$$\frac{\partial y}{\partial u} = v, \qquad \frac{\partial y}{\partial v} = u,$$

where we have used the fact that in partial differentiation with respect to u we regard v as a constant, while in partial differentiation with respect to v we regard u as a constant. Thus the rule for change of variable becomes

$$\frac{\partial F}{\partial u} = 2u \frac{\partial f}{\partial x} + v \frac{\partial f}{\partial y}$$

$$\frac{\partial F}{\partial v} = 2v \frac{\partial f}{\partial x} + u \frac{\partial f}{\partial y}.$$

These, then, are the required first order partial derivatives of F with respect to u and v expressed in terms of partial derivatives of f with respect to x and y.

Now, by definition.

$$\frac{\partial^2 F}{\partial u^2} = \frac{\partial}{\partial u}\left(\frac{\partial F}{\partial u}\right) = \frac{\partial}{\partial u}\left(2u \frac{\partial f}{\partial x} + v \frac{\partial f}{\partial y}\right).$$

Thus performing the indicated differentiation, and recalling that partial differentiation with respect to u regards v as a constant, we have

$$\frac{\partial^2 F}{\partial u^2} = 2 \frac{\partial f}{\partial x} + 2u \frac{\partial}{\partial u}\left(\frac{\partial f}{\partial x}\right) + v \frac{\partial}{\partial u}\left(\frac{\partial f}{\partial y}\right).$$

However, the operations of partial differentiation with respect to u, x and y are related by

$$\frac{\partial}{\partial u} \equiv 2u \frac{\partial}{\partial x} + v \frac{\partial}{\partial y},$$

so

$$\frac{\partial^2 F}{\partial u^2} = 2 \frac{\partial f}{\partial x} + 2u\left[2u \frac{\partial}{\partial x} + v \frac{\partial}{\partial y}\right]\left(\frac{\partial f}{\partial x}\right) + v\left[2u \frac{\partial}{\partial x} + v \frac{\partial}{\partial y}\right]\left(\frac{\partial f}{\partial y}\right)$$

$$= 2 \frac{\partial f}{\partial x} + 4u^2 \frac{\partial^2 f}{\partial x^2} + 2uv \frac{\partial^2 f}{\partial y \partial x} + 2uv \frac{\partial^2 f}{\partial x \partial y} + v^2 \frac{\partial^2 f}{\partial y^2}.$$

The stated twice differentiability of $f(x, y)$ means that $\partial^2 f/\partial x \partial y = \partial^2 f/\partial y \partial x$, and so

$$\frac{\partial^2 F}{\partial u^2} = 2 \frac{\partial f}{\partial x} + 4u^2 \frac{\partial^2 f}{\partial x^2} + v^2 \frac{\partial^2 f}{\partial y^2} + 4uv \frac{\partial^2 f}{\partial x \partial y}.$$

To determine $\partial^2 F/\partial v \partial u$ we start from the definition

$$\frac{\partial^2 F}{\partial v \partial u} = \frac{\partial}{\partial v}\left(\frac{\partial F}{\partial u}\right) = \frac{\partial}{\partial v}\left[2u \frac{\partial f}{\partial x} + v \frac{\partial f}{\partial y}\right].$$

Remembering that partial differentiation with respect to v regards u as a constant we see that

$$\frac{\partial^2 F}{\partial v \partial u} = 2u \frac{\partial}{\partial v}\left(\frac{\partial f}{\partial x}\right) + \frac{\partial f}{\partial y} + v \frac{\partial}{\partial v}\left(\frac{\partial f}{\partial y}\right).$$

However,

$$\frac{\partial}{\partial v} \equiv 2v \frac{\partial}{\partial x} + u \frac{\partial}{\partial y},$$

so

$$\frac{\partial^2 F}{\partial v \partial u} = 2u \left[2v \frac{\partial}{\partial x} + u \frac{\partial}{\partial y} \right] \left(\frac{\partial f}{\partial x} \right) + \frac{\partial f}{\partial y} + v \left[2v \frac{\partial}{\partial x} + u \frac{\partial}{\partial y} \right] \left(\frac{\partial f}{\partial y} \right)$$

$$= 4uv \frac{\partial^2 f}{\partial x^2} + 2u^2 \frac{\partial^2 f}{\partial y \partial x} + \frac{\partial f}{\partial y} + 2v^2 \frac{\partial^2 f}{\partial x \partial y} + uv \frac{\partial^2 f}{\partial y^2}.$$

As before, $\partial^2 f / \partial x \partial y = \partial^2 f / \partial y \partial x$, and so

$$\frac{\partial^2 F}{\partial v \partial u} = \frac{\partial f}{\partial y} + 4uv \frac{\partial^2 f}{\partial x^2} + uv \frac{\partial^2 f}{\partial y^2} + 2(u^2 + v^2) \frac{\partial^2 f}{\partial x \partial y}. \qquad \blacktriangle$$

PROBLEMS 32

1. The function $f(x, y)$ becomes the function $F(u, v)$ under the change of variable

    $$x = u^2 + v^2 \qquad \text{and} \qquad y = uv.$$

    Prove that

    $$\frac{1}{4} \left[\left(\frac{\partial F}{\partial u} \right)^2 + \left(\frac{\partial F}{\partial v} \right)^2 \right] = x \left[\left(\frac{\partial f}{\partial x} \right)^2 + \left(\frac{\partial f}{\partial y} \right)^2 \right] + 2y \left(\frac{\partial f}{\partial x} \right) \left(\frac{\partial f}{\partial y} \right).$$

    Show that

    $$\frac{\partial^2 F}{\partial u^2} = 2 \frac{\partial f}{\partial x} + 4u^2 \frac{\partial^2 f}{\partial x^2} + 8uv \frac{\partial^2 f}{\partial x \partial y} + 4v^2 \frac{\partial^2 f}{\partial y^2}.$$

2. The function $f(x, y)$ becomes the function $F(s, t)$ under the change of variable

    $$x = s^3 + 2s \qquad \text{and} \qquad y = st.$$

    Find $\partial F / \partial s$ and $\partial F / \partial t$ in terms of $\partial f / \partial x$ and $\partial f / \partial y$ and show that

    $$\frac{\partial^2 F}{\partial t \partial s} = \frac{\partial f}{\partial y} + (3s^3 + 2s) \frac{\partial^2 f}{\partial x \partial y} + st \frac{\partial^2 f}{\partial y^2}.$$

3. The function $f(x, y)$ becomes the function $F(u, v)$ under the change of variable

    $$x = u^2 - v^2 \qquad \text{and} \qquad y = st.$$

    Find $\partial F / \partial u$ and $\partial F / \partial v$, and show that

    $$\frac{\partial^2 F}{\partial u^2} = 2 \frac{\partial f}{\partial x} + 4u^2 \frac{\partial^2 f}{\partial x^2} + 4uv \frac{\partial^2 f}{\partial x \partial y} + v^2 \frac{\partial^2 f}{\partial y^2}.$$

4. The function $f(x, y)$ becomes the function $F(r, \theta)$ under the change of variable

$$x = r \cos \theta \quad \text{and} \quad y = r \sin \theta.$$

Use the results of Example 32.1 to show that

$$\frac{\partial^2 F}{\partial r^2} = \cos^2 \theta \, \frac{\partial^2 f}{\partial x^2} + 2 \sin \theta \cos \theta \, \frac{\partial^2 f}{\partial x \partial y} + \sin^2 \theta \, \frac{\partial^2 f}{\partial y^2}$$

and

$$\frac{\partial^2 F}{\partial \theta^2} + r \, \frac{\partial F}{\partial r} = r^2 \sin^2 \theta \, \frac{\partial^2 f}{\partial x^2} - 2r^2 \sin \theta \cos \theta \, \frac{\partial^2 f}{\partial x \partial y} + r^2 \cos^2 \theta \, \frac{\partial^2 f}{\partial y^2},$$

and hence that

$$\frac{\partial^2 F}{\partial r^2} + \frac{1}{r} \frac{\partial F}{\partial r} + \frac{1}{r^2} \frac{\partial^2 F}{\partial \theta^2} = \frac{\partial^2 f}{\partial x^2} + \frac{\partial^2 f}{\partial y^2}.$$

5. The function $f(x, y)$ becomes the function $F(u, v)$ under the change of variable

$$x = u^2 - v^2 \quad \text{and} \quad y = 2uv.$$

Show that

$$\left(\frac{\partial F}{\partial u} \right)^2 + \left(\frac{\partial F}{\partial v} \right)^2 = 4(u^2 + v^2) \left[\left(\frac{\partial f}{\partial x} \right)^2 + \left(\frac{\partial f}{\partial y} \right)^2 \right].$$

Prove that f is a function of y only if

$$u \frac{\partial F}{\partial u} - v \frac{\partial F}{\partial v} = 0.$$

6. The function $V(s, t)$ becomes the function $v(x, y)$ under the change of variable

$$s = \ln(x^2 + y^2) \quad \text{and} \quad t = e^{x^2 - y^2} \quad \text{for} \quad x > 0, \ y > 0.$$

Show that

$$\frac{1}{2x} \frac{\partial v}{\partial x} = e^{-s} \frac{\partial V}{\partial s} + t \frac{\partial V}{\partial t}$$

and

$$\frac{1}{2y} \frac{\partial v}{\partial y} = e^{-s} \frac{\partial V}{\partial s} - t \frac{\partial V}{\partial t}.$$

Hence show that if

$$y \frac{\partial v}{\partial x} + x \frac{\partial v}{\partial y} = 0,$$

then $\partial V/\partial s = 0$ and v is a function of $x^2 - y^2$.

7. The function $f(u, v)$ becomes the function $F(x, y)$ under the change of variable

$$u = \frac{x}{x^2 + y^2} \qquad \text{and} \qquad v = \frac{-y}{x^2 + y^2}.$$

Show that

$$\frac{\partial F}{\partial x} = (v^2 - u^2) \frac{\partial f}{\partial u} - 2uv \frac{\partial f}{\partial v}$$

and

$$\frac{\partial F}{\partial y} = 2uv \frac{\partial f}{\partial u} + (v^2 - u^2) \frac{\partial f}{\partial v}.$$

Hence show that if $f(u, v)$ is independent of v it follows that $F(x, y)$ satisfies the equation

$$2xy \frac{\partial F}{\partial x} + (y^2 - x^2) \frac{\partial F}{\partial y} = 0.$$

33 Antidifferentiation (integration)

Given a differentiable function $F(x)$, we already know that the process of finding its derivative $F'(x)$ is called differentiation. If we denote the derivative of $F(x)$ by $f(x)$, then

$$F'(x) = f(x)$$

or, equivalently,

$$\frac{dF}{dx} = f(x) .$$

The reverse of this process is called **antidifferentiation**, or **integration**, and given a function $f(x)$ it involves finding a function $F(x)$ whose derivative equals $f(x)$. The function $F(x)$ is then called an **antiderivative** of $f(x)$.

To illustrate matters let us find an antiderivative of $f(x)$ given that $f(x) = 4x^3$. We know from differentiation that

$$\frac{d}{dx}[x^4] = 4x^3,$$

so an antiderivative $F(x)$ is $F(x) = x^4$. However, as $d[c]/dx = 0$ for any constant c, it follows that other antiderivatives are

$$F_1(x) = x^4 - 7, \quad F_2(x) = x^4 + 1 \quad \text{and} \quad F_3(x) = x^4 + 91.$$

This suggests that antiderivatives are not unique, but that any two antiderivatives of $f(x)$ can only differ by an arbitrary constant. This conclusion is, indeed, true and it is contained in the following important result which we shall prove.

RELATIONSHIP BETWEEN ANTIDERIVATIVES

If $F(x)$ and $G(x)$ are antiderivatives of $f(x)$ for $a \leqslant x \leqslant b$, then

$$G(x) = F(x) + C,$$

where C is an arbitrary constant.

The proof of this result involves two steps. In the first step we show that $G'(x) = F'(x) = f(x)$. This follows because for $a \leqslant x \leqslant b$:

$$G'(x) = \frac{\mathrm{d}}{\mathrm{d}x} [F(x) + C] = F'(x) + \frac{\mathrm{d}}{\mathrm{d}x} [C] = F'(x) + 0 = f(x).$$

The second step involves showing that if $F(x)$ and $G(x)$ are any two anti-derivatives of $f(x)$, then they can only differ by a constant. Set $K(x) = G(x) - F(x)$ and suppose, if possible, that $K(x)$ is non-constant for $a \leqslant x \leqslant b$.

Then we can find an interval $\alpha \leqslant x \leqslant \beta$ inside $a \leqslant x \leqslant b$ in which $K(\alpha) \neq K(\beta)$. Now $F(x)$ and $G(x)$ are differentiable, so $K(x)$ is also differentiable, thus by the mean value theorem we can find some δ between α and β such that

$$K'(\delta) = \frac{K(\beta) - K(\alpha)}{\beta - \alpha}.$$

As $K(\alpha) \neq K(\beta)$ we conclude that $K'(\delta) \neq 0$. However, this is impossible, because we have already shown that $K'(x) = G'(x) - F'(x) = 0$ for all x such that $a \leqslant x \leqslant b$, and δ lies in this same interval.

This establishes a contradiction, so the assumption that $K(x)$ is non-constant for $a \leqslant x \leqslant b$ is false, and thus $K(x) = $ constant and the result is proved.

If $y = F(x)$ is an antiderivative of $f(x)$ it follows that $F(x)$ must be a solution of

$$\frac{\mathrm{d}y}{\mathrm{d}x} = f(x),$$

which has the equivalent differential form

$$\mathrm{d}y = f(x)\,\mathrm{d}x.$$

The operation of antidifferentiation is denoted by an integral sign $\int$, and the most general solution of the above equation is

$$y = \int f(x)\,\mathrm{d}x = F(x) + C.$$

Thus the expression $\int f(x)\,\mathrm{d}x$ denotes the antiderivative of the function $f(x)$ or, equivalently, the **indefinite integral** of $f(x)$, while the function $f(x)$ itself is called the **integrand** (the function whose antiderivative is to be determined or, equivalently, the function to be integrated).

CONNECTION BETWEEN ANTIDIFFERENTIATION AND DIFFERENTIATION

It follows directly from these definitions that

$$\int F'(x)\,\mathrm{d}x = F(x) + C \quad (C = \text{const.}),$$

while

$$\frac{d}{dx}\left[\int f(x)\,dx\right] = f(x).$$

The first result asserts that the operation of integration is the inverse of differentiation, while the second asserts that the operation of differentiation is the inverse of integration.

An illustration of the first of these two general results is provided by the fact that $x^4 + C$ is an antiderivative of $4x^3$. The second result is illustrated by setting $f(x) = \sin x$, for it then becomes

$$\frac{d}{dx}\left[\int \sin x\,dx\right] = \sin x.$$

The practical significance of these results lies in the fact that they allow us to find antiderivatives (indefinite integrals) by using tables of derivatives in reverse. The following list of integrals has been compiled by using in reverse the derivatives of functions established in previous sections.

A SHORT LIST OF INTEGRALS

1 $\quad \displaystyle\int k f(x)\,dx = k \int f(x)\,dx \quad (k = \text{const.}).$

2 $\quad \displaystyle\int [f(x) \pm g(x)]\,dx = \int f(x)\,dx \pm \int g(x)\,dx.$

3 $\quad \displaystyle\int x^n\,dx = \frac{x^{n+1}}{n+1} + C \quad (n \neq -1).$

4 $\quad \displaystyle\int \frac{dx}{x} = \ln |x| + C.$

5 $\quad \displaystyle\int a^x\,dx = \frac{a^x}{\ln a} + C \quad (a \neq 1, a > 0).$

6 $\quad \displaystyle\int e^{ax}\,dx = \frac{1}{a}\,e^{ax} + C \quad (a \neq 0).$

7 $\quad \displaystyle\int \sin ax\,dx = -\frac{1}{a}\cos ax + C \quad (a \neq 0).$

8   $\displaystyle\int \cos ax \, dx = -\frac{1}{a} \sin ax + C \quad (a \neq 0).$

9   $\displaystyle\int \sec^2 ax \, dx = \frac{1}{a} \tan ax + C \quad (a \neq 0).$

10   $\displaystyle\int \sec ax \tan ax \, dx = \frac{1}{a} \sec ax + C \quad (a \neq 0).$

11   $\displaystyle\int \operatorname{cosec}^2 ax \, dx = -\frac{1}{a} \cos ax + C \quad (a \neq 0).$

12   $\displaystyle\int \operatorname{cosec} ax \cot ax \, dx = -\frac{1}{a} \operatorname{cosec} ax + C \quad (a \neq 0).$

13   $\displaystyle\int \sinh ax \, dx = \frac{1}{a} \cosh ax + C \quad (a \neq 0).$

14   $\displaystyle\int \cosh ax \, dx = \frac{1}{a} \sinh ax + C. \quad (a \neq 0).$

15   $\displaystyle\int \operatorname{sech}^2 ax \, dx = \frac{1}{a} \tanh ax + C \quad (a \neq 0).$

16   $\displaystyle\int \operatorname{sech} ax \tanh ax \, dx = -\frac{1}{a} \operatorname{sech} ax + C \quad (a \neq 0).$

17   $\displaystyle\int \operatorname{cosec} ax \coth ax \, dx = -\frac{1}{a} \operatorname{cosech} ax + C \quad (a \neq 0).$

18· $\displaystyle\int \frac{dx}{\sqrt{(a^2 - x^2)}} = \arcsin \frac{x}{a} + C \quad (a > 0).$

19   $\displaystyle\int \frac{dx}{a^2 + x^2} = \frac{1}{a} \arctan \frac{x}{a} + C \quad (a \neq 0).$

20   $\displaystyle\int \frac{dx}{\sqrt{(a^2 + x^2)}} = \begin{cases} \operatorname{arsinh} \dfrac{x}{a} + C \\ \ln [x + \sqrt{(a^2 + x^2)}] + C \quad (a \neq 0). \end{cases}$

21   $\displaystyle\int \frac{dx}{\sqrt{(x^2 - a^2)}} = \begin{cases} \operatorname{arcosh} \dfrac{x}{a} + C & \text{if } x > a > 0 \\ \ln [x + \sqrt{(x^2 - a^2)}] + C & \text{if } |x| > a > 0. \end{cases}$

$$\mathbf{22} \int \frac{\mathrm{d}x}{a^2 - x^2} = \begin{cases} \dfrac{1}{a}\operatorname{artanh}\dfrac{x}{a} + C & \text{if } |x| < |a| \\[3mm] \dfrac{1}{2a}\ln\left|\dfrac{a+x}{a-x}\right| + C & \text{if } |x| < |a| \quad (a > 0). \end{cases}$$

Only the simplest antiderivatives (integrals) can be evaluated by direct appeal to entries in this list. In all other cases special techniques must be used, the most important of which will be discussed in subsequent sections. The example which now follows is a typical antiderivative capable of evaluation by direct appeal to the above list.

Example 33.1

Find

$$F(x) = \int \left(2x^2 + \frac{1}{4}\sin 3x\right)\mathrm{d}x.$$

Solution
From entry 2 in the list we have

$$F(x) = \int 2x^2\,\mathrm{d}x + \int \frac{1}{4}\sin 3x\,\mathrm{d}x,$$

and after using entry 1 this simplifies to

$$F(x) = 2\int x^2\,\mathrm{d}x + \frac{1}{4}\int \sin 3x\,\mathrm{d}x.$$

Setting $n = 2$ in entry 3 gives

$$\int x^2\,\mathrm{d}x = \frac{x^3}{3} + C_1,$$

with C_1 an arbitrary constant, while setting $a = 3$ in entry 7 shows that

$$\int \sin 3x\,\mathrm{d}x = -\frac{1}{3}\cos 3x + C_2,$$

where C_2 is another arbitrary constant.
Thus

$$F(x) = 2\left(\frac{x^3}{3} + C_1\right) + \frac{1}{4}\left(-\frac{1}{3}\cos 3x + C_2\right),$$

or

$$F(x) = \frac{2}{3}x^3 - \frac{1}{12}\cos 3x + \left(2\,C_1 + \frac{1}{4}C_2\right).$$

However, C_1 and C_2 are arbitrary constants, so the combination $2C_1 + \frac{1}{4}C_2$ is also an arbitrary constant, and we will simply denote it by C (we do not perform arithmetic on arbitrary constants). We have thus shown that

$$F(x) = \int \left(2x^2 + \frac{1}{4}\sin 3x\right)dx = \frac{2}{3}x^3 - \frac{1}{12}\cos 3x + C. \qquad \blacktriangle$$

Example 33.2

Find

$$F(x) = \int \frac{dx}{x^2 - 4}$$

for $|x| < 2$.

Solution
As it stands, this antiderivative does not appear in the above list. Entry 22, which is the closest in form, has the integrand $1/(a^2 - x^2)$ with $|x| < |a|$, whereas in this case the integrand is $1/(x^2 - 4)$ subject to the condition that $|x| < 2$.
 The difficulty is easily resolved, because $1/(x^2 - 4) = -1/(4 - x^2)$, so

$$F(x) = \int \frac{dx}{x^2 - 4} = -\int \frac{dx}{4 - x^2} = -\frac{1}{4}\ln\left(\frac{2+x}{2-x}\right) + C,$$

where we have made use of entry 22 with $a = 2$. $\qquad \blacktriangle$

 Routine algebraic manipulation, the use of trigonometric or hyperbolic identities, or the use of the definitions of hyperbolic functions can often reduce seemingly complicated integrals to results contained in the list. The three examples which follow illustrate this observation.

Example 33.3

Find

$$F(x) = \int \cosh^2 2x \, dx.$$

Solution
The integrand $\cosh^2 2x$ is not contained in the list, but it can be transformed into expressions which are. Using the identity

$$\cosh(A + B) = \cosh A \cosh B + \sinh A \sinh B,$$

and setting $A = B = 2x$, shows that

$$\cosh 4x = \cosh^2 2x + \sinh^2 2x.$$

However,

$$\cosh^2 2x - \sinh^2 2x = 1,$$

so

$$\cosh 4x = 2\cosh^2 2x - 1,$$

and thus

$$\cosh^2 2x = \frac{1}{2}(1 + \cosh 4x).$$

Thus

$$F(x) = \int \frac{1}{2}(1 + \cosh 4x)\,dx.$$

$$= \frac{1}{2}\int 1 \cdot dx + \frac{1}{2}\int \cosh 4x\,dx$$

$$= \frac{x}{2} + \frac{1}{8}\sinh 4x + C.$$

As $\sinh 4x = 2\sinh 2x\cosh 2x$, this result may also be written

$$F(x) = \int \cosh^2 2x\,dx = \frac{x}{2} + \frac{1}{4}\sinh 2x\cosh 2x + C. \qquad \blacktriangle$$

Example 33.4

Find

$$F(x) = \int [\sqrt{(x-1)} - 1][\sqrt{(x-1)} + 1]\,dx.$$

Solution
Multiplying the factors in the integrand gives

$$[\sqrt{(x-1)} - 1][\sqrt{(x-1)} + 1] = x - 2,$$

so

$$F(x) = \int [\sqrt{(x-1)} - 1][\sqrt{(x-1)} + 1]\,dx$$

$$= \int x\,dx - 2\int 1 \cdot dx$$

$$= \frac{x^2}{2} - 2x + C.$$

Notice that this result is only true for $x \geqslant 1$, because only if $x \geqslant 1$ are the terms $\sqrt{(x-1)}$ in the integrand real. $\qquad \blacktriangle$

Example 33.5

Find

$$F(x) = \int \left(\frac{e^{2x} - 1}{e^{2x} + 1} \right) \cosh x \, dx.$$

Solution
Multiplying the numerator and denominator of the integrand by e^{-x} gives

$$\left(\frac{e^{2x} - 1}{e^{2x} - 1} \right) \cosh x = \left(\frac{e^x - e^{-x}}{e^x + e^{-x}} \right) \cosh x.$$

However,

$$\cosh x = \frac{e^x + e^{-x}}{2},$$

so

$$\left(\frac{e^{2x} - 1}{e^{2x} + 1} \right) \cosh x = \left(\frac{e^x - e^{-x}}{e^x + e^{-x}} \right) \left(\frac{e^x + e^{-x}}{2} \right)$$

$$= \frac{e^x - e^{-x}}{2} = \sinh x.$$

Thus

$$F(x) = \int \left(\frac{e^{2x} - 1}{e^{2x} + 1} \right) \cosh x \, dx$$

$$= \int \sinh x \, dx$$

$$= \cosh x + C. \qquad \blacktriangle$$

The last two examples illustrate the need for better methods for finding antiderivatives then by appealing directly to entries in the table.

Example 33.6

Find $F(x) = \int \sinh(3x - 5) \, dx.$

Solution
This integral does not appear as an entry in the list, but $\int \sinh ax \, dx$ and $\int \cosh ax \, dx$ are listed. To use these entries we make use of the hyperbolic identity

$$\sinh(A - B) = \sinh A \cosh B - \cosh A \sinh B$$

with $A = 3x$ and $B = 5$ to obtain

$$\sinh(3x - 5) = \sinh 3x \cosh 5 - \cosh 3x \sinh 5.$$

Then it follows that

$$F(x) = \int \sinh(3x - 5)\,dx$$

$$= \int (\sinh 3x \cosh 5 - \cosh 3x \sinh 5)\,dx$$

$$= \cosh 5 \int \sinh 3x\,dx - \sinh 5 \int \cosh 3x\,dx$$

$$= \frac{1}{3}\cosh 5 \cosh 3x - \frac{1}{3}\sinh 5 \sinh 3x + C$$

$$= \frac{1}{3}\cosh(3x - 5) + C$$

where we have used the identity

$$\cosh(A - B) = \cosh A \cosh B - \sinh A \sinh B$$

with $A = 3x$, $B = 5$.

Thus the required result is

$$F(x) = \int \sinh(3x - 5)\,dx = \frac{1}{3}\cosh(3x - 5) + C.$$

The simple form of the solution coupled with the close relationship it bears to the integrand (apart from the factor 1/3, the solution is the derivative of the integrand) suggests there should be a simpler way by which to obtain this result. This is, indeed, the case and the appropriate method, called integration by substitution, will be discussed in the next section.　▲

Example 33.7

Find

$$F(x) = \int x(1 + x^2)^5\,dx.$$

Solution
The integrand $x(1 + x^2)^5$ is not contained in the list, but expanding $(1 + x^2)^5$ gives

$$(1 + x^2)^5 = 1 + 5x^2 + 10x^4 + 10x^6 + 5x^8 + x^{10},$$

so

$$x(1 + x^2)^5 = x + 5x^3 + 10x^5 + 10x^7 + 5x^9 + x^{11}.$$

We may now apply entry 3 to each term in this expression to obtain

$$F(x) = \int x(1+x^2)^5 \, dx = \frac{x^2}{2} + \frac{5}{4}x^4 + \frac{10}{6}x^6 + \frac{10}{8}x^8 + \frac{5}{10}x^{10} + \frac{1}{12}x^{12} + C,$$

or

$$F(x) = \int x(1+x^2)^5 \, dx = \frac{1}{2}x^2 + \frac{5}{4}x^4 + \frac{5}{3}x^6 + \frac{5}{4}x^8 + \frac{1}{2}x^{10} + \frac{1}{12}x^{12} + C.$$

If we now set $C = \frac{1}{12} + C'$, where C' is another arbitrary constant, this result can be written

$$\int x(1+x^2)^5 \, dx = \frac{1}{12}(1 + 6x^2 + 15x^4 + 20x^6 + 15x^8 + 6x^{10} + x^{12}) + C'$$

The expression in parentheses is simply $(1+x^2)^6$ so we have shown that

$$F(x) = \int x(1+x^2)^5 \, dx = \frac{(1+x^2)^6}{12} + C'.$$

As in Example 33.6, the final form of the solution is so simple that it suggests that a more direct approach should be possible. One such approach will be discussed in the next section. ▲

PROBLEMS 33

Evaluate the following integrals.

1. $\int (x^2 + 3x - 1) \, dx.$

2. $\int \left(\frac{x-3}{x^3}\right) dx.$

3. $\int (x^{1/2} + 3x^{1/4}) \, dx.$

4. $\int (e^{7x} + 1) \, dx.$

5. $\int (\cos 4x + 2\sqrt{x}) \, dx.$

6. $\int \left(\frac{x^3 + 5x + 3}{x^2}\right) dx.$

7. $\displaystyle\int \frac{4}{x^2+9}\,dx.$

8. $\displaystyle\int \sin x \cos x\,dx.$ (Hint: use $\sin 2x = 2\sin x \cos x$.)

9. $\displaystyle\int x(1+x^2)^3\,dx.$

10. $\displaystyle\int \frac{5}{\sqrt{(4-x^2)}}\,dx.$

11. $\displaystyle\int \frac{3}{\sqrt{(9-4x^2)}}\,dx.$

12. $\displaystyle\int \frac{dx}{x^2-10}.$

13. $\displaystyle\int \left(\frac{\sqrt{x}-x^{2/3}}{x^{1/3}}\right)dx.$

14. $\displaystyle\int (\sqrt{x}+1)(x-\sqrt{x}+1)\,dx.$

15. Use the approach of Example 33.3 to find

$$\int \sinh^2 x\,dx.$$

16. Modify the approach of Example 33.3 to find

$$\int \cos^2 2x\,dx.$$

17. Modify the approach of Example 33.3 to find

$$\int \sin^2 2x\,dx.$$

18. Make use of the definition of $\sinh x$ to find

$$\int e^x \sinh x\,dx.$$

19. Use the approach of Example 33.6 to find

$$\int \cosh(7x+3)\,dx.$$

20. Modify the approach of Example 33.6 to find

$$\int \sin(2x-1)\,dx.$$

Integration by substitution 34

It is usually the case that an integral $\int f(x) \, dx$ cannot be integrated as it stands because its integrand $f(x)$ is more complicated than any of those listed in the short list of integrals given in Section 33. In many cases, however, if the variable x is replaced by a suitable function of x, say by $u = U(x)$, the integral in terms of u is simpler and can be evaluated by direct appeal to the list of integrals. The result of this substitution is to give a result in terms of u, but by writing $u = U(x)$ we return to the original variable x and so obtain the required result. For obvious reasons, this method of evaluating integrals (anti-derivatives) is called **integration by substitution**.

There are five basic steps in integration by substitution.

1 Choose a suitable substitution $u = U(x)$.

2 Use the substitution $u = U(x)$ to eliminate x as far as possible from $f(x)$.

3 Differentiate the substitution $u = U(x)$ with respect to x and write the result in the differential form

$$du = U'(x) \, dx.$$

Use this result to express the differential dx in the original integral in terms of the differential du by writing

$$dx = \frac{1}{U'(x)} \, du.$$

4 In the original integral replace $f(x)$ by the result obtained in step 2, dx by $du/U'(x)$, and express any remaining terms involving x in terms of u. Then integrate to obtain a solution in terms of u.

5 To arrive at the solution in terms of the original variable x, substitute $u = U(x)$ into the solution found in step 4.

Example 34.1

Find

$$\int \cosh(4x - 9) \, dx.$$

Solution
Step 1
An obvious choice of substitution is $u = 4x - 9$.
Step 2
In terms of $u = 4x - 9$, the integrand $\cosh(4x - 9)$ becomes $\cosh u$.
Step 3
Differentiating $u = 4x - 9$ and writing the result in differential form gives

$$du = 4\,dx,$$

and so

$$dx = \frac{1}{4}\,du.$$

Step 4
Substituting into the original integral shows that

$$\int \cosh(4x - 9)\,dx = \int \frac{\cosh u}{4}\,du = \frac{1}{4}\int \cosh u\,du$$

$$= \frac{1}{4}\sinh u + C.$$

Step 5
To arrive at the required result in terms of the original variable x we now substitute $u = 4x - 9$ into the solution found in step 4 to obtain

$$\int \cosh(4x - 9)\,dx = \frac{1}{4}\sinh(4x - 9) + C. \qquad\blacktriangle$$

We now consider a slightly more complicated example, which was first evaluated in Example 33.7.

Example 34.2

Find

$$\int x(1 + x^2)^5\,dx.$$

Solution
Step 1
As the integrand involves a power of $1 + x^2$ let us attempt to simplify it by making the substitution

$$u = 1 + x^2.$$

Step 2
Using the substitution $u = 1 + x^2$ in the integrand $x(1 + x^2)^5$ gives $x\,u^5$. For the time being we do not try to express x in terms of u, in the hope that this will be unnecessary after the incorporation of dx into the result.

Step 3
Differentiating $u = 1 + x^2$ with respect to x and writing the result in differential form gives

$$\frac{du}{dx} = 2x,$$

and so

$$du = 2x\,dx,$$

or

$$dx = \frac{1}{2x}\,du.$$

Step 4
Combining steps 2 and 3 shows that

$$\int x(1 + x^2)^5\,dx = \int x\,u^5\,\frac{du}{2x} = \frac{1}{2}\int u^5\,du$$

$$= \frac{1}{12}\,u^6 + C.$$

This shows that we were fully justified in not trying to eliminate x from the result xu^5, because it cancelled when dx was expressed in terms of du.

Step 5
To arrive at the solution in terms of the original variable x we substitute $u = 4x - 9$ into the solution found in step 4 to obtain

$$\int x(1 + x^2)^5\,dx = \frac{1}{12}(1 + x^2)^6 + C. \qquad\qquad \blacktriangle$$

For the sake of conciseness, in the remaining examples we will omit the reference to steps 1–5.

Example 34.3

Find

$$\int \frac{\sin\sqrt{x}}{\sqrt{x}}\,dx.$$

Solution
The best choice of substitution is not immediately apparent. However, as $\sin\sqrt{x}$ is complicated, let us attempt to simplify the integral by using the substitution $\sqrt{x} = X$, or $x = X^2$, when

$$\frac{\sin\sqrt{x}}{\sqrt{x}} = \frac{\sin X}{X}.$$

Now differentiating $x = X^2$ with respect to x gives

$$\frac{\mathrm{d}x}{\mathrm{d}X} = 2X,$$

so in differential from we have

$$\mathrm{d}x = 2X\,\mathrm{d}X.$$

Thus collecting results shows that

$$\int \frac{\sin\sqrt{x}}{\sqrt{x}}\,\mathrm{d}x = \int \frac{\sin X}{X}\,2X\,\mathrm{d}X$$

$$= 2\int \sin X\,\mathrm{d}X$$

$$= -2\cos X + C.$$

Finally, writing $X = \sqrt{x}$ we see that

$$\int \frac{\sin\sqrt{x}}{\sqrt{x}}\,\mathrm{d}x = -2\cos\sqrt{x} + C. \qquad\qquad \blacktriangle$$

In the next example the substitution involved is a slightly more complicated one of the form $u(x) = v(y)$.

Example 34.4

Find

$$\int \frac{x(x^2 + 2)}{\sqrt{(5 + x^2)}}\,\mathrm{d}x.$$

Solution
Here also the choice of substitution is not at once apparent. So recognizing that the term $\sqrt{(5 + x^2)}$ is the most complicated one in the integrand, let us attempt to simplify the result by writing $u^2 = 5 + x^2$.

It then follows that in terms of u, the factor $(x^2 + 2)$ in the numerator becomes $(u^2 - 3)$, and for the time being we leave the factor x in the numerator unchanged. Thus we see that

$$\frac{x(x^2 + 2)}{\sqrt{(5 + x^2)}} = \frac{x(u^2 - 3)}{u}.$$

Now differentiating the substitution $u^2 = 5 + x^2$ with respect to x gives

$$2u\,\frac{\mathrm{d}u}{\mathrm{d}x} = 2x,$$

and in differential form this becomes

$$dx = \frac{u}{x} \, du.$$

Combining results gives

$$\frac{x(x^2 + 2)}{\sqrt{(5 + x^2)}} \, dx = \frac{x(u^2 - 3)}{u} \cdot \frac{u}{x} \, du$$

$$= (u^2 - 3) \, du.$$

Consequently we have

$$\int \frac{x(x^2 + 2)}{\sqrt{(5 + x^2)}} \, dx = \int (u^2 - 3) \, du$$

$$= \frac{1}{3} u^3 - 3u + C.$$

Returning to the original variable by writing $u^2 = 5 + x^2$, and $u = \sqrt{(5 + x^2)}$ gives the result

$$\int \frac{x(x^2 + 2)}{\sqrt{(5 + x^2)}} \, dx = \frac{1}{3} (5 + x^2)^{3/2} - 3(5 + x^2)^{1/2} + C$$

$$= \frac{(5 + x^2)^{1/2}(x^2 - 4)}{3} + C. \qquad \blacktriangle$$

When the integrand $f(x)$ is the quotient of two algebraic expressions, the denominator often contains a term of the form $ax^2 + bx + c$, sometimes raised to a fractional power. It is then useful to re-express this in the form $ax^2 + bx + c = a[(x + \alpha)^2 + k]$, where k is a constant, either positive or negative, and α and k depend on a, b and c. This then suggests making the change of variable $X = x + \alpha$.

To find how α and k depend on a, b and c, set

$$ax^2 + bx + c \equiv a[(x + \alpha)^2 + k]$$

and require this to be true for **all** x (it must be an **identity**). This is only possible if corresponding powers of x on either side of the identity have the same coefficients. Expanding the right-hand side gives

$$ax^2 + bx + c \equiv a[x^2 + 2\alpha x + \alpha^2 + k],$$

so equating corresponding coefficients gives

1 *coefficients of x^2* :

$$a = a;$$

2 *coefficients of x:*

$$b = 2a\alpha, \quad \text{so} \quad \alpha = b/2a;$$

3 *constant terms:*

$$c = a(\alpha^2 + k) = a\left(\frac{b^2}{4a^2} + k\right) = \frac{b^2}{4a} + ak,$$

so

$$k = \frac{c}{a} - \frac{b^2}{4a^2}.$$

This process is called **completing the square**, and we have proved that if
$$ax^2 + bx + c = a[(x + \alpha)^2 + k],$$

then

$$\alpha = \frac{b}{2a} \quad \text{and} \quad k = \frac{c}{a} - \frac{b^2}{4a^2}.$$

Example 34.5

Re-express

$$3 + 2x - x^2$$

by completing the square.

Solution
Identifying coefficients shows that
$$a = -1, \quad b = 2 \quad \text{and} \quad c = 3.$$
Thus

$$\alpha = \frac{b}{2a} = -1 \quad \text{and} \quad k = \frac{c}{a} - \frac{b^2}{4a^2} = -4,$$

so

$$3 + 2x - x^2 = -[(x-1)^2 - 4]$$
$$= 4 - (x-1)^2.$$
▲

Example 34.6

Find

$$\int \frac{dx}{(3 + 2x - x^2)^{1/2}}.$$

Solution
Using the result of Example 34.5 shows that

$$\int \frac{dx}{(3 + 2x - x^2)^{1/2}} = \int \frac{dx}{\sqrt{(4 - (x-1)^2)}}.$$

Setting $X = x - 1$, so that $dX = dx$, reduces this to

$$\int \frac{dx}{(3 + 2x - x^2)^{1/2}} = \int \frac{dX}{\sqrt{(4 - X^2)}}.$$

Appeal to entry 18 in the table in Section 33 shows that

$$\int \frac{dx}{(3 + 2x - x^2)^{1/2}} = \arcsin \frac{X}{2} + C,$$

but $X = x - 1$, so

$$\int \frac{dx}{(3 + 2x - x^2)^{1/2}} = \arcsin \left(\frac{x-1}{2} \right) + C. \qquad \blacktriangle$$

When choosing a substitution it is essential that it is **compatible** with $f(x)$. Thus if, for example, $f(x)$ contains the expression $\sqrt{(1 - x^2)}$ any change from the variable x to the variable u is only permissible if $|u| \leqslant 1$, for only then will $\sqrt{(1 - x^2)}$ remain real. The substitutions given in Table 5 are often useful.

Table 5 Substitution be used in $\int f(x)\, dx$

If $f(x)$ contains the term	Try using the substitution
$\sqrt{(a^2 - x^2)}$	$x = a \sin u$ or $x = a \cos u$
$\sqrt{(x^2 - a^2)}$	$x = a \cosh u$ or $x = a \sec u$
$\sqrt{(x^2 + a^2)}$	$x = a \sinh u$
$x^2 + a^2$	$x = a \tan u$

Example 34.7

Find

$$\int \frac{x - 1}{\sqrt{(a^2 - x^2)}}\, dx.$$

Solution
We first rewrite the integral in the form

$$\int \frac{x - 1}{\sqrt{(a^2 - x^2)}}\, dx = \int \frac{x}{\sqrt{(a^2 - x^2)}}\, dx - \int \frac{dx}{\sqrt{(a^2 - x^2)}}.$$

The last integral corresponds to entry 18 in the table, so

$$\int \frac{x - 1}{\sqrt{(a^2 - x^2)}}\, dx = \int \frac{x}{\sqrt{(a^2 - x^2)}}\, dx - \arcsin \frac{x}{a} + C. \qquad (A)$$

Let us now evaluate the first integral by using the substitution $x = a \sin u$, from which it follows that

$$dx = a \cos u\, du.$$

Thus

$$\int \frac{x}{\sqrt{(a^2 - x^2)}}\, dx = \int \frac{a \sin u}{a\sqrt{(1 - \sin^2 u)}}\, a \cos u\, du$$

$$= a \int \frac{\sin u \cos u}{\cos u}\, du$$

$$= a \int \sin u\, du = -a \cos u + D,$$

where D is an arbitrary constant. To obtain the solution in terms of x we first use the trigonometric identity $\sin^2 u + \cos^2 u = 1$, from which it follows that

$$\int \frac{x}{\sqrt{(a^2 - x^2)}}\, dx = -a\sqrt{(1 - \sin^2 u)} + D. \tag{B}$$

Then, using the result $\sin u = x/a$, it follows that

$$\int \frac{x}{\sqrt{(a^2 - x^2)}}\, dx = -(a^2 - x^2)^{1/2} + D.$$

Finally, incorporating result (B) into (A) and combining the two arbitrary constants to form another arbitrary constant K brings us to the result

$$\int \frac{x - 1}{\sqrt{(a^2 - x^2)}}\, dx = -\left[(a^2 - x^2)^{1/2} + \arcsin \frac{x}{a}\right] + K. \qquad \blacktriangle$$

When an integral contains an integrand $f(x)$ in the form of a quotient with only sums of sine and cosine functions in its numerator and denominator, the following special substitution will reduce it to a quotient of polynomials to which some of the earlier substitutions may be applied.

THE $t = \tan x/2$ SUBSTITUTION

When in the integral $\int f(x)\, dx$ the integrand is of the form

$$f(x) = \frac{N(x)}{D(x)},$$

with $N(x)$ and $D(x)$ sums involving only $\sin x$ and $\cos x$, make the substitutions

$$t = \tan \frac{x}{2}, \quad \sin x = \frac{2t}{1 + t^2}, \quad \cos x = \frac{1 - t^2}{1 + t^2} \quad \text{and} \quad dx = \frac{2dt}{1 + t^2}.$$

The compatibility of these substitutions follows from the easily verified facts that

$$\sin^2 x + \cos^2 x = \left(\frac{2t}{1+t^2}\right)^2 + \left(\frac{1-t^2}{1+t^2}\right)^2 = 1,$$

and

$$\tan x = \frac{2 \tan x/2}{1 - \tan^2 x/2} = \frac{2t}{1-t^2}.$$

The result

$$dx = \frac{2\, dt}{1+t^2}$$

follows by differentiating $\tan x = 2t/(t - t^2)$ and using the result that $\sec^2 x = 1 + \tan^2 x$.

Example 34.8

Find

$$\int \frac{dx}{5 + 4 \cos x}.$$

Solution
Making the substitutions

$$t = \tan \frac{x}{2}, \quad \cos x = \frac{1-t^2}{1+t^2} \quad \text{and} \quad dx = \frac{2\, dt}{1+t^2}$$

reduces the integral to

$$\int \frac{dx}{5 + 4 \cos x} = 2 \int \frac{dt}{9 + t^2}$$

$$= \frac{2}{3} \arctan \frac{t}{3} + C.$$

Thus writing $t = \tan x/2$ we arrive at the solution

$$\int \frac{dx}{5 + 4 \cos x} = \frac{2}{3} \arctan \left[\frac{1}{3} \tan \frac{x}{2} \right] + C. \qquad \blacktriangle$$

If an integral contains an integrand $f(x)$ in the form of a quotient in which the numerator and denominator only contain sums of even powers of sine and cosine functions a different substitution is advantageous.

THE $T = \tan x$ SUBSTITUTION

When in the integral $\int f(x)\, dx$ the integrand $f(x)$ is of the form

$$f(x) = \frac{N(x)}{D(x)},$$

with $N(x)$ and $D(x)$ sums of even powers of $\sin x$ and $\cos x$, make the substitutions

$$T = \tan x, \quad \sin^2 x = \frac{T^2}{1+T^2}, \quad \cos^2 x = \frac{1}{1+T^2} \quad \text{and} \quad dx = \frac{dT}{1+T^2}.$$

The compatibility of these substitutions is easily verified by arguments similar to those used to check the substitutions involving $t = \tan x/2$.

Example 34.9

Find

$$\int \frac{dx}{4\cos^2 x + \sin^2 x}.$$

Solution
Making the substitutions

$$T = \tan x, \quad \sin^2 x = \frac{T^2}{1+T^2}, \quad \cos^2 x = \frac{1}{1+T^2} \quad \text{and} \quad dx = \frac{dt}{1+T^2}$$

reduces the integral to

$$\int \frac{dx}{4\cos^2 x + \sin^2 x} = \int \frac{dT}{4+T^2}$$

$$= \frac{1}{2} \arctan \frac{T}{2} + C$$

$$= \frac{1}{2} \arctan \left[\frac{1}{2} \tan x\right] + C \qquad \blacktriangle$$

PROBLEMS 34

Evaluate the following integrals by means of a suitable substitution.

1. $\displaystyle\int \frac{6}{3x+9}\,dx.$

2. $\displaystyle\int \frac{3}{2-x}\,dx.$

3. $\displaystyle\int \cosh(6x+3)\,dx.$

4. $\displaystyle\int (x+5)^{2/3}\,dx.$

5. $\int \sin(3 - 2x)\,dx.$

6. $\int \sinh(1 - 4x)\,dx.$

7. $\int (5x + 4)^5\,dx.$

8. $\int x^2(1 + x^3)^7\,dx.$

9. $\int x(1 - 2x^2)^5\,dx.$

10. $\int \dfrac{x^2}{\sqrt{(2x^3 - 5)}}\,dx.$

11. $\int \dfrac{\cos x}{3 \sin x + 5}\,dx$

12. $\int \dfrac{4 \sin x}{2 \cos x + 7}\,dx.$

13. $\int x \exp(4 - x^2)\,dx.$

14. $\int \dfrac{5x}{2x^2 + 3}\,dx.$

15. $\int \dfrac{dx}{\sqrt{(5x - 3)}}.$

16. $\int \dfrac{x}{\sqrt{(1 + x^4)}}\,dx.$

17. $\int \dfrac{x^2}{\sqrt{(x^6 - 1)}}\,dx.$

18. $\int \dfrac{\ln x}{x}\,dx.$

19. $\int \dfrac{\ln 3x}{2x}\,dx.$

20. $\displaystyle\int \frac{\sin(\ln x)}{x}\,dx.$

21. $\displaystyle\int \frac{x+1}{\sqrt{(x^2+1)}}\,dx.$

22. $\displaystyle\int \frac{x+1}{\sqrt{(1-x^2)}}\,dx.$

23. $\displaystyle\int \frac{dx}{x(\ln x)^2}.$

24. $\displaystyle\int \frac{dx}{\sqrt{e^x}}.$

25. $\displaystyle\int \frac{dx}{\sqrt{e^{3x}}}.$

26. $\displaystyle\int \frac{1}{[\exp(2x-1)]^{1/2}}\,dx.$

27. $\displaystyle\int \frac{1}{2x^2-x+1}\,dx.$

28. $\displaystyle\int \frac{1}{x^2+4x-1}\,dx.$

29. $\displaystyle\int \frac{1}{(x^2+x+1)^{1/2}}\,dx.$

30. $\displaystyle\int \frac{1}{(x^2+2x-4)^{1/2}}\,dx.$

31. $\displaystyle\int \frac{1}{(4+2x-x^2)^{1/2}}\,dx.$

32. $\displaystyle\int \frac{1}{(4-2x-x^2)^{1/2}}\,dx.$

33. $\displaystyle\int \frac{1}{(x-2x^2)^{1/2}}\,dx.$

34. $\displaystyle\int \frac{1}{(4x^2+x)^{1/2}}\,dx.$

35. $\displaystyle \int \frac{2x}{(1+4x-x^2)^{1/2}} \, dx.$

36. $\displaystyle \int \frac{dx}{x\sqrt{(x^2+1)}} \, .$

37. $\displaystyle \int \frac{dx}{x\sqrt{(x^2-1)}} \, .$

38. $\displaystyle \int \frac{x^2}{\sqrt{(1-x^2)}} \, dx.$

39. $\displaystyle \int \frac{\sinh\sqrt{x}\,\operatorname{sech}^4\sqrt{x}}{\sqrt{x}} \, dx.$ (Hint: set $u = \cosh\sqrt{x}$.)

40. $\displaystyle \int \sqrt{[(x-1)(2-x)]} \, dx.$ (Hint: set $x = 1 + \sin^2 u$.)

41. $\displaystyle \int \frac{\sec^2 x}{1+3\tan^2 x} \, dx.$

42. $\displaystyle \int \frac{1}{(1+\cos x)^2} \, dx.$

43. $\displaystyle \int \frac{\sin x}{\sin x + \cos x} \, dx.$

44. $\displaystyle \int \frac{dx}{\cos^2 x + 9\sin^2 x} \, .$

45. $\displaystyle \int \frac{dx}{4\cos^2 x - \sin^2 x} \, dx.$

46. $\displaystyle \int \frac{\sin^2 x}{\cos^2 x + 9\sin^2 x} \, dx.$

47. $\displaystyle \int \frac{dx}{4+\cos^2 x} \, .$

48. $\displaystyle \int \frac{\tan x}{\tan x - 1} \, dx.$

Some useful standard forms

35

Three special cases, or **standard forms** as they are often called, are discussed in this section. Each result follows by first differentiating a commonly occurring functional form, and then using the result in reverse to determine an antiderivative.

The three basic results from which we start are:

$$\frac{d}{dx}[\{f(x)\}^n] = nf'(x)[f(x)]^{n-1};$$

$$\frac{d}{dx}[\ln|f(x)|] = \frac{f'(x)}{f(x)};$$

$$\frac{d}{dx}[e^{f(x)}] = f'(x)\,e^{f(x)}.$$

Reading each of these results in reverse gives the three useful standard forms of antiderivative:

1 $\int f'(x)[f(x)]^{n-1}\,dx = \frac{1}{n}[f(x)]^n + C;$

2 $\int \frac{f'(x)}{f(x)}\,dx = \ln|f(x)| + C;$

3 $\int f'(x)\,e^{f(x)}dx = e^{f(x)} + C.$

Example 35.1

Find

$$\int \sin 3x \cos^5 3x\,dx.$$

Solution

Apart from a numerical factor, this integral is of the form shown in (1), with $f(x) = \cos 3x$ and $n - 1 = 5$, so $n = 6$.

Now as

$$\frac{d}{dx}[\cos 3x] = -3\sin 3x,$$

and the multiplier of $\cos^5 3x$ in the integrand is only $\sin 3x$, it follows that if we set $n = 6$ and $f(x) = \cos 3x$ in antiderivative 1, we must divide the result by -3 to arrive at the required result. Thus we have

$$\int \sin 3x \cos^5 3x\, dx = -\frac{1}{18}\cos^6 3x + C. \qquad\qquad \blacktriangle$$

Example 35.2

Find

$$\int \tan x\, dx.$$

Solution
Writing

$$\int \tan x\, dx = \int \frac{\sin x}{\cos x}\, dx,$$

and comparing the result with antiderivative 2, shows it to be of the form

$$-\int \frac{f'(x)}{f(x)}\, dx$$

with $f(x) = \cos x$.
   Thus it follows at once that

$$\int \tan x\, dx = -\ln|\cos x| + C. \qquad\qquad \blacktriangle$$

Example 35.3

Find

$$\int \sin x \cos x\, e^{\sin^2 x}\, dx.$$

Solution
Apart from a numerical factor, this integral is of the form shown in 3 with $f(x) = \sin^2 x$. However,

$$\frac{d}{dx} [\sin^2 x] = 2 \sin x \cos x,$$

so when setting $f(x) = \sin^2 x$ in antiderivative 3 it will be necessary to divide the result by 2 in order to arrive at the required result. Thus we find that

$$\int \sin x \cos x \, e^{\sin^2 x} \, dx = \frac{1}{2} e^{\sin^2 x} + C.$$

We remark in passing that sometimes an elementary trigonometric identity will convert an integral into one of these elementary standard forms. Thus, for example, making use of the trigonometric identity

$$\sin^2 x = \frac{1}{2} (1 - \cos 2x),$$

together with the above result, shows that

$$\int \sin x \cos x \exp \left[\frac{1}{2} (1 - \cos 2x) \right] dx = \int \sin x \cos x \, e^{\sin^2 x} \, dx$$

$$= \frac{1}{2} e^{\sin^2 x} + C. \qquad \blacktriangle$$

PROBLEMS 35

Find the following integrals.

1. $\int \cos 4x \sin^6 4x \, dx.$

2. $\int \sin 2x \cos^3 2x \, dx.$

3. $\int \sinh 3x \cosh^7 3x \, dx.$

4. $\int \cosh 5x \sinh^4 5x \, dx.$

5. $\int \operatorname{sech}^2 x \tanh^3 x \, dx.$

6. $\int (x + 3)(x^2 + 6x + 1)^7 \, dx.$

7. $\int (3x^2 - 2)(3x^3 - 6x + 1)^4 \, dx.$

8. $\displaystyle\int \frac{x+2}{x^2+4x+1}\,\mathrm{d}x.$

9. $\displaystyle\int \frac{4x-1}{2x^2-x+1}\,\mathrm{d}x.$

10. $\displaystyle\int \cot 4x\,\mathrm{d}x.$

11. $\displaystyle\int \tanh 3x\,\mathrm{d}x.$

12. $\displaystyle\int \coth 6x\,\mathrm{d}x.$

13. $\displaystyle\int x^3\,\mathrm{e}^{x^4}\,\mathrm{d}x.$

14. $\displaystyle\int \cos 2x\,\mathrm{e}^{\sin 2x}\,\mathrm{d}x.$

15. $\displaystyle\int (x+1)\exp(x^2+2x-3)\,\mathrm{d}x.$

16. $\displaystyle\int \sec^2 2x\,\mathrm{e}^{\tan 2x}\,\mathrm{d}x.$

17. $\displaystyle\int \sin x \cos x \exp\left[\frac{1}{2}(1+\cos 2x)\right]\mathrm{d}x.$

18. $\displaystyle\int \frac{1+\tan^2 x}{\tan x}\,\mathrm{d}x.$

36 Integration by parts

No general method exists for the integration of the product of two functions. However, the method of integration by parts which we now derive is the one which comes the closest to meeting this requirement, and it provides a powerful and extremely useful integration technique.

To derive the method we start from the derivative of the product of two differentiable functions $u(x)$ and $v(x)$,

$$\frac{d}{dx}[u(x)\,v(x)] = u(x)\frac{d}{dx}[v(x)] + v(x)\frac{d}{dx}[u(x)].$$

Integrating this result and rearranging terms then gives the following formula for **integration by parts of an indefinite integral**:

$$\int u(x)\frac{d}{dx}[v(x)]\,dx = u(x)\,v(x) - \int v(x)\frac{d}{dx}[u(x)]\,dx.$$

Since, in differential form,

$$du = \frac{d}{dx}[u(x)]\,dx \qquad \text{and} \qquad dv = \frac{d}{dx}[v(x)]\,dx,$$

the formula for integration by parts is often written in the simplified form

$$\int u\,dv = uv - \int v\,du,$$

and it is in this easily remembered but less precise form that it is most frequently found in textbooks.

The idea underlying this method is that the integral

$$\int v(x)\frac{d}{dx}[u(x)]\,dx$$

appearing on the right-hand side of the formula is often simpler than the original integral

$$\int u(x)\frac{d}{dx}[v(x)]\,dx.$$

The method of integration by parts is not always applicable, and when it is it may be necessary to apply it more than once in order to arrive at the required result. This happens, for example, when applying it to certain types of integrals with integrands depending on trigonometric or hyperbolic functions, and elsewhere.

When applying the method to the integral $\int f(x)\,dx$, the problem is to choose a suitable pair of functions $u(x)$ and $v(x)$ such that

$$f(x) = u(x)\frac{d}{dx}[v(x)].$$

The guiding principle to be adopted is that the functions $u(x)$ and $v(x)$ must be chosen so that the integral

$$\int v(x)\frac{d}{dx}[u(x)]\,dx$$

is **simpler** than the original integral.

Example 36.1

Find

$$\int x\sin x\,dx.$$

Solution
We wish to write the integrand in the form

$$x\sin x = u(x)\frac{d}{dx}[v(x)].$$

Thus if we choose to set $u(x) = x$, it follows that $v(x)$ must be such that

$$\frac{dv}{dx} = \sin x,$$

so

$$v(x) = \int \sin x\,dx = -\cos x.$$

We omit the arbitrary constant of integration at this intermediate stage, and simply add it after the integral on the right-hand side of the formula for integration by parts has been evaluated.

Substituting $u(x) = x$, $v(x) = -\cos x$ into the general formula for integration by parts

$$\int u(x)\frac{d}{dx}[v(x)]\,dx = u(x)\,v(x) - \int v(x)\frac{d}{dx}[u(x)]\,dx$$

gives

$$\int x \sin x \, dx = -x \cos x - \int (-\cos x) \frac{d}{dx} [x] \, dx$$

$$= -x \cos x + \int \cos x \, dx$$

$$= -x \cos x + \sin x + C,$$

where the arbitrary constant C has now been added. Thus by using integration by parts we have shown that

$$\int x \sin x \, dx = \sin x - x \cos x + C.$$

Before leaving this problem let us examine the consequences of making the **wrong** choice for $u(x)$. Suppose, for example, we had set $u(x) = \sin x$, then $v(x)$ would need to be chosen such that

$$\frac{dv}{dx} = x,$$

so then

$$v(x) = \int x \, dx = \frac{1}{2} x^2.$$

Substituting $u(x) = \sin x$, $v(x) = \frac{1}{2} x^2$ into the general formula for integration by parts gives

$$\int x \sin x = \frac{x^2}{2} \sin x - \frac{1}{2} \int x^2 \cos x \, dx.$$

This result is correct, but the integral on the right-hand side is harder than the original integral. This tells us that we have made the wrong choice for $u(x)$.   ▲

Example 36.2

Find

$$\int (2x^2 + x - 4) \ln x \, dx.$$

Solution
As

$$\frac{d}{dx} [\ln x] = \frac{1}{x},$$

let us try setting $u(x) = \ln x$ and

$$\frac{\mathrm{d}v}{\mathrm{d}x} = 2x^2 + x - 4.$$

Integrating to find v gives

$$v(x) = \int (2x^2 + x - 4)\,\mathrm{d}x = \frac{2}{3}x^3 + \frac{1}{2}x^2 - 4x,$$

and substituting for $u(x)$ and $v(x)$ in the general formula for integration by parts brings us to the result

$$\int (2x^2 + x - 4)\ln x \,\mathrm{d}x = \left(\frac{2}{3}x^3 + \frac{1}{2}x^2 - 4x\right)\ln x - \int \left(\frac{2}{3}x^3 + \frac{1}{2}x^2 - 4x\right)\frac{1}{x}\,\mathrm{d}x$$

$$= \left(\frac{2}{3}x^3 + \frac{1}{2}x^2 - 4x\right)\ln x - \int \left(\frac{2}{3}x^2 + \frac{1}{2}x - 4\right)\mathrm{d}x$$

$$= \left(\frac{2}{3}x^3 + \frac{1}{2}x^2 - 4x\right)\ln x - \frac{2}{9}x^3 - \frac{1}{4}x^2 + 4x + C. \quad \blacktriangle$$

Example 36.3

Find

$$\int \ln |x| \,\mathrm{d}x.$$

Solution
At first, examination of the integral suggests no obvious way in which to choose $u(x)$ and $v(x)$, because the integrand is simply $\ln |x|$. However, if we write it as

$$(\ln |x|) \cdot 1$$

then this can be rewritten as

$$\ln |x| \frac{\mathrm{d}}{\mathrm{d}x}[x].$$

Thus

$$\int \ln |x| \,\mathrm{d}x = \int \ln |x| \frac{\mathrm{d}[x]}{\mathrm{d}x}\,\mathrm{d}x,$$

so in the notation of the general formula for integration by parts, $u(x) = \ln |x|$ and $v(x) = x$. Hence substituting into the formula gives

$$\int \ln |x| \,\mathrm{d}x = x \ln |x| - \int x \cdot \frac{1}{x}\,\mathrm{d}x$$

$$= x \ln |x| - x + C. \qquad \blacktriangle$$

Example 36.4

Find

$$\int x^2 \sinh x \, dx.$$

Solution
To simplify the integration when using integration by parts it is necessary to choose $u(x)$ so that the integral

$$\int v(x) \frac{d}{dx} [u(x)] \, dx$$

is simpler than the original expression. This suggests setting $u(x) = x^2$, so that $v(x)$ must satisfy

$$\frac{dv}{dx} = \sinh x,$$

so

$$v(x) = \int \sinh x \, dx = \cosh x.$$

Substituting $u(x) = x^2$, $v(x) = \cosh x$ into the general formula for integration by parts gives

$$\int x^2 \sinh x \, dx = x^2 \cosh x - 2 \int x \cosh x \, dx.$$

We now use integration by parts again on the integral on the right-hand side with $u(x) = x$, so that $v(x)$ must satisfy

$$\frac{dv}{dx} = \cosh x,$$

corresponding to

$$v(x) = \int \cosh x \, dx = \sinh x.$$

Thus substituting into the general formula for integration by parts gives

$$\int x^2 \sinh x \, dx = x^2 \cosh x - 2 \left[x \sinh x - \int \sinh x \, dx \right]$$

$$= x^2 \cosh x - 2x \sinh x + 2 \cosh x + C.$$

Consequently, two applications of integration by parts has shown that

$$\int x^2 \sinh x \, dx = x^2 \cosh x - 2x \sinh x + 2 \cosh x + C. \qquad \blacktriangle$$

Example 36.5

Find

$$\int e^{2x} \sin 3x \, dx.$$

Solution
Let us set $u(x) = e^{2x}$ so that

$$\frac{dv}{dx} = \sin 3x,$$

corresponding to

$$v(x) = -\frac{1}{3} \cos 3x.$$

Then substituting into the general formula for integration by parts gives

$$\int e^{2x} \sin 3x \, dx = -\frac{1}{3} e^{2x} \cos 3x + \frac{2}{3} \int e^{2x} \cos 3x \, dx. \qquad (A)$$

To proceed further we now use integration by parts again, but this time on the integral on the right-hand side of (A) with $u(x) = e^{2x}$, so that $v(x)$ must satisfy

$$\frac{dv}{dx} = \cos 3x.$$

Thus integration shows that

$$v(x) = \int \cos 3x \, dx = \frac{1}{3} \sin 3x.$$

When integration by parts is applied to the last term in (A) the resulting form for (A) becomes

$$\int e^{2x} \sin 3x \, dx = -\frac{1}{3} e^{2x} \cos 3x + \frac{2}{3} \left(\frac{1}{3} e^{2x} \sin 3x - \frac{2}{3} \int e^{2x} \sin 3x \, dx \right) + C.$$

At first sight it would appear that integration by parts has been unsuccessful, because two applications of the method has returned us to the original form of integral. However, on closer inspection, we see that the multiplier of the integral is different on each side of the equation, so combining terms and simplifying the result gives

$$\int e^{2x} \sin 3x \, dx = \frac{1}{13} e^{2x} (2 \sin 3x - 3 \cos 3x) + C. \qquad \blacktriangle$$

The integral in Example 36.5 is a special case of what is called a **reduction formula** for an integral. In general, if an integral contains a parameter n, its complexity will decrease as n decreases. If we signify the dependence of the integral on n by denoting it by I_n, a reduction formula is a formula which relates I_n to I_m with $m < n$. Successive applications of a reduction formula cause the value of n in the original integral to be reduced step by step. This process usually reduces the evaluation of the original integral to the evaluation of a simple standard integral. The idea is illustrated in the three examples which now follow.

Example 36.6

Given that

$$I_n = \int (\ln |x|)^n \, dx \quad \text{for} \quad n \geqslant 0,$$

show that I_n satisfies the reduction formula

$$I_n = x(\ln |x|)^n - n I_{n-1} .$$

Solution
Write

$$(\ln |x|)^n = (\ln |x|)^n \cdot 1 = (\ln |x|)^n \frac{d}{dx} [x],$$

so that

$$I_n = \int (\ln |x|)^n \, dx = \int (\ln |x|)^n \frac{d}{dx} [x] \cdot dx.$$

It then follows from the formula for integration by parts that

$$I_n = x(\ln |x|)^n - \int x \frac{d}{dx} [\{\ln |x| \}^n] \, dx$$

$$= x(\ln |x|)^n - \int xn(\ln |x|)^{n-1} \cdot \frac{1}{x} \, dx$$

$$= x(\ln |x|)^n - n \int (\ln |x|)^{n-1} dx.$$

However, replacing n by $n-1$ in I_n shows that

$$I_{n-1} = \int (\ln |x|)^{n-1} dx,$$

so it follows that

$$I_n = x(\ln |x|)^n - n I_{n-1}.$$

Notice that after each application of this reduction formula the parameter n steps down by 1.

Starting from $n = N$ (say), N successive applications of this reduction formula will reduce the evaluation of I_N to the determination of

$$I_0 = \int 1 \cdot dx = x.$$

For example, setting $n = 1$ we have

$$I_1 = x \ln |x| - I_0 = x \ln |x| - x + C,$$

which was the result found in Example 36.3.   ▲

The next example shows how sometimes some algebraic manipulation is necessary before a result obtained by means of integration by parts can be related to the original integral.

Example 36.7

Given that

$$I_n = \int (1 - x^3)^n dx \quad \text{for} \quad n \geq 0,$$

show that I_n satisfies the reduction formula

$$(n + 1)I_n = x(1 - x^3)^n + 3n I_{n-1}.$$

Solution
Write

$$(1 - x^3)^n = (1 - x^3)^n \cdot 1,$$

$$= (1 - x^3)^n \frac{d}{dx} [x].$$

Then

$$I_n = \int (1 - x^3)^n \frac{d}{dx} [x] dx,$$

so applying the general formula for integration by parts gives

$$I_n = x(1 - x^3)^n - \int x \, n(1 - x^3)^{n-1}(-3x^2) \, dx$$

$$= x(1 - x^3)^n + 3n \int x^3(1 - x^3)^{n-1} \, dx.$$

As it stands, the integral on the right-hand side is not expressible in terms of I_n. However, if we set

$$x^3 = (x^3 - 1) + 1$$

in the integral the above result becomes

$$I_n = x(1 - x^3)^n + 3n \int [(x^3 - 1) + 1](1 - x^3)^{n-1} \, dx$$

$$= x(1 - x^3)^n - 3n \int (1 - x^3)^n \, dx + 3n \int (1 - x^3)^{n-1} \, dx.$$

Now,

$$I_n = \int (1 - x^3)^n \, dx \quad \text{and} \quad I_{n-1} = \int (1 - x^3)^{n-1} \, dx,$$

so

$$I_n = x(1 - x^3)^n - 3n \, I_n + 3n \, I_{n-1},$$

and thus

$$(1 + 3n) I_n = x(1 - x^3)^n + 3n \, I_{n-1}.$$

Notice that each application of this reduction formula will reduce the value of the parameter n by 1.   ▲

The last example shows how the use of trigonometric identities is sometimes necessary when deriving a reduction formula.

Example 36.8

Given that

$$I_n = \int \sin^n x \, dx \quad \text{for} \quad n \geqslant 0,$$

show that I_n satisfies the reduction formula

$$n I_n = (n - 1) I_{n-2} - \sin^{n-1} x \cos x.$$

Solution

Write I_n as

$$I_n = \int \sin^{n-1} x \sin x \, dx,$$

and use the fact that

$$\frac{d}{dx} [-\cos x] = \sin x$$

to rewrite the result as

$$I_n = \int \sin^{n-1} x \frac{d}{dx} [-\cos x] \, dx.$$

Applying integration by parts with $u(x) = \sin^{n-1}$ and $v(x) = -\cos x$ gives

$$I_n = -\cos x \sin^{n-1} x - \int (-\cos x)(n-1)(\sin^{n-2} x)(\cos x) \, dx$$

or

$$I_n = -\cos x \sin^{n-1} x + (n-1) \int \cos^2 x \sin^{n-2} x \, dx.$$

To relate the integral on the right-hand side to I_n we use the trigonometric identity $\cos^2 x = 1 - \sin^2 x$ to arrive at the result

$$I_n = -\cos x \sin^{n-1} x + (n-1) \int (1 - \sin^2 x) \sin^{n-2} x \, dx$$

$$= -\cos x \sin^{n-1} x + (n-1) \int \sin^{n-2} x \, dx - (n-1) \int \sin^n x \, dx$$

$$= -\cos x \sin^{n-1} x + (n-1) I_{n-2} - (n-1) I_n.$$

Combining terms we then find that

$$n I_n = (n-1) I_{n-2} - \sin^{n-1} x \cos x.$$

Notice that when this reduction formula is applied, the parameter n steps down by 2. This is typical of reduction formulas involving trigonometric functions. ▲

PROBLEMS 36

Use integration by parts to evaluate the following integrals.

1. $\int x \cos x \, dx.$

2. $\int x\,e^x\,dx.$

3. $\int x\,e^{-x}\,dx.$

4. $\int e^x \sin x\,dx.$

5. $\int e^{2x} \cos x\,dx.$

6. $\int x \ln |x|\,dx.$

7. $\int \dfrac{\ln |x|}{x^2}\,dx.$

8. $\int x \sin^2 x\,dx.$

9. $\int x \arctan x\,dx.$

10. $\int x^2 e^x\,dx.$

11. $\int \ln(x^2 + 1)\,dx.$

12. $\int \cos(\ln |x|)\,dx.$

13. $\int x \arcsin x\,dx.$

14. $\int x^2 \sin 3x\,dx.$

15. $\int \sin(\ln |x|)\,dx.$

16. $\int \dfrac{x}{2^x}\,dx.$

17. Given that

$$I_n = \int (1 - x^5)^n \, dx \quad \text{for} \quad n \geqslant 0,$$

prove that I_n satisfies the reduction formula

$$(1 + 5n)I_n = x(1 - x^5) + 5n\,I_{n-1}.$$

18. Given that

$$I_n = \int \cos x(1 + \sin^2 x)^n \, dx \quad \text{for} \quad n \geqslant 0,$$

show that I_n satisfies the reduction formula

$$(1 + 2n)I_n = \sin x(1 + \sin^2 x)^n + 2n\,I_{n-1}.$$

19. Given that

$$I_n = \int \sec^n x \, dx \quad \text{for} \quad n \geqslant 0,$$

by using the result that

$$\sec^n x = \sec^{n-2} x \frac{d}{dx}[\tan x],$$

prove that I_n satisfies the reduction formula

$$(n - 1)I_n = \sec^{n-2} x \tan x + (n - 2)I_{n-2}.$$

20. Given that

$$I_n = \int x \cos^n x \, dx \quad \text{for} \quad n \geqslant 0,$$

by writing the integrand in the form

$$x \cos^n x = x \cos^{n-1} x \frac{d}{dx}[\sin x],$$

show that I_n satisfies the reduction formula

$$n^2 I_n = n x \cos^{n-1} x \sin x + \cos^n x + n(n - 1)I_{n-2}.$$

So far we have seen how to evaluate integrals in which the integrand is of the form $1/(ax + b)$ or $1/(ax^2 + bx + c)$. These are special cases of an integrand of the form

$$\frac{N(x)}{D(x)},$$

in which $N(x)$ and $D(x)$ are both arbitrary polynomials. Such expressions are called **rational functions** of x. To evaluate the integral of a general rational function

$$\int \frac{N(x)}{D(x)}\, dx$$

it is necessary to decompose $N(x)/D(x)$ into a sum of simple rational functions to which, if the degree of $N(x)$ equals or exceeds the degree of $D(x)$, there must be added a polynomial. Each term resulting from such a decomposition can then be integrated by one of the techniques discussed so far. This process of decomposition is called expressing $N(x)/D(x)$ in terms of **partial fractions.**

STEPS IN A PARTIAL FRACTION DECOMPOSITION

Step 1
Factorize $D(x)$ into a product of real linear and quadratic factors and write it in the form

$$D(x) = (a_1 x + b_1)^{r_1} \ldots (a_M x + b_M)^{r_M} (A_1 x^2 + B_1 x + C_1)^{S_1} \ldots (A_N x^2 + B_N x + C_N)^{S_N}.$$

Here the coefficients a_i, b_i, A_i, B_i and C_i are real, r_i is the number of times the linear factor $(a_i x - b_i)$ occurs (its multiplicity is r_i) and s_i is the number of times the quadratic factor $(A_i x^2 + B_i x + C_i)$ occurs (its multiplicity is s_i).

Notice that as the factors of $D(x)$ are required to be real, the quadratic factors will all be such that they have complex conjugate roots (they will be the product of two complex conjugate linear factors).

Step 2
To each linear factor $(ax - b)^r$ include in the decomposition the terms

$$\frac{P_1}{ax + b} + \frac{P_2}{(ax + b)^2} + \dots + \frac{P_r}{(ax + b)^r},$$

with the P_i undetermined coefficients (constants).
Step 3
To each quadratic factor $(Ax^2 + Bx + C)^s$ include in the decomposition the terms

$$\frac{Q_1 x + R_1}{(Ax^2 + Bx + C)} + \frac{Q_2 x + R_2}{(Ax^2 + Bx + C)^2} + \dots + \frac{Q_s x + R_s}{(Ax^2 + Bx + C)^s},$$

with the Q_i and R_i undetermined coefficients (constants).
Step 4
If the degree of the denominator is n and the degree of numerator is $n + p$, with $p \geqslant 0$, include in the decomposition the polynomial

$$T_0 + T_1 x + T_2 x^2 + \dots + T_p x^p,$$

with the T_i undetermined coefficients (constants).
   If the degree of the denominator exceeds that of the numerator no such terms are necessary.
Step 5
Equate $N(x)/D(x)$ to the sum of all the terms obtained in steps 2 to 4.
Step 6
Multiply the result of step 5 by $D(x)$ and determine the undetermined coefficients P_i, Q_i, R_i and T_i by equating the coefficients of corresponding powers of x on equal sides of the expression. This will lead to a set of simultaneous equations from which the coefficients may be found.
Comment
If the degree of $N(x)$ is greater than or equal to the degree of $D(x)$, so that step 4 requires the inclusion of a polynomial in the partial factors decomposition, it is often simpler to obtain it by long division than by the method just outlined.

Example 37.1

Find

$$\int \frac{x + 4}{2x^2 + 9x + 10} \, dx.$$

Solution
Step 1

$$2x^2 + 9x + 10 = (x + 2)(2 + 5),$$

so the denominator comprises two linear factors, each with multiplicity 1.
Step 2
Include in the partial fraction decomposition the terms

$$\frac{A}{x+2} + \frac{B}{2x+5}.$$

Steps 3 and 4
These steps contribute no terms to the partial fraction decomposition.
Step 5
Set

$$\frac{x+4}{(x+2)(2x+5)} = \frac{A}{x+2} + \frac{B}{2x+5}.$$

Step 6
Multiplication of the result of step 5 by $(x+2)(2x+5)$ gives

$$x+4 = A(2x+5) + B(x+2). \tag{A}$$

Equating the coefficients of x on each side of (A) gives

$$1 = 2A + B.$$

Equating the constant terms (the coefficients of x^0) on each side of (A) gives

$$4 = 5A + 2B.$$

Solving these two simultaneous equations for A and B we find

$$A = 2 \quad \text{and} \quad B = -3,$$

so

$$\frac{x+4}{2x^2+9x+10} = \frac{2}{x+2} - \frac{3}{2x+5}.$$

Integrating the partial fraction decomposition gives

$$\int \frac{x+4}{2x^2+9x+10} \, dx = \int \frac{2}{x+2} \, dx - \int \frac{3}{2x+5} \, dx$$

$$= 2 \ln |x+2| - 3 \ln |2x+5| + C.$$

There is a short-cut method for finding the undetermined coefficients associated with the terms introduced in step 2. This is sometimes called the **cover-up rule**, and we illustrate how it works by returning to step 5.
Starting from the result

$$\frac{x+4}{(x+2)(2x+5)} = \frac{A}{x+2} + \frac{B}{(2x+5)},$$

in order to determine A we multiply by the factor $(x+2)$ associated with A to obtain

$$\frac{x+4}{2x+5} = A + \frac{B(x+2)}{(2x+5)}.$$

Then setting $x = -2$ (to make the multiplier of B zero) gives

$$\frac{-2+4}{-4+5} = A = 2.$$

Similarly, to determine B we multiply by the factor $(2x+5)$ associated with B to obtain

$$\frac{x+4}{x+2} = A\frac{(2x+5)}{(x+2)} + B.$$

Then setting $x = -5/2$ (to make the multiplier of A zero) gives

$$\frac{-5/2+4}{-5/2+2} = B = -3.$$

This is called the cover-up rule because when finding A it amounts to 'covering-up' the factor $x+2$ in the denominator on left and setting $x = -2$ in the terms that remain on the left to find A, and similarly for B.   ▲

Example 37.2

Find

$$\int \frac{3x-1}{x^2+4x+4}\,dx.$$

Solution
Step 1

$$D(x) = x^2 + 4x + 4 = (x+2)^2,$$

so the sole linear factor $x+2$ appears with multiplicity 2.
Step 2
Since $D(x) = (x+2)^2$, we must include in the partial fraction decomposition the terms

$$\frac{A}{x+2} + \frac{B}{(x+2)^2}.$$

Steps 3 and 4
These contribute no terms to the partial function decomposition.
Step 5

$$\frac{3x-1}{(x+2)^2} = \frac{A}{x+2} + \frac{B}{(x+2)^2}.$$

Step 6
Multiplication of the result of step 5 by $(x+2)^2$ gives

$$3x - 1 = A(x+2) + B.$$

Equating coefficients of x on either side of this result gives

$$3 = A.$$

Equating the constant terms (the coefficients of x^0) on either side of this result gives

$$-1 = 2A + B,$$

so solving for A and B we find that

$$A = 3, \quad B = -7$$

and consequently

$$\frac{3x - 1}{x^2 + 4x + 4} = \frac{3}{x + 2} - \frac{7}{(x + 2)^2}.$$

Thus

$$\int \frac{3x - 1}{x^2 + 4x + 4} \, dx = \int \frac{3}{x + 2} \, dx - \int \frac{7}{(x + 2)^2} \, dx$$

$$= 3 \ln |x + 2| + \frac{7}{x + 2} + C.$$

Notice that had the cover-up rule been used in this case it would only have led to the determination of A. This is because it only applies to linear factors with multiplicity 1.   ▲

Example 37.3

Find

$$\int \frac{2x^2 - 1}{(x^2 + 1)^2} \, dx.$$

Solution
Step 1
This has already been accomplished.
Step 2
There are no terms to be included from this step as there are no real linear factors in the denominator.
Step 3
Owing to the sole quadratic factor $x^2 + 1$ which occurs in the denominator with multiplicity 2 we must include in the partial fraction decomposition terms of the form

$$\frac{Ax + B}{x^2 + 1} + \frac{Cx + D}{(x^2 + 1)^2}.$$

Step 4
There are no terms to be included from this step.
Step 5
Set

$$\frac{2x^2 - 1}{(x^2 + 1)^2} = \frac{Ax + B}{x^2 + 1} + \frac{Cx + D}{(x^2 + 1)^2}.$$

Step 6

Multiply the expression in step 5 by $(x^2 + 1)^2$ to obtain

$$2x^2 - 1 = (Ax + B)(x^2 + 1) + Cx + D.$$

Equating the coefficients of x^3 on either side of this result gives

$$0 = A.$$

Equating the coefficients of x^2 on either side of this result gives

$$2 = B.$$

Equating the coefficients of x on either side of this result gives

$$0 = A + C, \quad \text{so} \quad C = 0.$$

Equating the constant terms (the coefficients of x^0) on either side of this result gives

$$-1 = B + D, \quad \text{so} \quad D = -3,$$

and so

$$\frac{2x^2 - 1}{(x^2 + 1)^2} = \frac{2}{x^2 + 1} - \frac{3}{(x^2 + 1)^2}.$$

Thus

$$\int \frac{2x^2 - 1}{(x^2 + 1)^2} \, dx = 2 \int \frac{dx}{x^2 + 1} - 3 \int \frac{dx}{(x^2 + 1)^2}$$

$$= 2 \arctan x - 3 \int \frac{dx}{(x^2 + 1)^2}$$

To evaluate the last integral we set $x = \tan \theta$, so that $dx = \sec^2 \theta \, d\theta$, and then

$$\int \frac{dx}{(x^2 + 1)^2} = \int \frac{\sec^2 d\theta}{(\tan^2 \theta + 1)^2} = \int \frac{\sec^2 \theta}{\sec^4 \theta} \, d\theta = \int \cos^2 \theta \, d\theta.$$

Using the identity $\cos^2 \theta = \frac{1}{2}(1 + \cos 2\theta)$ this becomes

$$\int \frac{dx}{(x^2 + 1)^2} = \frac{1}{2} \int (1 + \cos 2\theta) \, d\theta$$

$$= \frac{\theta}{2} + \frac{1}{4} \sin 2\theta + C.$$

However, $\theta = \arctan x$ and $\sin 2\theta = 2 \sin \theta \cos \theta$, so

$$\int \frac{dx}{(x^2 + 1)^2} = \frac{1}{2} \arctan x + \frac{1}{2} \sin \theta \cos \theta + C.$$

To find θ and $\cos \theta$ in terms of x we proceed as follows. Let us consider a right-angled triangle with angle θ. Then it follows that as $x = \tan \theta$, the side opposite the angle θ is of length x and the side adjacent to it is of length 1. Consequently, $\sin\theta = x/[\sqrt{(1+x^2)}]$ and $\cos\theta = 1/[\sqrt{(1+x^2)}]$, so that

$$\int \frac{dx}{(x^2+1)^2} = \frac{1}{2}\arctan x + \frac{x}{2(1+x^2)} + C.$$

Combining results then shows that

$$\int \frac{(2x^2-1)}{(x^2+1)^2}\,dx = \frac{1}{2}\arctan x - \frac{3x}{2(1+x^2)} + C. \qquad \blacktriangle$$

Example 37.4

Find

$$\int \frac{x^4 - x^2 + 2x + 1}{(x+1)(x^2+2x+2)}\,dx.$$

Solution
Step 1
This has already been accomplished.
Step 2
Because of the factor $(x+1)$ we must include in the partial fraction decomposition the term $A/(x+1)$.
Step 3
As the factor $x^2 + 2x + 2$ which only occurs once in the denominator cannot be expressed as the product of two real linear factors, it follows that we must include in the partial fraction decomposition the term

$$\frac{Bx+C}{x^2+2x+2}.$$

Step 4
The degree of the numerator exceeds that of the denominator by 1 ($p = 1$), so we must include in the partial fraction decomposition the polynomial

$$Dx + E.$$

Step 5
Combining steps 2 to 5 shows we must set

$$\frac{x^4 - x^2 + 2x + 1}{(x+1)(x^2+2x+2)} = \frac{A}{x+1} + \frac{Bx+C}{x^2+2x+2} + Dx + E.$$

Step 6
Multiplying the result in step 5 by $(x+1)(x^2+2x+2)$ gives

$$x^4 - x^2 + 2x + 1 = A(x^2+2x+2) + (Bx+c)(x+1)$$
$$+ (Dx+E)(x+1)(x^2+2x+2).$$

Equating the coefficients of x^4 on either side of this result gives

$$1 = D.$$

Equating the coefficients of x^3 on either side of this result gives

$$0 = 3D + E.$$

Equating coefficients of x^2 on either side of this result gives

$$-1 = A + B + 4D + 3E.$$

Equating coefficients of x on either side of this result gives

$$2 = 2A + B + C + 2D + 4E.$$

Equating constant terms (the coefficients of x^0) on either side of this result gives

$$1 = 2A + C + 2E.$$

Solving the five simultaneous for the unknown constants we find that

$$A = -1, \quad B = 5, \quad C = 9, \quad D = 1, \quad E = -3,$$

so

$$\frac{x^4 - x^2 + 2x + 1}{(x+1)(x^2 + 2x + 2)} = \frac{-1}{x+1} + \frac{5x+9}{x^2 + 2x + 2} + x - 3.$$

Thus

$$\int \frac{x^4 - x^2 + 2x + 1}{(x+1)(x^2 + 2x + 2)} \, dx = -\int \frac{dx}{x+1} + \int \frac{5x+9}{x^2 + 2x + 2} \, dx + \int x \, dx - \int 3 \, dx$$

$$= -\ln|x+1| + \int \frac{5x+9}{x^2 + 2x + 2} \, dx + \frac{x^2}{2} - 3x.$$

To evaluate

$$\int \frac{5x+9}{x^2 + 2x + 2} \, dx$$

we first complete the square in the denominator and write the integral as

$$\int \frac{5x+9}{(x+1)^2 + 1} \, dx.$$

Setting $u = x + 1$, so that $du = dx$, this becomes

$$\int \frac{u+4}{u^2 + 1} \, dx = \int \frac{5u}{u^2 + 1} \, du + 4 \int \frac{dx}{u^2 + 1}$$

$$= \frac{5}{2} \ln|u^2 + 1| + 4 \arctan u + C$$

$$= \frac{5}{2} \ln|x^2 + 2x + 2| + 4 \arctan(x+1) + C.$$

Thus, after combining terms, we arrive at the result

$$\int \frac{x^4 - x^2 + 2x + 1}{(x+1)(x^2 + 2x + 2)}\, dx = \frac{5}{2} \ln |x^2 + 2x + 2| + 4 \arctan(x + 1)$$

$$+ \frac{x^2}{2} - \ln |x + 1| - 3x + C.$$

The determination of the partial fractions would have been simpler had we first divided the denominator into the numerator to arrive at the polynomial $x - 3$, and then proceeded to the determination of the partial fraction decomposition of the remainder. The argument would then have proceeded as follows.

Expanding the denominator gives

$$(x + 1)(x^2 + 2x + 2) = x^3 + 3x^2 + 4x + 2,$$

so

$$
x^3 + 3x^2 + 4x + 2 \,\overline{\left)\, x^4 + 0 \cdot x^3 - x^2 + 2x + 1 \right.}
$$

$$
\begin{array}{r}
x - 3 \\
\hline
x^4 + 3x^3 + 4x^2 + 2x \\
\hline
- 3x^3 - 5x^2 + 1 \\
- 3x^3 - 9x^2 - 12x - 6 \\
\hline
4x^2 + 12x + 7 \quad,
\end{array}
$$

and thus

$$\frac{x^4 - x^2 + 2x + 1}{(x+1)(x^2 + 2x + 2)} = x - 3 + \frac{4x^2 + 12x + 7}{(x+1)(x^2 + 2x + 2)}.$$

An application of the partial fraction expansion method to the last term, which is now much simpler, gives (with less effort)

$$\frac{4x^2 + 12x + 7}{(x+1)(x^2 + 2x + 2)} = \frac{5x + 9}{x^2 + 2x + 2} - \frac{1}{x + 1}. \qquad \blacktriangle$$

Thereafter, the integration proceeds as before.

The approach to the integration of rational functions may be summarized as follows:

1 $\displaystyle \int \frac{dx}{ax + b} = \frac{1}{a} \ln |ax + b| + C;$

2 $\displaystyle \int \frac{dx}{(ax+b)^n} = \frac{-1}{a(n-1)} \frac{1}{(ax+b)^{n-1}} + C \quad (n > 1);$

3 $\displaystyle \int \frac{Ax + B}{(ax^2 + bx + c)^n}\, dx$ should be rewritten as

$$\left(\frac{A}{2a}\right) \int \frac{2ax + b}{(ax^2 + bx + c)^n}\, dx + \left(B - \frac{Ab}{2a}\right) \int \frac{dx}{(ax^2 + bx + c)^n}.$$

Then in this form use should then be made of the following results,

$$\int \frac{2ax+b}{(ax^2+bx+c)^n}\,dx = \frac{-1}{(n-1)}\frac{1}{(ax^2+bx+c)^{n-1}}+C \quad (n\neq 1),$$

$$\int \frac{2ax+b}{ax^2+bx+c}\,dx = \ln|ax^2+bx+c|+C \quad (n=1).$$

When $n=1$,

$$\int \frac{dx}{ax^2+bx+c} = \frac{1}{a}\int \frac{dx}{(x+b/(2a))^2+(c/a-b^2/(4a^2))},$$

and when $n>1$ a reduction formula should be used.

PROBLEMS 37

Evaluate the following integrals after making use of the method of partial fractions.

1. $\displaystyle\int \frac{4x+5}{(2x+1)(1-x)}\,dx.$

2. $\displaystyle\int \frac{7x-1}{x^2-1}\,dx.$

3. $\displaystyle\int \frac{dx}{(x+2)(x^2-1)}.$

4. $\displaystyle\int \frac{1-4x-x^2}{(x-1)(x+1)^2}\,dx.$

5. $\displaystyle\int \frac{x+2}{(2x+1)^3}\,dx.$

6. $\displaystyle\int \frac{x^2+x-1}{(x+1)^3}\,dx.$

7. $\displaystyle\int \frac{x^3+2x^2-x+1}{x^2-x+2}\,dx.$

8. $\displaystyle\int \frac{2x^3-x^2+1}{x^2+x+1}\,dx.$

9. $\displaystyle\int \frac{x^3+x^2-2}{(x^2+4)^2}\,dx.$

10. $\displaystyle\int \frac{x^3 + 3x^2 - x - 1}{(x+1)^2(2x^2 + 2x + 1)}\,\mathrm{d}x.$

11. $\displaystyle\int \frac{3x^2 - 4}{(x-1)^2(x-2)^2}\,\mathrm{d}x.$

12. $\displaystyle\int \frac{x^4}{(x+1)^2}\,\mathrm{d}x.$

13. $\displaystyle\int \frac{x^2 - 5x + 1}{(x^2 - 4)(x+1)}\,\mathrm{d}x.$

14. $\displaystyle\int \frac{x^2 + x + 2}{x^2 + x + 1}\,\mathrm{d}x.$

15. $\displaystyle\int \frac{x+2}{(x+1)(x+x+3)}\,\mathrm{d}x.$

16. $\displaystyle\int \frac{3x - 1}{(x+1)^4}\,\mathrm{d}x.$

The definite integral   38

We have seen that an antiderivative, or indefinite integral as it is often called, is a **function**. In this section we define the **definite integral** which will be seen to be a **number**. The connection between these two types of integral will be established when we prove the fundamental theorem of the integral calculus.

For the sake of simplicity, we choose to interpret the definite integral geometrically by relating it to the area below a curve. More general definitions are possible, and are indeed necessary in certain circumstances, though they are unnecessary for our purposes.

Consider a function $f(x)$ defined for $a \leqslant x \leqslant b$, a typical example of which is shown in Fig. 84, and let us find the area I of the shaded region between the curve $y = f(x)$, the x–axis and the lines $x = a$ at the left and $x = b$ at the right. Two different ways of arriving at the result are shown in Fig. 85. In Fig. 85(a) area I is estimated as the sum of the areas of the n shaded rectangular strips of widths $\Delta_1, \Delta_2, ..., \Delta_n$ and heights $\underline{f_1}, \underline{f_2}, ..., \underline{f_n}$. Here $\underline{f_i}$ is taken to be the least value of $f(x)$ in the strip Δ_i, so it follows that

$$\Delta_1 \underline{f_1} + \Delta_2 \underline{f_2} + ... + \Delta_n \underline{f_n} \leqslant I$$

or, using the summation notation,

$$\sum_{i=1}^{n} \underline{f_i} \Delta_i \leqslant I.$$

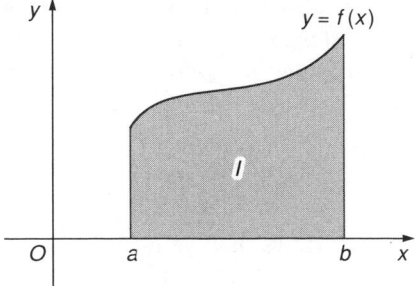

Fig. 84

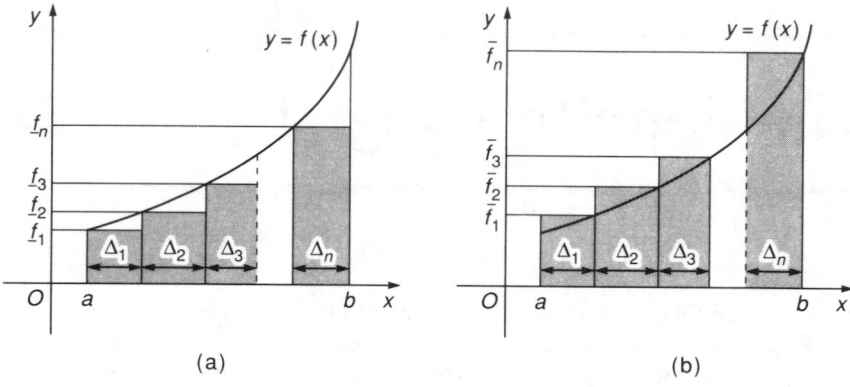

Fig. 85

The expression on the left of this inequality is called the **lower approximating sum** over the interval $a \leqslant x \leqslant b$.

Similarly, in Fig. 85(b) the area I is estimated as the sum of the areas of the n shaded rectangular strips of widths Δ_i where this time the heights of the strips $\bar{f}_1, \bar{f}_2, ..., \bar{f}_n$ are taken to be the greatest values of $f(x)$ in $\Delta_1, \Delta_2, ..., \Delta_n$. It then follows that

$$I \leqslant \bar{f}_1 \Delta_1 + \bar{f}_2 \Delta_2 + ... \bar{f}_n \Delta_n$$

or, in terms of the summation notation

$$I \leqslant \sum_{i=1}^{n} \bar{f}_i \Delta_i .$$

The expression on the right of this inequality is called the **upper approximating sum** over the interval $a \leqslant x \leqslant b$.

If the limits

$$I_1 = \lim_{n \to \infty} \sum_{i=1}^{n} \underline{f}_i \Delta_i \quad \text{and} \quad I_2 = \lim_{n \to \infty} \sum_{i=1}^{n} \bar{f}_i \Delta_i$$

exist as the number of strips increases and all the widths $\Delta_i \to 0$, and $I_1 = I_2 = I$, we say that $f(x)$ is **integrable** over the interval $a \leqslant x \leqslant b$ and that the value of the **definite integral** of $f(x)$ from a to b equals I. This definite integral is denoted by modifying the indefinite integral notation by adding the **lower limit** a and **upper limit** b to the integral sign and writing

$$I = \int_a^b f(x) \, dx.$$

A more careful argument shows that we may define this same integral as

$$I = \int_a^b f(x) \, dx = \lim_{n \to \infty} \sum_{i=1}^{n} f(\xi_i) \, \Delta_i,$$

where ξ_i is any point inside the ith interval Δ_i. Such an integral is called the **Riemann integral** of $f(x)$ between the lower limit $x = a$ and the upper limit $x = b$.

Clearly, if $f(x)$ is continuous for $a \leqslant x \leqslant b$, it follows that $I_1 = I_2 = I$, and we may determine I as the limit of either the lower or upper approximating sums.

To show that this definition can actually be used to evaluate a definite integral involving a simple function, let us determine

$$I = \int_a^b f(x)\,dx,$$

where

$$f(x) = x^2.$$

For simplicity, we shall divide the interval $a \leqslant x \leqslant b$ into n equal parts, so the width of each strip is

$$\Delta = \left(\frac{b-a}{n}\right).$$

Then x_r, the left end point of the rth interval, is given by

$$x_r = a + r\left(\frac{b-a}{n}\right), \quad \text{for} \quad r = 0, 1, ..., n.$$

As x^2 is a monotonic increasing function, it follows that in each interval its minimum value occurs at the left-hand end point and its maximum value at the right-hand end point. So in the rth interval the minimum value m_r and maximum value M_r of $f(x) = x^2$ are

$$m_r = x_{r-1}^2 \quad \text{and} \quad M_r = x_r^2, \quad \text{for} \quad r = 1, 2, ..., n$$

Thus if the lower approximating sum with n strips is denoted by $\underline{s}_n$, then

$$\underline{s}_n = \sum_{r=1}^{n} \Delta\, M_r = \Delta \sum_{r=1}^{n} x_{r-1}^2.$$

Similarly, if the upper approximating sum with n strips is denoted by $\overline{S}_n$ then

$$\overline{S}_n = \sum_{r=1}^{n} \Delta\, M_r = \Delta \sum_{r=1}^{n} x_r^2.$$

The geometrical interpretations of these sums are shown in Fig. 86 with the lower sum being represented by the shaded strips in Fig. 86(a) and the upper sum being represented by the shaded strips in Fig. 86(b).

Inserting the expressions for x_r and Δ gives

$$\underline{s}_n = \left(\frac{b-a}{n}\right) \sum_{r=1}^{n} \left[a + (r-1)\left(\frac{b-a}{n}\right)\right]^2$$

and

$$\overline{S}_n = \left(\frac{b-a}{n}\right) \sum_{r=1}^{n} \left[a + r\left(\frac{b-a}{n}\right)\right]^2.$$

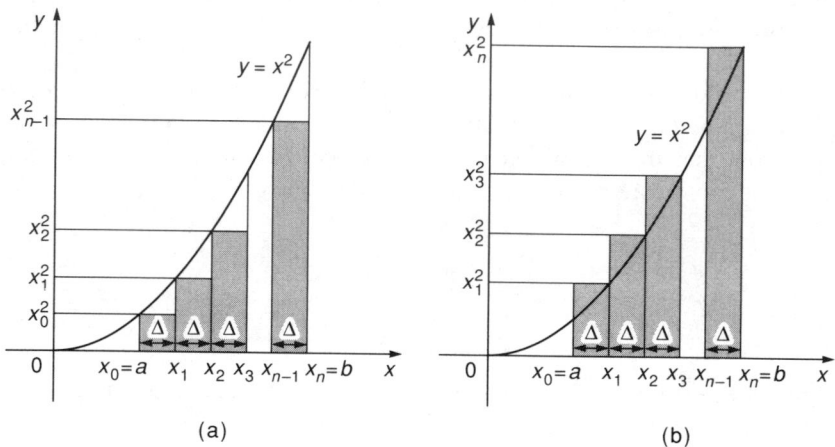

(a)   (b)

Fig. 86

Expanding $\underline{s}_n$ we obtain

$$\underline{s}_n = \left(\frac{b-a}{n}\right) \sum_{r=1}^{n} \left[a^2 + 2a\left(\frac{b-a}{n}\right)(r-1) + (r-1)^2\left(\frac{b-a}{n}\right)^2 \right],$$

so that

$$\underline{s}_n = \left(\frac{b-a}{n}\right)\left[\sum_{r=1}^{n} a^2 + 2a\left(\frac{b-a}{n}\right)\sum_{r=1}^{n}(r-1) + \left(\frac{b-a}{n}\right)^2 \sum_{r=1}^{n}(r-1)^2 \right],$$

or

$$\underline{s}_n = \left(\frac{b-a}{n}\right)\left[na^2 + 2a\left(\frac{b-a}{n}\right)\sum_{r=1}^{n}(r-1) + \left(\frac{b-a}{n}\right)^2 \sum_{r=1}^{n}(r-1)^2 \right].$$

We know from elementary algebra that

$$\sum_{r=1}^{n}(r-1) = \underbrace{0 + 1 + 2 + \dots + (n-1)}_{n \text{ terms}} = \frac{n}{2}(n-1) \qquad \text{(arithmetic series)}$$

and

$$\sum_{r=1}^{n}(r-1)^2 = \underbrace{0^2 + 1^2 + 2^2 + \dots + (n-1)^2}_{n \text{ terms}} = \frac{n(n-1)(2n-1)}{6} \qquad \text{(sum of squares).}$$

Using these results in $\underline{s}_n$ reduces it to

$$\underline{s}_n = \left(\frac{b-a}{n}\right)\left(na^2 + a(b-a)(n-1) + \left(\frac{b-a}{n}\right)^2 \frac{n(n-1)(2n-1)}{6}\right).$$

Taking the limit as $n \to \infty$, so the number of strips tends to infinity as their width $\Delta \to 0$, we have

$$\lim_{n \to \infty} \underline{s}_n = \lim_{n \to \infty} \left[(b-a)a^2 + a(b-a)^2\left(\frac{n-1}{n}\right) + (b-a)^3 \frac{n(n-1)(2n-1)}{6n^2}\right]$$

$$= (b-a)a^2 + a(b-a)^2 + (b-a)^3 \frac{1}{3}$$

$$= (b-a)\left(ab + \frac{1}{3}b^2 - \frac{2}{3}ab + \frac{1}{3}a^2\right)$$

$$= (b-a)\left(\frac{b^2 + ab + a^2}{3}\right)$$

$$= \frac{1}{3}(b^3 - a^3) \ .$$

A similar calculation shows that

$$\lim_{n \to \infty} \overline{S}_n = \frac{1}{3}(b^3 - a^3),$$

and thus the limit of I of both the lower and upper approximating sums is the same, and hence

$$I = \int_a^b x^2 \, dx = \frac{1}{3}(b^3 - a^3).$$

The expression on the right-hand side is the value of required definite integral.
   This use of the definition has served two quite different purposes:
1 it has shown that the definition has practical significance since it can be used to evaluate a definite integral; and
2 it will have convinced the reader that a better method is needed by which to evaluate definite integrals.
However, before developing such a method, let us use the definition to establish a number of fundamental properties of definite integrals.

GENERAL PROPERTIES OF DEFINITE INTEGRALS

1 If $f(x)$ is integrable for $a \leqslant x \leqslant b$ and $k = $ constant, then

$$\int_a^b kf(x) \, dx = k \int_a^b f(x) \, dx.$$

This result follows directly from the definition, because the constant factor k may be removed from inside to outside the summation, and hence from inside to outside the integral.

2 If $f(x)$ and $g(x)$ are integrable for $a \leqslant x \leqslant b$, then

$$\int_a^b (f(x) \pm g(x)) \, dx = \int_a^b f(x) \, dx \pm \int_a^b g(x) \, dx \text{ (linearity of the definite integral)}.$$

This result follows from the definition by separating terms involving f and g in the summations and hence in the integral.

3 If $f(x)$ is integrable for $a \leqslant x \leqslant b$ and c is such that $a < c < b$, then

$$\int_a^c f(x) \, dx + \int_c^b f(x) \, dx = \int_a^b f(x) \, dx.$$

This result asserts that the definite integral of $f(x)$ over the interval $a \leqslant x \leqslant b$ is the sum of the integral of $f(x)$ over any two adjacent subintervals into which $a \leqslant x \leqslant b$ is divided. The result follows from the interpretation of the definite integral as an area. It uses the fact that if the area below $y = f(x)$ for $a \leqslant x \leqslant b$ is divided into two parts, then the total area is the sum of the areas of each of the separate parts.

4 If $f(x)$ is integrable for $a \leqslant x \leqslant b$ and c is any internal point of this interval, then

$$\int_{c-}^{c+} f(x) \, dx = 0,$$

where $c-$ is the limit as c is approached from the left and $c+$ is the limit as it is approached from the right. This result asserts the obvious fact that the integral of $f(x)$ over a strip of finite height and zero width is zero.

5 If $f(x)$ is continuous and integrable for $a \leqslant x \leqslant c-$ and also for $c+ < x \leqslant b$, but it is discontinuous with a finite jump at $x = c$, then

$$\int_a^b f(x) \, dx = \int_a^{c-} f(x) \, dx + \int_{c+}^b f(x) \, dx.$$

This result asserts that if $f(x)$ is discontinuous at the point $x = c$ inside the interval $a \leqslant x \leqslant b$, then the integral over $a \leqslant x \leqslant b$ is the sum of the integrals over the intervals in which $f(x)$ is continuous. When proving this result, use is made of property 4 above to 'cut out' the discontinuity of $f(x)$ at $x = c$.

6 If $f(x)$ is integrable for $a \leqslant x \leqslant b$, then

$$\int_a^b f(x) \, dx = -\int_b^a f(x) \, dx.$$

This result asserts that reversing the limits of integration reverses the sign of the integral. The property follows from the fact that the interval widths (increments) Δ_i in the definition of a definite integral have a sign which is positive when x increases and negative when it decreases.

7 Areas determined by a definite integral have a positive sign when they lie above the x–axis and a negative sign when they lie below it. This is so because when integrating $f(x)$ from a to b, each strip width Δ_i is positive. However, the element of area associated with any width Δ_i will have the sign of $f(x)$ in the interval Δ_i.

8 The role of the symbol x in the definite integral

$$I = \int_a^b f(x)\,\mathrm{d}x$$

is simply to tell us that integration of function f with respect to its argument is to be carried out starting with the argument equal to a and ending with the argument equal to b. The symbol x representing the argument does not appear in the result, so any other symbol may be used in place of x with precisely the same meaning, and thus

$$I = \int_a^b f(x)\,\mathrm{d}x = \int_a^b f(t)\,\mathrm{d}t = \ldots = \int_a^b f(\theta)\,\mathrm{d}\theta.$$

For this reason, the symbols $x, t, \ldots, \theta$ appearing as the argument of f in the definite integral are called **dummy variables**.

The last result of importance in this section is a theorem which will be needed later when establishing the connection between definite and indefinite integrals. Let $f(x)$ be continuous for $a \le x \le b$, and let M and m be the respective maximum and minimum values attained by $f(x)$ in this interval. Consideration of Fig. 87 shows that

$$m(b-a) \le \int_a^b f(x)\,\mathrm{d}x \le M(b-a),$$

because area $S_1 = m(b-a)$ and area $S_2 = M(b-a)$, while the area below the curve, which is intermediate between S_1 and S_2, is $\int_a^b f(x)\,\mathrm{d}x$. Let us rewrite this result as

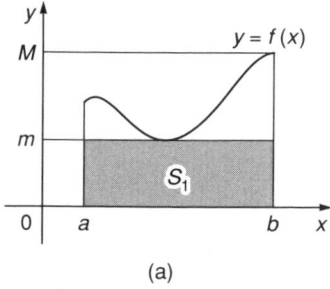 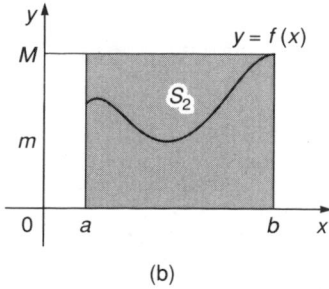

(a)   (b)

Fig. 87

$$m \leqslant \frac{1}{b-a} \int_a^b f(x)\,dx \leqslant M.$$

Now, as $f(x)$ is continuous, it follows from the intermediate value theorem (Section 15) that $f(x)$ must assume every value between m and M at least once, and so for some value of x it must equal the value of the integral. Thus there must be at least one value of x, say $x = \xi$, with $a < \xi < b$, such that

$$f(\xi) = \frac{1}{b-a} \int_a^b f(x)\,dx.$$

This result is called the **mean value theorem** for integrals, and it will be used in the next section when proving the fundamental theorem of integral calculus.

It is possible to verify this theorem in a special case, since we have already proved that

$$\int_a^b x^2\,dx = \frac{1}{3}(b^3 - a^3).$$

Thus in this case, as $f(x) = x^2$, it follows that

$$\frac{1}{b-a} \int_a^b f(x)\,dx = \frac{1}{b-a} \int_a^b x^2\,dx = \left(\frac{1}{b-a}\right)\frac{1}{3}(b^3 - a^3) = \frac{1}{3}(b^2 + ab + a^2).$$

However, by the mean value theorem, this result should equal $f(\xi) = \xi^2$ for some ξ such that $a < \xi < b$. This is indeed the case, because as $a < b$ we have

$$a^2 < \frac{1}{3}(b^2 + ab + a^2) < b^2,$$

and thus

$$\xi = \frac{1}{\sqrt{3}}(b^2 + ab + a^2)^{1/2},$$

with $a < \xi < b$.

The fundamental theorem of integral calculus and the evaluation of definite integrals

We now establish the fundamental connection between definite integrals and antiderivatives (indefinite integrals). Let a continuous function $f(t)$ be defined for $a \leqslant t \leqslant b$ and let x be any point inside the interval. Then if we regard a definite integral as a function of its upper limit, which we write as x, a function $F(x)$ may be defined as

$$F(x) = \int_a^x f(t)\, dt,$$

where t is a dummy variable.

Now let us differentiate $F(x)$ with respect to x, which is equivalent to differentiating the integral with respect to its upper limit x. By definition we have

$$F'(x) = \lim_{h \to 0} \left[\frac{F(x+h) - F(x)}{h} \right]$$

$$= \lim_{h \to 0} \left\{ \frac{1}{h} \left[\int_a^{x+h} f(t)\, dt - \int_a^x f(t)\, dt \right] \right\}.$$

However, from the third property of the definite integrals in Section 38 this may be rewritten as

$$F'(x) = \lim_{h \to 0} \left\{ \frac{1}{h} \int_a^{x+h} f(t)\, dt \right\}.$$

Applying the mean value theorem for integrals to the expression inside the limit gives

$$F'(x) = \lim_{h \to 0} \{ f(\xi) \},$$

where ξ is such that $x < \xi < x + h$ (it is some value of t intermediate between x and $x + h$). In the limit as $h \to 0$, we thus have $\xi \to x$, and so

$$F'(x) = f(x).$$

This has proved that $F(x)$ is an antiderivative of $f(x)$, so it follows from this that

$$F(x) = \int_a^x f(t)\,dt + C,$$

where C is an arbitrary constant.

Now setting $x = b$ in $F(x)$ we have

$$F(b) = \int_a^b f(t)\,dt + C,$$

while setting $x = a$ gives

$$F(a) = \int_a^a f(t)\,dt + C = C.$$

Thus differencing these results we find that

$$\int_a^b f(t)\,dt = F(b) - F(a).$$

This key result is called the **fundamental theorem of integral calculus**. It establishes the connection between the definite integral of a function f with respect to its argument taken over the interval $[a, b]$, and an antiderivative (indefinite integral) of f. Notice the important fact that the arbitrary constant of integration present in $F(x)$ cancels out when considering the difference $F(b) - F(a)$. On account of this, in practice the arbitrary constant of integration is always omitted from the antiderivative of $f(x)$ when evaluating a definite integral. We have thus arrived at the following result.

Fundamental theorem of integral calculus
Let $F(x)$ be an antiderivative of $f(x)$, then

$$\int_a^b f(x)\,dx = F(b) - F(a).$$

Any methods for finding antiderivatives which have already been discussed may be used to evaluate definite integrals. However, care must be taken with the limits on a definite integral when using integration by substitution or integration by parts.

DEFINITE INTEGRALS USING INTEGRATION BY SUBSTITUTION

When a definite integral

$$\int_a^b f(x)\,dx$$

is to be evaluated, the lower limit a and the upper limit b are the limits to be applied to the argument x of function $f(x)$. If this definite integral is to be evaluated by substitution, say by setting $u = U(x)$, with $U(x)$ some function of x, then when changing to the variable u under the integral sign, as described in Section 34, the limits on the integral must also be changed so that they refer to the new argument u. Thus the lower limit will become $u = U(a)$ and the upper limit will become $u = U(b)$.

INTEGRATION BY PARTS AND DEFINITE INTEGRALS

The development of integration by parts for indefinite integrals in Section 36 started from the formula for differentiating a product $u(x)v(x)$,

$$\frac{d}{dx}[u(x)v(x)] = u(x)\frac{d}{dx}[v(x)] + v(x)\frac{d}{dx}[u(x)].$$

If we integrate this over the interval $a \leqslant x \leqslant b$ it becomes

$$\int_a^b \frac{d}{dx}[u(x)v(x)]\,dx = \int_a^b u(x)\frac{d}{dx}[v(x)]\,dx + \int_a^b v(x)\frac{d}{dx}[u(x)]\,dx,$$

so as an antiderivative of $d/dx\,[u(x)v(x)]$ is $u(x)v(x)$, it follows from the fundamental theorem of integral calculus that

$$u(b)v(b) - u(a)v(a) = \int_a^b u(x)\frac{d}{dx}[v(x)]\,dx + \int_a^b v(x)\frac{d}{dx}[u(x)]\,dx.$$

Using the standard concise notation

$$[u(x)v(x)]\bigg|_a^b = u(b)v(b) - u(a)v(a),$$

and rearranging terms, we obtain the next formula.

The formula for integration by parts of a definite integral

$$\int_a^b u(x)\frac{d}{dx}[v(x)]\,dx = [u(x)v(x)]\bigg|_a^b - \int_a^b v(x)\frac{d}{dx}[u(x)]\,dx$$

or, in a more concise but less explicit notation

$$\int_a^b u\,dv = (uv)\bigg|_a^b - \int_a^b v\,du.$$

Notice that this differs from the formula for integration by parts of an indefinite integral by the inclusion of limits on both the integrals and on the $u(x)v(x)$ term.

Example 39.1

Find

$$\int_a^b x^2 \, dx.$$

Solution
An antiderivative of x^2 is $\frac{1}{3}x^3$, so

$$\int_a^b x^2 \, dx = \left(\frac{1}{3}x^3\right)_{x=b} - \left(\frac{1}{3}x^3\right)_{x=a}$$

$$= \frac{1}{3}(b^3 - a^3).$$

This is, of course, in agreement with the result obtained earlier in which we started from first principles and used upper and lower approximating sums.

▲

Example 39.2

Find

$$I_1 = \int_0^{\pi/2} \sin x \, dx \quad \text{and} \quad I_2 = \int_{-\pi/2}^{\pi/2} \sin x \, dx.$$

Solution
An antiderivative of $\sin x$ is $-\cos x$, so

$$I_1 = \int_0^{\pi/2} \sin x \, dx = (-\cos x)\Big|_0^{\pi/2}$$

$$= -\cos\frac{\pi}{2} - (-\cos 0) = 0 + 1 = 1$$

while

$$I = \int_{-\pi/2}^{\pi/2} \sin x \, dx = (-\cos x)\Big|_{-\pi/2}^{\pi/2}$$

$$= -\cos\frac{\pi}{2} - \left[-\cos\left(-\frac{\pi}{2}\right)\right]$$

$$= 0 + 0 = 0.$$

The vanishing of the definite integral I_2 is because $\sin x$ is an odd function, so the integral over the interval $-\pi/2 \leqslant x \leqslant 0$ is the negative of the integral over $0 \leqslant x \leqslant \pi/2$, causing the two results to cancel. The areas concerned in I_1 and I_2 are shown in Fig. 88.

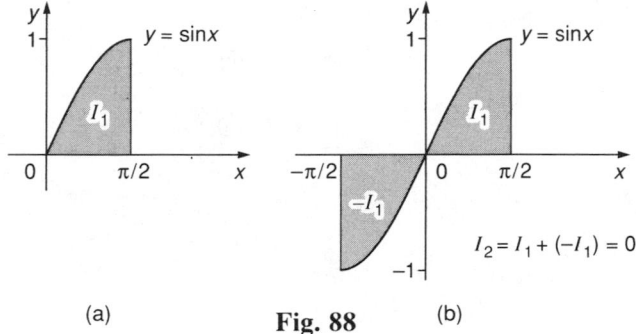

(a)   **Fig. 88**   (b)

▲

Example 39.3

Find

$$\int_{\pi/3}^{\pi/2} \frac{dx}{\sqrt{(4-x^2)}}.$$

Solution
An antiderivative of $(4-x^2)^{1/2}$ is arcsin $(x/2)$, so

$$\int_{\pi/3}^{\pi/2} \frac{dx}{\sqrt{(4-x^2)}} = \left(\arcsin\frac{x}{2}\right)_{x=\pi/2} - \left(\arcsin\frac{x}{2}\right)_{x=\pi/3}$$

$$= \arcsin\frac{\pi}{4} - \arcsin\frac{\pi}{6}$$

$$= 0.903\,34 - 0.551\,07 = 0.352\,27.$$ ▲

Example 39.4

Find

$$\int_{5}^{9} \cosh\left(\frac{1}{4}x - 1\right) dx.$$

Solution
Integrate by using the substitution $u = \frac{1}{4}x - 1$, so $du = \frac{1}{4}dx$, and thus

$$dx = 4\,du.$$

The limits on the definite integral are limits on x, so as $u = \frac{1}{4}x - 1$, the lower limit $x = 5$ becomes the lower limit $u = 5/4 - 1 = 1/4$, while the upper limit $x = 9$ becomes the upper limit $u = 9/4 - 1 = 5/4$. Thus

$$\int_{5}^{9} \cosh\left(\frac{1}{4}x - 1\right) dx = \int_{1/4}^{5/4} 4\cosh u\,du$$

$$= (4 \sinh u) \Big|_{1/4}^{5/4}$$

$$= 4(\sinh 5/4 - \sinh 1/4) = 5.397\,22. \quad \blacktriangle$$

Example 39.5

Find

$$\int_1^2 \ln (1 + x^2)\,dx.$$

Solution

Writing the integral as

$$\ln(1 + x^2) \cdot 1 = \ln(1 + x^2) \frac{d}{dx} [x]$$

and applying the formula for integration by parts for a definite integral with $u(x) = \ln(1 + x^2)$ and $v(x) = x$ gives

$$\int_1^2 \ln(1 + x^2)\,dx = [x \ln(1 + x^2)] \Big|_1^2 - \int_1^2 x \frac{d}{dx} [\ln(1 + x^2)]\,dx$$

$$= 2 \ln 5 - \ln 2 - \int_1^2 \frac{2x^2}{1 + x^2}\,dx$$

However, using either long division or partial fractions shows that

$$\frac{2x^2}{1 + x^2} = 2 - \frac{2}{1 + x^2}.$$

Thus

$$\int_1^2 \ln(1 + x^2)\,dx = 2 \ln 5 - \ln 2 - \int_1^2 2\,dx + \int_1^2 \frac{2}{1 + x^2}\,dx$$

$$= 2 \ln 5 - \ln 2 - [2x] \Big|_1^2 + [2 \arctan x] \Big|_1^2$$

$$= 2 \ln 5 - \ln 2 - 2 + 2 \arctan 2 - 2 \arctan 1$$

$$= 1.169\,23 \qquad\qquad \blacktriangle$$

Example 39.6

Show that if

$$J_n = \int_0^{\pi/2} x^n \cos x\,dx \quad \text{for} \quad n \geqslant 0,$$

then J_n satisfies the reduction formula

$$J_n = \left(\frac{\pi}{2}\right)^n - n(n-1)J_{n-2}, \quad \text{for} \quad n \geqslant 2.$$

Use the result to find J_4.

Solution
Writing the integrand as

$$x^n \frac{d}{dx}[\sin x],$$

and applying the formula for integration by parts for definite integrals with $u(x) = x^n$ and $v(x) = \sin x$, gives

$$J_n = \int_0^{\pi/2} x^n \cos x \, dx$$

$$= [x^n \sin x]\Big|_0^{\pi/2} - n \int_0^{\pi/2} x^{n-1} \sin x \, dx$$

$$= \left(\frac{\pi}{2}\right)^n - n \int_0^{\pi/2} x^{n-1} \sin x \, dx$$

However,

$$\int_0^{\pi/2} x^{n-1} \sin x \, dx = \int_0^{\pi/2} x^{n-1} \frac{d}{dx}[-\cos x] \, dx,$$

so again using integration by parts, but this time with $u(x) = x^{n-1}$ and $v(x) = -\cos x$, gives

$$\int_0^{\pi/2} x^{n-1} \sin dx = [-x^{n-1} \cos x]\Big|_0^{\pi/2} + (n-1) \int_0^{\pi/2} x^{n-2} \cos x \, dx$$

$$= 0 + (n-1) \int_0^{\pi/2} x^{n-2} \cos x \, dx$$

$$= (n-1)J_{n-2}.$$

Combining results we obtain the required reduction formula

$$J_n = \left(\frac{\pi}{2}\right)^n - n(n-1)J_{n-2}, \quad \text{for} \quad n \geqslant 2.$$

We now make use of this reduction formula in reverse to find J_4. Setting $n = 0$ in the integral defining J_n gives

$$J_0 = \int_0^{\pi/2} \cos x \, dx = (\sin x)\Big|_0^{\pi/2} = 1.$$

Next, writing $n = 2$ in the reduction formula, we find that

$$J_2 = \left(\frac{\pi}{2}\right)^2 - 2 \cdot 1 \, J_0 = \frac{\pi^2}{4} - 2.$$

Finally, to find J_4, we set $n = 4$ in the reduction formula to obtain

$$J_4 = \left(\frac{\pi}{2}\right)^4 - 4 \cdot 3 \, J_2.$$

Substituting the expression for J_2 obtained above we arrive at the required result

$$J_4 = \frac{\pi^4}{16} - 3\pi^2 + 24. \qquad \blacktriangle$$

We conclude this section by considering three simple but extremely important integrals we will use repeatedly when we come to discuss Fourier series. Although these integrals can all be evaluated by using integration by parts, it will be more helpful when working with Fourier series if we evaluate them by using some standard trigonometric identities.

Example 39.7

Prove that

$$\int_{-\pi}^{\pi} \sin mx \, \cos nx \, \mathrm{d}x = 0$$

for all integers $m, n = 0, 1, 2, \ldots$.

Solution
We start from the identities

$$\sin(A + B) = \sin A \cos B + \cos A \sin B$$

and

$$\sin(A - B) = \sin A \cos B - \cos A \sin B.$$

Adding the results gives

$$\sin(A + B) + \sin(A - B) = 2 \sin A \cos B.$$

Thus setting $A = mx$, $B = nx$ this becomes

$$\sin[(m + n)x] + \sin[(m - n)x] = 2 \sin mx \cos nx,$$

and so

$$\int_{-\pi}^{\pi} \sin mx \cos nx \, \mathrm{d}x = \frac{1}{2} \int_{-\pi}^{\pi} \sin[(m + n)x] \, \mathrm{d}x + \frac{1}{2} \int_{-\pi}^{\pi} \sin[(m - n)]x \, \mathrm{d}x.$$

Now if $m \neq n$ and $m \neq 0$

$$\int_{-\pi}^{\pi} \sin mx \cos nx \, dx = \left(-\frac{1}{2} \frac{\cos[(m+n)x]}{m+n}\right)\Big|_{-\pi}^{\pi} + \left(-\frac{1}{2} \frac{\cos[(m-n)x]}{m-n}\right)\Big|_{-\pi}^{\pi} = 0,$$

because the cosine is an even function, so

$$[\cos(m+n)\pi] = \cos(m+n)(-\pi)]$$

and

$$\cos[m-n)\pi] = \cos[(m-n)(-\pi)].$$

The result is certainly true when $m = 0$ for then the integrand is identically zero, so we have proved that

$$\int_{-\pi}^{\pi} \sin mx \cos nx \, dx = 0$$

for $m, n = 0, 1, 2, \ldots$.   ▲

Example 39.8

Prove that

$$\int_{-\pi}^{\pi} \sin mx \sin nx \, dx = \begin{cases} 0 & \text{for} \quad m \neq n \\ \pi & \text{for} \quad m = n \neq 0. \end{cases}$$

Solution
This time we start from the trigonometric identities

$$\cos(A+B) = \cos A \cos B - \sin A \sin B$$

and

$$\cos(A-B) = \cos A \cos B + \sin A \sin B.$$

Subtracting the first result from the second gives

$$\cos(A-B) - \cos(A+B) = 2 \sin A \sin B,$$

so setting $A = mx$ and $B = nx$ gives

$$\cos[(m-n)x] - \cos[(m+n)x] = 2 \sin mx \sin nx.$$

Thus

$$\int_{-\pi}^{\pi} \sin mx \sin nx \, dx = \frac{1}{2} \int_{-\pi}^{\pi} \cos[(m-n)x] \, dx - \frac{1}{2} \int_{-\pi}^{\pi} \cos[(m+n)x] \, dx$$

and provided $m \neq n \neq 0$

$$\int_{-\pi}^{\pi} \sin mx \cos nx \, dx = \left(\frac{1}{2} \frac{\sin[(m-n)x]}{m-n}\right)\Big|_{-\pi}^{\pi} - \left(\frac{1}{2} \frac{\sin[(m+n)x]}{m+n}\right)\Big|_{-\pi}^{\pi} = 0,$$

because the sine of any integral multiple of π is zero.

The result is obviously true if $m = 0$ or $n = 0$ for then the integrand is identically zero, so it only remains for us to consider the case in which $m = n \neq 0$. Our identity becomes

$$\sin^2 nx = \frac{1}{2}(1 - \cos 2nx),$$

from which we see that

$$\int_{-\pi}^{\pi} \sin^2 nx \, dx = \int_{-\pi}^{\pi} \frac{1}{2}(1 - \cos 2nx) \, dx$$

$$= \frac{1}{2}\int_{-\pi}^{\pi} 1 \cdot dx - \frac{1}{2}\int_{-\pi}^{\pi} \cos 2nx \, dx$$

$$= \pi - \left(\frac{1}{4n}\sin 2nx\right)\bigg|_{-\pi}^{\pi}$$

$$= \pi,$$

because the sine of any integral multiple of π is zero.

Thus we have proved that

$$\int_{-\pi}^{\pi} \sin mx \sin nx \, dx = \begin{cases} 0 & \text{for} \quad m \neq n \\ \pi & \text{for} \quad m = n \neq 0. \end{cases} \qquad \blacktriangle$$

Example 39.9

Prove that

$$\int_{-\pi}^{\pi} \cos mx \cos nx \, dx = \begin{cases} 0 & \text{for} \quad m \neq n \\ \pi & \text{for} \quad m = n \neq 0 \\ 2\pi & \text{for} \quad m = n = 0. \end{cases}$$

Solution
Consider first the case $m = n = 0$. The integral then reduces to

$$\int_{-\pi}^{\pi} 1 \cdot dx = 2\pi,$$

which establishes the last result.

We again use the identities

$$\cos(A + B) = \cos A \cos B - \sin A \sin B$$

and

$$\cos(A - B) = \cos A \cos B + \sin A \sin B,$$

but this time we add them to obtain

$$\cos(A - B) + \cos(A + B) = 2\cos A \cos B.$$

Setting $A = mx, B = nx$, the last result becomes

$$\cos[(m - n)x] + \cos[(m + n)x] = 2\cos mx \cos nx,$$

and so

$$\int_{-\pi}^{\pi} \cos mx \cos nx \, dx = \frac{1}{2}\int_{-\pi}^{\pi} \cos[(m - n)x] \, dx + \frac{1}{2}\int_{-\pi}^{\pi} \cos[(m + n)x] \, dx.$$

Thus if $m \neq n$

$$\int_{-\pi}^{\pi} \cos mx \cos nx \, dx = \left(\frac{1}{2}\frac{\sin[(m - n)x]}{m - n}\right)\Bigg|_{-\pi}^{\pi} + \left(\frac{1}{2}\frac{\sin[(m + n)x]}{m + n}\right)\Bigg|_{-\pi}^{\pi} = 0,$$

because the sine of an integral multiple of π is zero.

Finally, if $m = n \neq 0$ we need to consider the integral

$$\int_{-\pi}^{\pi} \cos^2 nx \, dx.$$

However, if $m = n$ our identity reduces to

$$\cos^2 nx = \frac{1}{2}(1 + \cos 2nx),$$

so

$$\int_{-\pi}^{\pi} \cos nx \, dx = \int_{-\pi}^{\pi} \frac{1}{2}(1 + \cos 2nx) \, dx$$

$$= \frac{1}{2}\int_{-\pi}^{\pi} 1 \cdot dx + \left(\frac{1}{2}\frac{\sin 2nx}{2n}\right)\Bigg|_{-\pi}^{\pi}$$

$$= \pi,$$

because the sine of an integral multiple of π is zero. Thus we have proved the result that

$$\int_{-\pi}^{\pi} \cos mx \cos nx \, dx = \begin{cases} 0 & \text{for } m \neq n \\ \pi & \text{for } m = n \neq 0 \\ 2\pi & \text{for } m = n \neq 0. \end{cases} \qquad \blacktriangle$$

PROBLEMS 39

Evaluate the following definite integrals.

1. $\displaystyle\int_{1}^{2} (x^3 - 2x + 3) \, dx.$

2. $\displaystyle\int_1^3 (1 + \sinh x)\,dx.$

3. $\displaystyle\int_1^{\pi/2} (2x + 3\cos x)\,dx.$

4. $\displaystyle\int_0^4 (x^{1/3} + x^{1/4})\,dx.$

5. $\displaystyle\int_1^{1/3} \frac{dx}{\sqrt{(2 + 5x^2)}}.$

6. $\displaystyle\int_0^1 \frac{dx}{\sqrt{(2 + x^2)}}.$

7. $\displaystyle\int_0^2 \frac{dx}{2x + 5}.$

8. $\displaystyle\int_1^3 \frac{dx}{5 - x}.$

9. $\displaystyle\int_{-2}^2 \frac{dx}{\sqrt{(5 + 4x + x^2)}}.$

10. $\displaystyle\int_{-4}^{-6} \frac{dx}{\sqrt{(1 + 4x - x^2)}}.$

11. $\displaystyle\int_2^8 \sqrt{(x - 2)}\,dx.$

12. $\displaystyle\int_1^4 \sqrt{(x - 1)}\,dx.$

13. $\displaystyle\int_0^{\pi/4} \frac{dx}{x^2 + 1}.$

14. $\displaystyle\int_{-4}^{-2} \frac{dx}{x^2 - 1}.$

15. $\displaystyle\int_0^1 \frac{dx}{x^2 + 4x + 5}.$

16. $\displaystyle\int_3^4 \frac{dx}{x^2 - 3x + 2}.$

17. $\displaystyle\int_0^1 \frac{y^2}{1+y^6}\,\mathrm{d}y$.

18. $\displaystyle\int_2^{1/\sqrt{2}} \frac{\mathrm{d}t}{\sqrt{(1-t^2)}}$.

19. $\displaystyle\int_0^{\pi/4} \cos^2\theta\,\mathrm{d}\theta$.

20. $\displaystyle\int_0^{\pi/4} \sin^2\theta\,\mathrm{d}\theta$.

21. $\displaystyle\int_{-\pi/4}^{\pi/4} \tan x\,\mathrm{d}x$.

22. $\displaystyle\int_0^1 \frac{e^x}{1+e^{2x}}\,\mathrm{d}x$.

23. $\displaystyle\int_0^{\pi/3} \sin^2 4x\,\mathrm{d}x$.

24. $\displaystyle\int_0^1 \frac{\mathrm{d}x}{\sqrt{(1+x^2)}}$.

25. $\displaystyle\int_0^1 \frac{\mathrm{d}x}{1+e^x}$.

26. $\displaystyle\int_0^1 \ln(1+x)\,\mathrm{d}x$.

27. $\displaystyle\int_0^1 \sqrt{(1+x^2)}\,\mathrm{d}x$.

28. $\displaystyle\int_0^{1/2} \sqrt{\left(\frac{x}{1-x}\right)}\,\mathrm{d}x$.

29. $\displaystyle\int_0^4 \frac{\mathrm{d}x}{1+\sqrt{(2x+1)}}$.

30. $\displaystyle\int_0^1 \arcsin x\,\mathrm{d}x$.

31. $\displaystyle\int_0^1 \arctan x\, dx.$

32. $\displaystyle\int_0^1 x \arcsin x\, dx.$

33. $\displaystyle\int_0^1 x \arctan x\, dx.$

34. $\displaystyle\int_0^2 x^2\sqrt{(4-x^2)}\, dx.$

35. $\displaystyle\int_0^{\pi/2} x \sin x\, dx.$

36. $\displaystyle\int_0^{\pi/4} x \cos x\, dx.$

37. $\displaystyle\int_0^1 x\, e^{2x}\, dx.$

38. $\displaystyle\int_0^2 x^2 e^{-x}\, dx.$

39. $\displaystyle\int_2^3 x^2 \ln x\, dx.$

40. $\displaystyle\int_1^2 \frac{x}{(x+1)(x+2)^2}\, dx.$

41. $\displaystyle\int_2^3 \frac{dx}{(x^2-1)^2}\, dx.$

42. $\displaystyle\int_0^2 \frac{2+x}{x(1+x^2)}\, dx.$

43. $\displaystyle\int_0^1 \frac{2-x^2}{(1+x)(1+x^2)}\, dx.$

44. $\displaystyle\int_0^{1/2} \frac{dx}{1-x^4}.$

45. Set

$$J_n = \int_0^{\pi/2} \sin^n x\, dx \quad \text{for} \quad n \geqslant 0,$$

and show that J_n satisfies the reduction formula

$$J_n = \left(\frac{n-1}{n}\right)J_{n-2} \quad \text{for} \quad n \geqslant 2.$$

Use this result to determine J_2, J_4 and J_6.

46. Set

$$J_n = \int_0^{\pi/2} \cos^n x \, dx \quad \text{for} \quad n \geqslant 0,$$

and show that J_n satisfies the reduction formula

$$J_n = \left(\frac{n-1}{n}\right)J_{n-2} \quad \text{for} \quad n \geqslant 2.$$

Use this result to determine J_2, J_4 and J_6.

47. Set

$$J_n = \int_0^{\pi/2} x \cos^n x \, dx \quad \text{for} \quad n \geqslant 0,$$

and show that J_n satisfies the reduction formula

$$n^2 J_n = n(n-1)J_{n-2} - 1 \quad \text{for} \quad n \geqslant 2.$$

Use this result to determine J_3 and J_4.

48. Set

$$J_n = \int_0^{\pi/4} \sec^n x \, dx \quad \text{for} \quad n \geqslant 0,$$

and show that J_n satisfies the reduction formula

$$(n-1) J_n = 2^{(n-2)/2} + (n-2) J_{n-2} \quad \text{for} \quad n \geqslant 2.$$

Use this result to determine J_4 and J_6.

40   Improper integrals

There is an important group of definite integral which has not yet been considered, containing what are called **improper integrals**. These are definite integrals in which either the integrand becomes infinite at some point in the interval of integration, or in which the length of the interval of integration itself is infinite in length; some integrals are improper in both of these ways. The question to be answered in such cases is whether or not the integral has a finite value. If the value of the integral can be shown to be a finite number I, the integral is said to be **convergent**, and to **converge** to the value I. If the value of the integral is infinite, or undefined, then the integral is said to be **divergent**.

The two basic types of improper integral are illustrated in Fig. 89. In Fig. 89(a) the integrand $f(x)$ becomes infinite at $x = c$ (an asymptote to $y = f(x)$) inside the interval of integration $a \leqslant x \leqslant b$, while in Fig. 89(b) the interval of integration is $a \leqslant x < \infty$ and the x–axis is an asymptote to $y = f(x)$ as $x \to \infty$.

We say the improper integral illustrated in Fig. 89(a) **converges** to the value I if

$$I = \lim_{\varepsilon \to 0} \int_{a}^{c-\varepsilon} f(x)\,dx + \lim_{\delta \to 0} \int_{c+\delta}^{b} f(x)\,dx$$

exists and is finite when ε and δ tend to zero through positive values. If either or both of these limits is infinite, or undefined, we say the improper integral is **divergent**.

If the infinity of the integrand occurs at the left-hand end point $x = a$, the above limiting process is modified in an obvious manner by setting

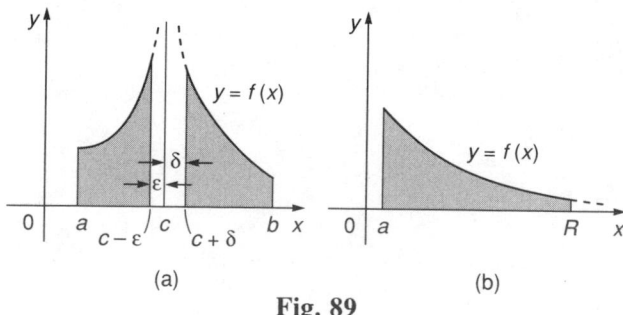

(a)   (b)

Fig. 89

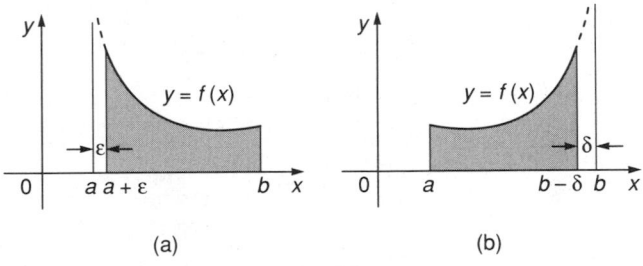

Fig. 90

$$I = \lim_{\varepsilon \to 0} \int_{a+\varepsilon}^{b} f(x)\,dx,$$

where ε tends to zero through positive values. Here also we say the integral converges to the value I if this limit exists and is finite. If, however, the limit is infinite or undefined we say the integral is divergent. The way in which the limiting operation is performed is illustrated in Fig. 90(a).

Similarly, if the infinity of the integrand occurs at the right-hand end point $x = b$, as in Fig. 90(b), we set

$$I = \lim_{\delta \to 0} \int_{a}^{b-\delta} f(x)\,dx,$$

where δ tends to zero through positive values. Again, the integral will be said to be convergent to the value I if this limit exists and is finite, and it will be said to be divergent if the limit is infinite or undefined.

The improper integral of the other type which is illustrated in Fig. 89(b) will be said to converge to the value I if

$$I = \lim_{R \to \infty} \int_{a}^{R} f(x)\,dx$$

exists and is finite. If the value of the limit is infinite, or undefined, the improper integral will be said to be divergent.

Example 40.1

Examine the convergence of

$$\int_{0}^{1} \frac{dx}{\sqrt{(1-x^2)}}.$$

Solution
This is an improper integral because the integrand $1/\sqrt{(1-x^2)}$ becomes infinite at the upper limit $x = 1$, as illustrated in Fig. 90(b).

Thus to determine its convergence properties we must examine

$$I = \lim_{\delta \to 0} \int_0^{1-\delta} \frac{dx}{\sqrt{(1-x^2)}}.$$

An antiderivative of $1/\sqrt{(1-x^2)}$ is arcsin x, so

$$I = \lim_{\delta \to 0} \left[(\arcsin x) \Big|_0^{1-\delta} \right]$$

$$= \lim_{\delta \to 0} [\arcsin(1-\delta) - \arcsin 0]$$

$$= \lim_{\delta \to 0} [\arcsin(1-\delta)] = \pi/2.$$

Thus I is finite and equal to $\pi/2$, so the integral converges to this value, and hence

$$\lim_{\delta \to 0} \int_0^1 \frac{dx}{\sqrt{(1-x^2)}} = \frac{\pi}{2}. \qquad \blacktriangle$$

Example 40.2

Examine the convergence of

$$I = \int_1^\infty \frac{dx}{1+x^2}.$$

Solution
This is an improper integral because although the integrand remains finite, the interval of integration is infinite in length; as in Fig. 89(b).
Thus to determine the convergence properties we must examine

$$I = \lim_{R \to \infty} \int_1^R \frac{dx}{1+x^2}.$$

An antiderivative of $1/(1+x^2)$ is arctan x, so

$$I = \lim_{R \to \infty} \left[(\arctan x) \Big|_1^R \right]$$

$$= \lim_{R \to \infty} [\arctan R - \arctan 1]$$

$$= \lim_{R \to \infty} [\arctan R] - \pi/4$$

$$= \pi/2 - \pi/4 = \pi/4.$$

Thus I is finite and equal to $\pi/4$, so the integral converges to this value, and hence

$$\int_1^\infty \frac{dx}{1+x^2} = \pi/4.$$ ▲

Example 40.3

Examine the convergence of

$$I = \int_0^1 \frac{dx}{x}.$$

Solution
This is an improper integral because the integrand $1/x$ becomes infinite at the lower limit $x = 0$, as illustrated in Fig. 90(a).

Thus to determine the convergence properties we must examine

$$I = \lim_{\varepsilon \to 0} \int_\varepsilon^1 \frac{dx}{x}.$$

An antiderivative of $1/x$ is $\ln|x|$, so

$$I = \lim_{\varepsilon \to 0} \left[(\ln|x|) \Big|_\varepsilon^1 \right]$$

$$= \lim_{\varepsilon \to 0} [\ln 1 - \ln \varepsilon]$$

$$= \lim_{\varepsilon \to 0} [- \ln \varepsilon] = \infty.$$

Thus this integral is divergent. ▲

Example 40.4

Examine the convergence of

$$I = \int_{\pi/2}^\infty \cos x \, dx.$$

Solution
This is an improper integral because although $\cos x$ is bounded for all x, the interval of integration is infinite, as in Fig. 89(b).

Thus we must consider the behaviour of

$$I = \lim_{R \to \infty} \int_{\pi/2}^R \cos x \, dx.$$

An antiderivative of $\cos x$ is $\sin x$, so

$$I = \lim_{R \to \infty} \left[(\sin x) \Big|_{\pi/2}^{R} \right]$$

$$= \lim_{R \to \infty} [\sin R - 1].$$

However, $\lim_{R \to \infty} \sin R$ does not exist (the function oscillates boundedly between ± 1) so the integral is divergent. ▲

Example 40.5

Examine the convergence of

$$I = \int_0^{\infty} x\,e^{-x}\,dx.$$

Solution
This is an improper integral because the interval of integration is infinite, as in Fig. 89(b).
   Thus we must consider the behaviour of

$$I = \lim_{R \to \infty} \int_0^R x\,e^{-x}\,dx.$$

Integrating by parts we find that

$$\int_0^R x\,e^{-x}\,dx = \int_0^R x\frac{d}{dx}[-e^{-x}]\,dx$$

$$= (-x\,e^{-x})\Big|_0^R + \int_0^R e^{-x}\,dx$$

$$= -R\,e^{-R} + 1 - e^{-R}.$$

Now an application of L'Hôpital's rule (Section 26) shows that

$$\lim_{R \to \infty} R\,e^{-R} = \lim_{R \to \infty} \frac{R}{e^R} = 0,$$

so

$$I = \lim_{R \to \infty} [-R\,e^{-R} + 1 - e^{-R}]$$

$$= 0 + 1 - 0 = 1.$$

   Thus this integral is convergent and it converges to the value 1, so we may write

$$\int_0^{\infty} x\,e^{-x}\,dx = 1.$$ ▲

PROBLEMS 40

Investigate the convergence of the following improper integrals.

1. $\displaystyle\int_1^\infty \frac{dx}{x^2}$.

2. $\displaystyle\int_0^1 \frac{dx}{\sqrt{x}}$.

3. $\displaystyle\int_0^2 \frac{dx}{\sqrt{(2-x)}}$.

4. $\displaystyle\int_0^4 \frac{dx}{(x-2)^2}$.

5. $\displaystyle\int_1^\infty \frac{dx}{4+x^2}$.

6. $\displaystyle\int_2^\infty \frac{\ln x}{x}\,dx$.

7. $\displaystyle\int_0^3 \frac{x}{\sqrt{(9-x^2)}}$.

8. $\displaystyle\int_1^\infty e^{-x}\sin x\,dx$.

9. $\displaystyle\int_0^\infty \frac{dx}{(x+2)(x+5)}$.

10. $\displaystyle\int_{-1/2}^{1/2} \left(\frac{1+2x}{1-2x}\right)^{1/2}dx$.

11. $\displaystyle\int_1^\infty \frac{dx}{x^\lambda}$,   for $\lambda > 0$.

12. $\displaystyle\int_{-\infty}^\infty x\,e^{-x^2}dx$.

13. $\displaystyle\int_0^2 \frac{dx}{1-x^2}$.

14. $\displaystyle\int_0^{1/2} \frac{dx}{x\ln x}$.

41   Numerical integration

The integrands of many definite integrals are sufficiently complicated that an antiderivative cannot be found, so their value cannot be determined analytically. In such cases the value of the integral must be determined numerically. In this section we describe two methods for the numerical integration of a definite integral. The slightly simpler and far less accurate of the two methods is called the **trapezoidal rule**. The second and far more accurate method, which computationally takes no longer, is called **Simpson's rule**. These are only two of a large class of methods for the numerical integration of definite integrals which collectively are called **quadrature formulas**. The term quadrature formula is simply a synonym for numerical integration formula.

TRAPEZOIDAL RULE WITH n EQUAL STRIPS

To derive the formula for this rule when used to evaluate

$$I = \int_a^b f(x)\,dx,$$

the interval of integration $a \leqslant x \leqslant b$ is first divided into n equal strips (divisions) of width h, with

$$h = (b - a)/n \qquad (n \text{ an integer}).$$

If x_r is the left-hand end point of the rth strip, it then follows that

$$x_r = a + (r - 1)h, \quad \text{with} \quad r = 1, 2, ..., n.$$

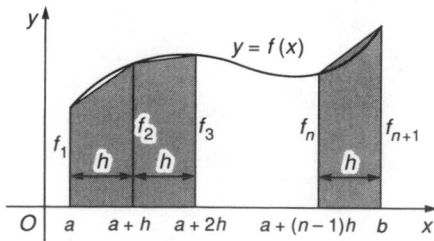

Fig. 91

Now set

$$f_r = f(x_r), \quad \text{with} \quad r = 1, 2, ..., n, n+1,$$

so the f_r are the functional values assumed by $f(x)$ at the ends of the strips, with $f_1 = f(a)$ and $f_{n+1} = f(b)$.

Now approximate the graph of $y = f(x)$ for $a \leqslant x \leqslant b$ by the polygonal line shown in Fig. 91. The approximate value of the definite integral I (interpreted as the area below the curve) is then seen to be given by the sum of the areas of the n shaded trapezia.

The area of the rth trapezium is $\frac{1}{2} h(f_r + f_{r+1})$, so

$$I \approx \frac{1}{2} h(f_1 + f_2) + \frac{1}{2} h(f_2 + f_3) + \ldots + \frac{1}{2} h(f_{n-1} + f_n) + \frac{1}{2} h(f_n + f_{n+1}),$$

or

$$I = h\left(\frac{1}{2} f_1 + f_2 + f_3 + \ldots + f_n + \frac{1}{2} f_{n+1}\right).$$

This is the trapezoidal rule, and the numbers $\frac{1}{2}, 1, 1, 1, ..., 1, \frac{1}{2}$ multiplying the ordinates f_i are called the **weight coefficients for the trapezoidal rule**.

The magnitude of the error involved can be estimated by means of the error estimate given in the following rule, though we will not discuss its derivation.

Trapezoidal rule
To evaluate

$$I = \int_a^b f(x)\,dx$$

using n equal width strips set

$$h = (b-a)/n, \quad x_r = a + (r-1)h \quad \text{and} \quad f_r = f(x_r),$$

with $r = 1, 2, ..., n+1$. Then

$$I \approx h\left(\frac{1}{2} f_1 + f_2 + f_3 + \ldots + f_n + \frac{1}{2} f_{n+1}\right).$$

If the error involved is E_T, so that

$$I = h\left(\frac{1}{2} f_1 + f_2 + \ldots + f_n + \frac{1}{2} f_{n+1}\right) + E_T,$$

an estimate of the magnitude of E_T is given by

$$\left|E_T\right| \leqslant \frac{h^2(b-a)}{12} M_T,$$

where $M_T = \max \left|d^2 f/dx^2\right|$ for $a \leqslant x \leqslant b$.

SIMPSON'S RULE

In the derivation of this rule the interval $a \leqslant x \leqslant b$ is divided into an even number of strips n, so

$$h = (b - a)/n \qquad (n \text{ an even integer}).$$

A parabola (quadratic function) is then fitted so that it passes through the functional values at the two end points and mid-point of successive pairs of adjacent intervals (strips), and each of the $n/2$ quadratic expressions so obtained is then integrated analytically. We omit the details, but the rule that results is Simpson's rule. This rule, together with its error estimate, is stated below.

Simpson's rule
To evaluate

$$I = \int_a^b f(x)\,dx$$

using an even number n of equal width strips set

$$h = (b - a)/n, \quad x_r = a + (r - 1)h \quad \text{and} \quad f_r = f(x_r),$$

with $r = 1, 2, ..., n + 1$. Then

$$I \approx \frac{h}{3}\left(f_1 + 4f_2 + 2f_3 + 4f_4 + 2f_5 + ... + 4f_n + f_{n+1}\right).$$

If the error involved is E_S, so that

$$I = \frac{h}{3}\left(f_1 + 4f_2 + 2f_3 + ... + 4f_n + f_{n+1}\right) + E_S,$$

an estimate of the magnitude of E_S is given by

$$\left| E_S \right| \leqslant \frac{h^4(b - a)}{180} M_S,$$

where

$$M_S = \max \left| d^4 f/dx^4 \right| \quad \text{for} \quad a \leqslant x \leqslant b.$$

The numbers 1, 4, 2, 4, 2, ..., 4, 1 multiplying the ordinates f_i are called the **weight coefficients for Simpson's rule**.

Example 41.1

Find

$$I = \int_1^2 x \ln x \, dx$$

by the trapezoidal rule and Simpson's rule using four strips in each case. Estimate the magnitude of the error involved when using each rule and compare the results of the numerical integrations with the analytical result.

Solution
The lower limit $a = 1$, the upper limit $b = 2$ and there are four strips ($n = 4$) so $h = (b - a)/n = 0.25$ and $x_r = 1 + (r - 1)/4$ (Table 6).

Table 6

r	x_r	$f_r = x_r \ln x_r$	Trapezoidal weights and products		Simpson weights and products	
(1)	(2)	(3)	(4)	(5)	(6)	(7)
1	1.0	0	0.5	0	1	0
2	1.25	0.278 93	1	0.278 93	4	1.115 72
3	1.5	0.608 20	1	0.608 20	2	1.216 40
4	1.75	0.979 33	1	0.979 33	4	3.917 32
5	2.0	1.386 29	0.5	0.693 15	1	1.386 29

Let

$$\sum_T = \text{sum of column 5 and } \sum_S = \text{sum of column 7,}$$

so that

$$\sum_T = 2.559\,61 \quad \text{and} \quad \sum_S = 7.635\,73.$$

Then

$$I_{\text{trapezoid}} = h \sum_T = 0.25 \times 2.559\,61 = 0.639\,90$$

and

$$I_{\text{Simpson}} = \frac{h}{3} \sum_S = \frac{0.25}{3} \times 7.635\,73 = 0.636\,31.$$

Thus the trapezoidal estimate is seen to differ from the Simpson estimate by an amount of order 0.003.

To estimate the magnitude of the actual errors involved in each case we proceed as follows:

$$f(x) = x \ln x, \quad \frac{df}{dx} = 1 + \ln x, \quad \frac{d^2 f}{dx^2} = \frac{1}{x}$$

$$\frac{d^3 f}{dx^3} = -\frac{1}{x^2} \quad \text{and} \quad \frac{d^4 f}{dx^4} = \frac{2}{x^3}.$$

Now $M_T = \max |d^2 f/dx^2|$ for $1 \leqslant x \leqslant 2$, so

$$M_T = \max_{1 \leqslant x \leqslant 2} |1/x| = 1,$$

while

$$M_S = \max |d^4 f/dx^4| \quad \text{for} \quad 1 \leqslant x \leqslant 2,$$

so

$$M_S = \max_{1 \leqslant x \leqslant 2} |2/x^3| = 2.$$

Thus

$$\left|E_\mathrm{T}\right| \leqslant \frac{(0.25)^2}{12} \times 1 = 0.005\,21$$

while

$$\left|E_\mathrm{S}\right| \leqslant \frac{(0.25)^4}{180} \times 2 = 0.000\,09.$$

Consequently,

$$I = 0.639\,90 \pm 0.005\,21 \text{ (trapezoidal estimate)}$$

and

$$I = 0.636\,31 \pm 0.000\,09 \text{ (Simpson estimate)}.$$

The actual value found by integration by parts is

$$I = \int_1^2 x \ln x \, \mathrm{d}x = \left(\frac{x^2}{2} \ln x - \frac{x^2}{4}\right)\bigg|_1^2 = 0.636\,29. \qquad \blacktriangle$$

The values of M_S and M_T used in the error estimates are not always as easily determined as in the above example. Thus, in practice, M_T is often replaced by the average of the values of $\left|\mathrm{d}^2 f/\mathrm{d}x^2\right|$ at the points x_r in $a \leqslant x \leqslant b$. Similarly, M_S is often replaced by the average of the values of $\left|\mathrm{d}^4 f/\mathrm{d}x^4\right|$ at the points x_r in $a \leqslant x \leqslant b$.

When a quadrature rule is used on a computer the analytical estimate of the magnitude of the error is usually omitted. In its place the accuracy is estimated by comparing the value obtained using a given strip width h and the one obtained by doubling the number of strips (h becomes $h/2$).

PROBLEMS 41

1. Using the trapezium rule and Simpson's rule, each with eight strips, and working to five decimal places, estimate ln 3 by evaluating

$$\int_1^3 \frac{\mathrm{d}x}{x}.$$

Compare your results with the tabulated value of ln 3 = 1.098 61.

2. Using the trapezium rule and Simpson's rule, each with six strips, and working to five decimal places, find

$$\int_1^4 \ln(1 + x^2) \, \mathrm{d}x.$$

Compare your results with the analytical result obtained by using integration by parts.

3. Define the function $f(x)$ by

$$f(x) = \begin{cases} 1 & \text{if} \quad x = 0 \\ \dfrac{\sin x}{x} & \text{for} \quad x \neq 0 \end{cases}$$

Using Simpson's rule, first with four strips and then with eight strips, and working to five decimal places, find

$$\int_0^5 f(x)\,dx.$$

Compare your result with the tabulated value of 1.549 93. The function

$$\text{Si}(x) = \int_0^x \frac{\sin t}{t}\,dt,$$

for which you have found Si(5) is called the **sine integral**.

4. Using the trapezoidal rule and Simpson's rule, each with eight strips, find

$$\int_0^2 x\,e^x\,dx.$$

Compare your results with the analytical result obtained by using integration by parts.

5. Using Simpson's rule, first with four strips and then with eight strips, find

$$\int_0^\pi \frac{x\sin 3x}{\sqrt{(1+x^2)}}\,dx.$$

Compare the results with the value 0.358 56 obtained by means of a high accuracy quadrature formula. Suggest why there is such a large difference between the values with four and eight strips.

6. Using Simpson's rule with eight strips, and working to five decimal places, find

$$\int_{-1}^2 \left(\frac{3+x}{3-x}\right)^{1/2}\,dx.$$

By writing the integrand as

$$\left(\frac{3+x}{3-x}\right)^{1/2} = \left[\frac{(3+x)^2}{(3-x)(3+x)}\right]^{1/2} = \frac{3+x}{\sqrt{(9-x^2)}},$$

evaluate the integral analytically and hence find the exact value of the integral.

7. Using Simpson's rule with six strips, and working to five decimal places, find

$$\int_0^{3\pi/4} |\sin x| \sqrt{(1 + \cos^2 x)} \, dx.$$

Compare the result with the value 1.910 05 obtained by means of a high accuracy quadrature formula.

8. Using Simpson's rule with eight strips, and working to five decimal places, find

$$\int_0^{2\pi} \sqrt{x} \sin x \, dx.$$

Compare the result with the value − 1.894 69 obtained by means of a high accuracy quadrature formula.

Geometrical applications of definite integrals   42

DETERMINATION OF AREAS

The definite integral was introduced in Section 38 in terms of the area between a curve $y = f(x)$, the x-axis and the lines $x = a$ and $x = b$, with due regard to the sign of the area (areas above the x-axis are positive, and those below it are negative).

Because of this interpretation, it follows that if $f(x) \geqslant g(x)$ for $a \leqslant x \leqslant b$, the area A contained between the two curves $y = f(x)$ and $y = g(x)$ is given by

$$A = \int_a^b [f(x) - g(x)] \, dx$$

$$= \int_a^b f(x) \, dx - \int_a^b g(x) \, dx.$$

The sign convention for areas in terms of definite integrals means that A will be the actual area between the curves because $f(x) - g(x) \geqslant 0$, so A will be positive.

Example 42.1

Find the area enclosed between the line $y = x + 2$ and the parabola $y = x^2 - 4$ for $-2 \leqslant x \leqslant 3$.

Solution
The area A between the two curves is shown in Fig. 92. As the line $y = x + 2$ lies above the parabola $y = x^2 - 4$ for $-2 \leqslant x \leqslant 3$, it follows that

$$A = \int_{-2}^3 [x + 2 - (x^2 - 4)] \, dx$$

$$= \int_{-2}^3 (6 + x - x^2) \, dx$$

$$= 125/6. \qquad \blacktriangle$$

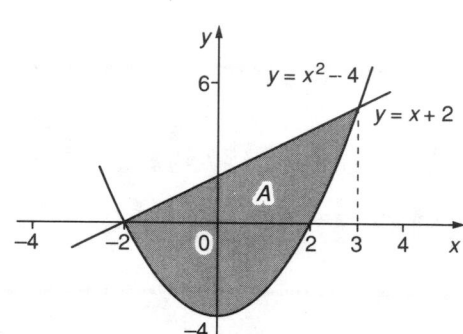

Fig. 92

ARC LENGTH

The length of an arc of a curve $y = f(x)$ between $x = a$ and $x = b$ may be determined in terms of a definite integral. The situation is illustrated in Fig. 93, in which P and Q are two adjacent points on the curve $y = f(x)$ whose x-coordinates differ by Δx. If Δs is the length of the chord PQ, it follows from Pythagoras' theorem that

$$(\Delta s)^2 = (\Delta x)^2 + (\Delta y)^2.$$

Then, as $\Delta x \to 0$, so $\Delta s \to \mathrm{d}s$ the differential element of arc length along the curve. Dividing by $(\Delta x)^2$ and letting $\Delta x \to 0$ this becomes

$$\left(\frac{\mathrm{d}s}{\mathrm{d}x}\right)^2 = 1 + \left(\frac{\mathrm{d}y}{\mathrm{d}x}\right)^2,$$

where s is the arc length along the curve.

As $\mathrm{d}y/\mathrm{d}x = f'(x)$, it follows that in terms of differentials,

$$\mathrm{d}s = \sqrt{\{1 + [f'(x)]^2\}}\ \mathrm{d}x.$$

Integrating along the curve from A to B gives

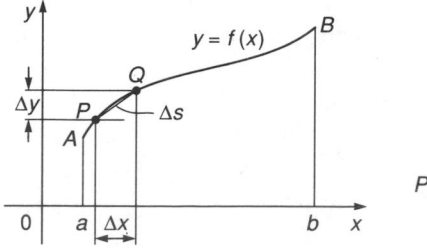

Fig. 93

$$s = \int_A^B ds = \int_a^b \sqrt{\{1 + [f'(x)]^2\}}\, dx.$$

We have thus arrived at the following result.

Formula for arc length
The arc length s along the curve $y = f(x)$ from $x = a$ to $x = b$ is given by

$$s = \int_a^b \sqrt{\{1 + [f'(x)]^2\}}\, dx.$$

Example 42.2

Find the length of the arc of the curve $x^2 + y^2 = a^2$ in the first quadrant from $x = \alpha$ to $x = \beta$, where $0 \leqslant \alpha < \beta \leqslant a$.

Solution
The curve $x^2 + y^2 = a^2$ is a circle of radius a, centred on the origin, as shown in Fig. 94. Writing this in the form $y = f(x)$, with $f(x) = \sqrt{(a^2 - x^2)}$, differentiation with respect to x gives

$$f'(x) = -x/\sqrt{(a^2 - x^2)},$$

and thus

$$\sqrt{\{1 + [f'(x)]^2\}} = \frac{a}{\sqrt{(a^2 - x^2)}}.$$

Using this result in the above formula gives

$$s = \int_\alpha^\beta \frac{a}{\sqrt{(a^2 - x^2)}}\, dx = \left(a \arcsin \frac{x}{a} \right)\Big|_\alpha^\beta,$$

and so

$$s/a \left(\arcsin \frac{\beta}{a} - \arcsin \frac{\alpha}{a} \right) = \left(\frac{\pi}{2} - \theta_2 \right) - \left(\frac{\pi}{2} - \theta_1 \right) = (\theta_1 - \theta_2),$$

as would be expected. If $\alpha = 0$ and $\beta = a$ this reduces to $s = a\pi/2$ which is simply the arc length of a quadrant of a circle.

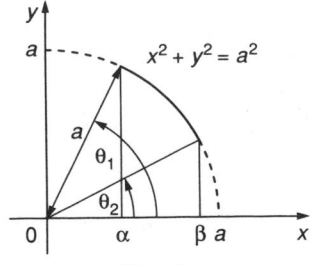

Fig. 94

The formula for arc length along a curve is easily adapted to the case in which the curve is specified in terms of a parameter θ. Let a curve be specified in the parametric form $x = X(\theta)$ and $y = Y(\theta)$, where θ is a parameter, and suppose we wish to determine the length of the arc of this curve between the points on the curve corresponding to $\theta = \alpha$ to $\theta = \beta$.

Starting from the result

$$ds = \sqrt{\left[1 + \left(\frac{dy}{dx}\right)^2\right]}\, dx,$$

and using the results from parametric differentiation (Section 21)

$$\frac{dy}{dx} = \frac{dy}{d\theta}\frac{d\theta}{dx} = Y'(\theta)/X'(\theta)$$

together with

$$dx = X'(\theta)\, d\theta,$$

shows that

$$ds = \sqrt{\{1 + [Y'(\theta)/X'(\theta)]^2\}}\, X'(\theta)\, d\theta.$$

Thus the formula for the arc length between the points on the curve corresponding to $\theta = \alpha$ to $\theta = \beta$ becomes

$$s = \int_{\alpha}^{\beta} \sqrt{\{1 + [Y'(\theta)/X'(\theta)]^2\}}\, X'(\theta)\, d\theta.$$

Example 42.3

Find the length of the cycloid

$$x = a(\theta - \sin\theta) \quad \text{and} \quad y = a(1 - \cos\theta)$$

between the points on the curve corresponding to $\theta = 0$ and $\theta = 2\pi$.

Solution
The section *OPA* of the cycloid in question is shown in Fig. 95, to which point *O* corresponds to $\theta = 0$, point *P* to $\theta = \pi$ and point *A* to $\theta = 2\pi$.

Now

$$X'(\theta) = a(1 - \cos\theta) \quad \text{and} \quad Y'(\theta) = a\sin\theta,$$

so substituting into the formula for arc length gives

$$s = \int_{0}^{2\pi} \sqrt{\left[1 + \left(\frac{\sin\theta}{1 - \cos\theta}\right)^2\right]}\, a(1 - \cos\theta)\, d\theta$$

$$= a \int_{0}^{2\pi} \sqrt{\left[\frac{2 - 2\cos\theta}{(1 - \cos\theta)^2}\right]}(1 - \cos\theta)\, d\theta$$

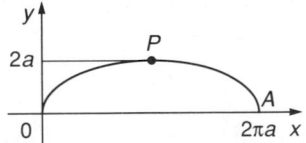

Fig. 95

$$= a \int_0^{2\pi} \sqrt{[2 - 2 \cos \theta]} \, d\theta.$$

Using the result $1 - \cos \theta = 2 \sin^2 \frac{1}{2} \theta$ brings this to the form

$$s = 2a \int_0^{2\pi} \sin \frac{1}{2} \theta \, d\theta,$$

$$= \left(-4a \cos \frac{1}{2} \theta \right) \Bigg|_0^{2\pi} = 8a,$$

and so the required length of the arc OPA is seen to be

$$s = 8a. \qquad \blacktriangle$$

AREA OF A SURFACE OF REVOLUTION

If an arc of a curve $y = f(x)$ lying between $x = a$ and $x = b$ is rotated about the x-axis it generates a **surface of revolution** about the x-axis as shown in Fig. 96. The area S of this surface or revolution comprises the sum of all strips of differential area dS contained between parallel planes normal to the x-axis and separated by the differential dx. The strip dS has a circular cross-section of radius $|y| = |f(x)|$. We denote the radius by $|f(x)|$ rather than $f(x)$ because a radius of a circle is always considered to be non-negative.

If the differential element of arc length along this strip is ds it follows that

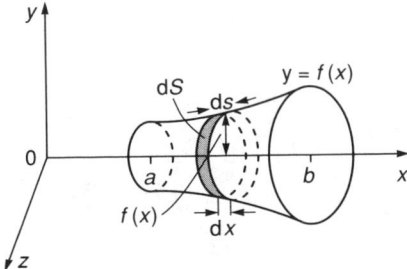

Fig. 96

$$dS = (\text{circumference of strip}) \times ds$$

so

$$dS = 2\pi \ |f(x)| \ ds.$$

Now we have already seen that

$$ds = \sqrt{\{1 + [f'(x)]^2\}} \ dx,$$

so

$$dS = 2\pi \ |f(x)| \ \sqrt{\{1 + [f'(x)]^2\}} \ dx.$$

Thus integrating from $x = a$ to $x = b$ gives

$$S = 2\pi \int_a^b |f(x)| \ \sqrt{\{1 + [f'(x)]^2\}} \ dx.$$

We have established the following result.

Formula for the area of a surface of revolution about the x-axis
The area S of a surface of revolution obtained by rotating the curve $y = f(x)$ about the x-axis between $x = a$ and $x = b$ is

$$S = 2\pi \int_a^b |f(x)| \ \sqrt{\{1 + [f'(x)]^2\}} \ dx.$$

Example 42.4

Find the area of the surface of revolution obtained when the curve $x^2 + y^2 = a^2$ is rotated about the x-axis between $x = \alpha$ and $x = a$, with $0 \leqslant \alpha < a$.

Solution
The curve $x^2 + y^2 = a^2$ is a circle of radius a centred on the origin. Thus rotating it about the x-axis will generate a spherical surface centred on the origin of radius a. The portion of this surface contained between $x = \alpha$ and $x = a$ is a **spherical cap**, as shown in Fig. 97.

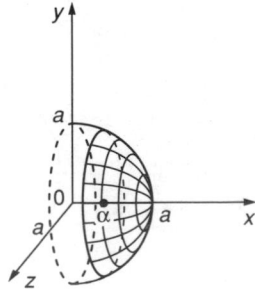

Fig. 97

We know from Example 42.2 that

$$\sqrt{\{1 + [f'(x)]^2\}} = \frac{a}{\sqrt{(a^2 - x^2)}}.$$

Thus as

$$|f(x)| = \sqrt{(a^2 - x^2)},$$

it follows from the above formula that

$$S = 2\pi \int_\alpha^a |f(x)| \sqrt{\{1 + [f'(x)]^2\}} \, dx$$

$$= 2\pi \int_\alpha^a [\sqrt{(a^2 - x^2)}] \frac{a}{\sqrt{(a^2 - x^2)}} \, dx$$

$$= 2\pi a \int_\alpha^a dx,$$

and so

$$S = 2\pi \, a(a - \alpha).$$

As would be expected, if $\alpha = 0$ the spherical cap becomes a hemispherical surface with area $A = 2\pi a^2$.   ▲

Note that a surface of revolution may also be generated if the arc of the curve $y = f(x)$ in Fig. 96 is rotated about the y-axis. An analogous argument then establishes the following result.

Formula for the area of a surface of revolution about the y-axis
The area S of a surface of revolution obtained by rotating the curve $x = g(x)$ about the y-axis between $y = c$ and $y = d$ is

$$S = 2\pi \int_c^d |g(y)| \sqrt{\{1 + [g'(y)]^2\}} \, dy.$$

This situation is illustrated in Fig. 98.

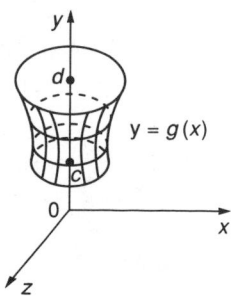

Fig. 98

VOLUME OF A SURFACE OF REVOLUTION

Let us determine the volume V contained within the surface of revolution generated by rotating $y = f(x)$ about the x-axis between $x = a$ and $x = b$. This is often called the **volume of revolution** of $y = f(x)$ about the x-axis between $x = a$ and $x = b$.

The situation is illustrated in Fig. 96, from which it can be seen that the volume V will be the sum of the differential elements of volume dV (slices) contained between planes normal to the x-axis and separated by the differential dx.

Then clearly,

$$dV = \pi y^2 dx$$

or, as $y = f(x)$,

$$dV = \pi \, [f(x)]^2 \, dx.$$

Integrating from $x = a$ to $x = b$ gives

$$V = \pi \int_a^b [f(x)]^2 \, dx.$$

We thus arrive at our last result.

Formula for a volume of revolution
The volume V contained within the surface of revolution generated by rotating the curve $y = f(x)$ about the x-axis between $x = a$ and $x = b$ is

$$V = \pi \int_a^b [f(x)]^2 \, dx.$$

Example 42.5

Find the volume contained within the surface of revolution generated by rotating the curve $x^2 + y^2 = a^2$ about the x-axis between $x = \alpha$ and $x = a$, with $0 \leqslant \alpha < a$.

Solution
We are required to find the volume contained within the spherical cap shown in Fig. 97. As $y^2 = a^2 - x^2$ it follows from the above formula that

$$V = \pi \int_\alpha^a (a^2 - x^2) \, dx$$

$$= \pi \, a^2(a - \alpha) - \frac{\pi}{3} (a^3 - \alpha^3).$$

Thus the required volume

$$V = \frac{\pi}{3}(2a^3 - 3\alpha a^2 + \alpha^3).$$

Notice that when $a = 0$ this reduces to the volume of a hemisphere $2\pi a^3/3$, as would be expected.   ▲

PROBLEMS 42

1.   Find the area between the curves $y = 3 + \sin 2x$ and $y = \frac{1}{2}\cos x$ from $x = 0$ to $x = \pi$.

2.   Find the area between the curves $y = \sin x$ and $y = \cos x$ from $x = 0$ to $x = \pi$. (Hint: remember that $\sin x \ngtr \cos x$ for all x in $0 \leqslant x \leqslant \pi$.)

3.   Find the length of arc along the curve $y = \cosh x$ from $x = 1$ to $x = 3$.

4.   Find the length of arc along the curve $y = 2x^{3/2} + 1$ from $x = 0$ to $x = 1$.

5.   Find the length of arc along the curve $y = \ln|(1 + \sin x)/\cos x|$ from $x = 0$ to $x = \pi/4$.

6.   Find the length of arc along the curve $y = \dfrac{x^5}{10} + \dfrac{1}{6x^3}$ from $x = 1$ to $x = 3$.

7.   The four pointed star-shaped curve defined in terms of the parameter θ by $x = a\cos^3\theta$ and $y = a\sin^3\theta$ is called an **astroid**. Show that if the arc length s along the curve is required to increase with θ, then by making a suitable choice of sign in the square root, $\mathrm{d}s/\mathrm{d}\theta = 3/2$. Hence find the length of the arc of this astroid between the two adjacent 'points' on the star corresponding to $\theta = 0$ and $\theta = \pi/2$, and deduce the total length of the curve.

8.   Find the area of the surface of revolution obtained by rotating $y = \cosh x$ about the x-axis between $x = 1$ and $x = 2$.

9.   Find the area of the surface of revolution generated when $y = x^3$ is rotated about the x-axis from $x = 1$ to $x = 2$.

10. Find the area of the surface of revolution generated when $y = 3 - x$ is rotated about the y-axis from $x = 1$ to $x = 3$.

11. Find the volume contained within the surface of revolution generated when $y = \cosh x$ is rotated about the x-axis from $x = 0$ to $x = 2$.

12. Find the volume contained within the surface of revolution generated when $y = \sin x$ is rotated about the x-axis from $x = \pi/4$ to $x = \pi/2$.

13. Find the volume contained within the surface of revolution generated when $y = \arcsin x$ is rotated about the x-axis from $x = 0$ to $x = 1$.

14. Find the volume contained within the surface of revolution generated when $y = \operatorname{arsinh} x$ is rotated about the x-axis from $x = 2$ to $x = 4$.

43 Centre of mass of a plane lamina (centroid)

To understand the notion of the **centre of mass** (CM) (or **centre of gravity** (CG)) of a two-dimensional (plane) lamina, we start by considering a distribution of n point masses $m_1, m_2, ..., m_n$ in the plane. Imagine the plane in which the masses are located to be horizontal, weightless and rigid. Then the **moment** of these masses about a line L in the plane measures their combined turning effect about the line L. The **magnitude** M_L of the moment is defined to be

$$M_L = m_1 d_1 + m_2 d_2 + ... + m_n d_n,$$

where d_i is the perpendicular distance of m_i from L, with d_i taken to be positive when m_i lies on one side of the line and negative when it lies on the other (the choice of which side is positive is arbitrary).

An immediate consequence of this definition is seen to be that if the masses are distributed symmetrically about L then $M_L = 0$, because the moment of each mass to one side of L will be cancelled by the moment of a corresponding mass on the opposite side. Any mass lying on L will not, of course, contribute to M_L since its distance from L will be zero.

There will be a moment of magnitude M_L about any line L in the plane due to the n masses $m_1, m_2, ..., m_n$. The centre of mass of these particles is that point in the plane at which all the masses may be concentrated into a single mass $M = m_1 + m_2 + ... + m_n$ such that the moment of M about L equals M_L.

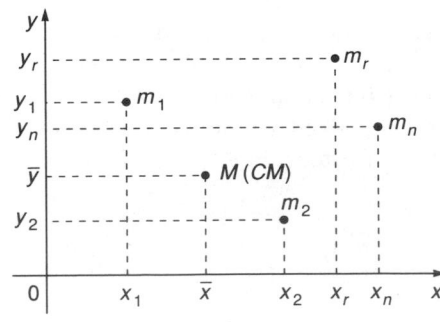

Fig. 99

Let the mass m_i be located at the point (x_i, y_i) in the (x, y)-plane for $i = 1, 2, ..., n$, as illustrated in Fig. 99. Then the moment about any line L in the plane may be resolved into two separate moments at right angles to one another, with one about the x-axis and the other about the y-axis.

The moment M_x of the masses about the x-axis is

$$M_x = m_1 y_1 + m_2 y_2 + ... + m_n y_n,$$

and the moment M_y of the masses about the y-axis is

$$M_y = m_1 x_1 + m_2 x_2 + ... + m_n x_n.$$

The moment of the combined mass $M = m_1 + m_2 + ... + m_n$ located at the centre of gravity which we take to be at the point $(\bar{x}, \bar{y})$ is $M\bar{y}$ about the x-axis and $M\bar{x}$ about the y-axis. Thus, from the definition of the centre of mass,

$$M\bar{y} = m_1 y_1 + m_2 y_2 + ... + m_n y_n$$

and

$$M\bar{x} = m_1 x_1 + m_2 x_2 + ... + m_n x_n,$$

and thus the centre of mass is located at the point $(\bar{x}, \bar{y})$, where

$$\bar{x} = \frac{m_1 x_1 + m_2 x_2 + ... + m_n x_n}{M} \quad \text{and} \quad \bar{y} = \frac{m_1 y_1 + m_2 y_2 + ... + m_n y_n}{M}.$$

When a continuous distribution of mass is involved these discrete sums become definite integrals. Consider the plane lamina shown in Fig. 100 which has a mass distribution in the x-direction of $\rho(x)$ per unit area of the lamina, with $f(x)$ and $g(x)$ such that $f(x) \geq g(x)$ for $a \leq x \leq b$. The area of the shaded rectangular strip of width Δx is $[f(x_i) - g(x_i)] \Delta x$, so as the mass distribution per unit area is $\rho(x)$, the mass of this strip is

$$\rho(x_i) [f(x_i) - g(x_i)] \Delta x.$$

By symmetry, the centre of mass of the rectangular strip must be located at its mid-point $\frac{1}{2} [f(x_i) + g(x_i)]$, so the moment of this strip about the x-axis is

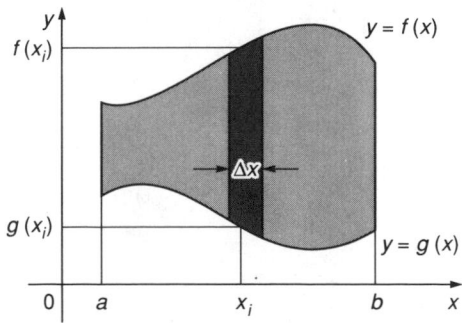

Fig. 100

$$\frac{1}{2} \rho (x_i) [f(x_i) - g(x_i)] [f(x_i) + g(x_i)] \Delta x.$$

Integrating from $x = a$ to $x = b$ we find that in the limit as $\Delta x \to 0$,

$$M_x = \frac{1}{2} \int_a^b \rho (x) \{[f(x)]^2 - [g(x)]^2\} \, dx.$$

A similar argument shows that the moment of the lamina about the y-axis is

$$M_y = \int_a^b x\rho (x) [f(x) - g(x)] \, dx,$$

while the total mass of the lamina is seen to be

$$M = \int_a^b \rho (x) [f(x) - g(x)] \, dx.$$

Thus the centre of mass is located at

$$\bar{x} = \frac{M_y}{M} \quad \text{and} \quad \bar{y} = \frac{M_x}{M}.$$

We have arrived at the following result.

Formula for the centre of mass of a plane lamina
Let a plane lamina with a mass distribution in the x-direction of $\rho (x)$ per unit area occupy the region between the curves $y = f(x)$ and $y = g(x)$, and the lines $x = a$ and $x = b$, with $f(x) \leqslant g(x)$, for $a \leqslant x \leqslant b$. Then if,

$$M_x = \frac{1}{2} \int_a^b \rho (x) \{[f(x)]^2 - [g(x)]^2\} \, dx,$$

$$M_y = \int_a^b x\rho (x) [f(x) - g(x)] \, dx,$$

and

$$M = \int_a^b \rho (x) [f(x) - g(x)] \, dx,$$

the centre of mass of the lamina is located at the point $(\bar{x}, \bar{y})$, where

$$\bar{x} = \frac{M_y}{M} \quad \text{and} \quad \bar{y} = \frac{M_x}{M}.$$

Example 43.1

Find the centre of mass of a plane lamina in the form of an equilateral triangle of side $2a$ with a uniform mass distribution $\rho (x) = \rho_0 = $ constant.

Solution

From symmetry, the centre of mass must lie on one of the medians of the equilateral triangle. To take advantage of this, let us locate the (x, y) axes as shown in Fig. 101. The upper edge of the triangle then has the equation $y = a - x/\sqrt{3}$ and the lower edge the equation $y = -a + x/\sqrt{3}$, for $0 \leqslant x \leqslant a\sqrt{3}$.

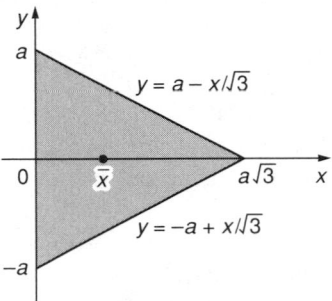

Fig. 101

Let the centre of mass be located at the point $(\bar{x}, 0)$. Then using the notation of the rule for the determination of the centre of mass, $f(x) = a - x/\sqrt{3}$, $g(x) = -a + x/\sqrt{3}$ and $\rho(x) = \rho_0$, so

$$M_y = \rho_0 \int_0^{a\sqrt{3}} x \left[\left(a - \frac{1}{\sqrt{3}} x \right) - \left(-a + \frac{1}{\sqrt{3}} x \right) \right] dx$$

$$= 2\rho \int_0^{a\sqrt{3}} x \left(a - \frac{1}{\sqrt{3}} x \right) dx$$

$$= \rho_0 a^3$$

while

$$M = \rho_0 \int_0^{a\sqrt{3}} \left[\left(a - \frac{1}{\sqrt{3}} x \right) - \left(-a + \frac{1}{\sqrt{3}} x \right) \right] dx$$

$$= 2\rho_0 \int_0^{a\sqrt{3}} \left(a - \frac{1}{\sqrt{3}} x \right) dx$$

$$= \rho_0 a^2 \sqrt{3}.$$

Thus

$$\bar{x} = \frac{M_y}{M} = \frac{\rho_0 a^3}{\rho_0 a^3 \sqrt{3}} = \frac{a}{\sqrt{3}},$$

so the centre of mass is located at $(a/\sqrt{3}, 0)$.   ▲

It often happens that the method of calculation used to determine the location of the centre of mass of a plane lamina needs to be applied to situations in which only a planar area is involved without any associated distribution of mass. This may be accomplished by means of the rule set out above for the determination of the centre of mass by setting $\rho = 1$. In such circumstances we speak of the **centroid** of the area instead of its centre of mass. Thus from Example 43.1 we see that the centroid of an equilateral triangle is located one-third of the distance along a median measured from the base.

Example 43.2

A lamina in the form of the equilateral triangle shown in Fig. 101 has a mass distribution $\rho(x) = \rho_0(1 + kx)$ per unit area in the x-direction, with ρ_0 and k constants. Find the position of its centre of mass.

Solution
As the mass distribution only changes in the x-direction and it is symmetrical about the x-axis, the centre of mass must lie on the x-axis.

Using the notation of the rule for the determination of the centre of mass we see that, as in Example 43.1, $f(x) = a - x/\sqrt{3}$, $g(x) = -a + x/\sqrt{3}$, but now $\rho(x) = \rho_0(1 + kx)$. Thus

$$M_y = \rho_0 \int_0^{a\sqrt{3}} x(1 + kx)\left[\left(a - \frac{1}{\sqrt{3}}x\right) - \left(-a + \frac{1}{\sqrt{3}}x\right)\right]dx$$

$$= \frac{1}{2}\rho_0 a^3(2 + ak\sqrt{3})$$

and

$$M = \rho_0 \int_0^{a\sqrt{3}} (1 + kx)\left[\left(a - \frac{1}{\sqrt{3}}x\right) - \left(-a + \frac{1}{\sqrt{3}}x\right)\right]dx$$

$$= \rho_0 a^2(\sqrt{3} + ak).$$

Thus

$$\bar{x} = \frac{M_y}{M} = \frac{1}{2}a\left(\frac{2 + ak\sqrt{3}}{\sqrt{3} + ak}\right),$$

and so the centre of mass of this non-uniform triangular lamina is located on the x-axis at the point $(\bar{x}, 0)$,   ▲

PROBLEMS 43

Find the location of the centre of mass of each of the laminas shown in problems 1 to 8 when the mass distribution in the lamina is uniform with $\rho(x) = \rho_0$.

1.

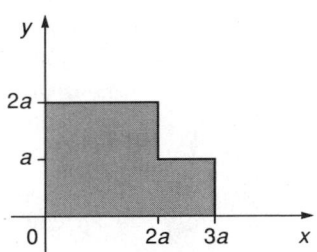

2.

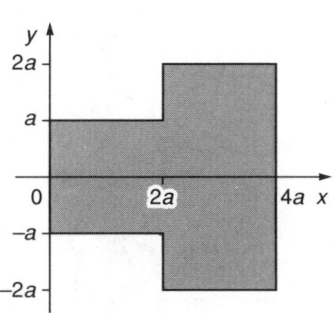

3.

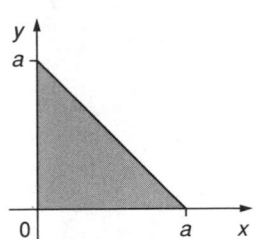

4.

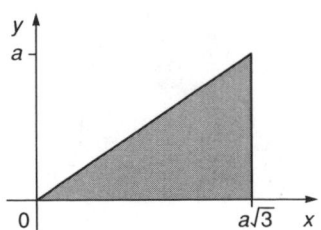

5.

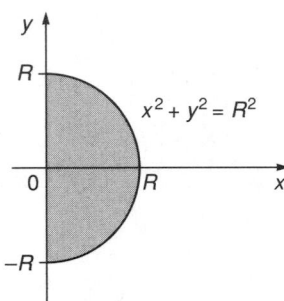

6.

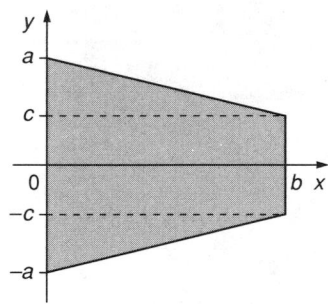

7.

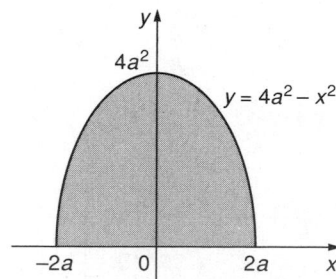

8.

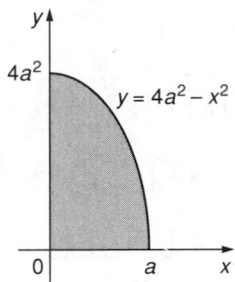

9.   Find the centre of mass of the trapezoidal lamina in problem 6 if the mass
     distribution per unit area in the x-direction is $p(x) = p_0(1 + kx)$.
10. Find the centre of mass of the parabolic lamina in problem 7 if the mass
     distribution per unit area in the x-direction is $p(x) = p_0(1 + kx)$.

Application of integration to the hydrostatic pressure on a plate

44

If an element of area ΔS is located horizontally at a depth h below the surface of a liquid, the force acting downwards on it equals the weight of the column of liquid above ΔS Thus if the density of the liquid is ρ, this weight is $F = \rho\, h\Delta S$. Pascal's law asserts that this force is independent of the orientation of the element of area ΔS so it may be horizontal, vertical or at an arbitrary inclination, and the fluid force will be the same. Forces due to liquid pressure are called **hydrostatic forces**, and the force per unit area $F/\Delta S$ is called the **hydrostatic pressure** in the liquid at the depth h. This means that if the element of area is completely immersed in liquid, the forces on either side of it will be equal and opposite. If, however, ΔS only has liquid on one side, the hydrostatic force will not be balanced by an equal and opposite one on the other side.

If a plate is thought of as forming the side wall of a tank containing liquid, there will be a distribution of hydrostatic pressure over the plate. The **centre of pressure** of the plate is the point on the plate at which a single force equal to the total force acting on the plate may be applied with the same external effect as the one produced by the hydrostatic pressure distribution. This means that the moment of this single force about any line L in the plate equals the sum of the moments about L produced by the hydrostatic pressure acting on each element of the plate.

When the location of the centroid of a vertical submerged plate is known, the determination of the total force F acting on a side in contact with the fluid is easily calculated. The force F is given by

$$F = \rho\, Sd, \tag{A}$$

where ρ is the fluid density, S is the area of the plate and d is the depth of the centroid of the plate below the surface.

To see why this is, let us calculate the total force acting on the vertical plate of arbitrary shape and area S shown in Fig. 102. The force ΔF acting normal to the horizontal strip AB of area ΔS located at a depth $h - y$ below the surface is

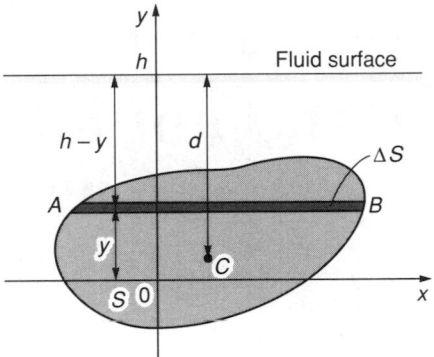

Fig. 102

$$\Delta F = \rho \, (h - y) \, \Delta S,$$

where ρ is the density of the fluid. Thus, summing all such forces acting on the plate and letting $\Delta S \to 0$, the force F is seen to be given by the integral

$$F = \int_{\text{Plate}} \rho \, (h - y) \, dS,$$

so

$$F = \rho \int_{\text{Plate}} (h - y) \, dS. \tag{B}$$

Here $\int_{\text{Plate}}$ means integration of $(h - y) \, dS$ over the entire plate.

However, from the definition of the centroid of an area, it follows that

$$\int_{\text{Plate}} (h - y) \, dS = Sd,$$

where d is the distance of the centroid C below the surface of the fluid. Combining these results then gives the required formula

$$F = \rho \, Sd.$$

If the location of the centroid is unknown, the determination of F will require the direct evaluation of integral (B) over the plate. To illustrate both the convenience of formula (A), and the way in which integral (B) is to be evaluated, the force F is obtained by each method in the two examples which follow.

Example 44.1

An equilateral triangular plate of side $2a$ is completely immersed in fluid and located in a vertical plane with a vertex at a depth h below the surface of the

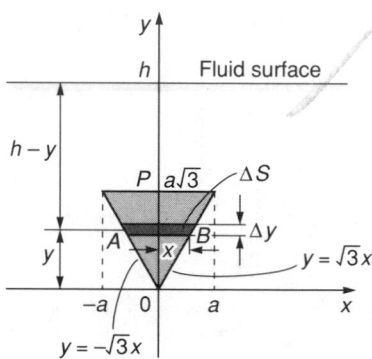

Fig. 103

fluid as shown in Fig. 103. Find the force acting on one side of the plate and the location of its centre of pressure.

Solution
Finding F by formula (A)
The area of the plate is $S = a^2\sqrt{3}$, and we know from Example 43.1 that the centroid is located at a distance $a/\sqrt{3}$ below the point P in Fig. 103. Thus the depth of the centroid below the fluid surface is $d = h - 2a/\sqrt{3}$. Applying formula (A) we find that

$$F = \rho\, a^2\sqrt{3}\,(h - 2a/\sqrt{3})$$

and so

$$F = \rho\, a^2\,(h\sqrt{3} - 2a).$$

Finding F by integral (B)
The equations of the inclined sides of the triangle are $y = \sqrt{3}x$ and $0 \le x \le a$ and $y = -\sqrt{3}x$ for $-a \le x \le 0$.
   The area of the strip AB is

$$\Delta S = 2x\Delta y$$

but $x = y/\sqrt{3}$

$$\Delta S = \frac{2}{\sqrt{3}}\, y\, \Delta y.$$

As the strip is at a depth $h - y$ it follows that the force acting on it is

$$\Delta F = \rho\,(h - y)\cdot\frac{2}{\sqrt{3}}\, y\, \Delta y.$$

   Integrating this result from $y = 0$ to $y = a\sqrt{3}$ (i.e. over the plate) and letting $\Delta y \to 0$ shows that the total force F acting on one side of the plate is given by the definite integral

$$F = \frac{2\rho}{\sqrt{3}} \int_0^{a\sqrt{3}} y(h - y)\, dy$$

$= \rho\, a^2(h\sqrt{3} - 2a)$. (The result given by formula (A).)

To determine the location of the centre of pressure we now proceed as follows. The moment ΔM_L of the force ΔF about the line L is

$$\Delta M_L = (h - y)\, \Delta F$$

$$= \frac{2\rho}{\sqrt{3}}\, y(h - y)^2\, \Delta y.$$

Integrating this result from $y = 0$ to $y = a\sqrt{3}$ (over the plate) and letting $\Delta y \to 0$ shows that the total moment M_L about the line L produced by the distributed hydrostatic forces is given by the definite integral

$$M_L = \frac{2\rho}{\sqrt{3}} \int_0^{a\sqrt{3}} y(h - y)^2\, dy$$

$$= \frac{1}{2}\, \rho\, a^2(3\sqrt{3}a^2 - 8ah + 2\sqrt{3}h^2).$$

We see from symmetry that the centre of pressure must lie on the y-axis, so let it be located at the point $(0, \bar{y})$. Then the moment about L produced by the total force F concentrated at the centroid is $F(h - \bar{y})$, so

$$F(h - \bar{y}) = M_L.$$

Substituting for F and M_L and solving for $\bar{y}$ gives

$$\bar{y} = \frac{h}{8} + \frac{3\sqrt{3}a}{4} - \frac{\sqrt{3}\, h^2}{8(\sqrt{3}h - 2a)},$$

In the special case in which the top of the triangular plate coincides with the surface of the fluid $h = a\sqrt{3}$. The force F and position of the centre of pressure $\bar{y}$ then reduce to

$$F = \rho\, a^3 \quad \text{and} \quad \bar{y} = \frac{\sqrt{3}a}{2}. \qquad \blacktriangle$$

Example 44.2

Find the total force acting on a plane circular window of radius R in the vertical side of a swimming pool, if the window is completely immersed with its centre at a depth h below the surface of the water. Determine the location of the centre of pressure.

Solution
Finding F from formula (A)
The area of the window is $S = \pi R^2$, and as by symmetry its centroid is at its centre it follows that the centroid is at a distance $d = h$ below the surface of the water, and so

$$F = \rho\, \pi R^2 h.$$

Finding F from integral (B)

The situation is illustrated in Fig. 104 where, for reasons of symmetry, the axes have been located as shown. The equation of the rim of the window is $x^2 + y^2 = R^2$, so $x = \sqrt{(R^2 - y^2)}$. If we consider the shaded strip of width $2x$ and thickness Δy, its area

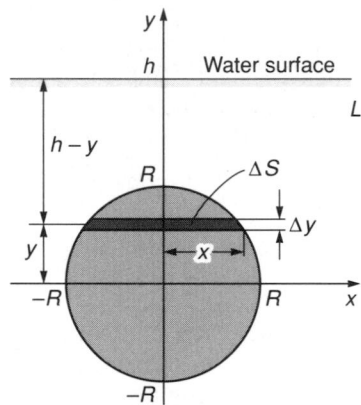

Fig. 104

$$\Delta S = 2x\Delta y = 2\sqrt{(R^2 - y^2)}\,\Delta y,$$

so as it is at a depth $h - y$ below the surface, the force acting on it is

$$\Delta F = \rho\,(h - y) \times 2\sqrt{(R^2 - y^2)}\,\Delta y,$$

where ρ is the density of the water.

Letting $\Delta y \to 0$, and combining the effects of all such strips we see that the total force F acting on the window is given by the definite integral

$$F = 2\rho \int_{-R}^{R} (h - y)\,\sqrt{(R^2 - y^2)}\,dy,$$

and so

$$F = 2\rho h \int_{-R}^{R} \sqrt{(R^2 - y^2)}\,dy - 2\rho \int_{-R}^{R} y\,\sqrt{(R^2 - y^2)}\,dy.$$

Only the first integral need be evaluated since the second one is zero. To see this we first recall the interpretation of a definite integral in terms of signed areas. With this in mind, we see that as the integrand $y\sqrt{(R^2 - y^2)}$ is an **odd function**, and the limits are **symmetric** about the origin, it follows that the integral is equivalent to the sum of two equal areas with opposite signs, and so vanishes.

Setting $y = R \sin \theta$ in the remaining integral gives

$$F = 2\rho\, hR \int_{-\pi/2}^{\pi/2} \sqrt{(1 - \sin^2\theta)}\, \cos\theta\; d\theta$$

$$= 2\rho\, hR^2 \int_{-\pi/2}^{\pi/2} \cos^2\theta\; d\theta.$$

As $\cos^2\theta = \dfrac{1}{2}(1 + \cos 2\theta)$ this may be rewritten as

$$F = \rho\, hR^2 \int_{-\pi/2}^{\pi/2} (1 + \cos 2\theta)\, d\theta,$$

and on integration this becomes

$$F = \rho\, \pi R^2 h.$$

To determine the location of the centre of pressure of the window we proceed as follows. The moment of strip about the line L in surface is

$$\Delta M_L = \Delta F(h - y),$$

so

$$\Delta M_L = 2\rho\,(h - y)^2 \sqrt{(R^2 - y^2)}\, \Delta y.$$

Summing over all strips and letting $\Delta y \to 0$ we find that the total moment about L is

$$M_L = 2\rho \int_{-R}^{R} (h - y)^2 \sqrt{(R^2 - y^2)}\, dy$$

$$= 2\rho\, h^2 \int_{-R}^{R} \sqrt{(R^2 - y^2)}\, dy - 4\rho\, h \int_{-R}^{R} y\sqrt{(R^2 - y^2)}\, dy + 2\rho \int_{-R}^{R} y^2 \sqrt{(R^2 - y^2)}\, dy.$$

However, we have already seen that

$$2 \int_{-R}^{R} \sqrt{(R^2 - y^2)}\, dy = \pi R^2,$$

and that the second integral is zero, so we only need determine the last integral. Thus

$$M_L = \rho\, \pi R^2 h^2 + 2\rho \int_{-R}^{R} y^2 \sqrt{(R^2 - y^2)}\, dy.$$

Setting $y = R \sin\theta$ gives

$$M_L = \rho\, \pi R^2 h^2 + 2\rho\, R^4 \int_{-\pi/2}^{\pi/2} \sin^2\theta \cos^2\theta\; d\theta.$$

Using integration by parts this reduces to

$$M_L = \rho \, \pi \, R^2 h^2 + \frac{1}{4} \rho \, \pi \, R^4$$

$$= \frac{1}{4} \rho \, \pi \, R^2 (4h^2 + R^2).$$

If the centre of pressure is at a distance d below the surface it then follows that

$$M_L = F d,$$

or

$$\frac{1}{4} \rho \, \pi \, R^2 (4h^2 + R^2) = \rho \, \pi \, R^2 h d,$$

and thus

$$d = h + \frac{R^2}{4h}. \qquad\qquad \blacktriangle$$

PROBLEMS 44

1. Find the location of the centre of pressure of a rectangular plate of width $2a$ and depth $2b$ when suspended vertically in a fluid of density ρ with its top edge of length $2a$ horizontal and its centre a depth h below the surface of the fluid.
2. Find the location of the centre of pressure of a triangular plate of arbitrary shape suspended vertically in a fluid of density ρ with one edge in the surface of the fluid.
3. Find the location of the centre of pressure of a semicircular plate of radius R suspended vertically in a fluid of density ρ with its bounding diameter in the surface.
4. Find the centre of pressure of a semicircular plate of radius R in the vertical plane submerged in a fluid of density ρ with its bounding diameter horizontal and at a depth h below the surface.

Moments of inertia

45

We begin by considering a system of n point masses $m_1, m_2, ..., m_n$ situated at perpendicular distances $d_1, d_2, ..., d_n$ from a straight line L. Then the quantity

$$I_L = m_1 d_1^2 + m_2 d_2^2 + ... + m_n d_n^2$$

is called the **moment of inertia** of the system of particles about L. If $M = m_1 + m_2 + ... + m_n$ is the total mass of the n particles, the length k_L defined by

$$M k_L^2 = I_L,$$

or equivalently by

$$k_L = (I_L / M)^{1/2},$$

is called the **radius of gyration** of the particles about the line L.

These ideas may be applied directly to continuous bodies by replacing the summation involved in the determination of I_L by an appropriate integral.

Thus if an element of mass Δm_i of a rigid body lies at a perpendicular distance r_i from a given line L, the moment of inertia of the body about L is

$$I_L = \lim_{\substack{\Delta m_i \to 0 \\ n \to \infty}} \sum_{i=1}^{n} r_i^2 \Delta m_i = \int_{\text{body}} r^2 dm,$$

where $\int_{\text{body}}$ represents integration over the region occupied by the body.

Example 45.1

Find the moment of inertia and radius of gyration about the y-axis of a thin rod of length a in the interval $0 \leqslant x \leqslant a$ if the mass per unit length of the rod is given by

$$\rho(x) = m\left(1 + \frac{2x}{a}\right).$$

Solution
The situation is shown in Fig. 105. The mass of the element AB of length Δx located at a distance x from 0 is

$$\Delta m = m\left(1 + \frac{2x}{a}\right)\Delta x,$$

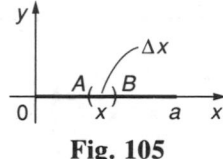

Fig. 105

so its moment of inertia about the y-axis is

$$\Delta I_y = mx^2 \left(1 + \frac{2x}{a}\right)\Delta x.$$

Thus letting $\Delta x \to 0$ and integrating over the length of the rod gives

$$I_y = m \int_0^a x^2 \left(1 + \frac{2x}{a}\right)dx$$

$$= \frac{5ma^3}{6}.$$

Now the total mass of the rod is

$$M = \int_0^a m \left(1 + \frac{2x}{a}\right)dx$$

$$= 2am,$$

so the radius of gyration about the y-axis is

$$k_y = (I_y/M)^{1/2} = a\sqrt{\frac{5}{12}}.$$

Example 45.2

Find the moment of inertia and radius of gyration of a disc of radius a and mass M about an axis L through its centre which is normal to its plane.

Solution
The area of the disc is πa^2 so its mass per unit area $\rho = M/\pi a^2$.

If we now divide the disc into annular rings and consider the one extending from r to $r + \Delta r$, where r is the radius of the inside of the annulus, as the area of the annulus is $2\pi r\Delta r$ its mass will be

$$\Delta M = (M/\pi a^2)\, 2\pi r\Delta r.$$

As this is at a distance r from the axis L, its moment of inertia about L will be

$$\Delta I_L = \frac{2M}{a^2}\, r^3 \Delta r.$$

Thus letting $\Delta r \rightarrow 0$ and integrating over the disc from $r=0$ to $r=a$ gives

$$I_L = \frac{2M}{a^2} \int_0^a r^3 dr = \frac{1}{2} Ma^2.$$

The radius of gyration

$$k_L = (I_L / M)^{1/2} = a/\sqrt{2}. \qquad\qquad \blacktriangle$$

PROBLEMS 45

1. Find the moment of inertia and radius of gyration of a thin rod of length $2a$ and mass M about an axis normal to its mid-point.
2. Find the moment of inertia and radius of gyration of a thin rod of length $2a$ and mass M about an axis normal to its length and distant $a/2$ from one end.
3. Find the moment of inertia and radius of gyration about the y-axis of the rod of length a illustrated in the diagram which extends from $x=-a/2$ to $x=a/2$ and has a mass per unit length of $\rho(x)=m\left(1+\dfrac{2x}{a}\right)$.

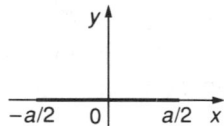

4. Find the moment of inertia and radius of gyration of the disc in Example 45.2 if its density per unit area is $\rho(x) = m(1 + r/a)$.
5. Find the moment of inertia of a uniform square lamina of mass M and side a about an edge.
6. Find the moment of inertia of an annular lamina of mass M with inner radius R_1 and outer radius R_2 about a line L through its centre which is normal to its plane.

46   Sequences

Before discussing series, it is necessary to give some brief consideration to the notion of a sequence and its limit. In the calculus a **sequence** is an arrangement of terms, either numbers or functions, in a definite order. Thus, $1, 1/2, (1/2)^2, (1/2)^3, \ldots$, is a sequence of numbers and $(1 + x/1)$, $(1 + x/2)^2$, $(1 + x/3)^3, \ldots$, is a sequence of functions. Changing the order of the terms in a sequence changes the sequence.

As the terms in a sequence occur in a definite order they may be numbered $1, 2, \ldots$, and then the natural order of the integers will determine the ordering of terms in the sequence. It is convenient to denote the nth term of a sequence, usually called the **general term**, by u_n in which the suffix n indicates the location of the term in the sequence. Thus if $u_n = (1/2)^n$ we see we have the nth term of the numerical sequence illustrated above. In the main we will only be concerned with **infinite sequences**, which are sequences with an infinite number of terms. In such cases we will be interested in the behaviour of u_n as $n \to \infty$, so the terms at the start of the sequence are usually unimportant. For this reason an infinite sequence is often denoted by $\{u_n\}$, it being understood that n can increase without bound with the starting point of the sequence being unimportant.

If there is a need for an explicit statement of the term with which a sequence begins and the one with which it ends we write $\{u_n\}_{n=M}^{N}$, meaning the finite sequence (finitely many terms) $u_M, u_{M+1}, \ldots, u_N$.

Some typical examples of sequences are listed below.

Infinite sequences of numbers

1 $1, 2^2, 3^2, 4^2, \ldots$; $\{u_n\}$ with the general term $u_n = n^2$;

2 $1, 1/2!, 1/3!, 1/4!, \ldots$; $\{u_n\}$; with general term $u_n = 1/n!$;

3 $\dfrac{1}{1 \cdot 2}, \dfrac{-1}{2 \cdot 3}, \dfrac{1}{3 \cdot 4}, \dfrac{-1}{4 \cdot 5}, \ldots$; $\{u_n\}$ with general term $u_n = \dfrac{(-1)^{n+1}}{n(n+1)}$;

4 $\dfrac{(2 \cdot 1)\cos(\pi)}{(3 \cdot 1) + 1}, \dfrac{(2 \cdot 2)\cos(2\pi)}{(3 \cdot 2) + 1}, \dfrac{(2 \cdot 3)\cos(3\pi)}{(3 \cdot 3) + 1}, \ldots$; $\{u_n\}$ with general term $u_n = \dfrac{2n\cos(n\pi)}{3n + 1}$.

Infinite sequences of functions

5 $1, x, x^2, x^3, \ldots$; $\{u_n\}$ with general term $u_n = x^n$;

6 $(1 + x^2) \cos \pi$, $(2 + x^4) \cos(2\pi)$, $(3 + x^6) \cos(3\pi)$, ... ; $\{u_n\}$ with general term $u_n = (n + x^{2n}) \cos(n\pi)$;

7 $\left(\dfrac{1}{1 + 1}\right) \sin x$; $\left(\dfrac{2}{1 + 2^2}\right) \sin 2x$, $\left(\dfrac{3}{1 + 3^2}\right) \sin 3x$, ... , $\{u_n\}$ with general term

$$u_n = \left(\frac{n}{1 + n^2}\right) \sin nx.$$

Of particular importance when we come to consider series will be the idea of the limit of a sequence. A sequence $\{u_n\}$ will be said to have the **limit** L if once n has exceeded a suitably large number N, say, all the remaining terms in the sequence are arbitrarily close to L. When this condition is satisfied we say the sequence $\{u_n\}$ **converges** to the limit L and write

$$\lim_{n \to \infty} u_n = L.$$

When a limit exists it is unique. Any sequence which is not convergent will be said to be **divergent**.

The idea of a limit of a sequence can be made mathematically rigorous as follows. Let $\varepsilon > 0$ be some arbitrarily small real number. Then $\{u_n\}$ has the limit L if it is possible to find a number N such that

$$\left| u_n - L \right| < \varepsilon \quad \text{for} \quad n > N.$$

We will not make use of this rigorous definition, but merely consider cases in which the limit can be found by inspection.

The numerical sequence in 1 above is divergent, because $u_n = 2^n$ increases without bound as $n \to \infty$. The numerical sequences in both 2 and 3 converge to the limit $L = 0$ because

$$\lim_{n \to \infty} \frac{1}{n!} = 0 \quad \text{and} \quad \lim_{n \to \infty} \frac{(-1)^{n+1}}{n(n+1)} = 0.$$

To examine the behaviour of u_n as $n \to \infty$ in 4 we need to use the fact that $\cos(n\pi) = (-1)^n$. Thus the general term of the sequence becomes

$$u_n = \frac{(-1)^n \, 2n}{3n + 1}.$$

If the sign of u_n is disregarded we see that the factor $2n/(3n + 1) \to 2/3$ as $n \to \infty$. However, $(-1)^n$ is positive when n is even and negative when it is odd, so as $n \to \infty$ the general term u_n alternates ever more closely between $2/3$ and $-2/3$. Thus this sequence does not have a limit and so is divergent.

The behaviour of sequences of functions of x depends on the value of x. Thus in 5 the sequence will converge to the value $L = 0$ if $|x| < 1$, for

$$\lim_{n \to \infty} x^n = 0 \quad \text{if} \quad |x| < 1.$$

However, the sequence will diverge if $|x| > 1$ for then the nth term $u_n = x^n$ increases without bound, and alternates in sign if x is negative. The sequence converges to the value $L = 1$, if $x = 1$ for then every term is identically equal to 1, but it diverges if $x = -1$, for then the terms oscillate boundedly between ± 1.

The sequence in 6 is divergent, because the multiplier $(n + x^{2n})$ in the general term increases without bound as $n \to \infty$, while $\cos(n\pi) = (-1)^n$ simply alternates in sign. Finally, in 7 the sequence is seen to converge to the limit $L = 0$, because the multiplier $n/(1 + n^2) \to 0$ as $n \to \infty$, while $\sin nx$ oscillates boundedly between ± 1.

PROBLEMS 46

In the following problems the form of the general term u_n in an infinite sequence $\{u_n\}$ is given. Determine by inspection which of the sequences is convergent and, where appropriate, give the limit.

1. $u_n = n^2/(n^2 + 3)$.

2. $u_n = (-1)^n n/(2n^2 + n + 1)$.

3. $u_n = (-1)^n$.

4. $u_n = \dfrac{[2(-1)^n + 1]n}{3n + 2}$.

5. $u_n = \dfrac{(-1)^n}{(n+2)(n+3)}$.

6. $u_n = x^n \sin(2n + 1)\dfrac{\pi}{2}$.

7. $u_n = \left(\dfrac{3n}{2n+4}\right)\sin nx$.

8. $u_n = \left(\dfrac{n^2}{n^3 + 1}\right)\cos nx$.

9. $u_n = \cos n^2 x$.

10. $u_n = e^x/n!$.

Infinite numerical series   47

An infinite series with numerical terms is an expression of the form

$$a_1 + a_2 + a_3 + \ldots + a_n + \ldots,$$

in which the **terms** a_n of the series are positive or negative numbers and are infinite in number. We use the summation notation to write this more concisely as

$$\sum_{n=1}^{\infty} a_n,$$

where a_n is called the nth term, or general term, of the series. When speaking about an arbitrary infinite series this notation is often contracted to $\sum a_n$.

A **finite series** is one with a finite number of terms and, for example, when using the summation notation, the finite series $a_3 + a_4 + \ldots + a_{20}$ would be written

$$\sum_{n=3}^{20} a_n.$$

The **summation index** n is a **dummy index**, in the sense that it may be replaced by any other symbol without changing the meaning of the summation, and thus

$$\sum_{n=1}^{\infty} a_n = \sum_{r=1}^{\infty} a_r = \ldots = \sum_{s=1}^{\infty} a_s.$$

The following are four examples of infinite series with numerical terms:
Series (a):

$$1 - \frac{2}{3} + \left(\frac{2}{3}\right)^2 - \left(\frac{2}{3}\right)^3 + \ldots = \sum_{n=1}^{\infty} \left(\frac{-2}{3}\right)^{n-1}.$$

Series (b):

$$1 + \frac{1}{2} + \frac{1}{3} + \frac{1}{4} + \ldots = \sum_{n=1}^{\infty} \frac{1}{n}.$$

Series (c):

$$\ln 2 + \ln \frac{3}{2} + \ln \frac{4}{3} + \ldots = \sum_{n=1}^{\infty} \ln \left(\frac{n+1}{n} \right).$$

Series (d):

$$\frac{1}{1 \cdot 2} + \frac{1}{2 \cdot 3} + \frac{1}{3 \cdot 4} + \ldots = \sum_{n=1}^{\infty} \frac{1}{n(n+1)}.$$

The connection between the sum of an infinite series and the limit of a sequence may be established as follows. Consider the infinite series of numerical terms

$$\sum_{n=1}^{\infty} a_n,$$

and set

$$S_n = a_1 + a_2 + a_3 + \ldots + a_n = \sum_{r=1}^{n} a_r.$$

Notice the use of the dummy summation index r in the last expression, which tells us to sum the terms a_r starting with $r = 1$ and ending with $r = n$. Had we used n as the summation index there would have been confusion between the fixed number of terms to be added (namely n) and the numbering of the individual terms in the series.

We call S_n the nth **partial sum** of the series

$$\sum_{n=1}^{\infty} a_n,$$

because it is the sum of the first n terms. The numbers $S_1, S_2, \ldots$, form a **sequence** $\{S_n\}$ with general term S_n. We say the infinite series converges to the sum L if

$$\lim_{n \to \infty} S_n = L.$$

If this limit does not exist the series will be said to be divergent.

The question of the convergence or divergence of a finite series cannot arise, because the sum of a finite number of terms must be finite, so all finite series converge.

In general, the sum of an infinite series with numerical terms cannot be expressed in **closed form** (that is, it cannot be expressed as a specific number) and so must be estimated numerically. Thus before any numerical calculations are performed on a series it is necessary to know that the series converges. Various tests called **convergence tests** are available for this purpose. As a general rule they do not give information about the sum of a series, but merely about whether or not the series is convergent.

Sometimes an infinite series can be summed analytically, either by use of a simple algebraic device (trick), or by appeal to the sum of the **geometric series**

$$1 + r + r^2 + \ldots + r^{n-1} = \sum_{s=0}^{n-1} r^s = \frac{1 - r^n}{1 - r}.$$

Inspection of example (a) above shows that

$$S_n = 1 + \left(\frac{-2}{3}\right) + \left(\frac{-2}{3}\right)^2 + \ldots + \left(\frac{-2}{3}\right)^{n-1} = \sum_{s=0}^{n-1} \left(\frac{-2}{3}\right)^s,$$

but this is the sum of a geometric series with n terms in which $r = -2/3$, so

$$S_n = \frac{1 - (-2)^n}{1 - (-2/3)} = \frac{3}{5} [1 - (-2/3)^n].$$

As $\lim_{n \to \infty} (-2/3)^n = 0$, it follows that

$$\lim_{n \to \infty} S_n = \lim_{n \to \infty} \frac{3}{5} [1 - (2/3)^n] = \frac{3}{5},$$

so series (a) converges to the sum $S = 3/5$.

Apart from the general observation that the terms of series (b) tend to zero rather slowly, at this stage we are not in a position to infer anything about the convergence or divergence of this series. We will see later that the fact that the nth term of a series tends to zero is not a sufficient condition to ensure the convergence of a series.

Using the property of logarithms enables us to write the nth partial sum of series (c) as

$$S_n = \ln 2 + \ln \frac{3}{2} + \ln \frac{4}{3} + \ldots + \ln \left(\frac{n+1}{n}\right)$$

$$= \ln \left[\frac{2 \cdot 3 \cdot 4 \ldots (n+1)}{1 \cdot 2 \cdot 3 \ldots n}\right]$$

$$= \ln (n+1).$$

Thus this series is divergent, because

$$\lim_{n \to \infty} S_n = \lim_{n \to \infty} \ln (n+1) = \infty.$$

To examine the convergence of series (d) we write

$$\frac{1}{r(r-1)} = \left(\frac{1}{r} - \frac{1}{r+1}\right).$$

so that the nth partial sum becomes

$$S_n = \frac{1}{1 \cdot 2} + \frac{1}{2 \cdot 3} + \frac{1}{3 \cdot 4} + \ldots + \frac{1}{n(n+1)}$$

$$= \left(\frac{1}{1} - \frac{1}{2}\right) + \left(\frac{1}{2} - \frac{1}{3}\right) + \left(\frac{1}{3} - \frac{1}{4}\right) + \ldots + \left(\frac{1}{n} - \frac{1}{n+1}\right),$$

and after removing the brackets and cancelling terms this becomes

$$S_n = 1 - \frac{1}{n+1}.$$

This process is called the **telescoping** of a series. Thus we have

$$\lim_{n \to \infty} S_n = \lim_{n \to \infty} \left(1 - \frac{1}{n+1}\right) = 1$$

so this series converges to the sum 1.

Before discussing convergence tests, let us first examine the behaviour of series (b) more closely. Consider the partial sum S_{2^n} involving the first 2^n terms of the series, so

$$S_{2^n} = 1 + \frac{1}{2} + \frac{1}{3} + \ldots + \frac{1}{2^n}.$$

Then

$$S_{2^n} = 1 + \frac{1}{2} + \left(\frac{1}{3} + \frac{1}{4}\right) + \left(\frac{1}{5} + \frac{1}{6} + \frac{1}{7} + \frac{1}{8}\right) + \ldots + \left(\frac{1}{2^{n-1}+1} + \ldots + \frac{1}{2^n}\right),$$

and so by underestimating terms in the brackets we find that

$$S_{2^n} > 1 + \frac{1}{2} + \underbrace{\left(\frac{1}{4} + \frac{1}{4}\right)}_{1/2} + \underbrace{\left(\frac{1}{8} + \frac{1}{8} + \frac{1}{8} + \frac{1}{8}\right)}_{1/2} + \ldots + \underbrace{\left(\frac{1}{2^n} + \frac{1}{2^n} + \ldots + \frac{1}{2^n}\right)}_{1/2}$$

leading to the result

$$S_{2^n} > 1 + \underbrace{\frac{1}{2} + \frac{1}{2} + \ldots + \frac{1}{2}}_{n \text{ terms}}.$$

Thus

$$S_{2^n} > 1 + \frac{n}{2},$$

but

$$\lim_{n \to \infty} \left(1 + \frac{n}{2}\right) = \infty$$

so

$$\lim S_{2^n} = \infty$$

and we have proved that the series (b) is divergent. The series in (b), namely the series

$$1 + \frac{1}{2} + \frac{1}{3} + \frac{1}{4} + \ldots = \sum_{n=1}^{\infty} \frac{1}{n},$$

is called the **harmonic series**. It has many uses, one of which is to serve as a basis for comparison with other series. If a series of positive terms $\sum a_n$ is such that $a_n \geq 1/n$, then term for term, $\sum a_n$ exceeds or equals $\sum 1/n$. However, $\sum 1/n$ is divergent, so $\sum a_n$ must also be divergent.

This is a typical example of what is called a **comparison test**, and as stated is a test for divergence.

Example 47.1

Determine the convergence property of

$$\sum_{n=1}^{\infty} \frac{2n^2}{3n^3 + 1}.$$

Solution
The general term

$$u_n = \frac{2n^2}{3n^3 + 1} = \frac{2}{3n + (1/n^2)},$$

so

$$u_n > \frac{2}{3n},$$

and thus

$$\sum_{n=1}^{\infty} \frac{2n^2}{3n^3 + 1} > \frac{2}{3} \sum_{n=1}^{\infty} \frac{1}{n}.$$

However, the series on the right is divergent (it is the harmonic series) so

$$\sum_{n=1}^{\infty} \frac{2n^2}{3n^3 + 1}$$

is divergent.   ▲

A general comparison test for divergence may be formulated in the following obvious manner.

Comparison test for divergence
If a series of positive terms $\sum a_n$ is known to be divergent, and another series of positive terms $\sum b_n$ is such that $b_n \geq a_n$ then $\sum b_n$ is also divergent.

An important property of a convergent series is that if $\sum a_n$ is convergent, then $\lim_{n \to \infty} a_n = 0$. This follows from the fact that if $\sum a_n$ converges to the limit L, then

$$\sum_{n=1}^{\infty} a_n = \lim_{n \to \infty} S_n = L,$$

but

$$S_n = S_{n-1} + a_n,$$

and as

$$\lim_{n \to \infty} S_n = \lim S_{n-1} = L,$$

we must have

$$L = \lim_{n \to \infty} S_n = \lim_{n \to \infty} (S_{n-1} + a_n) = L + \lim_{n \to \infty} a_n,$$

showing that if $\sum a_n$ is convergent then

$$\lim_{n \to \infty} a_n = 0.$$

An example of this result may be seen in series (a) above, in which $a_n = (-2/3)^n$.

The converse of this result is not necessarily true, for even if the nth term of an infinite series tends to zero, the series may still diverge. An example of this is to be found in the harmonic series in (b) in which $a_n = 1/n$. Here $\lim_{n \to \infty} 1/n = 0$, yet the series is divergent. This general result gives us the nth term test for divergence.

nth term test for divergence
If in the series $\sum a_n$

$$\lim_{n \to \infty} a_n \neq 0,$$

then the series is divergent.

Example 47.2

Determine the convergence properties of

$$\sum_{n=1}^{\infty} \frac{2n}{5n+3}.$$

Solution
As

$$a_n = \frac{2n}{5n+3}$$

we see that

$$\lim_{n \to \infty} a_n = \lim_{n \to \infty} \frac{2n}{5n+3} = \frac{2}{5} \neq 0,$$

so the series diverges by the nth term test.   ▲

It follows from the definition of the limit of a sequence that when a series is convergent, its sum is unique. Other properties of series which follow from the general properties of limits, and from the definition of the limit of a sequence in particular, are set out below.

SIMPLE PROPERTIES OF SERIES

Let $\sum a_n$ and $\sum b_n$ be two convergent series with the respective sums A and B, and let k be a real number. Then

$$1 \sum_{n=1}^{\infty} k\,a_n = k\,A;$$

$$2 \sum_{n=1}^{\infty} (a_n + b_n) = A + B;$$

$$3 \sum_{n=1}^{\infty} (a_n - b_n) = A - B.$$

Example 47.3

Sum the series

(i) $\displaystyle\sum_{n=0}^{\infty} 5\left(\frac{1}{4}\right)^n$,

(ii) $\displaystyle\sum_{n=0}^{\infty} \left[\left(\frac{1}{2}\right)^n + \left(\frac{1}{3}\right)^n\right]$;

(iii) $\displaystyle\sum_{n=0}^{\infty} \left[\left(\frac{1}{2}\right)^n + \left(\frac{-1}{2}\right)^n\right]$.

Solution

(i) $\displaystyle\sum_{n=0}^{\infty} 5\left(\frac{1}{4}\right)^n = 5 \sum_{n=0}^{\infty} \left(\frac{1}{4}\right)^n = 5 \lim_{n \to \infty} \left[\frac{1-(1/4)^n}{1-(1/4)}\right] = \frac{20}{3}.$

(ii) $\displaystyle\sum_{n=0}^{\infty} \left[\left(\frac{1}{2}\right)^n + \left(\frac{1}{3}\right)^n\right] = \sum_{n=0}^{\infty} \left(\frac{1}{2}\right)^n + \sum_{n=0}^{\infty} \left(\frac{1}{3}\right)^n$

$$= \lim_{n \to \infty} \left[\frac{1-(1/2)^n}{1-(1/2)}\right] + \lim_{n \to \infty} \left[\frac{1-(1/3)^n}{1-(1/3)}\right]$$

$$= 2 + \frac{3}{2} = \frac{7}{2}.$$

(iii) $\displaystyle\sum_{n=0}^{\infty} \left[\left(\frac{1}{2}\right)^n + \left(\frac{-1}{2}\right)^n \right] = \sum_{n=0}^{\infty} \left(\frac{1}{2}\right)^n + \sum_{n=0}^{\infty} \left(\frac{-1}{2}\right)^n$

$$= \lim_{n \to \infty} \left[\frac{1 - (1/2)^n}{1 - (1/2)} \right] + \lim_{n \to \infty} \left[\frac{1 - (-1/2)^n}{1 + (1/2)} \right]$$

$$= 2 + \frac{2}{3} = \frac{8}{3}. \qquad\qquad \blacktriangle$$

The series

$$\sum_{n=1}^{\infty} (-1)^{n+1} a_n$$

with $a_n > 0$ for all n is called an **alternating series** (the signs of the terms alternate between $+$ and $-$). The convergence properties of these series are easily determined by using the following test.

Alternating series test
If in the alternating series

$$\sum_{n=1}^{\infty} (-1)^{n+1} a_n$$

the terms $a_n > 0$ are such that $a_{n+1} < a_n$ and

$$\lim_{n \to \infty} a_n = 0,$$

then the series converges. Furthermore, if the sum of the series is approximated by the nth partial sum

$$S_n = a_1 - a_2 + a_3 - \dots + (-1)^n a_n,$$

the magnitude of the error cannot exceed a_{n+1}.

Proof
The sum of the first $2n$ terms is

$$S_{2n} = a_1 - a_2 + a_3 - a_4 + \dots + a_{2n-1} - a_{2n}$$

$$= (a_1 - a_2) + (a_3 - a_4) + \dots + (a_{2n-1} - a_{2n}) > 0,$$

because each bracketed pair of terms is positive since $a_{n+1} < a_n$. Furthermore,

$$S_{2n} = a_1 - (a_2 - a_3) - (a_4 - a_5) - \dots - (a_{2n-2} - a_{2n-1}) - a_{2n} < a_1,$$

since each bracketed pair of terms is positive and $a_{2n} > 0$. Thus we have the estimate

$$0 < S_{2n} < a_1, \quad \text{for all} \quad n.$$

Now

$$S_{2n+1} = S_{2n} + a_{2n+1}$$

and if the series is convergent to the sum S

$$\lim_{n \to \infty} S_{2n+1} = \lim_{n \to \infty} S_{2n} = S,$$

so we must have

$$\lim_{n \to \infty} a_{2n+1} = 0.$$

This same argument shows that the magnitude of the error made when the sum is approximated by S_n cannot exceed a_{n+1}, so the result is proved.

Example 47.4

Determine the convergence properties of:

(i) $\displaystyle\sum_{n=1}^{\infty} \frac{(-1)^{n+1}}{n}$;

(ii) $\displaystyle\sum_{n=1}^{\infty} (-1)^{n+1} \left(\frac{n}{2n+1} \right)$; and

(iii) $\displaystyle\sum_{n=1}^{\infty} \frac{(-1)^{n+1}}{n!}$.

When a series is convergent, estimate the magnitude of the error made if it is approximated by its nth partial sum.

Solution

(i) This is an alternating series with $a_n = 1/n$. As $1/(n+1) < 1/n$ it follows that $a_{n+1} < a_n$, and $\lim_{n \to \infty} (1/n) = 0$, so the series is convergent. If the sum S is approximated by

$$S_n = 1 - \frac{1}{2} + \frac{1}{3} - \frac{1}{4} + \ldots + \frac{(-1)^n}{n} ,$$

then it follows from the last part of the alternating series test that

$$|S - S_n| < \frac{1}{n+1} .$$

Thus the series converges very slowly, and to attain an accuracy of 0.001 when summing the series numerically would require 1000 terms.

(ii) This is an alternating series but

$$\lim_{n \to \infty} a_n = \lim_{n \to \infty} \left(\frac{n}{2n+1} \right) = \frac{1}{2} ,$$

so the series diverges by the nth term test for divergence.

(iii) This is an alternating series with $a_n = 1/n!$, so as

$$\frac{1}{(n+1)!} < \frac{1}{n!}$$

we have $a_{n+1} < a_n$. Furthermore,

$$\lim_{n \to \infty} a_n = \lim_{n \to \infty} \frac{1}{n!} = 0,$$

so the series is convergent. The magnitude of the error made when the sum S is approximated by the nth partial sum

$$S_n = 1 - \frac{1}{2!} + \frac{1}{3!} + \dots + \frac{(-1)^{n+1}}{n!}$$

is such that

$$|S - S_n| < \frac{1}{n!}.$$

This series converges rapidly, and even if the sum is approximated by only five terms the magnitude of the error will not exceed $1/6! = 1/720$.

▲

In general, series contain both positive and negative terms, but they are not necessarily alternating series so other tests for convergence are needed. The nature of some tests for convergence make it important to distinguish between different types of series containing positive and negative terms. This is accomplished by introducing the idea of absolute and conditional convergence. If a series $\sum a_n$ containing both positive and negative terms is convergent, and the sum of the absolute values $\sum |a_n|$ is also convergent, the series $\sum a_n$ will be said to be **absolutely convergent**. If, however, the series $\sum a_n$ is convergent, but the series $\sum |a_n|$ is divergent, the series $\sum a_n$ will be said to be **conditionally convergent**.

Example 47.5

Determine the convergence properties of

(i) $\displaystyle\sum_{n=1}^{\infty} \frac{(-1)^{n+1}}{n}$; and

(ii) $\displaystyle\sum_{n=1}^{\infty} (-1)^{n+1} \left(\frac{1}{5}\right)^n$.

Solution
(i)   We have seen in Example 47.4(i) that this series is convergent. However, the sum of the absolute values is

$$\sum_{n=1}^{\infty} \left| \frac{(-1)^n}{n} \right| = \sum_{n=1}^{\infty} \frac{1}{n} ,$$

which is the harmonic series, and so is divergent. Thus the series

$$\sum_{n=1}^{\infty} \frac{(-1)^{n+1}}{n}$$

is conditionally convergent.

(ii)   As $a_n = (1/5)^n$ and

$$(1/5)^{n+1} < (1/5)^n,$$

it follows that $a_{n+1} < a_n$. In addition

$$\lim_{n \to \infty} a_n = \lim_{n \to \infty} \left(\frac{1}{5} \right)^n = 0,$$

so the series is convergent by the alternating series test. However,

$$\sum_{n=1}^{\infty} \left| (-1)^n \left(\frac{1}{5} \right)^n \right| = \sum_{n=1}^{\infty} \left(\frac{1}{5} \right)^n,$$

and this is a convergent geometric series because $r = 1/5 < 1$, so the series

$$\sum_{n=1}^{\infty} (-1)^{n+1} \left(\frac{1}{5} \right)^n$$

is absolutely convergent.   ▲

Two important properties of absolutely convergent series which we state but do not prove are the following.

BRACKETING AND REARRANGEMENT OF TERMS IN SERIES

If the series $\sum a_n$ is absolutely convergent, then
1 groups of terms may be bracketed without altering the sum;
2 terms may be rearranged without altering the sum.

To see that bracketing and rearrangement of terms in a conditionally convergent series is not permissible we need only consider the following example. We have shown that the series

$$S = 1 - \frac{1}{2} + \frac{1}{3} - \frac{1}{4} + \frac{1}{5} \ldots$$

is conditionally convergent and we are denoting its sum by S. Let us rearrange the order of the terms and then group them by bracketing as follows:

$$S = 1 - \frac{1}{2} - \frac{1}{4} + \frac{1}{3} - \frac{1}{6} - \frac{1}{8} + \frac{1}{5} - \frac{1}{10} - \frac{1}{12} + \ldots$$

$$= \left(1 - \frac{1}{2}\right) - \frac{1}{4} + \left(\frac{1}{3} - \frac{1}{6}\right) - \frac{1}{8} + \left(\frac{1}{5} - \frac{1}{10}\right) + \frac{1}{12} + \dots$$

$$= \frac{1}{2}\left(1 - \frac{1}{2} + \frac{1}{3} - \frac{1}{4} + \frac{1}{5} - \frac{1}{6} + \dots\right)$$

$$= \frac{1}{2} S.$$

This shows that if these operations are permissible $S = \frac{1}{2} S$, which is only possible if $S = 0$. However, $S \neq 0$, so the operations on the series which led to this conclusion are not permissible.

A direct extension of the idea of a comparison theorem is contained in the following obvious test for convergence.

Comparison test for convergence

If the series of positive terms $\sum a_n$ is convergent, and the series $\sum b_n$ is such that $|b_n| \leqslant a_n$, then the series $\sum b_n$ is absolutely convergent.

Example 47.6

Use the comparison test to determine the convergence properties of

$$\sum_{n=1}^{\infty} [3(-1)^n + 1]\left(\frac{1}{6n+1}\right)\left(\frac{1}{5}\right)^n.$$

Solution
Setting

$$b_n = [3(-1)^n + 1]\left(\frac{1}{6n+1}\right)\left(\frac{1}{5}\right)^n,$$

and using the fact that

$$3(-1)^n + 1 = \begin{cases} 4 & \text{for even } n \\ -2 & \text{for odd } n, \end{cases}$$

we see that

$$b_n < \left(\frac{4}{6n+1}\right)\left(\frac{1}{5}\right)^n.$$

However, $4/(6n+1) < 1$, so

$$b_n < \left(\frac{1}{5}\right)^n.$$

If in the comparison test we set

$$a_n = (1/5)^n,$$

the series

$$\sum_{n=1}^{\infty} a_n = \sum_{n=1}^{\infty} \left(\frac{1}{5}\right)^n$$

is convergent since it is a geometric series with $r = 1/5 < 1$. Then since $\left| b_n \right| < a_n$ it follows from the comparison test that $\sum_{n=1}^{\infty} b_n$ is convergent. ▲

We now give a useful and simple test for absolute convergence.

Ratio test
If a series $\sum_{n=1}^{\infty} a_n$ is such that $a_n \neq 0$, and

$$\lim_{n \to \infty} \left| \frac{a_{n+1}}{a_n} \right| = L,$$

then

1 the series $\sum a_n$ is absolutely convergent if $L < 1$;

2 the series $\sum a_n$ is divergent if $L > 1$;

3 the test provides no information about the convergence or divergence of $\sum a_n$ if $L = 1$.

Proof
Suppose the ratio $\left| a_{n+1}/a_n \right|$ is always defined and that

$$\lim_{n \to \infty} \left| \frac{a_{n+1}}{a_n} \right| = L$$

with $L < 1$. Then for some fixed number r, such that $L < r < 1$ it follows from the existence of the limit that for some suitably large integer N

$$\left| a_{n+1} \right| < r \left| a_n \right| \quad \text{if} \quad n > N.$$

Thus we have

$$\left| a_{N+2} \right| < r \left| a_{N+1} \right|, \; \left| a_{N+3} \right| < r \left| a_{N+2} \right| < r^2 \left| a_{N+1} \right|, \dots,$$

so that in general

$$\left| a_{N+m+1} \right| < r^m \left| a_{N+1} \right|.$$

Writing

$$\sum_{n=1}^{\infty} a_n = \sum_{n=1}^{N} a_n + \sum_{n=N+1}^{\infty} a_n,$$

so that

$$R_N = \sum_{n=N+1}^{\infty} a_n$$

is the **remainder** after N terms, we have

$$R_N = \sum_{n=N+1}^{\infty} a_n < \sum_{n=N+1}^{\infty} \left| a_n \right| < \left| a_{N+1} \right| (1 + r + r^2 + \ldots).$$

The bracketed expression is a geometric series with $r < 1$, and so it is convergent. Thus, if $L < 1$, $\sum a_n$ must be absolutely convergent. If $r > 1$ $\lim_{n \to \infty} \left| a_n \right| \neq 0$, and thus $\lim_{n \to \infty} a_n \neq 0$, so $\sum a_n$ is divergent. When $L = 1$ it follows that $r = 1$ and then the test provides no information.

Example 47.7

Test the following series for convergence by using the ratio test:

(i) $\displaystyle\sum_{n=1}^{\infty} \frac{(-1)^{n+1}}{n!}$;

(ii) $\displaystyle\sum_{n=1}^{\infty} \frac{(-1)^{n+1}}{n^2}$.

Solution

(i) Setting $a_n = \dfrac{(-1)^{n+1}}{n!}$ we have

$$\frac{a_{n+1}}{a_n} = \frac{-n!}{(n+1)!} = \frac{-1}{n+1}.$$

so

$$\left| \frac{a_{n+1}}{a_n} \right| = \left| \frac{-1}{n+1} \right| = \frac{1}{n+1}.$$

Now

$$L = \lim_{n \to \infty} \left| \frac{a_{n+1}}{a_n} \right| = \lim_{n \to \infty} \left(\frac{1}{n+1} \right) = 0,$$

so as $L < 1$ the series is absolutely convergent. Thus we have shown that both

$$\sum_{n=1}^{\infty} \frac{(-1)^{n+1}}{n!} \quad \text{and} \quad \sum_{n=1}^{\infty} \frac{1}{n!}$$

are convergent.

(ii) Setting

$$a_n = \frac{(-1)^{n+1}}{n^2}$$

we have

$$\frac{a_{n+1}}{a_n} = \frac{-n^2}{(n+1)^2},$$

so

$$\left|\frac{a_{n+1}}{a_n}\right| = \left|\frac{-n^2}{(n+1)^2}\right| = \frac{n^2}{(n+1)^2}.$$

Now

$$L = \lim_{n \to \infty} \left|\frac{a_{n+1}}{a_n}\right| = \lim_{n \to \infty} \left[\frac{n^2}{(n+1)^2}\right] = 1,$$

so as $L = 1$ the test fails and we are unable to determine whether or not the series is absolutely convergent on the basis of this test.

We know from the alternating series test that the series is convergent, but as yet we are unable to determine whether or not it is absolutely convergent (it is). ▲

A test which can be proved in a manner analogous to that used for the ratio test is as follows.

nth root test

If the series $\displaystyle\sum_{n=1}^{\infty} a_n$ is such that $a_n \neq 0$, and

$$\lim_{n \to \infty} \left|a_n\right|^{1/n} = L,$$

then

1 the series $\sum a_n$ is absolutely convergent if $L < 1$;

2 the series $\sum a_n$ is divergent if $L > 1$;

3 the test provides no information about the convergence or divergence of $\sum a_n$ if $L = 1$.

Example 47.8

Test for convergence the series

$$\sum_{n=1}^{\infty} \left(\frac{-n}{3n+1}\right)^n = -\frac{1}{4} + \left(\frac{2}{7}\right)^2 - \left(\frac{3}{10}\right)^3 + \dots .$$

Solution
Set

$$a_n = \left(\frac{-n}{3n+1}\right)^n,$$

then

$$|a_n| = \left(\frac{n}{3n+1}\right)^n,$$

so

$$|a_n|^{1/n} = \frac{n}{3n+1}.$$

Now

$$L = \lim_{n \to \infty} |a_n|^{1/n} = \lim_{n \to \infty} \left(\frac{n}{3n+1}\right) = \frac{1}{3}$$

so as $L < 1$ the series is absolutely convergent.   ▲

For our last test we describe the integral test which, although it is only applicable to series of positive terms, is both powerful and useful.

Integral test
Let $f(x)$ be a positive, continuous and decreasing function for $x \geq 1$ and set $a_n = f(n)$. Then the series

$$\sum_{n=1}^{\infty} a_n$$

converges or diverges as the improper integral

$$\int_1^{\infty} f(x)\,dx$$

converges or diverges.

Proof
Consider the diagrams in Fig. 106. Then, using the interpretation of the definite integral as an area, we have the obvious area inequalities

$$\sum_{r=2}^{n} f(r) \leq \int_1^n f(x)\,dx \leq \sum_{r=1}^{n-1} f(r) \leq \sum_{r=1}^{n} f(r).$$

Here, the summation to the left of the integral is the area of the shaded rectangles in Fig. 106(a), while the sum to the immediate right is the area of the shaded rectangles in Fig. 106(b). The summation to the extreme right has one additional term which further reinforces the inequality.

As $a_r = f(r)$ this becomes

$$\sum_{r=2}^{n} a_r \leq \int_1^n f(x)\,dx \leq \sum_{r=1}^{n} a_r.$$

The summation on the right only differs from the one on the left by the single term a_1, so the series and the integral converge or diverge together as $n \to \infty$.

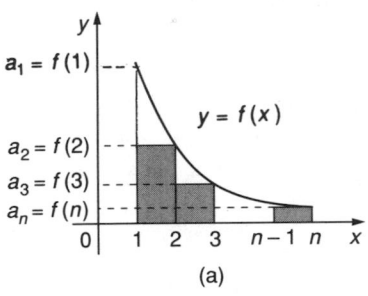
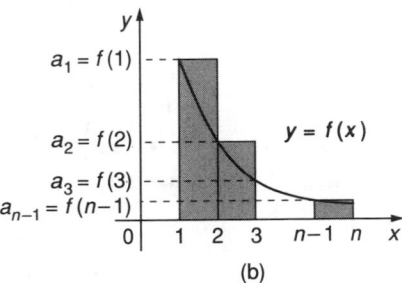

(a)   (b)

Fig. 106

Example 47.9

Determine the convergence properties of the series

$$\sum_{n=1}^{\infty} \frac{1}{n^p},$$

where p is a parameter in the range $0 < p < \infty$. Such series are often called p-series.

Solution
The general term of the series is

$$a_n = \frac{1}{n^p},$$

so we set $f(x) = 1/x^p$, for then $a_n = f(n)$ as required by the integral test. Now $f(x)$ is defined for $1 \leqslant x < \infty$, is continuous and decreases to zero as $x \to \infty$, so the integral test may be used:

$$\int_1^n f(x)\,dx = \int_1^n \frac{dx}{x^p} = \left(\frac{1}{1-p}\right)\left(\frac{1}{x^{p-1}} - 1\right).$$

If $0 < p < 1$, we see from this that

$$\lim_{n \to \infty} \int_1^n \frac{dx}{x^p} = \lim_{n \to \infty} \left\{\left(\frac{1}{1-p}\right)\left(\frac{1}{x^{p-1}} - 1\right)\right\} = \infty,$$

so the integral, and hence the series, diverge.
    If $p > 1$, then

$$\lim_{n \to \infty} \int_1^n \frac{dx}{x^p} = \lim_{n \to \infty} \left\{\left(\frac{1}{1-p}\right)\left(\frac{1}{x^{p-1}} - 1\right)\right\}$$

$$= \frac{1}{p-1},$$

which is finite, so the integral, and hence the series, converge.

If $p = 1$

$$\lim_{n \to \infty} \int_1^n \frac{dx}{x} = \lim_{n \to \infty} (\ln n - \ln 1) = \infty,$$

so the integral, and hence the series, diverge.

The p-series

$$\sum_{n=1}^{\infty} \frac{1}{n^p}$$

diverges for $0 < p \leqslant 1$ and converges for $p > 1$.   ▲

This result may be used to complete the determination of the convergence properties of the series

$$\sum_{n=1}^{\infty} \frac{(-1)^{n+1}}{n^2},$$

first attempted in Example 47.7(ii). The ratio test failed, but we know from the alternating series test that the series is convergent. It will be absolutely convergent if the series

$$\sum_{n=1}^{\infty} \frac{1}{n^2}$$

is convergent. This is, indeed, the case because it is a p-series with $p > 1$, so

$$\sum_{n=1}^{\infty} \frac{(-1)^{n+1}}{n^2}$$

is absolutely convergent.

PROBLEMS 47

Investigate the convergence of the following series.

1. $\displaystyle\sum_{n=1}^{\infty} \frac{4n^2 + 2}{5n^2 + 6}$.

2. $\displaystyle\sum_{n=1}^{\infty} \left(1 + \frac{1}{n}\right)^n$.

3. $\displaystyle\sum_{n=1}^{\infty} \left(\frac{3}{4}\right)^n$.

4. $\displaystyle\sum_{n=1}^{\infty} \left[\left(\frac{1}{3}\right)^n + \left(\frac{6}{5}\right)^n\right]$.

5. $\displaystyle\sum_{n=1}^{\infty} \frac{1}{\sqrt{n}}$.

6. $\displaystyle\sum_{n=0}^{\infty} \left(\frac{2^n + 3^n}{6^n} \right)$.

7. $\displaystyle\sum_{n=0}^{\infty} (-1)^n$.

8. $\displaystyle\sum_{n=1}^{\infty} \left(\frac{3^n + 1}{3^n} \right)$.

9. $\displaystyle\sum_{n=1}^{\infty} \frac{1}{n} \left(\frac{1}{2} \right)^n$.

10. $\displaystyle \ln 2 + \sum_{n=2}^{\infty} \ln \left(\frac{n+1}{n-1} \right)$.

11. $\displaystyle\sum_{n=1}^{\infty} \frac{1}{n(n+2)}$.

12. $\displaystyle\sum_{n=1}^{\infty} \frac{1}{(2n-1)(2n+1)}$.

13. $\displaystyle\sum_{n=1}^{\infty} \frac{n}{2^n}$.

14. $\displaystyle\sum_{n=1}^{\infty} \frac{n}{3n-1}$.

15. $\displaystyle\sum_{n=1}^{\infty} \frac{2n-1}{(\sqrt{2})^n}$.

16. $\displaystyle\sum_{n=1}^{\infty} \frac{(-1)^{n+1}}{2n-1}$.

17. $\displaystyle\sum_{n=1}^{\infty} \frac{(-1)^{n+1}}{\sqrt{n}}$.

18. $\displaystyle\sum_{n=1}^{\infty} \frac{(-1)^{n+1} n}{2^n}$.

19. $\displaystyle\sum_{n=1}^{\infty} (-1)^{(n^2+n)/2} \frac{n}{3^n}$.

20. $\displaystyle\sum_{n=1}^{\infty} \frac{(-1)^{n+1}(3n+1)}{n(n+1)}$.

21. $\dfrac{1}{\sqrt{4}} + \dfrac{1}{\sqrt{7}} + \dfrac{1}{\sqrt{10}} + \dots$.

22. $\displaystyle\sum_{n=1}^{\infty} \left(\dfrac{n+1}{4n-1} \right)^{n}$.

23. $\displaystyle\sum_{n=1}^{\infty} \left(\dfrac{n}{4n-1} \right)^{2n-1}$.

24. $\displaystyle\sum_{n=1}^{\infty} \dfrac{n}{(n+1)^3}$.

25. $\displaystyle\sum_{n=1}^{\infty} \dfrac{n}{1+n^2}$.

26. $\displaystyle\sum_{n=1}^{\infty} \dfrac{1}{(2n+1)^2 - 1}$.

27. $\displaystyle\sum_{n=1}^{\infty} \dfrac{n}{n^4 + 1}$.

28. $\displaystyle\sum_{n=1}^{\infty} \dfrac{\sin na}{n^2}$.

29. $\displaystyle\sum_{n=2}^{\infty} \left[\dfrac{-1}{\ln(2n+1)} \right]^{n}$.

30. $\displaystyle\sum_{n=2}^{\infty} \left(\dfrac{\ln n}{n} \right)^{n}$.

Power series   48

A power series in $x - x_0$ is an expression of the form

$$a_0 + a_1(x - x_0) + a_2(x - x_0)^2 + \ldots + a_n(x - x_0)^n + \ldots,$$

in which the **coefficients** a_n of the power series are numbers and x_0 is some given numerical value of the variable x. The power series is said to be **expanded** about the **point** x_0. For any fixed numerical value of x this infinite series in powers of $x - x_0$ will become an infinite numerical series of the type considered in the previous section, and so will either converge or diverge. Thus a power series in $x - x_0$ will define a function of x for all x in the interval in which the series converges. In terms of the summation notation we can write the power series as

$$\sum_{n=0}^{\infty} a_n(x - x_0)^n,$$

and if the function to which this infinite series converges is denoted by $f(x)$, often called its **sum function**, we may write

$$f(x) = \sum_{n=0}^{\infty} a_n(x - x_0)^n.$$

The interval in which this power series will converge will depend on the coefficients a_n, the point (number) x_0 about which the series is expanded and x itself. To determine the convergence properties let us apply the ratio test to the power series, in which the nth term is $a_n(x - x_0)^n$ and the $(n+1)$th term is $a_{n+1}(x - x_0)^{n+1}$.

Then we know from the ratio test that the power series will converge if

$$\lim_{n \to \infty} \left| \frac{a_{n+1}(x - x_0)^{n+1}}{a_n(x - x_0)^n} \right| < 1,$$

which is equivalent to

$$\lim_{n \to \infty} \left\{ \left| \frac{a_{n+1}}{a_n} \right| \left| x - x_0 \right| \right\} < 1$$

or, since $\left| x - x_0 \right|$ is not involved in the limit process, to

$$\lim_{n \to \infty} \left\{ \left| \frac{a_{n+1}}{a_n} \right| \right\} \left| x - x_0 \right| < 1.$$

Assuming that $\left| a_{n+1}/a_n \right|$ is always defined, that is $a_n \neq 0$, we find after division that

$$\left| x - x_0 \right| < \lim_{n \to \infty} \left| \frac{a_n}{a_{n+1}} \right|.$$

If we now define the number r to be

$$r = \lim_{n \to \infty} \left| \frac{a_n}{a_{n+1}} \right|,$$

we see that the power series converges absolutely (the ratio test is a test for absolute convergence) if

$$\left| x - x_0 \right| < r.$$

This inequality defines the interval

$$x_0 - r < x < x_0 + r$$

in which the power series is absolutely convergent. The number r is called the **radius of convergence** of the power series, and the interval $x_0 - r < x < x_0 + r$ is called the **interval of convergence**. As the ratio test fails when $L = 1$, it is not possible to say on the basis of the above argument whether or not the series converges at the end points of the interval of convergence.

If necessary, the convergence properties of the series at the end points of the interval of convergence must be investigated separately (by using other tests when $x = x_0 \pm r$).

For any x outside the interval of convergence a power series will diverge. Thus the meaning of the interval of convergence can be illustrated diagrammatically as in Fig. 107, in which the behaviour of the series at the points P and Q requires special investigation.

When it is more convenient, the nth root test may also be used to determine the radius and interval of convergence of a power series, for this test is also a test for absolute convergence. The same form of argument then shows that the radius of convergence r is given by

$$r = \lim_{n \to \infty} \left| 1/a_n \right|^{1/n}.$$

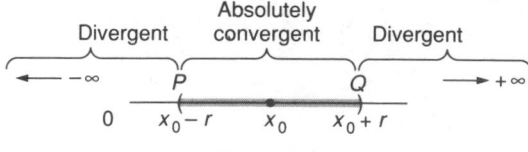

Fig. 107

We have arrived at the following fundamental results.

Radius and interval of convergence of a power series
Let the power series

$$\sum_{n=0}^{\infty} a_n (x - x_0)^n$$

be such that $a_n \neq 0$. Then the radius of convergence of the series is given by

$$r = \lim_{n \to \infty} \left| \frac{a_n}{a_{n+1}} \right|,$$

or by

$$r = \lim_{n \to \infty} \left| \frac{1}{a_n} \right|^{1/n},$$

and the series will be absolutely convergent in the interval of convergence

$$x_0 - r < x < x_0 + r.$$

Example 48.1

Find the radius and interval of convergence of

$$x - \frac{x^2}{2} + \frac{x^3}{3} - \frac{x^4}{4} + \dots = \sum_{n=1}^{\infty} (-1)^{n+1} \frac{x^n}{n}.$$

Solution
This series is expanded about the point $x_0 = 0$ (the origin) and the nth coefficient

$$a_n = \frac{(-1)^{n+1}}{n}.$$

Thus

$$\left| \frac{a_n}{a_{n+1}} \right| = \left| \frac{(-1)^{n+1}}{n} \cdot \frac{(n+1)}{(-1)^{n+2}} \right| = \frac{n+1}{n},$$

and so the radius of convergence

$$r = \lim_{n \to \infty} \left| \frac{a_n}{a_{n+1}} \right| = \lim_{n \to \infty} \left(\frac{n+1}{n} \right) = 1.$$

Consequently, the interval of convergence (the interval in which the series is absolutely convergent) is

$$-1 < x < 1.$$

The series will diverge if $|x| > 1$, but we need to examine separately its behaviour when $x = \pm 1$. When $x = 1$ the series is seen to be convergent by the alternating series test, but when $x = -1$ it becomes the harmonic series, and so is divergent. Thus the series is convergent for $-1 < x \leqslant 1$, and divergent outside this interval. ▲

Example 48.2

Find the radius and interval of convergence of

$$1 - x + \frac{x^2}{2!} - \frac{x^3}{3!} + \ldots = \sum_{n=0}^{\infty} (-1)^n \frac{x^n}{x!}.$$

Solution
The series is expanded about the point $x_0 = 0$ and the nth coefficient

$$a_n = \frac{(-1)^n}{n!}.$$

Thus

$$\left| \frac{a_n}{a_{n+1}} \right| = \left| \frac{(-1)^n (n+1)!}{(-1)^{n+1}} \right| = \frac{1 \cdot 2 \cdot 3 \ldots n(n+1)}{1 \cdot 2 \cdot 3 \ldots n} = n + 1,$$

and so the radius of convergence

$$r = \lim_{n \to \infty} \left| \frac{a_n}{a_{n+1}} \right| = \infty.$$

Thus this series is absolutely convergent for all x, as the interval of convergence is $-\infty < x < \infty$. ▲

Example 48.3

Find the radius and interval of convergence of

$$1 - \frac{1}{2^2} (x - 1) + \frac{1}{2^4} (x - 1)^2 - \frac{1}{2^6} (x - 1)^3 + \ldots = \sum_{n=0}^{\infty} \frac{(-1)^n}{2^{2n}} (x - 1)^n.$$

Solution
The series is expanded about the point $x_0 = 1$ and the nth coefficient

$$a_n = \frac{(-1)^n}{2^{2n}}.$$

Thus

$$\left| \frac{a_n}{a_{n+1}} \right| = \left| \frac{(-1)^n 2^{2(n+1)}}{(-1)^{n+1} 2^{2n}} \right| = 4,$$

and so the radius of convergence

$$r = \lim_{n \to \infty} \left| \frac{a_n}{a_{n+1}} \right| = 4.$$

As $x_0 = 1$ and $r = 4$, it follows that the interval of convergence is

$$-3 < x < 5.$$

We leave as an exercise the task of showing that the series diverges at the end points of this interval.

Example 48.4

Find the radius and interval of convergence of

$$1 + \frac{x^2}{2!} + \frac{x^4}{4!} + \ldots = \sum_{n=0}^{\infty} \frac{x^{2n}}{(2n)!}.$$

Solution
This series is expanded about the point $x_0 = 0$, but it only contains even powers of x, so the nth coefficient

$$a_n = \begin{cases} \dfrac{1}{(2n)!}, & \text{if } n \text{ is even} \\[2mm] 0, & \text{if } n \text{ is odd.} \end{cases}$$

The ratio test which gave rise to the formula for r requires $a_n \neq 0$, so it cannot be applied directly.

To overcome the difficulty, set $z = x^2$, for then the series becomes the power series in z

$$1 + \frac{z}{2!} + \frac{z^2}{4!} + \ldots = \sum_{n=0}^{\infty} \frac{z^n}{(2n!)},$$

in which all the coefficients of z^n are non-zero.

This series is expanded about the point $z_0 = 0$, and its nth coefficient is

$$a_n = \frac{1}{(2n)!},$$

so

$$\left| \frac{a_n}{a_{n+1}} \right| = \frac{[2(n+1)]!}{(2n)!} = (2n+1)(2n+2).$$

Thus

$$r = \lim_{n \to \infty} \left| \frac{a_n}{a_{n+1}} \right| = \lim_{n \to \infty} [(2n+1)(2n+2)] = \infty,$$

so the radius of convergence with respect to z is infinite, but $z = x^2$, so the radius of convergence with respect to x is also infinite. Thus the series converges for $-\infty < x < \infty$.   ▲

Example 48.5

Find the radius and interval of convergence of

$$\sum_{n=0}^{\infty} (-1)^n \left(\frac{n+1}{5n+3} \right)^n (x-2)^n.$$

Solution
The series is expanded about the point $x_0 = 2$ and the nth coefficient

$$a_n = (-1)^n \left(\frac{n+1}{5n+3} \right)^n.$$

The form of a_n suggests that we make use of the formula for the radius of convergence based on the nth root test. Thus

$$r = \lim_{n \to \infty} \left| \frac{1}{a_n} \right|^{1/n}$$

$$= \lim_{n \to \infty} \left| (-1)^n \left(\frac{5n+3}{n+1} \right)^n \right|^{1/n}$$

$$= \lim_{n \to \infty} \left(\frac{5n+3}{n+1} \right) = 5.$$

As the series is expanded about the point $x_0 = 2$, it follows that the interval of convergence is

$$-3 < x < 7.$$ ▲

PROBLEMS 48

Find the radius and interval of convergence for each of the following power series.

1. $\displaystyle\sum_{n=0}^{\infty} x^n.$

2. $\displaystyle\sum_{n=0}^{\infty} \frac{x^n}{3^n(n+1)}.$

3. $\displaystyle\sum_{n=1}^{\infty} \frac{x^n}{n \cdot 2^n}.$

4. $\displaystyle\sum_{n=1}^{\infty} \frac{(x-1)^n}{(2n-1)\cdot 2^n}$.

5. $\displaystyle\sum_{n=1}^{\infty} \frac{(x+1)^n}{n\cdot 4^{n-1}}$.

6. $\displaystyle\sum_{n=1}^{\infty} \frac{(x-2)^n}{n^2}$.

7. $\displaystyle\sum_{n=1}^{\infty} n!\,x^n$.

8. $\displaystyle\sum_{n=1}^{\infty} \frac{n!}{n^n}\, x^n$.

9. $\displaystyle\sum_{n=1}^{\infty} \frac{x^n}{n^n}$.

10. $\displaystyle\sum_{n=1}^{\infty} \left(\frac{n}{n+1}\right)\left(\frac{x}{2}\right)^n$.

11. $\displaystyle\sum_{n=0}^{\infty} \frac{(x+2)^n}{n!}$.

12. $\displaystyle\sum_{n=1}^{\infty} \frac{10^n x^n}{\sqrt{n}}$.

13. $\displaystyle\sum_{n=1}^{\infty} \frac{(x-4)^n}{\sqrt{(n+1)}}$.

14. $\displaystyle\sum_{n=1}^{\infty} \frac{x^n}{n\cdot 2^n}$.

15. $\displaystyle\sum_{n=0}^{\infty} \frac{2^n x^n}{\sqrt{[(4n+1)/5^n]}}$.

16. $\displaystyle\sum_{n=0}^{\infty} \frac{2^n x^n}{(2n+1)^2\sqrt{(3n)}}$.

17. $\displaystyle\sum_{n=1}^{\infty} \left(1+\frac{1}{n}\right)^{n^2} (x+2)^n$.

18. $\displaystyle\sum_{n=1}^{\infty} (-1)^{n+1}\left(\frac{2n-1}{3n-2}\right)^{2n} (x-1)^n$.

19. $\displaystyle\sum_{n=1}^{\infty} \frac{(-1)^{n+1} x^{2n-1}}{5^n\sqrt{(n+1)}}$.

20. $\displaystyle\sum_{n=1}^{\infty} \frac{(x-1)^{2n-1}}{2n-1}$.

21. $\displaystyle\sum_{n=1}^{\infty} \frac{(x-3)^n}{n \cdot 5^n}$.

22. $\displaystyle\sum_{n=1}^{\infty} n^n (x+5)^n$.

23. $\displaystyle\sum_{n=1}^{\infty} \frac{x^{2n}}{(2n)^2 \, 2^{2n}}$.

24. $\displaystyle\sum_{n=1}^{\infty} \frac{x^{2n-1}}{3^n}$.

25. $\displaystyle\sum_{n=0}^{\infty} \frac{(n+1)^5}{2n+1} x^{2n}$.

26. $\displaystyle\sum_{n=1}^{\infty} x^{n!}$.

Taylor and Maclaurin series

In the previous section we saw how a power series defines a function, and how to determine the interval of convergence of the function represented by this series. We will now consider the converse of this situation, by discovering how a given function may be expressed in the form of a power series expanded about some convenient point.

Let $f(x)$ be a function which may be differentiated arbitrarily many times at $x = x_0$, and let us seek to represent $f(x)$ in the form of the power series

$$f(x) = \sum_{n=0}^{\infty} a_n (x - x_0)^n.$$

Our task is then to determine the coefficients a_n in terms of the given function $f(x)$. For the sake of simplicity, instead of using the summation notation, we will work with the series in the form

$$f(x) = a_0 + a_1(x - x_0) + a_2(x - x_0)^2 + a_3(x - x_0)^3 + \dots .$$

Setting $x = x_0$ shows that

$$a_0 = f(x_0).$$

Differentiating the series gives

$$f^{(1)}(x) = a_1 + 2a_2(x - x_0) + 3a_3(x - x_0)^2 + \dots ,$$

where, as usual, $f^{(1)}(x) = df/dx$.

Again setting $x = x_0$ we find from this that

$$a_1 = f^{(1)}(x_0).$$

A further differentiation yields

$$f^{(2)}(x) = 2a_2 + 2 \cdot 3a_3(x - x_0) + \dots ,$$

so once again setting $x = x_0$ we obtain the

$$a_2 = \frac{1}{2} f^{(2)}(x_0) = \frac{1}{2!} f^{(2)}(x_0).$$

A repetition of this process shows that

$$a_n = \frac{1}{n!} f^{(n)}(x_0),$$

where $f^{(n)}(x_0) = (d^n f / dx^n)_{x = x_0}$.

Substituting these coefficients into the original series gives

$$f(x) = f(x_0) + (x - x_0) f^{(1)}(x_0) + \frac{(x - x_0)^2}{2!} f^{(2)}(x_0) + \dots + \frac{(x - x_0)^n}{n!} f^{(n)}(x_0) + \dots ,$$

or

$$f(x) = \sum_{n = 0}^{\infty} \frac{(x - x_0)^n f^{(n)}(x_0)}{n!} ,$$

where, for convenience, we define $f^{(0)}(x_0) = f(x_0)$.

This power series expansion of $f(x)$ is called the **Taylor series expansion** of $f(x)$ about the point x_0. When $x_0 = 0$ the Taylor series expansion reduces to the **Maclaurin series expansion** of $f(x)$ (a Maclaurin series is always an expansion about the origin)

$$f(x) = \sum_{n = 0}^{\infty} \frac{x^n f^{(n)}(0)}{n!} .$$

Taylor and Maclaurin series

Let $f(x)$ be differentiable arbitrarily many times at $x = x_0$. Then the Taylor series expansion of $f(x)$ about the point x_0 is

$$f(x) = f(x_0) + (x - x_0) f^{(1)}(x_0) + \frac{(x - x_0)^2}{2!} f^{(2)}(x_0) + \dots + \frac{(x - x_0)^n}{n!} f^{(n)}(x_0) + \dots ,$$

or

$$f(x) = \sum_{n = 0}^{\infty} \frac{(x - x_0)^n f^{(n)}(x_0)}{n!} .$$

When the expansion of $f(x)$ is about the origin ($x_0 = 0$) the series is called the Maclaurin series expansion of $f(x)$ and it has the form

$$f(x) = f(0) + x f^{(1)}(0) + \frac{x^2}{2!} f^{(2)}(0) + \dots + \frac{x^n}{n!} f^{(n)}(0) + \dots ,$$

or

$$f(x) = \sum_{n = 0}^{\infty} \frac{x^n f^{(n)}(0)}{n!} .$$

The four examples which follow illustrate the determination of Maclaurin series.

Example 49.1

Find the Maclaurin series expansion of $\sin x$.

Solution

We must set $f(x) = \sin x$ and determine the values of successive derivatives of $f(x)$ at $x = 0$. Substitution of these values into the general Maclaurin series given above will then yield the required expansion. We have

$$f(0) = \sin 0 = 0,$$

$$f^{(1)}(x) = \cos x \quad, \quad \text{so} \quad f^{(1)}(0) = 1,$$

$$f^{(2)}(x) = -\sin x \quad, \quad \text{so} \quad f^{(2)}(0) = 0,$$

$$f^{(3)}(x) = -\cos x, \quad \text{so} \quad f^{(3)}(0) = -1.$$

Because of the differentiability properties of the sine and cosine functions, further differentiations will simply repeat the pattern of coefficients given above. So, for example, $f^{(4)}(0) = 0$, $f^{(5)}(0) = 1$, $f^{(6)}(0) = 0$ and $f^{(7)}(0) = -1$.

Thus, we see that $f^{(n)}(0) = 0$ when n is even, but that $f^{(n)}(0)$ alternates between $+1$ and -1 when n is odd. Substituting the values of $f^{(n)}(0)$ into the general Maclaurin series shows that the Maclaurin series for $\sin x$ is

$$\sin x = x - \frac{x^3}{3!} + \frac{x^5}{5!} - \frac{x^7}{7!} + \frac{x^9}{9!} - \cdots .$$

To write this more concisely by means of the summation convention we use the fact that if n is an integer, $2n$ must be an even number, and thus $2n + 1$ is an odd number. It then follows that as the expansion only contains odd powers of x and the signs alternate, the above result may also be written as

$$\sin x = \sum_{n=0}^{\infty} (-1)^n \frac{x^{2n+1}}{(2n+1)!}.$$

The radius of convergence of this series is easily shown to be $r = \infty$, so it is absolutely convergent for $-\infty < x < \infty$.   ▲

Example 49.2

Find the Maclaurin series for e^x.

Solution

Setting $f(x) = e^x$, and using the fact that

$$\frac{d^n}{dx^n}[e^x] = e^x,$$

we find that $f(0) = 1$ and, in general, $f^{(n)}(0) = 1$.

Thus, substituting the values of $f^{(n)}(0)$ into the general Maclaurin series gives as the Maclaurin series for e^x

$$e^x = 1 + x + \frac{x^2}{2!} + \frac{x^3}{3!} + \cdots ,$$

or

$$e^x = \sum_{n=0}^{\infty} \frac{x^n}{n!} \quad \text{(remember, by definition, } 0! = 1\text{)}.$$

This series has an infinite radius of convergence, so it is absolutely convergent for $-\infty < x < \infty$. Thus replacing x by $-x$ we see that the Maclaurin series for e^{-x} is

$$e^{-x} = 1 - x + \frac{x^2}{2!} - \frac{x^3}{3!} + \dots ,$$

or

$$e^{-x} = \sum_{n=0}^{\infty} (-1)^n \frac{x^n}{n!}.$$ ▲

Example 49.3

Find the Maclaurin series for $\ln(1 + x)$.

Solution
Setting $f(x) = \ln(1 + x)$ we have

$$f(0) = 0,$$

$$f^{(1)}(x) = \frac{1}{1 + x} \quad , \quad \text{so} \quad f^{(1)}(0) = 1,$$

$$f^{(2)}(x) = \frac{-1}{(1 + x)^2}, \quad \text{so} \quad f^{(2)}(0) = -1,$$

$$f^{(3)}(x) = \frac{1 \cdot 2}{(1 + x)^3} \quad , \quad \text{so} \quad f^{(3)}(0) = 2!$$

and, in general,

$$f^{(n)}(x) = \frac{(-1)^{n+1}(n-1)!}{(1 + x)^n}, \quad \text{so} \quad f^{(n)}(0) = (-1)^{n+1}(n-1)!,$$

for $n = 1, 2, 3, \dots$.
Substituting these values of $f^{(n)}(0)$ into the general Maclaurin series shows that the Maclaurin series for $\ln(1 + x)$ is

$$\ln(1 + x) = x - \frac{x^2}{2} + \frac{x^3}{3} - \frac{x^4}{4} + \dots + \frac{(-1)^{n+1}}{n} + \dots ,$$

or

$$\ln(1 + x) = \sum_{n=1}^{\infty} \frac{(-1)^{n+1} x^n}{n}.$$

This series was examined in Example 48.1, where it was shown to converge for $-1 < x \leqslant 1$.   ▲
Although the general term in the Maclaurin series considered so far has been easy to find by inspection, this is usually not the case. The last example shows how the successive derivatives of $f(x)$ often follow no simple pattern, so that then each term of the Maclaurin series must be found by direct calculation.

Example 49.4

Find the Maclaurin series for tan x.

Solution
We have

$$f(x) = \tan x, \quad \text{so} \quad f(0) = 0$$
$$f^{(1)}(x) = \sec^2 x, \quad \text{so} \quad f^{(1)}(0) = 1$$
$$f^{(2)}(x) = 2\sec^2 x \tan x, \quad \text{so} \quad f^{(2)}(0) = 0$$
$$f^{(3)}(x) = 4\sec^2 x \tan^2 x + 2\sec^4 x, \quad \text{so} \quad f^{(3)}(0) = 2$$
$$f^{(4)}(x) = 8\sec^2 x \tan^3 x + 16\sec^4 x \tan x, \quad \text{so} \quad f^{(4)}(0) = 0.$$

Continuing in this fashion we find (after tedious calculations) that $f^{(5)}(0) = 16$, $f^{(6)}(0) = 0$ and $f^{(7)}(0) = 272$. Thus substituting into the general Maclaurin series shows that the Maclaurin series for tan x is

$$\tan x = x + \frac{2}{3!} x^3 + \frac{16}{5!} x^5 + \frac{272}{7!} x^7 + \ldots ,$$

or

$$\tan x = x + \frac{1}{3} x^3 + \frac{2}{15} x^5 + \frac{17}{315} x^7 + \ldots . \qquad \blacktriangle$$

A series expansion of a function about the origin (a Maclaurin series) is not always convenient, and an expansion about some other point may be required. In many cases a function does not even possess a Maclaurin series expansion because it is not differentiable at the origin. This happens, for example, in the case of a function as simple as $f(x) = 1/x$. This has no Maclaurin series expansion but it may be expanded as a Taylor series about any point other than the origin.

This is also true of the function $f(x) = \ln x$, because it is not differentiable at the origin. The problem did not arise in Example 49.3, because the function expanded as a Maclaurin series was $\ln(1 + x)$ which is differentiable when $x = 0$.

Example 49.5

Find the Taylor series expansion of cos x about the point a.

Solution
To determine the required Taylor series we must set $f(x) = \cos x$ and $x_0 = a$, and then compute the derivatives $f^{(n)}(a)$, prior to substituting them into the general Taylor series expansion.

We have

$$f(x) = \cos x, \quad \text{so} \quad f(a) = \cos a,$$
$$f^{(1)}(x) = -\sin x, \quad \text{so} \quad f^{(1)}(a) = -\sin a,$$

$$f^{(2)}(x) = -\cos x, \quad \text{so} \quad f^{(2)}(a) = -\cos a$$
$$f^{(3)}(x) = \sin x, \quad \text{so} \quad f^{(3)}(a) = \sin a.$$

Hereafter, further differentiation simply repeats this pattern of coefficients, as in Example 49.1. Thus substituting into the general Taylor series expansion shows that the Taylor series expansion of $\cos x$ about the point a is

$$\cos x = \cos a - \frac{\sin a}{1!}(x-a) - \frac{\cos a}{2!}(x-a)^2 + \frac{\sin a}{3!}(x-a)^3 + \frac{\cos a}{4!}(x-a)^4 - \dots .$$

This series is easily shown to be absolutely convergent, so we may rearrange terms without altering its sum. As a result we may write

$$\cos x = \cos a\left[1 - \frac{(x-1)^2}{2!} + \frac{(x-a)^4}{4!} - \dots\right] - \sin a\left[(x-a) - \frac{(x-a)^3}{3!} + \frac{(x-a)^5}{5!} - \dots\right],$$

or

$$\cos x = \cos a \sum_{n=0}^{\infty} \frac{(-1)^n(x-a)^{2n}}{(2n)!} - \sin a \sum_{n=0}^{\infty} \frac{(-1)^n(x-a)^{2n+1}}{(2n+1)!}.$$

As a special case, by setting $a = 0$ we obtain from this the Maclaurin series expansion of $\cos x$

$$\cos x = \sum_{n=0}^{\infty} \frac{(-1)^n x^{2n}}{(2n)!}. \qquad\qquad \blacktriangle$$

As a final example let us find by means of a Taylor series an expansion which could also be obtained by use of the binomial theorem.

Example 49.6

Find the Taylor series expansion of $(2+x)^{-1/2}$ about the point 1.

Solution
To develop the required Taylor series we must set $f(x) = (2+x)^{1/2}$ and $x_0 = 1$, and then compute the derivatives $f^{(n)}(1)$, prior to substituting them into the general form of the Taylor series.
We have

$$f(x) = \frac{1}{(2+x)^{1/2}}, \quad \text{so} \quad f(1) = \frac{1}{3^{1/2}},$$

$$f^{(1)}(x) = -\frac{1}{2}\cdot\frac{1}{(2+x)^{3/2}}, \quad \text{so} \quad f^{(1)}(1) = -\frac{1}{2}\cdot\frac{1}{3^{3/2}},$$

$$f^{(2)}(x) = \frac{1}{2}\cdot\frac{3}{2}\cdot\frac{1}{(2+x)^{5/2}}, \quad \text{so} \quad f^{(2)}(1) = \frac{1\cdot3}{2^2 3^{5/2}},$$

$$f^{(3)}(x) = -\frac{1}{2}\cdot\frac{3}{2}\cdot\frac{5}{2}\cdot\frac{1}{(2+x)^{7/2}}, \quad \text{so} \quad f^{(3)}(1) = \frac{-1\cdot3\cdot5}{2^3 3^{7/2}},$$

and an inspection of the general pattern of the results together with some experimentation shows that

$$f^{(n)}(1) = (-1)^n \frac{1 \cdot 3 \cdot 5 \dots (2n-1)}{2^n 3^{(2n+1)/2}}.$$

Substituting the values for $f^{(n)}(1)$ into the general form of the Taylor series and setting $x_0 = 1$ shows that the required Taylor series expansion of $(2+x)^{-1/2}$ about the point 1 is

$$(2+x)^{-1/2} = \frac{1}{3^{1/2}} - \frac{1}{2 \cdot 3^{3/2}} \frac{(x-1)}{1!} + \frac{1 \cdot 3}{2^2 \cdot 3^{5/2}} \frac{(x-1)^2}{2!}$$

$$- \frac{1 \cdot 3 \cdot 5}{2^3 \cdot 3^{7/2}} \frac{(x-1)^3}{3!} + \dots + (-1)^n \frac{1 \cdot 3 \cdot 5 \dots (2n-1)}{2^2 \cdot 3^{(2n+1)/2}} \frac{(x-1)^n}{2!} + \dots.$$

This result could also have been obtained by means of the binomial theorem. First we introduce the term $(x-1)$ into the function $(2+x)^{-1/2}$ by writing it as

$$\frac{1}{(2+x)^{1/2}} = \frac{1}{[3+(x-1)]^{1/2}} = \frac{1}{3^{1/2}} \frac{1}{\left[1+\left(\dfrac{x-1}{3}\right)\right]^{1/2}},$$

$$= \frac{1}{3^{1/2}}(1+a)^{-1/2},$$

with $a = (x-1)/3$. Expanding this expression by the binomial theorem (Section 6) gives

$$\frac{1}{(2+x)^{1/2}} = \frac{1}{3^{1/2}}\left(1 - \frac{1}{2}a + \frac{1 \cdot 3}{2 \cdot 4}a^2 - \frac{1 \cdot 3 \cdot 5}{2 \cdot 4 \cdot 6}a^3 + \dots\right).$$

Substituting for a we obtain

$$\frac{1}{(2+x)^{1/2}} = \frac{1}{3^{1/2}}\left[1 - \frac{1}{2 \cdot 3}(x-1) + \frac{1 \cdot 3}{2^2 \cdot 3^2}\frac{(x-1)^2}{2!} - \frac{1 \cdot 3 \cdot 5}{2^3 \cdot 3^3}\frac{(x-1)^3}{3!} + \dots\right]$$

$$= \frac{1}{3^{1/2}} - \frac{1}{2 \cdot 3^{3/2}}(x-1) + \frac{1 \cdot 3}{2^2 \cdot 3^{5/2}}\frac{(x-1)^2}{2!} - \frac{1 \cdot 3 \cdot 5}{2^2 \cdot 3^{7/2}}\frac{(x-1)^3}{3!} + \dots,$$

which agrees with the previous result.   ▲

So far, our development of functions in terms of Taylor and Maclaurin series has been **formal**, in the sense that although we now know how to relate a power series to a given function, we have not actually proved that the function and its series are equal.

The justification for this is provided by writing the Taylor series of $f(x)$ about the point x_0 in the form

$$f(x) = f(x_0) + (x-x_0)f^{(1)}(x_0) + (x-x_0)^2\frac{f^{(2)}(x_0)}{2!} + \dots$$

$$+ (x - x_0)^{n-1} \frac{f^{(n-1)}(x_0)}{(n-1)!} + R_n(x),$$

where $R_n(x)$ is the **remainder** after n terms, and then showing that

$$\lim_{n \to \infty} R_n(x) = 0$$

for x in the interval of convergence. When expressed in this form, the result is called **Taylor's theorem**, from which **Maclaurin's theorem** follows by setting $x_0 = 0$.

The precise form of the remainder term $R_n(x)$ is given below in the statement of the Taylor and Maclaurin theorems.

Taylor and Maclaurin theorems
If $f(x)$ is differentiable n times, then the Taylor series expansion of $f(x)$ about the point x_0 can be written

$$f(x) = f(x_0) + (x - x_0)f^{(1)}(x_0) + (x - x_0)^2 \frac{f^{(2)}(x_0)}{2!} + (x - x_0)^3 \frac{f^{(3)}(x_0)}{3!} + \dots$$

$$+ (x - x_0)^{n-1} \frac{f^{(n-1)}(x_0)}{(n-1)!} + R_n(x),$$

where the remainder term

$$R_n(x) = \frac{(x - x_0)^n f^{(n)}(\xi)}{n!},$$

with ξ some number between x_0 and x. The above result reduces to the corresponding Maclaurin series expansion and remainder term when $x_0 = 0$.

We omit the proof of this result, though we remark that it follows by constructing a special function related to $f(x)$ to which Rolle's theorem may be applied.

Although the precise determination of the number ξ is usually impossible, the remainder term is still valuable because it may be used to estimate of the magnitude of the error made when $f(x)$ is represented by the polynomial

$$T_n(x) = f(x_0) + (x - x_0)f^{(1)}(x_0) + (x - x_0)^2 \frac{f^{(2)}(x_0)}{2!} + \dots + (x - x_0)^n \frac{f^{(n)}(x_0)}{n!}.$$

For obvious reasons $T_n(x)$ is called the **Taylor polynomial** of degree n obtained when $f(x)$ is expanded about the point x_0. It is the polynomial approximation to $f(x)$ obtained when its Taylor series is truncated after $n + 1$ terms. When the expansion is about the origin, the Taylor polynomial of degree n represents the corresponding polynomial approximation obtained when the Maclaurin series is truncated after $n + 1$ terms.

Example 49.7

Find the Taylor polynomial of degree 3 which approximates $e^{-x/2}$ when the expansion is about the point 1. Determine the magnitude of the error involved when x lies in the interval $-2 \leqslant x \leqslant 2$.

Solution
We set $f(x) = e^{-x/2}$ and $x_0 = 1$. Then we have

$$f(x) = e^{-x/2}, \quad \text{so} \quad f(1) = e^{-1/2},$$

$$f^{(1)}(x) = \frac{-1}{2} e^{-x/2}, \quad \text{so} \quad f^{(1)}(1) = \frac{-1}{2} e^{-1/2},$$

$$f^{(2)}(x) = \frac{1}{4} e^{-x/2}, \quad \text{so} \quad f^{(2)}(1) = \frac{1}{4} e^{-1/2},$$

$$f^{(3)}(x) = \frac{-1}{8} e^{-x/2}, \quad \text{so} \quad f^{(3)}(x) = \frac{-1}{8} e^{-x/2},$$

and

$$f^{(4)}(x) = \frac{1}{16} e^{-x/2}, \quad \text{so} \quad f^{(4)}(\xi) = \frac{1}{16} e^{-\xi/2}, \quad -2 \leqslant \xi \leqslant 2.$$

Substituting into Taylor's theorem we find that

$$e^{-x/2} = e^{-1/2} - \frac{e^{-1/2}}{2} \cdot \frac{(x-1)}{1!} + \frac{e^{-1/2}}{4} \frac{(x-1)^2}{2!} - \frac{e^{-1/2}}{8} \frac{(x-1)^3}{3!} + \frac{e^{-\xi/2}}{16} \frac{(x-1)^4}{4!},$$

so the Taylor polynomial $T_3(x)$ of degree 3 approximating $e^{-x/2}$ when expanded about the point 1 is

$$T_3(x) = e^{-1/2} \left[1 - \frac{1}{2}(x-1) + \frac{1}{8}(x-1)^2 - \frac{1}{48}(x-1)^3 \right],$$

and the remainder term

$$R_4(x) = \frac{e^{-\xi/2}}{16 \cdot 4!} (x-1)^4, \quad \text{for} \quad -2 \leqslant \xi \leqslant 2 \quad \text{and} \quad \xi \neq 1.$$

To estimate the magnitude of the error made when $e^{-x/2}$ is represented by $T_3(x)$ with $-2 \leqslant x \leqslant 2$, we proceed as follows. The function $e^{-x/2}$ is a strictly decreasing function of x, so on the interval $-2 \leqslant x \leqslant 2$ its maximum value occurs at the left end point of the interval where it equals e. The maximum value of the non-negative function $(x-1)^4$ on the interval $-2 \leqslant x \leqslant 2$, occurs at the left end-point at which it equals $(-3)^4 = 81$. Thus we have the over-estimate

$$R_4(x) < \left(\frac{e}{16} \right) \left(\frac{81}{4!} \right) = 0.573\,39.$$

In point of fact this is a gross over-estimate of the error, as may be seen from Table 7.

Table 7

x	$T_3(x)$	$e^{-x/2}$
-2	2.539 84	2.718 28
-1	1.617 41	1.648 72
0	0.998 25	1

| 1 | 0.606 53 | 0.606 53 |
| 2 | 0.366 45 | 0.367 88 |

The greatest error of 0.178 44 occurs when $x = -2$, but even here it is well within the error estimate. ▲

It can be shown that within its radius of convergence, the differentiation and integration of the power series (Taylor or Maclaurin series) representing a function $f(x)$ will yield the power series for $d[f(x)]/dx$ and $\int f(x)\,dx$, respectively. We now state this important result formally, though we will not prove it.

Differentiation and integration of power series
Let $f(x)$ be given by the power series

$$f(x) = \sum_{n=0}^{\infty} a_n(x - x_0)^n$$

with the radius of convergence r, so it is absolutely convergent for $x_0 - r < x < x_0 + r$. Then term-by-term differentiation and integration of the power series is permissible, and within the same interval of convergence $x_0 - r < x < x_0 + r$,

$$\frac{d[f(x)]}{dx} = \sum_{n=1}^{\infty} n\, a_n(x = x_0)^{n-1},$$

and

$$\int f(x)\,dx = \sum_{n=0}^{\infty} \frac{a_n}{n+1}(x - x_0)^{n+1} + C.$$

Example 49.8

Deduce the series expansion of $\cos x$ from the Maclaurin series expansion for $\sin x$.

Solution
We saw in Example 49.1 that

$$\sin x = x - \frac{x^3}{3!} + \frac{x^5}{5!} - \frac{x^7}{7!} + \frac{x^9}{9!} - \dots,$$

so as this is absolutely convergent for $-\infty < x < \infty$, it follows by differentiation that

$$\cos x = 1 - \frac{x^2}{2!} + \frac{x^4}{4!} - \frac{x^6}{6!} + \dots,$$

for $-\infty < x < \infty$. ▲

Example 49.9

Deduce the series expansion of $\ln(1+x)$ from the binomial expansion of $1/(1+x)$.

Solution
From the binomial theorem we have

$$\frac{1}{1+t} = 1 - t + t^2 - t^3 + \ldots + (-1)^n t^n + \ldots,$$

which we know to be absolutely convergent for $-1 < t < 1$. Thus we may integrate this result from 0 to x to obtain

$$\int_0^x \frac{dt}{1+t} = \int_0^x dt - \int_0^x t\,dt + \int_0^x t^2 dt - \int_0^x t^3 dt + \ldots + (-1)^n \int_0^x t^n dt + \ldots,$$

so

$$\ln(1+x) = x - \frac{x^2}{2} + \frac{x^3}{3} - \frac{x^4}{4} + \ldots + (-1)^n \frac{x^{n+1}}{n+1} + \ldots,$$

for $-1 < x < 1$, in agreement with the result obtained in Example 49.3.   ▲

Example 49.10

Deduce the series expansion of $\arctan x$ from the binomial expansion of $1/(1+x^2)$.

Solution
From the binomial theorem we have

$$\frac{1}{1+t^2} = 1 - t^2 + t^4 - t^6 + \ldots + (-1)^n t^{2n} + \ldots,$$

which is absolutely convergent for $-1 < t < 1$. Thus we may integrate this result from 0 to x to obtain

$$\int_0^x \frac{dt}{1+t^2} = \int_0^x dt - \int_0^x t^2 dt + \int_0^x t^4 dt + \ldots + (-1)^n \int_0^x t^{2n} dt + \ldots,$$

so

$$\arctan x = x - \frac{x^3}{3} + \frac{x^5}{5} - \frac{x^7}{7} + \ldots + (-1)^{n+1} \frac{x^{2n-1}}{2n-1} + \ldots,$$

for $-1 < x < 1$.   ▲

Often when working with Maclaurin series only the first few terms are required. In such circumstances, when the function $f(x)$ involved is the product of two functions with known Maclaurin series, the simplest way of finding first few terms of the required expansion of $f(x)$ may be by multiplication of the two series.

Example 49.11

Find the first three non-zero terms of the Maclaurin series expansion of
(i) $x \ln(1 + x^2)$;
(ii) $e^{-x} \sin 2x$.

Solution
(i) We saw in Example 49.3 that

$$\ln(1 + x) = x - \frac{x^2}{2} + \frac{x^2}{3} - \frac{x^4}{4} + \dots,$$

thus replacing x by x^2 gives

$$\ln(1 + x^2) = x^2 - \frac{x^4}{2} + \frac{x^6}{3} - \frac{x^8}{4} + \dots,$$

so

$$x \ln(1 + x^2) = x^3 - \frac{x^5}{2} + \frac{x^7}{3} + \dots,$$

for $-1 < x < 1$ (the interval of convergence of $\ln(1 + x)$ and thus of $\ln(1 + x^2)$).

(ii) We saw in Example 49.2 that

$$e^x = 1 + x + \frac{x^2}{2!} + \frac{x^3}{3!} + \dots,$$

for $-\infty < x < \infty$, so replacing x by $-x$ gives

$$e^{-x} = 1 - x + \frac{x^2}{2!} - \frac{x^3}{3!} + \dots,$$

for $-\infty < x < \infty$.
In Example 49.1 we found that

$$\sin x = x - \frac{x^3}{3!} + \frac{x^5}{5!} - \frac{x^7}{2!} + \dots,$$

for $-\infty < x < \infty$, so replacing x by $2x$ gives

$$\sin 2x = 2x - \frac{(2x)^3}{3!} + \frac{(2x)^5}{5!} - \dots,$$

or

$$\sin 2x = 2x - \frac{4}{3} x^3 + \frac{4}{15} x^5 - \dots,$$

for $-\infty < x < \infty$.
    Thus

$$e^{-x}\sin 2x = \left(1 - x + \frac{x^2}{2!} - \frac{x^3}{3!} + \ldots\right)\left(2x - \frac{4}{3}x^3 - \frac{4}{15}x^5 - \ldots\right),$$

so multiplying out the first few terms we have

$$e^{-x}\sin 2x = \left(2x - \frac{4}{3}x^3 + \frac{4}{15}x^5 - \ldots\right) + \left(-2x^2 + \frac{4}{3}x^4 - \frac{4}{15}x^6 + \ldots\right)$$

$$+ \left(x^3 - \frac{2}{3}x^5 + \frac{2}{15}x^7 - \ldots\right) + \left(-\frac{1}{3}x^4 + \frac{2}{9}x^6 - \frac{1}{45}x^8 + \ldots\right) + \ldots,$$

after which collecting terms gives the required result

$$e^{-x}\sin 2x = 2x - 2x^2 - \frac{1}{3}x^3 + \ldots.$$

When carrying out this operation care must always be taken to see that each function is expanded far enough to ensure that all terms of the required degree are contained in the answer.   ▲

Example 49.12

Use the Maclaurin series expansion of e^x to find the Maclaurin series expansions of $\sinh x$ and $\cosh x$.

Solution
We have from Example 49.2 that

$$e^x = 1 + x + \frac{x^2}{2!} + \frac{x^3}{3!} + \frac{x^4}{4!} + \ldots$$

for $-\infty < x < \infty$, so replacing x by $-x$ gives

$$e^{-x} = 1 - x + \frac{x^2}{2!} - \frac{x^3}{3!} + \frac{x^4}{4!} - \ldots,$$

for $-\infty < x < \infty$.
  Recalling that

$$\sinh x = \frac{e^x - e^{-x}}{2} \quad \text{and} \quad \cosh x = \frac{e^x + e^{-x}}{2},$$

it follows by addition and subtraction of these series that

$$\sinh x = x + \frac{x^3}{3!} + \frac{x^5}{5!} + \frac{x^7}{7!} + \ldots + \frac{x^{2n+1}}{(2n+1)!} + \ldots,$$

and

$$\cosh x = 1 + \frac{x^2}{2!} + \frac{x^4}{4!} + \frac{x^6}{6!} + \ldots + \frac{x^{2n}}{(2n)!} + \ldots,$$

for $-\infty < x < \infty$.   ▲

SOME USEFUL SERIES

1 $(1 \pm x)^{-1} = 1 \mp x + x^2 \mp x^3 \mp x^4 \mp \dots ,$

  for $-1 < x < 1$.

2 $(1 \pm x)^{1/2} = 1 \pm \dfrac{1}{2} x - \dfrac{1 \cdot 1}{2 \cdot 4} x^2 \pm \dfrac{1 \cdot 1 \cdot 3}{2 \cdot 4 \cdot 6} x^3 - \dfrac{1 \cdot 1 \cdot 3 \cdot 5}{2 \cdot 4 \cdot 6 \cdot 8} x^4 \pm \dots ,$

  for $-1 < x < 1$.

3 $(1 \pm x)^{1/2} = 1 \mp \dfrac{1}{2} x + \dfrac{1 \cdot 3}{2 \cdot 4} x^2 \mp \dfrac{1 \cdot 3 \cdot 5}{2 \cdot 4 \cdot 6} x^3 + \dfrac{1 \cdot 3 \cdot 5 \cdot 7}{2 \cdot 4 \cdot 6 \cdot 8} x^4 \mp \dots$

  for $-1 < x < 1$.

4 $e^x = 1 + x + \dfrac{x^2}{2!} + \dfrac{x^3}{3!} + \dfrac{x^4}{4!} + \dots + \dfrac{x^n}{n!} + \dots ,$

  for $-\infty < x < \infty$.

5 $e^{-x} = 1 - x + \dfrac{x^2}{2!} - \dfrac{x^3}{3!} + \dfrac{x^4}{4!} + \dots + (-1)^n \dfrac{x^n}{n!} + \dots ,$

  for $-\infty < x < \infty$.

6 $\sin x = x - \dfrac{x^3}{3!} + \dfrac{x^5}{5!} - \dfrac{x^7}{7!} + \dots + (-1)^{n+1} \dfrac{x^{2n-1}}{(2n-1)} + \dots ,$

  for $-\infty < x < \infty$.

7 $\cos x = 1 - \dfrac{x^2}{2!} + \dfrac{x^4}{4!} - \dfrac{x^6}{6!} + \dots + (-1)^n \dfrac{x^{2n}}{(2n)!} + \dots ,$

  for $-\infty < x < \infty$.

8 $\ln(1 + x) = x - \dfrac{x^2}{2} + \dfrac{x^3}{3} - \dfrac{x^4}{4} + \dots + (-1)^{n+1} \dfrac{x^n}{n} + \dots ,$

  for $-1 < x < 1$.

9 $\sinh x = x + \dfrac{x^3}{3!} + \dfrac{x^5}{5!} + \dfrac{x^7}{7!} + \dots + \dfrac{x^{2n+1}}{(2n-1)!} + \dots ,$

  for $-\infty < x < \infty$.

10 $\cosh x = 1 + \dfrac{x^2}{2!} + \dfrac{x^4}{4!} + \dfrac{x^6}{6!} + \dots + \dfrac{x^{2n}}{(2n)!} + \dots ,$

  for $-\infty < x < \infty$.

NEWTON'S METHOD: AN APPLICATION OF TAYLOR'S THEOREM

The solution of many problems in both science and engineering depend for their success on finding the zeros of a function $f(x)$. Let us make clear at the outset the relationship between the roots of an equation and the zeros of a function. The numbers $x_1, x_2, \dots$, which satisfy the equation

$$f(x) = 0$$

are called the **roots** of the equation. Thus the roots of the quadratic equation

$$ax^2 + bx + c = 0$$

can be found from the familiar quadratic formula

$$x = \frac{-b \pm \sqrt{(b^2 - 4ac)}}{2a}.$$

If, now, $f(x)$ is considered as a function, then these same numbers $x_1, x_2, \ldots$, which make $f(x)$ zero are called the **zeros** of $f(x)$. Thus the roots of $f(x) = 0$ are the zeros of $f(x)$.

Unfortunately, the roots of most functions cannot be found by means of a simple formula, so when they are required it is necessary to use numerical methods. Such a method is **Newton's method**, and it is based on a simple application of Taylor's theorem.

Suppose we wish to find a zero (there may be more than one) of the differentiable function $f(x)$. Then by graphing the function, or by experimentation to find two values of x between which $f(x)$ changes sign (its graph crosses the x-axis), it is possible to find an approximate zero x_0, say. Then if $x_0 + h$ is an exact zero (h is the correction we must add to x_0) it follows that

$$f(x_0 + h) = 0.$$

Now using Taylor's theorem with a remainder after one term (this is, in fact, the mean value theorem of Section 26) we may write

$$f(x_0 + h) = f(x_0) + h f'(\xi),$$

where $x_0 < \xi < x_0 + h$. However, $f(x_0 + h) = 0$, so

$$f(x_0) + h f'(\xi) = 0.$$

If we now approximate ξ by x_0 we find that the approximate correction

$$h_0 = -\frac{f(x_0)}{f'(x_0)}.$$

Thus a better approximation to the zero is

$$x_1 = x_0 + h_0.$$

This process may now be repeated using x_1 in place of x_0 and, as a result, an improved approximation to the zero will be

$$x_2 = x_1 + h_1, \text{ where } h_1 = -\frac{f(x_1)}{f'(x_1)}.$$

Repetition of this process is called **iteration**, and it is terminated when the magnitude of the difference $\left| x_r - x_{r+1} \right|$ between two successive **iterates** (x_r is called the rth iterate) becomes less than some preassigned small number, say 0.0001.

Newton's iterative scheme

Let $f(x)$ be a differentiable function, and let x_0 be an approximate zero of $f(x)$. Then the $(n+1)$th approximation to the exact zero (the $(n+1)$th iterate) is given by

$$x_{n+1} = x_n + h_n,$$

where

$$h_n = -\frac{f(x_n)}{f'(x_n)}.$$

Example 49.13

Find the positive zero of

$$f(x) = \sin x - \frac{1}{2}x.$$

Solution

The required zero occurs at the positive value of x at which the graphs $y = \sin x$ and $y = \frac{1}{2}x$ intersect. Inspection of Fig. 108 shows that intersection occurs for positive x at the approximate value $x = 2$. Thus in Newton's method we set $x_0 = 2$.

The calculation then proceeds as follows.

As

$$f(x) = \sin x - \frac{1}{2}x,$$

it follows that

$$f'(x) = \cos x - \frac{1}{2}.$$

Thus the iterative scheme becomes

$$x_{n+1} = x_n + h_n,$$

where

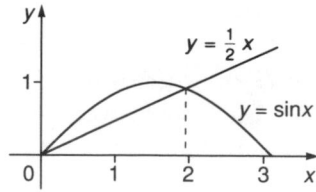

Fig. 108

$$h_n = -\left(\frac{\sin x_n - \frac{1}{2} x_n}{\cos x_n - \frac{1}{2}}\right).$$

First iteration

$$x_0 = 2, \quad \text{so} \quad h_0 = -\left(\frac{\sin 2 - \left(\frac{1}{2}\right) \cdot 2}{\cos 2 - \frac{1}{2}}\right) = -0.099\,004,$$

thus $x_1 = x_0 + h_0 = 1.900\,996$.

Second iteration

$$x_1 = 1.900\,996, \quad \text{so} \quad h_1 = -\left(\frac{\sin x_1 - \frac{1}{2} x_1}{\cos x_1 - \frac{1}{2}}\right) = -0.005\,484,$$

thus $x_2 = x_1 + h_1 = 1.895\,512$.

Third iteration

$$x_2 = 1.895\,512, \quad \text{so} \quad h_2 = -\left(\frac{\sin x_2 - \frac{1}{2} \dot{x}_2}{\cos x_2 - \frac{1}{2}}\right) = -0.000\,180,$$

thus $x_3 = x_2 + h_2 = 1.895\,494$.

Fourth iteration

$$x_3 = 1.895\,494, \quad \text{so} \quad h_3 = -\left(\frac{\sin x_3 - \frac{1}{2} x_3}{\cos x_3 - \frac{1}{2}}\right) = 2.67 \times 10^{-7},$$

thus $x_4 = x_3 + h_3 = 1.895\,494$.

We now have no change to six decimal places, so the zero to six decimal places is

$$x = 1.895\,494. \qquad \blacktriangle$$

DIFFICULTIES WITH NEWTON'S METHOD

If a bad choice is made for the initial approximation to the zero of $f(x)$ the method may either converge to a **different** zero (if there is more than one) or it may diverge, in which case successive iterates will increase rapidly in magnitude and will usually oscillate in sign. This is an indication that a better choice is needed for the initial approximation to the zero.

Consider, for example, the quadratic equation

$$50x^2 - 15x + 1 = 0,$$

which has the roots $x = 1/10$ and $x = 1/5$. Suppose the smaller of the two roots was required and a rough calculation suggested that a reasonable choice for x_0 was $x_0 = 0.15$. Then in this case the method would, indeed, converge to the value $x = 0.1$. However, had we made the choice $x_0 = 0.16$ it would have converged to the root $x = 0.2$.

PROBLEMS 49

In problems 1 to 20 find the first four non-zero terms in the Maclaurin series expansion of the given functions.

1. $f(x) = xe^x$.
2. $f(x) = \cos 2x$.
3. $f(x) = (1 + x)^\alpha$ (α real).
4. $f(x) = \cosh 3x$.
5. $f(x) = \sinh \dfrac{1}{2} x$.
6. $f(x) = \ln(3 + 2x)$.
7. $f(x) = \ln(1 + x^{1/2})$.
8. $f(x) = (1 + x^2)^{-1/2}$.
9. $f(x) = e^x \sin x$.
10. $f(x) = e^{2x} \sinh x$.
11. $f(x) = e^{-x} \ln(1 - x)$.
12. $f(x) = \dfrac{x}{\sqrt{(1 - x)}}$.
13. $f(x) = a^x$ ($a > 0$).
14. $f(x) = \sin^2 x$.
15. $f(x) = \tanh x$.
16. $f(x) = \sec x$.
17. $f(x) = \sin\left(x + \dfrac{\pi}{6}\right)$.
18. $f(x) = \ln[x + \sqrt{(1 + x^2)}]$.
19. $f(x) = \dfrac{x}{4 + x^2}$.
20. $f(x) = \dfrac{2x + 1}{(x - 1)^2}$.

In problems 21 to 26 find the first four terms of the Taylor series expansion of the function about the stated point.

21. $\ln x$ about the point 1.
22. $f(x) = 1/x$ about the point 1.
23. $f(x) = 1/x^2$ about the point -1.
24. $f(x) = e^x$ about the point -2.
25. $f(x) = \sqrt{x}$ about the point 4.
26. $f(x) = \cos x$ about the point $\pi/2$.

Use known series to express the integrands in problems 27 to 32 as series in
t. Then, by integrating term-by-term, find a series expansion for each of the
functions defined by an integral.

27. $\displaystyle\int_0^x \frac{\sin t}{t}\,dt.$

28. $\displaystyle\int_0^x \left(\frac{1-\cos t}{t^2}\right)dt.$

29. $\displaystyle\int_0^x \frac{\ln(1+2t)}{t}\,dt.$

30. $\displaystyle\int_0^x (1+t^2)^{1/3}\,dt.$

31. $\displaystyle\int_0^x \left(\frac{1-e^{-t^2}}{t^2}\right)dt.$

32. $\displaystyle\int_0^x \left(\frac{1-\cosh 2t}{t^2}\right)dt.$

33. Use known series to find the Maclaurin series for
$$f(x) = \ln\left(\frac{1+x}{1-x}\right).$$

34. Using known series find the first two non-zero terms of the Maclaurin
series for
$$f(x) = \sin x \sinh x.$$

35. Use known series to find the first three terms in the Maclaurin series
expansion of
$$f(x) = e^{\sin x}.$$

36. Use known series to find the first three non-zero terms in the Maclaurin
series expansion of
$$f(x) = e^{\cos x}.$$

37. Use known series to find the first three non-zero terms in the Maclaurin
series expansion of
$$f(x) = \sin^2 x.$$

(a) by multiplication of series, and (b) by using the trigonometric identity
$$\sin^2 x = \frac{1}{2}(1 - \cos 2x),$$

and compare the work involved.

38. Use known series to find the first three non-zero terms in the Maclaurin series expansion of

$$f(x) = e^{\cos^2 x}$$

(a) by multiplication of series, and (b) by using the trigonometric identity

$$\cos^2 x = \frac{1}{2}(1 + \cos 2x),$$

and compare the work involved.

In problems 39 to 46 use Newton's method with the stated initial approximation x_0 to find the zero of the given function accurately to four decimal places.

39. $f(x) = \sin x - \frac{2}{3}x$, with $x_0 = 1.5$.

40. $f(x) = \tan x - 3x$, with $x_0 = 1.2$.

41. $f(x) = x^3 + 2x^2 - x - 1$, with $x_0 = 1$.

42. $f(x) = (1 + x^2)\tan x - 4x$, with $x_0 = 1.3$.

43. $f(x) = x^4 + 4x^3 - 3x^2 + 1$, with $x_0 = -0.2$.

44. $f(x) = \sinh x - 3\cos x$, with $x_0 = 0.7$.

45. $f(x) = x^4 + 4x^3 - 3x^2 + 1$, with $x_0 = -6$.

46. $f(x) = 32x^2 - 12x + 1$, with (a) $x_0 = 0.1$, (b) $x_0 = 0.16$ and (c) $x_0 = 0.19$.

Compare the initial approximations and the value of the zero to which the method converges with the exact solutions $x = 1/8$ and $x = 1/4$.

47. By using the known series for e^θ, $\sin \theta$ and $\cos \theta$, verify that replacing θ by $i\theta$ in e^θ and then grouping the real and imaginary terms leads to the result

$$e^{i\theta} = \left(1 - \frac{\theta^2}{2!} + \frac{\theta^4}{4!} - \cdots\right) + i\left(\theta - \frac{\theta^3}{3!} + \frac{\theta^5}{5!} - \cdots\right],$$

and hence to the **Euler formula**

$$e^{i\theta} = \cos \theta + i \sin \theta,$$

from which it follows that

$$(e^{i\theta})^n = e^{in\theta} = \cos n\theta + i \sin n\theta.$$

Taylor's theorem for functions of two variables: stationary points and their identification 50

Taylor's theorem for an n times differentiable function $f(x)$ is

$$f(x) = f(x_0) + (x - x_0)f^{(1)}(x_0) + \frac{(x - x_0)^2}{2!}f^{(2)}(x_0) + \ldots$$

$$+ \frac{(x - x_0)^{n-1}}{(n-1)!}f^{(n-1)}(x) + \frac{(x - x_0)^n}{n!}f^{(n)}(\xi),$$

where ξ lies between x_0 and x. Let us use this result to derive the corresponding theorem for a suitably differentiable function $f(x, y)$ of two independent variables. Let $f(x, y)$ be differentiable at the adjacent points (x_0, y_0) and $(x_0 + h, y_0 + k)$, where h, k are numbers. Then if we regard $y = y_0 + k$ as fixed, we may expand $f(x_0 + h, y_0 + k)$ in terms of $x = x_0 + h$ by means of Taylor's theorem for one independent variable. Performing this expansion gives

$$f(x_0 + h, y_0 + k) = f(x_0, y_0 + k) + h\left(\frac{\partial f}{\partial x}\right)_{(x_0, y_0 + k)} + \frac{h^2}{2!}\left(\frac{\partial^2 f}{\partial x^2}\right)_{(x_0, y_0 + k)} + \ldots .$$

We now expand each term on the right-hand side in similar fashion, where now it is in terms of the variable $y = y_0 + k$. As a result we obtain

$$f(x_0, y_0 + k) = f(x_0, y_0) + k\left(\frac{\partial f}{\partial x}\right)_{(x_0, y_0)} + \frac{k^2}{2!}\left(\frac{\partial^2 f}{\partial x^2}\right)_{(x_0, y_0 + k)} + \ldots ,$$

$$\left(\frac{\partial f}{\partial x}\right)_{(x_0, y_0 + k)} = \left(\frac{\partial f}{\partial x}\right)_{(x_0, y_0)} + k\left(\frac{\partial^2 f}{\partial x \partial x}\right)_{(x_0, y_0)} + \frac{k^2}{2!}\left(\frac{\partial^3 f}{\partial^2 y \partial x}\right)_{(x_0, y_0)} + \ldots ,$$

$$\left(\frac{\partial^2 f}{\partial x^2}\right)_{(x_0, y_0 + k)} = \left(\frac{\partial^2 f}{\partial x^2}\right)_{(x_0, y_0)} + k\left(\frac{\partial^3 f}{\partial y \partial x^2}\right)_{(x_0, y_0)} + \ldots ,$$

and similar expressions for higher order partial derivatives.

Substituting these expressions into the original Taylor series, and collecting together derivatives of the same order, gives

$$f(x_0 + h, y_0 + k) = f(x_0, y_0) + \left[h \left(\frac{\partial f}{\partial x} \right)_{(x_0, y_0)} + k \left(\frac{\partial f}{\partial y} \right)_{(x_0, y_0)} \right]$$

$$+ \frac{1}{2!} \left[h^2 \left(\frac{\partial^2 f}{\partial x^2} \right)_{(x_0, y_0)} + 2hk \left(\frac{\partial^2 f}{\partial x \partial y} \right)_{(x_0, y_0)} + k^2 \left(\frac{\partial^2 f}{\partial y^2} \right)_{(x_0, y_0)} \right] + \ldots + \text{remainder term}$$

where use has been made of the fact that because the derivatives are continuous $\partial^2 f / \partial x \partial y = \partial^2 f / \partial y \partial x$.

To formulate Taylor's theorem for the function $f(x, y)$ of two variables in a concise form we need to introduce a new notation for repeated differentiation.

Let us agree to understand by the expression

$$\left[(x - x_0) \frac{\partial}{\partial x} + (y - y_0) \frac{\partial}{\partial y} \right]^r$$

the differentiation operation obtained by expanding the expression by the binomial theorem and interpreting products such as

$$\frac{\partial}{\partial x} \cdot \frac{\partial}{\partial y} \quad \text{and} \quad \frac{\partial}{\partial x} \cdot \frac{\partial}{\partial y} \cdot \frac{\partial}{\partial y}$$

as the differentiation operations

$$\frac{\partial^2}{\partial x \partial y} \quad \text{and} \quad \frac{\partial^3}{\partial x \partial y^2}.$$

Let us also use the convenient notation

$$\left[(x - x_0) \frac{\partial}{\partial x} + (y - y_0) \frac{\partial}{\partial y} \right]^r f(x_0, y_0)$$

to represent the result of applying the above differentiation operation to $f(x, y)$ and then setting $x = x_0$, $y = y_0$ **only in the derivatives**. Thus, for example,

$$\left[(x - x_0) \frac{\partial}{\partial x} + (y - y_0) \frac{\partial}{\partial y} \right]^2 f(x_0, y_0) = (x - x_0)^2 \left(\frac{\partial^2 f}{\partial x^2} \right)_{(x_0, y_0)}$$

$$+ 2(x - x_0)(y - y_0) \left(\frac{\partial^2 f}{\partial x \partial y} \right)_{(x_0, y_0)} + (y - y_0)^2 \left(\frac{\partial^2 f}{\partial y^2} \right)_{(x_0, y_0)}$$

Then, after taking account of the remainder terms, we arrive at the following form of Taylor's theorem.

Taylor's theorem for a function of two variables
Let $f(x, y)$ have continuous partial derivatives up to order n in some region containing the point (x_0, y_0). Then, for any point (x, y) in this same region,

$$f(x, y) = f(x_0, y_0) + \sum_{r=1}^{n-1} \frac{1}{r!} \left[(x - x_0) \frac{\partial}{\partial x} + (y - y_0) \frac{\partial}{\partial y} \right]^r f(x_0, y_0)$$

$$+ \frac{1}{n!} \left[(x - x_0) \frac{\partial}{\partial x} + (y - y_0) \frac{\partial}{\partial y} \right]^n f(\xi, \eta),$$

where ξ lies between x_0 and x and η between y_0 and y in the remainder term.

Example 50.1

Use Taylor's theorem to expand the function
$$f(x, y) = x^2 + 3x^2y^2 - 4y^2$$
about the point $(1, 2)$ up to and including terms of degree 2.

Solution
The Taylor series up to and including terms in x and y of degree 2 is

$$f(x, y) = f(x_0, y_0) + (x - x_0) \left(\frac{\partial f}{\partial x} \right)_{(x_0, y_0)} + (y - y_0) \left(\frac{\partial f}{\partial y} \right)_{(x_0, y_0)}$$

$$+ \frac{1}{2!} \left[(x - x_0)^2 \left(\frac{\partial^2 f}{\partial x^2} \right)_{(x_0, y_0)} + 2(x - x_0)(y - y_0) \left(\frac{\partial^2 f}{\partial x \partial y} \right)_{(x_0, y_0)} \right.$$

$$\left. + (y - y_0)^2 \left(\frac{\partial^2 f}{\partial y^2} \right)_{(x_0, y_0)} \right] + \dots .$$

However, in this example $x_0 = 1$, $y_0 = 2$ and $f(x, y) = x^2 + 3x^2y^2 - 4y^2$, so

$$\frac{\partial f}{\partial x} = 2x + 6xy^2, \quad \frac{\partial f}{\partial y} = 6x^2y - 8y,$$

$$\frac{\partial^2 f}{\partial x^2} = 2 + 6y^2, \quad \frac{\partial^2 f}{\partial x \partial y} = 12xy, \quad \frac{\partial^2 f}{\partial y^2} = 6x^2 - 8.$$

Thus at the point $(1, 2)$,

$$\frac{\partial f}{\partial x} = 26, \quad \frac{\partial f}{\partial y} = -4,$$

$$\frac{\partial f}{\partial x} = 26, \quad \frac{\partial^2 f}{\partial x \partial y} = 24, \quad \frac{\partial^2 f}{\partial y^2} = -2.$$

Substituting into the Taylor's series and neglecting the remainder after the derivatives of order 2 have been taken into account gives

$$f(x, y) = -3 + 26(x - 1) - 4(y - 2)$$

$$+ \frac{1}{2} [26(x - 1)^2 + 48(x - 1)(y - 2) - 2(y - 2)^2]. \quad \blacktriangle$$

The most important use of Taylor's theorem for a function of two variables to be considered here is the identification of the nature of the stationary points of a twice differentiable function $z = f(x, y)$.

By definition, the **stationary points** of $f(x, y)$ are the points at which

$$\frac{\partial f}{\partial x} = 0 \quad \text{and} \quad \frac{\partial f}{\partial y} = 0,$$

so they are points at which the **tangent plane** to the graph of $z = f(x, y)$ is **parallel** to the (x, y)-plane. This can occur at a **local maximum** as in

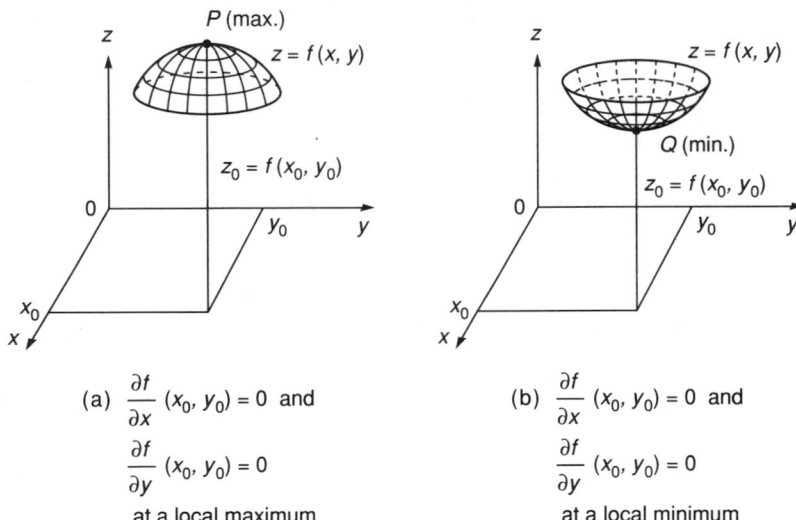

(a) $\dfrac{\partial f}{\partial x}(x_0, y_0) = 0$ and

$\dfrac{\partial f}{\partial y}(x_0, y_0) = 0$

at a local maximum

(b) $\dfrac{\partial f}{\partial x}(x_0, y_0) = 0$ and

$\dfrac{\partial f}{\partial y}(x_0, y_0) = 0$

at a local minimum

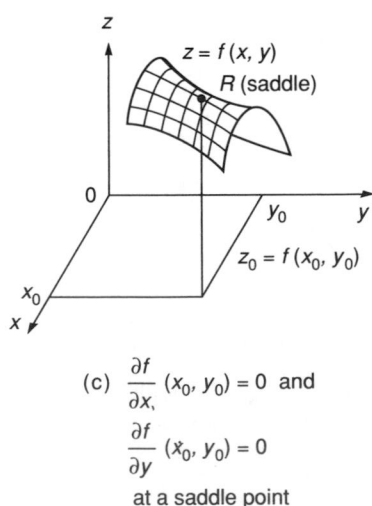

(c) $\dfrac{\partial f}{\partial x}(x_0, y_0) = 0$ and

$\dfrac{\partial f}{\partial y}(x_0, y_0) = 0$

at a saddle point

Fig. 109

Fig. 109(a), at a **local minimum** as in Fig. 109(b) or at a **saddle point** as in Fig. 109(c). We refer to P and Q as local maxima and minima, because there may be others elsewhere which are, respectively, larger or smaller.

When a stationary point occurs at (x_0, y_0) the characteristics which identify its nature are:

$$f(x, y) - f(x_0, y_0) = \begin{cases} \text{negative for a local maximum} \\ \text{positive for a local minimum} \\ \text{changes sign at a saddle point depending on} \\ \text{location of } (x, y) \text{ relative to } (x_0, y_0). \end{cases}$$

To examine the behaviour of $f(x, y) - f(x_0, y_0)$ at a stationary point we shall use Taylor's theorem with the remainder term corresponding to $n = 2$. Thus we will make use of the result

$$f(x, y) = f(x_0, y_0) + \left[(x - x_0) \left(\frac{\partial f}{\partial x} \right)_{(x_0, y_0)} + (y - y_0) \left(\frac{\partial f}{\partial y} \right)_{(x_0, y_0)} \right]$$

$$+ \frac{1}{2!} \left[(x - x_0)^2 \left(\frac{\partial^2 f}{\partial x^2} \right)_{(\xi, \eta)} + 2(x - x_0)(y - y_0) \left(\frac{\partial^2 f}{\partial x \partial y} \right)_{(\xi, \eta)} + (y - y_0)^2 \left(\frac{\partial^2 f}{\partial y^2} \right)_{(\xi, \eta)} \right]$$

where ξ lies between x_0 and x and η between y_0 and y.

Now if (x_0, y_0) is a stationary point,

$$\left(\frac{\partial f}{\partial x} \right)_{(x_0, y_0)} = \left(\frac{\partial f}{\partial y} \right)_{(x_0, y_0)} = 0,$$

so Taylor's theorem reduces to

$$f(x, y) - f(x_0, y_0) = \frac{1}{2!} \left[(x - x_0)^2 \left(\frac{\partial^2 f}{\partial x^2} \right)_{(\xi, \eta)} + 2(x - x_0)(y - y_0) \left(\frac{\partial^2 f}{\partial x \partial y} \right)_{(\xi, \eta)} \right.$$

$$\left. + (y - y_0)^2 \left(\frac{\partial^2 f}{\partial y^2} \right)_{(\xi, \eta)} \right]$$

To simplify the notation we now set

$$A = \left(\frac{\partial^2 f}{\partial x^2} \right)_{(\xi, \eta)}, \quad B = \left(\frac{\partial^2 f}{\partial x \partial y} \right)_{(\xi, \eta)} \quad \text{and} \quad C = \left(\frac{\partial^2 f}{\partial y^2} \right)_{(\xi, \eta)},$$

so that

$$f(x, y) - f(x_0, y_0) = \frac{1}{2} [h^2 A + 2hkB + k^2 C],$$

where $h = x - x_0$ and $k = y - y_0$.

After completing the square this becomes

$$f(x, y) - f(x_0, y_0) = \frac{1}{2} A \left[\left(h + \frac{B}{A} k \right)^2 + \left(\frac{AC - B^2}{A^2} \right) k^2 \right].$$

Now $(h + Bk/A)^2 > 0$ while $(AC - B^2)k^2/A^2 > 0$ if $k \neq 0$ and $AC - B^2 > 0$. If $k = 0$ this reduces to Ah^2 which will be positive if $A > 0$. Then if $A > 0$ and $AC - B^2 > 0$, we see that $f(x, y) - f(x_0, y_0) > 0$, so (x_0, y_0) must be a local minimum.

Similarly, if $A < 0$ and $AC - B^2 > 0$ it follows that (x_0, y_0) must be a local maximum.

If, however, $AC - B^2 < 0$ the expression $f(x, y) - f(x_0, y_0)$ can change sign depending on h and k, so this situation must correspond to a saddle point. Thus, close to (x_0, y_0), we may set $\xi = x_0$ and $\eta = y_0$ to arrive at the following test.

Identification of stationary points of f(x, y)

1 The point (x_0, y_0) is a local $\begin{Bmatrix} \text{maximum} \\ \text{minimum} \end{Bmatrix}$ of $f(x, y)$ if

(i) $\frac{\partial f}{\partial x}(x_0, y_0) = 0$; and $\frac{\partial f}{\partial y}(x_0, y_0) = 0$;

(ii) $\frac{\partial^2 f}{\partial x^2}(x_0, y_0) \frac{\partial^2 f}{\partial y^2}(x_0, y_0) - \left[\frac{\partial^2 f}{\partial x \partial y}(x_0, y_0) \right]^2 > 0$;

(iii) $\begin{cases} \dfrac{\partial^2 f}{\partial x^2}(x_0, y_0) < 0 \\ \dfrac{\partial^2 f}{\partial x^2}(x_0, y_0) > 0. \end{cases}$

2 The function $f(x, y)$ has a saddle point at (x_0, y_0) if, in addition to 1(i),

$$\frac{\partial^2 f}{\partial x^2}(x_0, y_0) \frac{\partial^2 f}{\partial y^2} - (x_0, y_0) - \left[\frac{\partial^2 f}{\partial x \partial y}(x_0, y_0) \right]^2 < 0.$$

3 If

$$\frac{\partial^2 f}{\partial x^2}(x_0, y_0) \frac{\partial^2 f}{\partial y^2}(x_0, y_0) - \left[\frac{\partial^2 f}{\partial x \partial y}(x_0, y_0) \right]^2 = 0$$

the test fails to identify the nature of the stationary point.

Example 50.2

Locate and identify the stationary points of

$$f(x, y) = 4 - x^2 + 4xy - y^2.$$

Solution
To locate the stationary points we must solve

$$\frac{\partial f}{\partial x} = 0 \quad \text{and} \quad \frac{\partial f}{\partial y} = 0.$$

We have

$$\frac{\partial f}{\partial x} = -2x + 4y.$$

$$\frac{\partial f}{\partial y} = 4x - 2y.$$

So $\partial f/\partial x = 0$ and $\partial f/\partial y = 0$ implies

$$-2x + 4y = 0, \quad \text{or} \quad x = 2y$$

and

$$4x - 2y = 0, \quad \text{or} \quad x = y/2.$$

The only solution to this pair of linear equations is $x = y = 0$. Thus $f(x, y)$ only has a stationary point at the origin $(0, 0)$.

To identify the nature of this stationary point we must first find the partial derivatives $\partial^2 f/\partial x^2$, $\partial^2 f/\partial x \partial y$ and $\partial^2 f/\partial y^2$. We have

$$\frac{\partial^2 f}{\partial x^2} = -2, \quad \frac{\partial^2 f}{\partial x \partial y} = 4 \quad \text{and} \quad \frac{\partial^2 f}{\partial y^2} = -2.$$

Thus

$$\frac{\partial^2 f}{\partial x^2} \frac{\partial^2 f}{\partial y^2} - \left(\frac{\partial^2 f}{\partial x \partial y} \right)^2 = (-2)(-2) - 4^2 = -12 < 0,$$

so by condition 2 the single stationary point of $f(x, y)$ located at the origin $(0, 0)$ must be a saddle point.   ▲

Example 50.3

Show that

$$f(x, y) = 13x^4 - 8x^3 y - 72x^2 + 24y^2 + 3$$

has five stationary points and identify their nature.

Solution
To locate the stationary points we must solve

$$\frac{\partial f}{\partial x} = 0 \quad \text{and} \quad \frac{\partial f}{\partial y} = 0.$$

We have

$$\frac{\partial f}{\partial x} = 52x^3 - 24x^2 y - 144x,$$

$$\frac{\partial f}{\partial y} = -8x^3 + 48y,$$

so $\partial f/\partial x = 0$ and $\partial f/\partial y = 0$ implies

$$13x^3 - 6x^2y - 36x = 0,$$
$$-x^3 + 6y = 0,$$

which must be solved simultaneously.

Substituting for y in the first equation using the second equation gives

$$13x^3 - 6x^2\left(\frac{x^3}{6}\right) - 36x = 0,$$

or

$$x(-x^4 + 13x^2 - 36) = 0.$$

Thus either $x = 0$ or

$$x^4 - 13x^2 + 36 = 0.$$

This is a biquadratic equation, so to solve it we set $x^2 = u$ and find that

$$u^2 - 13u + 36 = 0.$$

Thus using the quadratic formula gives

$$u = \frac{13 \pm \sqrt{(169 - 144)}}{2} = \frac{13 \pm 5}{2},$$

and so $u = 9$ and $u = 4$, and thus $x = \pm 3$ and $x = \pm 2$. However, $y = x^3/6$, so the stationary points are $(0, 0)$, $(2, 4/3)$, $(-2, -4/3)$, $(3, 9/2)$ and $(-3, -9/2)$.

Now we must use the test, so first we find the second order partial derivatives

$$\frac{\partial^2 f}{\partial x^2} = 156x^2 - 48xy - 144$$

$$\frac{\partial^2 f}{\partial x \partial y} = -24x^2$$

$$\frac{\partial^2 f}{\partial y^2} = 48.$$

At $(0, 0)$.

$$\frac{\partial^2 f}{\partial x^2}\frac{\partial^2 f}{\partial y^2} - \left(\frac{\partial^2 f}{\partial x \partial y}\right)^2 = -6912 < 0,$$

so $(0, 0)$ is a saddle point.

At $(2, 4/3)$ and $(-2, -4/3)$

$$\frac{\partial^2 f}{\partial x^2}\frac{\partial^2 f}{\partial y^2} - \left(\frac{\partial^2 f}{\partial x \partial y}\right)^2 = 7680 > 0, \text{ but } f_{xx} = 352 > 0,$$

so $(2, 4/3)$ and $(-2, -4/3)$ are local minima.

At $(3, 9/2)$ and $(-3, -9/2)$

$$\frac{\partial^2 f}{\partial x^2}\frac{\partial^2 f}{\partial y^2} - \left(\frac{\partial^2 f}{\partial x \partial y}\right)^2 = -17\,280 < 0,$$

so (3, 9/2) and (− 3, − 9/2) are saddle points.
  Thus, summarizing, we have:

  (0, 0) is a saddle point with $f(0, 0) = 3$;
  (2, 4/3) is a local minimum with $f(2, 4/3) = -359/3$;
  (− 2, 4/3) is a local minimum with $f(-2, -4/3) = -359/3$,
  (3, 9/2) is a saddle point with $f(3, 9/2) = -78$;
  (− 3, − 9/2) is a saddle point with $f(-3, -9/2) = -78$.   ▲

PROBLEMS 50

In problems 1 to 4, find the Taylor series expansion about the given point of each of the functions up to and including terms of degree 3.
1. $f(x, y) = e^x \cos y$ about the point (0, 0).
2. $f(x, y) = (1 + x)^{1+y}$ about the point (0, 0).
3. $f(x, y) = \exp(x + y)$ about the point (2, − 2).
4. $f(x, y) = \sin(x + y)$ about the point (0, $\pi/2$).
In the following problems locate and identify the nature of the stationary points.
5. $f(x, y) = x^2 + y^2 - 2x + 4y + 6$.
6. $f(x, y) = x^2 - y^2 - 2x + 4y + 6$.
7. $f(x, y) = 3 + 2x + 2y - 2x^2 - 2xy - y^2$.
8. $f(x, y) = x + x^2 + y^2 - 1$.
9. $f(x, y) = x^3 - y^3 + 3xy + 7$.
10. $f(x, y) = x - x^2 + 4x^2 y - xy^2$.
11. $f(x, y) = x^3 + 3xy^2 - 15x - 12y + 3$.
12. $f(x, y) = 2x^4 - 3x^2 y^2 + y^4 + 8x^2 + 3y^2$.
13. $f(x, y) = xy(3x + 6y - 2)$.

14. $f(x, y) = xy \exp\left[-\frac{1}{2}(x^2 + y^2)\right]$.

51 Fourier series

A **Fourier series** on the interval $-\pi \leqslant x \leqslant \pi$ is a way of representing a given function $f(x)$ in the form of a trigonometric series of the form

$$\frac{1}{2}a_0 + \sum_{n=1}^{\infty} (a_n \cos nx + b_n \sin nx),$$

in which the **Fourier coefficients** a_n and b_n are determined by the function $f(x)$.

It may be that $f(x)$ is defined outside the interval $-\pi \leqslant x \leqslant \pi$, called the **fundamental interval**, but the representation in terms of the Fourier series applies only to the fundamental interval.

The periodicity of the sine and cosine functions means that

$$\sin m(x+2\pi) = \sin mx \quad \text{and} \quad \cos n(x+2\pi) = \cos nx,$$

so the Fourier series itself will be periodic with period 2π. Remember that a function $g(x)$ is **periodic** with **period** X if

$$g(x+X) = g(x),$$

and X is the smallest number for which this is true.

In terms of Fourier series this means that since such a series is defined for all x, and not just in the fundamental interval, a Fourier series will repeat in each of the intervals

$$(2n-1)\pi < x < (2n+1)\pi, \text{ with } n = 0, \pm 1, \pm 2, \dots,$$

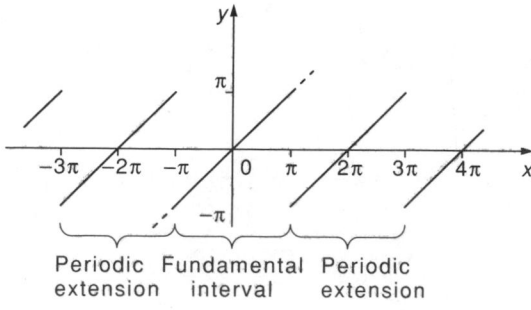

Periodic   Fundamental   Periodic
extension   interval   extension

Fig. 110

the same representation of $f(x)$ as in the fundamental interval. The Fourier series representation in each such interval outside the fundamental interval is called a **periodic extension** of the function defined in the fundamental interval. The function $f(x) = x$, together with some of its periodic extensions, is shown in Fig. 110, in which the behaviour of $f(x)$ outside the fundamental interval is shown by the dashed line. Thus $f(x) = x$ is not periodic, but when this function is represented by its Fourier series, the Fourier series representation will be periodic with period 2π. Naturally, if $f(x)$ is itself periodic with period 2π, the function and its Fourier series representation will coincide for all x.

To see how the Fourier coefficients a_n, b_n are to be found from $f(x)$ we need to make use of the results of Examples 39.7 to 39.9, which are repeated below for convenience.

Basic definite integrals

1 $\displaystyle\int_{-\pi}^{\pi} \sin mx \cos nx \, dx = 0;$

2 $\displaystyle\int_{-\pi}^{\pi} \sin mx \sin nx \, dx = \begin{cases} 0 & \text{for } m \neq n \\ \pi & \text{for } m = n \neq 0; \end{cases}$

3 $\displaystyle\int_{-\pi}^{\pi} \cos mx \cos nx \, dx = \begin{cases} 0 & \text{for } m \neq n \\ \pi & \text{for } m = n \neq 0 \\ 2\pi & \text{for } m = n = 0; \end{cases}$

for all integers $m, n = 0, 1, \ldots$.

These relationships between $\sin mx$ and $\cos nx$ are expressed in mathematical terms by saying that these functions are **orthogonal** over the interval $-\pi \leqslant x \leqslant \pi$.

To determine the coefficients a_n and b_n we first set

$$f(x) = \frac{1}{2}a_0 + \sum_{m=1}^{\infty} (a_m \cos mx + b_m \sin mx).$$

Then, to find a_n, we multiply this Fourier series representation by $\cos nx$ and integrate over the fundamental interval $-\pi \leqslant x \leqslant \pi$ to obtain

$$\int_{-\pi}^{\pi} f(x) \cos nx \, dx = \frac{1}{2}a_0 \int_{-\pi}^{\pi} \cos nx \, dx$$

$$+ \int_{-\pi}^{\pi} \cos nx \left[\sum_{m=1}^{\infty} (a_m \cos mx + b_m \sin mx) \right] dx.$$

$$= \frac{1}{2}a_0 \int_{-\pi}^{\pi} \cos nx \, dx + \sum_{m=1}^{\infty} a_m \left[\int_{-\pi}^{\pi} \cos mx \cos nx \, dx \right]$$

$$+ \sum_{m=1}^{\infty} b_m \left[\int_{-\pi}^{\pi} \sin mx \cos nx \, dx \right].$$

When $n = 0$ this reduces to

$$a_0 = \frac{1}{\pi} \int_{-\pi}^{\pi} f(x) \, dx,$$

since all the terms in the first summation vanish because of integral (3), while all the terms in the second summation vanish because of integral (1).

When $n \neq 0$, because of integral (3), all the terms in the first summation vanish with the exception of the one for which $m = n$, while once again all the terms in the second summation vanish, showing that

$$a_n = \frac{1}{\pi} \int_{-\pi}^{\pi} f(x) \cos nx \, dx,$$

for $n = 1, 2 \ldots$.

Examination of the expression determining a_0 shows that $\frac{1}{2} a_0$ is the **average value** of $f(x)$ over the interval $-\pi \leqslant x \leqslant \pi$.

To determine the coefficients b_n we use the same form of argument, but this time multiply the Fourier series by $\sin nx$ and again integrate over the fundamental interval $-\pi \leqslant x \leqslant \pi$ and as a result we obtain the formula

$$b_n = \frac{1}{\pi} \int_{-\pi}^{\pi} f(x) \sin nx \, dx,$$

for $n = 1, 2, \ldots$.

Combining these arguments brings us to the following fundamental result.

Fourier series representation of $f(x)$ over the interval $-\pi \leqslant x \leqslant \pi$
The function $f(x)$ defined in the interval $-\pi \leqslant x \leqslant \pi$ has the Fourier series representation

$$f(x) = \frac{1}{2} a_0 + \sum_{n=1}^{\infty} (a_n \cos nx + b_n \sin nx),$$

where the Fourier coefficients

$$a_n = \frac{1}{\pi} \int_{-\pi}^{\pi} f(x) \cos nx \, dx \quad \text{and} \quad b_n = \frac{1}{\pi} \int_{-\pi}^{\pi} f(x) \sin nx \, dx,$$

with $n = 0, 1, 2, \ldots$, in a_n and $n = 1, 2, \ldots$, in b_n.

Before considering some of the properties of Fourier series and, in particular, how we should interpret the equality sign in the above result, let us first construct the Fourier series representation for a simple function.

Example 51.1

Find the Fourier series of the function

$$f(x) = \begin{cases} -1 & \text{for } -\pi < x < 0 \\ 1 & \text{for } 0 < x < \pi. \end{cases}$$

Solution
We start by determining a_0, which it is usually best to calculate separately. In this case, $f(x)$ is defined differently on the intervals $-\pi < x < 0$ and $0 < x < \pi$, so we must replace the integral over the fundamental interval $-\pi \leqslant x \leqslant \pi$ used to define a_0 by the sum of an integral over the interval $-\pi \leqslant x \leqslant 0$ and one over $0 \leqslant x \leqslant \pi$ as follows:

$$a_0 = \frac{1}{\pi} \int_{-\pi}^{\pi} f(x)\, \mathrm{d}x$$

$$= \frac{1}{\pi} \int_{-\pi}^{0} (-1)\, \mathrm{d}x + \frac{1}{\pi} \int_{0}^{\pi} (1)\, \mathrm{d}x$$

$$= \frac{1}{\pi} (-\pi) + \frac{1}{\pi} (\pi) = 0$$

Then, to find a_n we have

$$a_n = \frac{1}{\pi} \int_{-\pi}^{\pi} f(x) \cos nx\, \mathrm{d}x$$

$$= \frac{1}{\pi} \int_{-\pi}^{0} (-1) \cos nx\, \mathrm{d}x + \frac{1}{\pi} \int_{0}^{\pi} (1) \cos nx\, \mathrm{d}x$$

$$= \frac{1}{\pi} \left[-\frac{1}{n} \sin nx \right]_{-\pi}^{0} + \frac{1}{\pi} \left[\frac{1}{n} \sin nx \right]_{0}^{\pi} = 0,$$

for $n = 1, 2, \ldots$. Notice that we could not have determined a_0 from this result because of the occurrence of the factor n in the denominator when the definite integrals are evaluated.
Similarly,

$$b_n = \frac{1}{\pi} \int_{-\pi}^{\pi} f(x) \cos nx\, \mathrm{d}x$$

$$= \frac{1}{\pi} \int_{-\pi}^{0} (-1) \sin nx\, \mathrm{d}x + \frac{1}{\pi} \int_{0}^{\pi} (1) \sin nx\, \mathrm{d}x$$

$$= \frac{1}{\pi} \left[\frac{1}{n} \cos nx \right]_{-\pi}^{0} + \frac{1}{\pi} \left[-\frac{1}{n} \cos nx \right]_{0}^{\pi}$$

$$= \frac{2}{n\pi}(1 - \cos n\pi),$$

for $n = 1, 2, \ldots$.

Now $\cos n\pi = (-1)^n$, so

$$b_n = \frac{2}{n\pi}[1 - (-1)^n],$$

and thus

$$b_n = \begin{cases} \dfrac{4}{n\pi} & \text{when } n \text{ is odd} \\[2mm] 0 & \text{when } n \text{ is even,} \end{cases}$$

for $n = 1, 2, \ldots$.

This type of behaviour, in which the even numbered coefficients are defined differently from the odd numbered ones, occurs frequently in Fourier series.

Since for any integer n the number $2n$ is even, it follows that the number $2n - 1$ is odd. Thus we have shown that

$$a_n = 0, \quad \text{for all} \quad n = 0, 1, 2, \ldots,$$

and

$$b_n = \frac{4}{(2n - 1)\pi}, \quad \text{for} \quad n = 1, 2, \ldots .$$

Inserting these Fourier coefficients into the Fourier series gives

$$f(x) = \frac{4}{\pi} \sum_{n=1}^{\infty} \frac{\sin(2n - 1)x}{2n - 1}$$

or, when expanded,

$$f(x) = \frac{4}{\pi}\left[\sin x + \frac{\sin 3x}{3} + \frac{\sin 5x}{5} + \cdots \right],$$

for $-\pi < x < \pi$.

In practice, when working with Fourier series, only a finite number of terms can be summed. To see how these finite sums approximate the original function, Fig. 111(a) shows the original function and Fig. 111(b) graphs of $S_N(x)$ for $N = 1, 2, 3$ and 4, where

$$S_N(x) = \frac{4}{\pi} \sum_{n=1}^{N} \frac{\sin(2n - 1)x}{2n - 1}.$$

Notice that although $f(x)$ was discontinuous at $x = 0$, and was not in fact even defined there, the Fourier series representation of $f(x)$ is defined at $x = 0$ where it passes through the mid-point of the discontinuity. This is characteristic of the behaviour of a Fourier series representation at a discontinuity.   ▲

The vanishing of the coefficients a_n in Example 51.1 illustrates an important general result in Fourier series which saves a considerable amount of work. It

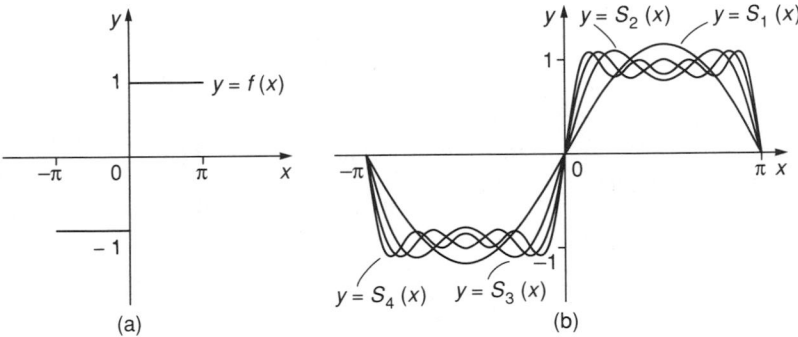

Fig. 111

is that the Fourier series of an **even** function only contains **cosine** terms (and possibly a constant term), so then $b_n = 0$ for $n = 1, 2, \ldots$, while the Fourier series of an **odd** function only contains **sine** terms, so then $a_n = 0$ for $n = 0, 1, 2, \ldots$.

To see why this is, consider the definite integral

$$I = \int_{-\pi}^{\pi} f(x)\,\mathrm{d}x,$$

in which $f(x)$ is an odd function, so $f(-x) = -f(x)$. We have

$$I = \int_{-\pi}^{0} f(x)\,\mathrm{d}x + \int_{0}^{\pi} f(x)\,\mathrm{d}x$$

so writing $x = -u$ in the first integral gives

$$I = -\int_{\pi}^{0} f(-u)\,\mathrm{d}u + \int_{0}^{\pi} f(x)\,\mathrm{d}x$$

$$= \int_{0}^{\pi} f(-u)\,\mathrm{d}u + \int_{0}^{\pi} f(x)\,\mathrm{d}x.$$

However, since $f(x)$ is odd, $f(-u) = -f(u)$, so substituting this into the first integral gives

$$I = -\int_{0}^{\pi} f(u)\,\mathrm{d}u + \int_{0}^{\pi} f(x)\,\mathrm{d}x,$$

but u is a dummy variable, so replacing it by x shows that $I = 0$.

To apply this to Fourier series we need to use the fact that the product of an even and an odd function is an odd function.

Thus if $f(x)$ is odd, $f(x) \cos nx$ is odd, so

$$a_n = \frac{1}{\pi} \int_{-\pi}^{\pi} f(x) \cos nx \, \mathrm{d}x = 0 \quad \text{for} \quad f(x) \text{ odd};$$

while if $f(x)$ is even, $f(x) \sin nx$ is odd, so

$$b_n = \frac{1}{\pi} \int_{-\pi}^{\pi} f(x) \sin nx \, dx = 0 \quad \text{for} \quad f(x) \text{ odd.}$$

The same form of argument also shows that if $f(x)$ is even, so that $f(-x) = f(x)$, then

$$a_n = \frac{1}{\pi} \int_{-\pi}^{\pi} f(x) \cos nx \, dx = \frac{2}{\pi} \int_{0}^{\pi} f(x) \cos nx \, dx,$$

while if $f(x)$ is odd,

$$b_n = \frac{1}{\pi} \int_{-\pi}^{\pi} f(x) \sin nx \, dx = \frac{2}{\pi} \int_{0}^{\pi} f(x) \sin nx \, dx.$$

The next example of a Fourier series provides an illustration of the expansion of an even function.

Example 51.2

Find the Fourier series of the function

$$f(x) = |x|, \quad \text{for} \quad -\pi \leqslant x \leqslant \pi.$$

Solution
The function $f(x) = |x|$ is an even function, so we need only determine the coefficients a_n because automatically $b_n = 0$, for $n = 1, 2, \ldots$. A graph of the function is shown in Fig. 112, together with the fundamental interval, two periodic extensions and the behaviour of the actual function $y = |x|$ outside the fundamental interval shown by the dashed lines.

As $|x|$ is defined as

$$|x| = \begin{cases} x & \text{if } x \geqslant 0 \\ -x & \text{if } x < 0, \end{cases}$$

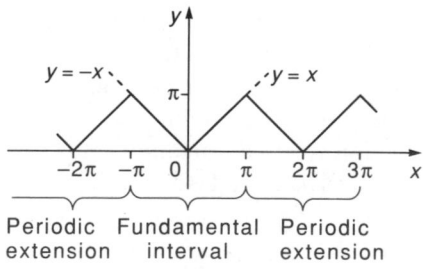

Periodic   Fundamental   Periodic
extension   interval   extension

Fig. 112

if we wish to determine a_n directly from its definition in terms of an integral we would need to replace the integral over $-\pi \leqslant x \leqslant \pi$ by the sum of one over $-\pi \leqslant x \leqslant 0$ and another over $0 \leqslant x \leqslant \pi$ to give

$$a_n = \frac{1}{\pi} \int_{-\pi}^{0} (-x) \cos nx \, dx + \frac{1}{\pi} \int_{0}^{\pi} x \cos nx \, dx,$$

for $n = 0, 1, 2, \ldots$.

However, this leads to unnecessary work for we know that if $f(x)$ is an even function

$$a_n = \frac{2}{\pi} \int_{0}^{\pi} f(x) \cos nx \, dx,$$

so we will use this result instead to give

$$a_n = \frac{2}{\pi} \int_{0}^{\pi} x \cos nx \, dx,$$

for $n = 0, 1, 2, \ldots$.

Setting $n = 0$ to determine a_0 first gives

$$a_0 = \frac{2}{\pi} \int_{0}^{\pi} x \, dx = \pi \, .$$

For $n \neq 0$ we have

$$a_n = \frac{2}{\pi} \int_{0}^{\pi} x \cos nx \, dx,$$

and integration by parts gives

$$a_n = \frac{2}{\pi} \left(\frac{x \sin nx}{n} + \frac{\cos nx}{n^2} \right) \Bigg|_{0}^{\pi}$$

$$= \frac{2}{\pi n^2} [\cos n\pi - 1]$$

$$= \frac{2}{\pi n^2} [(-1)^n - 1],$$

and so

$$a_n = \begin{cases} \dfrac{-4}{\pi n^2}, & \text{when } n \text{ is odd} \\[2mm] 0, & \text{when } n \text{ is even,} \end{cases}$$

for $n = 1, 2, 3, \ldots$.

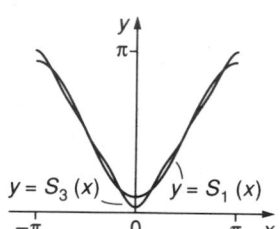

Fig. 113

Thus, arguing as in Example 51.1, we may write

$$a_n = \frac{-4}{\pi\,(2n-1)^2}\ ,$$

for $n = 1, 2, \dots$.

Substituting for a_0 and a_n, with $n = 1, 2, \dots$, into the Fourier series shows that

$$f(x) = \frac{\pi}{2} - \frac{4}{\pi} \sum_{n=1}^{\infty} \frac{\cos(2n-1)x}{(2n-1)^2}\ ,$$

for $-\pi \leqslant x \leqslant \pi$ or, when expanded,

$$f(x) = \frac{\pi}{2} - \frac{4}{\pi}\left(\frac{\cos x}{1^2} + \frac{\cos 3x}{3^2} + \frac{\cos 5x}{5^2} + \dots\right).$$

Figure 113 gives graphs of $S_1(x)$ and $S_3(x)$ where

$$S_N(x) = \frac{\pi}{2} - \frac{4}{\pi} \sum_{n=1}^{N} \frac{\cos(2n-1)x}{(2n-1)^2}\ .$$

These graphs show how with this function, which is everywhere continuous, even the low order approximation $S_3(x)$ provides a reasonable approximation to $f(x) = |x|$.   ▲

We now summarize the basic properties of Fourier series, but offer no proof of the important properties 3 and 4 which are stated here in a simplified form suitable for all practical purposes.

BASIC PROPERTIES

1 If $f(x)$ is an even function on the interval $-\pi \leqslant x \leqslant \pi$, then its Fourier series contains no sine functions (all $b_n = 0$).

2 If $f(x)$ is an odd function on the interval $-\pi \leqslant x \leqslant \pi$, then its Fourier series contains no cosine functions (all $a_n = 0$).

3 At points in the interval $-\pi \leqslant x \leqslant \pi$ at which $f(x)$ is continuous the Fourier series of $f(x)$ converges to $f(x)$.

4 At points in the interval $-\pi \leqslant x \leqslant \pi$ at which $f(x)$ is discontinuous the Fourier series of $f(x)$ converges to the average of the values of $f(x)$ to the immediate left and right of the discontinuity.

Example 51.3

Use Example 51.1 to deduce a series for $\pi/4$, and Example 51.2 to deduce a series for $\pi^2/8$.

Solution
From property 3 and Example 51.1 we know that the Fourier series

$$\frac{4}{\pi}\left[\sin x + \frac{\sin 3x}{3} + \frac{\sin 5x}{5} + \dots\right]$$

will converge to

$$f(x) = \begin{cases} -1 & \text{for } -\pi < x < 0 \\ 1 & \text{for } 0 < x < \pi \end{cases}$$

for any x at which $f(x)$ is continuous. Setting $x = \pi/2$ for which $f(x)$ is continuous and equal to 1, it follows that

$$1 = \frac{4}{\pi}\left[\sin\frac{\pi}{2} + \frac{\sin 3\pi}{3} + \frac{\sin 5\pi}{5} + \dots\right]$$

and so

$$\frac{\pi}{4} = 1 - \frac{1}{3} + \frac{1}{5} - \frac{1}{7} + \dots,$$

or

$$\frac{\pi}{4} = \sum_{n=1}^{\infty} \frac{(-1)^{n+1}}{(2n-1)}.$$

We remark in passing that this series is seen to be convergent by the alternating series test, though it converges very slowly and if it is terminated when $n = N$, say, the magnitude of the error will not exceed $1/(2N-1)$. Thus even if 1000 terms are taken, the magnitude of the error will be of the order of 0.0005.

Again from property 3, but this time using Example 51.2, we know that the Fourier series

$$\frac{\pi}{2} - \frac{4}{\pi}\sum_{n=1}^{\infty}\frac{\cos(2n-1)x}{(2n-1)^2},$$

will converge to $f(x) = |x|$ which is continuous for all x. Thus setting $x = 0$, when $f(0) = 0$ we find that

$$0 = \frac{\pi}{2} - \frac{4}{\pi}\sum_{n=1}^{\infty}\frac{1}{(2n-1)^2},$$

and so

$$\frac{\pi^2}{8} = \sum_{n=1}^{\infty}\frac{1}{(2n-1)^2}.$$

This series converges fairly quickly and, for example, summing the first 100 terms yields the estimate 1.231 20 for $\pi^2/8$ which is in error by 0.2% (low).

▲

Example 51.4

Find the Fourier series of the function

$$f(x) = \begin{cases} 0, & \text{for } -\pi \leqslant x \leqslant 0 \\ \sin 2x, & \text{for } 0 \leqslant x \leqslant \pi. \end{cases}$$

Solution
The graph of this function in its fundamental interval is shown in Fig. 114, from which it is easily seen that it is neither even, nor odd, so both sine and cosine terms will arise in its Fourier series.
The coefficient a_0 is given by

$$a_0 = \frac{1}{\pi} \int_0^\pi \sin 2x = 0,$$

while for $n \neq 0$,

$$a_n = \frac{1}{\pi} \int_0^\pi \sin 2x \cos nx \, dx.$$

This integral could be evaluated by means of integration by parts, but it is easier to proceed as follows. Using the trigonometric identity

$$\sin A \cos B = \frac{1}{2} [\sin(A+B) + \sin(A-B)],$$

and setting $A = 2x, B = nx$, we find after substituting the result into the integral for a_n that

$$a_n = \frac{1}{2\pi} \int_0^\pi \sin(2+n)x \, dx + \frac{1}{2\pi} \int_0^\pi \sin(2-n)x \, dx.$$

Integrating this gives

$$a_n = -\frac{1}{2\pi} \left[\frac{\cos(2+n)x}{(2+n)} \right]\Big|_0^\pi - \frac{1}{2\pi} \left[\frac{\cos(2-n)x}{(2-n)} \right]\Big|_0^\pi$$

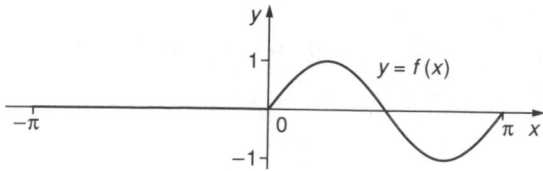

Fig. 114

$$= -\frac{1}{2\pi}\left[\frac{\cos(2+n)\pi - 1}{(2+n)}\right] - \frac{1}{2\pi}\left[\frac{\cos(2-n)\pi - 1}{(2-n)}\right],$$

which is valid provided $n \neq 2$, for then the denominator in the second term vanishes. Now $\cos(2+n)\pi = (-1)^{2+n} = (-1)^n$ and $\cos(2-n)\pi = (-1)^{2-n} = (-1)^{-n} = (-1)^n$, so

$$a_n = \frac{2[1+(-1)^{n+1}]}{\pi\,(2-n)(2+n)}, \quad \text{for } n \neq 2.$$

To find a_2 we return to the original integral for a_n and set $n = 2$ before integrating. Using the result $\sin 4x = 2\sin 2x \cos 2x$ we see that

$$a_2 = \frac{1}{2\pi}\int_0^\pi \sin 4x \, dx = 0,$$

so

$$a_n = \begin{cases} 0, & \text{for } n \text{ even} \\[2mm] \dfrac{4}{\pi\,(2-n)(2+n)}, & \text{for } n \text{ odd.} \end{cases}$$

Similarly,

$$b_n = \frac{1}{\pi}\int_0^\pi \sin 2x \sin nx \, dx$$

for $n = 1, 2, \ldots$.

Now

$$\sin A \sin B = \frac{1}{2}[\cos(A-B) - \cos(A+B)],$$

so setting $A = 2x, B = nx$ and using the result in the integral for b_n gives

$$b_n = \frac{1}{2\pi}\int_0^\pi \cos(n-2)x \, dx - \frac{1}{2\pi}\int_0^\pi \cos(n+2)x \, dx$$

$$= \frac{1}{2\pi}\left[\frac{\sin(n-2)x}{(n-2)}\right]\Big|_0^\pi - \frac{1}{2\pi}\left[\frac{\sin(n+2)x}{(n+2)}\right]\Big|_0^\pi = 0,$$

provided $n \neq 2$.

When $n = 2$

$$b_2 = \frac{1}{\pi}\int_0^\pi \sin^2 2x \, dx,$$

so as $\sin^2 2x = \frac{1}{2}(1 - \cos 4x)$ we have

$$b_2 = \frac{1}{2\pi}\int_0^\pi (1 - \cos 4x)\, dx = \frac{1}{2}.$$

Thus

$$b_n = \begin{cases} \dfrac{1}{2}, & \text{for } n = 2 \\ 0, & \text{for all other } n. \end{cases}$$

Combining results gives

$$f(x) = \frac{1}{2}\sin 2x + \frac{4}{\pi}\left[\frac{\cos x}{1 \cdot 3} - \frac{\cos 3x}{1 \cdot 5} - \frac{\cos 5x}{3 \cdot 7} - \frac{\cos 7x}{5 \cdot 9} - \cdots\right],$$

for $-\pi \leqslant x \leqslant \pi$.

A little experimentation shows that this may be written more concisely as

$$f(x) = \frac{1}{2}\sin 2x + \frac{4}{\pi}\sum_{n=1}^{\infty}\frac{\cos(2n-1)x}{(3-2n)(1+2n)},$$

for $-\pi \leqslant x \leqslant \pi$. ▲

The next example is more interesting since it shows how numerical series may be summed in terms of known functions by using a point at which the function $f(x)$ is continuous and one at which it is discontinuous.

Example 51.5

Find the Fourier series for the function

$$f(x) = e^x \quad \text{for} \quad -\pi < x < \pi.$$

Use the result to find numerical series for $\pi/\sinh\pi$ and $\pi\coth\pi$.

Solution

The function $f(x)$ is shown in Fig. 115 for $-\pi < x < \pi$, together with two of its periodic extensions, with the mid-point of the jump at $\cosh\pi$ shown as a dot.

We have

$$a_0 = \frac{1}{\pi}\int_{-\pi}^{\pi} e^x \mathrm{d}x = \frac{e^\pi - e^{-\pi}}{\pi} = \frac{2\sinh\pi}{\pi},$$

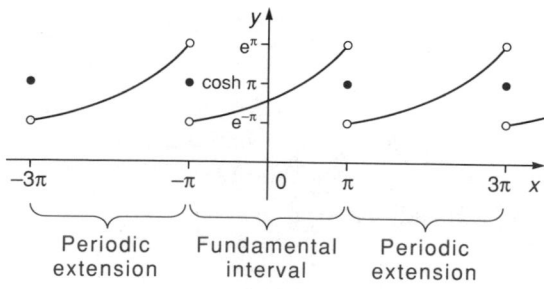

Fig. 115

and

$$a_n = \frac{1}{\pi} \int_{-\pi}^{\pi} e^x \cos nx \, dx, \quad \text{for} \quad n = 1, 2, \ldots .$$

Integrating by parts (twice) shows that

$$a_n = \frac{1}{\pi} \left[\frac{e^x}{1 + n^2} (\cos nx + n \sin nx) \right]_{-\pi}^{\pi}$$

$$= \frac{1}{\pi} \left[\frac{e^\pi}{1 + n^2} (\cos n\pi + n \sin n\pi) - \frac{e^{-\pi}}{1 + n^2} (\cos(-n\pi) + n \sin(-n\pi)) \right],$$

but $\cos(\pm n\pi) = (-1)^n$ and $\sin(\pm n\pi) = 0$, so

$$a_n = \frac{1}{\pi} \frac{(-1)^n}{1 + n^2} (e^\pi - e^{-\pi})$$

$$= \frac{(-1)^n}{1 + n^2} 2 \frac{\sinh \pi}{\pi}, \quad \text{for} \quad n = 1, 2, \ldots .$$

Similarly,

$$b_n = \frac{1}{\pi} \int_{-\pi}^{\pi} e^x \sin nx \, dx, \quad \text{for} \quad n = 1, 2, \ldots ,$$

so again integrating by parts (twice) shows that

$$b_n = \frac{1}{\pi} \left[\frac{e^x}{1 + n^2} (\sin nx - n \cos nx) \right]_{-\pi}^{\pi}$$

$$= -\frac{1}{\pi} \frac{(-1)^n n}{1 + n^2} (e^\pi - e^{-\pi})$$

$$= (-1)^{n+1} \cdot \frac{2n}{1 + n^2} \frac{\sinh \pi}{\pi}, \quad \text{for} \quad n = 1, 2, \ldots .$$

Substituting for a_n and b_n into the general form of the Fourier series gives

$$f(x) = \frac{\sinh \pi}{\pi} \left\{ 1 + 2 \sum_{n=1}^{\infty} (-1)^n \left(\frac{\cos nx - n \sin nx}{1 + n^2} \right) \right\},$$

for $-\pi \leqslant x \leqslant \pi$

The function $f(x) = e^x$ is continuous at $x = 0$, at which it has the value 1. Thus at $x = 0$ the Fourier series converges to 1 so that

$$1 = \frac{\sinh \pi}{\pi} \left\{ 1 + 2 \sum_{n=1}^{\infty} \frac{(-1)^n}{1 + n^2} \right\},$$

and thus

$$\frac{\pi}{\sinh \pi} = \pi \operatorname{cosech} \pi = 1 + 2 \sum_{n=1}^{\infty} \frac{(-1)^n}{1+n^2}.$$

However, the function $f(x)$ is discontinuous at $x = \pi$, at which point by property 4 the Fourier series converges to $\frac{1}{2}(e^\pi + e^{-\pi}) = \cosh \pi$. Thus setting $x = \pi$ in the Fourier series and using the fact that $\cos n\pi = (-1)^n$ we have

$$\cosh \pi = \frac{\sinh \pi}{\pi} \left\{ 1 + 2 \sum_{n=1}^{\infty} \frac{1}{1+n^2} \right\},$$

and so

$$\pi \coth \pi = 1 + 2 \sum_{n+1}^{\infty} \frac{1}{1+n^2}. \qquad \blacktriangle$$

The following property of Fourier series is both important and useful, since it often simplifies the determination of the Fourier coefficients.

Shift of interval in Fourier series
If a function $f(x)$ is defined on the fundamental interval $-\pi \leqslant x \leqslant \pi$ and by periodic extension outside it, then its Fourier series on the interval $k \leqslant x \leqslant k + 2\pi$, where k is arbitrary, is the same as its Fourier series on the fundamental interval.

This means that, provided $f(x)$ is defined for all x by periodic extension outside its fundamental interval $-\pi \leqslant x \leqslant \pi$, then its Fourier series in the shifted interval $k \leqslant x \leqslant k + 2\pi$ is

$$f(x) = \frac{1}{2} a_0 + \sum_{n=1}^{\infty} (a_n \cos nx + b_n \sin nx),$$

where

$$a_n = \frac{1}{\pi} \int_a^{a+2\pi} f(x) \cos nx \, dx = \frac{1}{\pi} \int_{-\pi}^{\pi} f(x) \cos nx \, dx,$$

for $n = 0, 1, 2, \ldots$, and

$$b_n = \frac{1}{\pi} \int_a^{a+2\pi} f(x) \sin nx \, dx = \frac{1}{\pi} \int_{-\pi}^{\pi} f(x) \sin nx \, dx,$$

for $n = 1, 2, \ldots$.
The proof of this result is simple. Let $h(x)$ be periodic with period 2π, and consider the integral

$$I = \int_a^{a+2\pi} h(x) \, dx.$$

Then since $h(x)$ is defined for all x we may use the property of definite integrals to write

$$I = \int_a^{a+2\pi} h(x)\,dx = \int_a^{-\pi} h(x)\,dx + \int_{-\pi}^{\pi} h(x)\,dx + \int_{\pi}^{a+2\pi} h(x)\,dx.$$

Setting $u = x + 2\pi$ in the first integral on the right-hand side gives

$$\int_a^{-\pi} h(x)\,dx = \int_{a+2\pi}^{\pi} h(u-2\pi)\,du = -\int_a^{a+2\pi} h(u-2\pi)\,dx.$$

Now the periodicity of $h(x)$ with period 2π means that

$$h(u-2\pi) = h(u),$$

so

$$\int_a^{-\pi} h(x)\,dx = -\int_{\pi}^{a+2\pi} h(u)\,du = -\int_{\pi}^{a+2\pi} h(x)\,dx,$$

where we have changed the dummy variable back from u to x. Thus using this result in the expression for I gives

$$I = \int_a^{a+2\pi} h(x)\,dx = -\int_{\pi}^{a+2\pi} h(x)\,dx + \int_{-\pi}^{\pi} h(x)\,dx + \int_{\pi}^{a+2\pi} h(x)\,dx$$

$$= \int_{-\pi}^{\pi} h(x)\,dx.$$

The required result then follows by first setting $h(x) = \frac{1}{\pi} f(x) \cos nx$, when it follows that

$$a_n = \frac{1}{\pi} \int_a^{a+2\pi} f(x) \cos nx \,dx = \frac{1}{\pi} \int_{-\pi}^{\pi} f(x) \cos nx \,dx,$$

and then setting $h(x) = \frac{1}{\pi} f(x) \sin nx$ to establish the corresponding result for b_n.

The last example makes use of a different approach by shifting the origin to simplify the task of finding a Fourier series.

Example 51.6

Find the Fourier series for the function $f(x)$ shown in Fig. 116, given that $f(x)$ is periodic with period 2π.

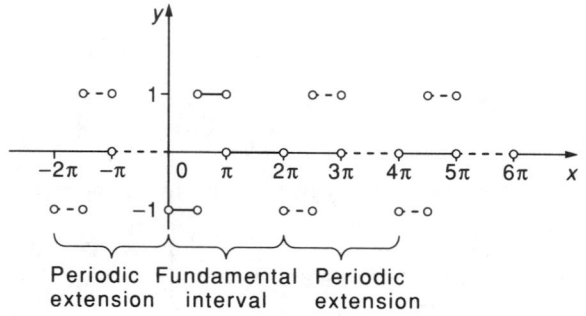

Periodic Fundamental Periodic
extension interval   extension

Fig. 116

Solution
The function $f(x)$ is neither even nor odd, but a shift of origin to the right by $\pi/2$ makes the new function $g(x)=f(x+\pi/2)$ the odd function shown on the interval $-\pi<x<\pi$ in Fig. 117.

As the new function $g(x)$ is odd, its Fourier series must be a sine series with

$$b_n = \frac{1}{\pi}\int_{-\pi/2}^{0}(-1)\sin nx\,dx + \frac{1}{\pi}\int_{0}^{\pi/2}(1)\sin nx\,dx$$

$$= \frac{2}{\pi}\int_{0}^{\pi/2}\sin nx\,dx$$

$$= -\frac{2}{\pi}\left(\frac{\cos nx}{n}\right)\Big|_{0}^{\pi/2}$$

$$= \frac{2}{\pi}\left[\frac{1-\cos(n\pi/2)}{n}\right],$$

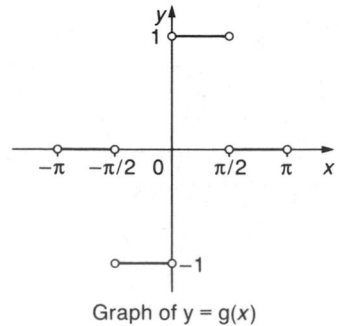

Graph of $y = g(x)$

Fig. 117

for $n = 1, 2, 3, \ldots$.

So

$$g(x) = \frac{2}{\pi} \sum_{n=1}^{\infty} \left[\frac{1 - \cos(n\pi/2)}{n} \right] \sin nx$$

$$= \frac{2}{\pi} \left[\sin x + \sin 2x + \frac{\sin 3x}{3} + \frac{\sin 5x}{5} + \frac{\sin 6x}{3} + \frac{\sin 7x}{7} + \frac{\sin 9x}{9} + \ldots \right],$$

for $-\pi < x < \pi$. The Fourier series for $f(x)$ now follows by replacing x by $x - \pi/2$ in this series. Simplification of $g(x - \pi/2)$ gives   ▲

$$f(x) = -\frac{2}{\pi} \left(\cos x + \sin 2x - \frac{\cos 3x}{3} + \frac{\cos 5x}{5} + \frac{\sin 6x}{3} - \frac{\cos 7x}{7} + \ldots \right).$$

PROBLEMS 51

1. Find the Fourier series for the function
$$f(x) = \begin{cases} 0, & \text{for } -\pi < x < 0 \\ 1, & \text{for } 0 < x < \pi. \end{cases}$$

2. Find the Fourier series for the function
$$f(x) = \begin{cases} 0, & \text{for } -\pi < x < -\pi/2 \\ 1, & \text{for } -\pi/2 < x < \pi/2. \\ 1, & \text{for } \pi/2 < x < \pi. \end{cases}$$

3. Find the Fourier series for the function
$$f(x) = \begin{cases} 0, & \text{for } -\pi < x < 0 \\ 1, & \text{for } 0 < x < \pi. \end{cases}$$

4. Find the Fourier series for the function
$$f(x) = \begin{cases} \pi + x, & \text{for } -\pi \leqslant x \leqslant 0 \\ \pi - x, & \text{for } 0 \leqslant x \leqslant \pi. \end{cases}$$

5. Find the Fourier series for the function
$$f(x) = \cos(x/3), \quad \text{for } -\pi \leqslant x \leqslant \pi,$$
and by choosing a suitable value of x sum the series
$$\sum_{n=1}^{\infty} \frac{(-1)^n}{(9n^2 - 1)}.$$

6. Find the Fourier series for the function
$$f(x) = x^2, \quad \text{for } -\pi \leqslant x \leqslant \pi,$$

and by choosing suitable values of x sum the series

(a) $\displaystyle\sum_{n=1}^{\infty} \frac{(-1)^{n+1}}{n^2}$; and

(b) $\displaystyle\sum_{n=1}^{\infty} \frac{1}{n^2}$.

7. Find the Fourier series of the function

$$f(x) = \begin{cases} 0, & \text{for } -\pi \leqslant x \leqslant 0 \\ \sin 3x, & \text{for } 0 \leqslant x \leqslant \pi. \end{cases}$$

8. Find the Fourier series for the function

$$f(x) = \begin{cases} 0, & \text{for } -\pi \leqslant x \leqslant 0 \\ \sin x, & \text{for } 0 \leqslant x \leqslant \pi. \end{cases}$$

9. Find the Fourier series for the function

$$f(x) = \begin{cases} 1, & \text{for } -\pi \leqslant x \leqslant 0 \\ \cos x, & \text{for } 0 \leqslant x \leqslant \pi. \end{cases}$$

10. Find the Fourier series for the function

$$f(x) = |\cos x|, \quad \text{for } -\pi \leqslant x \leqslant \pi.$$

11. Find the Fourier series for the function

$$f(x) = |\sin x|, \quad \text{for } -\pi < x < \pi.$$

12. Find the Fourier series for the function

$$f(x) = \begin{cases} \pi + x, & \text{for } -\pi \leqslant x \leqslant -\pi/2 \\ |x|, & \text{for } -\pi/2 \leqslant x \leqslant \pi/2 \\ \pi - x, & \text{for } \pi/2 \leqslant x \leqslant \pi. \end{cases}$$

Determinants

A **second order determinant** involves four elements a, b, c and d which may either be numbers (real or complex) or functions, and it is displayed by writing them as follows:

$$\begin{vmatrix} a & b \\ c & d \end{vmatrix}.$$

The **value** of this second order determinant is defined to be

$$\begin{vmatrix} a & b \\ c & d \end{vmatrix} = ad - bc.$$

Thus, by way of example, we have

$$\begin{vmatrix} 3 & -2 \\ 4 & 5 \end{vmatrix} = 3 \times 5 - (-2) \times 4 = 23,$$

$$\begin{vmatrix} 1+i & 1 \\ 2 & 2-i \end{vmatrix} = (1+i)(2-i) - 1 \times 2 = 1 + i,$$

and

$$\begin{vmatrix} x+1 & 3 \\ 2 & x-2 \end{vmatrix} = (x+1)(x-2) - 2 \times 3 = x^2 - x - 8.$$

More generally, an nth order determinant involves n^2 elements arranged in n rows and n columns. The **order** of the determinant is the number of elements (entries) in a row on a column. Equivalently, the order of a determinant is the number of elements in the diagonal line drawn from top left to bottom right in the determinant; this is called the **leading diagonal**. We use the convention that the symbol a_{ij} represents the element in a determinant which is located in the ith row and the jth column. Thus a_{32} represents the element in row 3 and column 2, while a_{14} represents the element in row 1 and column 4. This convention is illustrated in the following diagram:

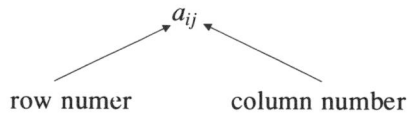

and the general nth order determinant is written

$$\begin{vmatrix} a_{11} & a_{12} & \dots & a_{1n} \\ a_{21} & a_{22} & \dots & a_{2n} \\ \cdot & \cdot & \cdot & \cdot \\ a_{n1} & a_{n2} & \dots & a_{nn} \end{vmatrix},$$

with the elements $a_{11}, a_{22}, \dots, a_{nn}$ comprising the leading diagonal.

Example 52.1

Construct the second order determinant with the elements $a_{11} = -1, a_{12} = 3$, $a_{21} = 4, a_{22} = 2$, and find its value.

Solution
The determinant is

$$\begin{vmatrix} -1 & 3 \\ 4 & 2 \end{vmatrix} = (-1) \times (2) - (3) \times (4) = -14. \qquad \blacktriangle$$

Example 52.2

Construct the third order determinant in which

$$a_{ij} = (1 + 3i) - j^2.$$

Solution
As the determinant is of order 3 it follows that $i = 1, 2, 3$ and $j = 1, 2, 3$. So calculating the elements we find $a_{11} = (1 + 3) - 1^2 = 3$, $a_{12} = (1 + 3) - 2^2 = 0$, $a_{13} = (1 + 3) - 3^2 = -5$, $a_{21} = (1 + 6) - 1^2 = 6$, $a_{22} = (1 + 6) - 2^2 = 3$, $a_{23} = (1 + 6) - 3^2 = -2$, $a_{31} = (1 + 9) - 1^2 = 9$, $a_{32} = (1 + 9) - 2^2 = 6$, $a_{33} = (1 + 9) - 3^2 = 1$, and so the determinant is

$$\begin{vmatrix} 3 & 0 & -5 \\ 6 & 3 & -2 \\ 9 & 6 & 1 \end{vmatrix}. \qquad \blacktriangle$$

We now turn our attention to the evaluation of an nth order determinant, which we will define (inductively) in terms of second order determinants. First, though, we need two simple definitions. The **minor** M_{ij} associated with the element a_{ij} in an nth order determinant is defined to be the determinant of order $n - 1$ obtained by removing the ith row and jth column of the original determinant.

Example 52.3

Find the minors of the third order determinant:

$$\begin{vmatrix} 1 & 2 & 0 \\ 3 & 1 & 4 \\ 1 & 0 & 2 \end{vmatrix}.$$

Solution

To find the minor M_{11} of this third order determinant we must delete the elements in row 1 and column 1 to obtain

$$M_{11} = \begin{vmatrix} 1 & 4 \\ 0 & 2 \end{vmatrix} = 2.$$

To find the minor M_{12} we must delete the elements in row 1 and column 2 to obtain

$$M_{12} = \begin{vmatrix} 3 & 4 \\ 1 & 2 \end{vmatrix} = 2.$$

Proceeding in similar fashion, we find that

$$M_{13} = \begin{vmatrix} 3 & 1 \\ 1 & 0 \end{vmatrix} = -1, \quad M_{21} = \begin{vmatrix} 2 & 0 \\ 0 & 2 \end{vmatrix} = 4, \quad M_{22} = \begin{vmatrix} 1 & 0 \\ 1 & 2 \end{vmatrix} = 2,$$

$$M_{23} = \begin{vmatrix} 1 & 2 \\ 1 & 0 \end{vmatrix} = -2, \quad M_{31} = \begin{vmatrix} 2 & 0 \\ 1 & 4 \end{vmatrix} = 8, \quad M_{32} = \begin{vmatrix} 1 & 0 \\ 3 & 4 \end{vmatrix} = 4,$$

$$M_{33} = \begin{vmatrix} 1 & 2 \\ 3 & 1 \end{vmatrix} = -5. \qquad\qquad \blacktriangle$$

Next we introduce the **cofactor** C_{ij} associated with the element a_{ij} in an nth order determinant. We define the cofactor C_{ij} in terms of the minor M_{ij} to be

$$C_{ij} = (-1)^{i+j} M_{ij}.$$

Notice that the factor $(-1)^{i+j}$ is $+1$ when $i+j$ is an even number and -1 when $i+j$ is an odd number. Thus the cofactor and minor of the element a_{ij} in an nth order determinant are identical when $i+j$ is even, and one is the negative of the other when $i+j$ is odd.

Example 52.4

Find the cofactors of the third order determinant:

$$\begin{vmatrix} 1 & 2 & 0 \\ 3 & 1 & 4 \\ 1 & 0 & 2 \end{vmatrix}.$$

Solution

This is the determinant whose minors were obtained in Example 52.3, where it was found that:

$$M_{11} = 2, \quad M_{12} = 2, \quad M_{13} = -1,$$

$$M_{21} = 4, \quad M_{22} = 2, \quad M_{23} = -2,$$
$$M_{31} = 8, \quad M_{32} = 4, \quad M_{33} = -5.$$

Thus as $c_{ij} = (-1)^{i+j} M_{ij}$, we see that

$$C_{11} = M_{11} = 2, \qquad C_{12} = -M_{12} = -2, \quad C_{13} = M_{13} = -1,$$
$$C_{21} = -M_{21} = -4, \quad C_{22} = M_{22} = 2, \qquad C_{23} = -M_{23} = 2,$$
$$C_{31} = M_{31} = 8, \qquad C_{32} = -M_{32} = -4, \quad C_{33} = M_{33} = -5. \qquad \blacktriangle$$

To understand the significance of cofactors we notice first that the cofactors of the second order determinant

$$\Delta = \begin{vmatrix} a_{11} & a_{12} \\ a_{21} & a_{22} \end{vmatrix} = a_{11}a_{22} - a_{12}a_{21}$$

are

$$C_{11} = a_{22}, \quad C_{12} = -a_{21}, \quad C_{21} = -a_{12}, \quad C_{22} = a_{11}.$$

Using these cofactors, the determinant Δ may be written in any one of the following four ways:

$$\Delta = \begin{cases} a_{11} \, C_{11} + a_{12} \, C_{12} \\ a_{11} \, C_{11} + a_{21} \, C_{21} \\ a_{21} \, C_{21} + a_{22} \, C_{22} \\ a_{12} \, C_{12} + a_{22} \, C_{22.} \end{cases}$$

Thus the value of the determinant is seen to be equal to the sum of the products of the elements and their cofactors in any row or column of the determinant.

The process of finding the value of a determinant by summing the products of the elements and their cofactors in row r is called **expanding** the determinant in terms of the elements of the rth row. Correspondingly, the process of finding the value of a determinant by summing the products of the elements and their cofactors in column s is called expanding the determinant in terms of the elements of the sth column.

Example 52.5

Expand the following determinant in four different ways:

$$\Delta = \begin{vmatrix} 3 & 7 \\ 2 & -1 \end{vmatrix}.$$

Solution
The cofactors are

$$C_{11} = -1, \quad C_{12} = -2, \quad C_{21} = -7, \quad C_{22} = 3.$$

Expanding in terms of the elements of row 1 gives

$$\Delta = 3C_{11} + 7C_{12} = (3) \times (-1) + (7) \times (-2) = -17.$$

Expanding in terms of the elements of row 2 gives

$$\Delta = 2C_{21} + (-1)C_{22} = (2) \times (-7) + (-1) \times (3) = -17.$$

Expanding in terms of the elements of column 1 gives

$$\Delta = 3C_{11} + 2C_{21} = (3) \times (-1) + (2) \times (-7) = -17.$$

Expanding in terms of the elements of column 2 gives

$$\Delta = 7C_{12} + (-1)C_{22} = (7) \times (-2) + (-1) \times (3) = -17. \qquad \blacktriangle$$

We now use this same rule to define the value of a third order determinant in terms of second order determinants. Thus, the value of a third order determinant is defined to be the sum of the products of the elements and their cofactors (second order determinants) in any row or column. This means there are $3 \times 2 = 6$ different ways of expanding a third order determinant.

Example 52.6

Expand the determinant

$$\Delta = \begin{vmatrix} 1 & 2 & 0 \\ 3 & 1 & 4 \\ 1 & 0 & 2 \end{vmatrix}$$

(i)   in terms of the elements in column 1;
(ii) in terms of the elements of row 2;
(iii) in terms of the elements of row 1.

Solution
This is the determinant whose cofactors were found in Example 52.4, so we will make use of them.
(i)   Expanding in terms of the elements of column 1 gives

$$\Delta = C_{11} + 3C_{21} + C_{31}$$
$$= 2 + (3) \times (-4) + 8 = -2.$$

(ii) Expanding in terms of the elements of row 2 gives

$$\Delta = 3C_{21} + C_{22} + 4C_{23}$$
$$= (3) \times (-4) + 2 + (4) \times (2) = -2.$$

(iii) Expanding in terms of the elements of row 1 gives

$$\Delta = C_{11} + 2C_{12}$$
$$= 2 + (2) \times (-2) = -2.$$

Notice the advantage of expanding in terms of a row or column containing some zero elements, because the cofactors corresponding to those elements need not be computed. $\qquad \blacktriangle$

The same rule applied to an nth order determinant determines its value in terms of n determinants of order $n-1$. Thus by repeated application of the rule the value of an nth order determinant may be evaluated in terms of second order determinants. The expansion rule which we now state in a formal manner is called the **Laplace expansion rule** for a determinant.

Expanding a determinant
The value of a determinant of any order is equal to the sum of the products of the elements of the determinant and their cofactors in any row or column.

Example 52.7

Expand the fourth order determinant:

$$\Delta = \begin{vmatrix} 1 & 8 & 2 & -3 \\ 3 & 0 & 2 & 0 \\ -1 & 2 & 1 & 2 \\ 1 & -1 & 2 & 1 \end{vmatrix}.$$

Solution
As the second row contains two zero elements, it will be best to expand Δ in terms of the elements of row 2. We have

$$\Delta = 3C_{21} + 2C_{23},$$

where

$$C_{21} = (-1)^{2+1} \begin{vmatrix} 8 & 2 & -3 \\ 2 & 1 & 2 \\ -1 & 2 & 1 \end{vmatrix} \quad \text{and} \quad C_{23} = (-1)^{2+3} \begin{vmatrix} 1 & 8 & -3 \\ -1 & 2 & 2 \\ 1 & -1 & 1 \end{vmatrix}.$$

Expanding these determinants in terms of elements of their first row gives

$$\begin{vmatrix} 8 & 2 & -3 \\ 2 & 1 & 2 \\ -1 & 2 & 1 \end{vmatrix} = 8 \cdot \underbrace{\begin{vmatrix} 1 & 2 \\ 2 & 1 \end{vmatrix}}_{C_{11}} + 2 \cdot (-1) \cdot \underbrace{\begin{vmatrix} 1 & 2 \\ -1 & 1 \end{vmatrix}}_{C_{12}} + (-3) \cdot \underbrace{\begin{vmatrix} 1 & 2 \\ 2 & 1 \end{vmatrix}}_{C_{13}}$$

$$= (8)(-3) - (2)(4) - (3)(5) = -47,$$

and

$$\begin{vmatrix} 1 & 8 & -3 \\ -1 & 2 & 2 \\ 1 & -2 & 1 \end{vmatrix} = 1 \cdot \underbrace{\begin{vmatrix} 2 & 2 \\ -1 & 1 \end{vmatrix}}_{C_{11}} + 8 \cdot (-1) \underbrace{\begin{vmatrix} -1 & 2 \\ 1 & 1 \end{vmatrix}}_{C_{12}} + (-3) \cdot \underbrace{\begin{vmatrix} -1 & 2 \\ 1 & -1 \end{vmatrix}}_{C_{13}}$$

$$= (1)(4) + (8)(3) - (3)(-1) = 31.$$

Thus, combining results we find that

$$\Delta = (3)(-1)(-47) + (2)(-1)(31) = 79.$$ ▲

Two simple determinants arise when either every element below the leading diagonal is zero, or when every element above it is zero. The first is called an **upper-triangular determinant** and the second is called a **lower-triangular determinant**.

Upper-triangular determinant of order n

$$\Delta = \begin{vmatrix} a_{11} & a_{12} & a_{13} & \cdots & a_{1n} \\ 0 & a_{22} & a_{23} & \cdots & a_{2n} \\ 0 & 0 & a_{33} & \cdots & a_{3n} \\ \cdot & \cdot & \cdot & \cdots & \cdot \\ 0 & 0 & 0 & \cdots & a_{nn} \end{vmatrix}.$$

Lower-triangular determinant of order n

$$\Delta = \begin{vmatrix} a_{11} & 0 & 0 & \cdots & 0 \\ a_{21} & a_{22} & 0 & \cdots & 0 \\ a_{31} & a_{32} & a_{33} & \cdots & 0 \\ \cdot & \cdot & \cdot & \cdots & \cdot \\ a_{n1} & a_{n2} & a_{n3} & \cdots & a_{nn} \end{vmatrix}.$$

Expanding an upper-triangular determinant in terms of the elements of its first column, and repeating the process with all the subsequent determinants that arise, shows that

$$\Delta = a_{11}a_{22}a_{33} \ldots a_{nn}.$$

The same result is true for a lower-triangular determinant, but to show this we need to expand it in terms of the elements in its last column.

Thus the value of an upper or lower-triangular determinant is equal to the product of the elements in its leading diagonal.

Example 52.8

Find the value of the following determinants:

(i) $\Delta = \begin{vmatrix} 1 & 3 & 1 \\ 0 & 0 & 2 \\ 0 & 0 & 5 \end{vmatrix}$;

(ii) $\Delta = \begin{vmatrix} 3 & 0 & 0 & 0 \\ 2 & 1 & 0 & 0 \\ 0 & 1 & -2 & 0 \\ 0 & 0 & 0 & 3 \end{vmatrix}$.

Solution
(i) $\Delta = (1)(0)(5) = 0$;

(ii) $\Delta = (3)(1)(-2)(3) = -18.$ ▲

We list below without formal proof a number of simple properties of determinants which simplify their manipulation.

Rules for the manipulation of determinants
1 If all the elements in a row or column of a determinant are zero, the value of the determinant is zero.
2 If two rows or two columns in a determinant are identical, the value of the determinant is zero.
3 If two rows or two columns in a determinant are interchanged, the determinant changes sign.
4 If all the elements in any row or column of a determinant are multiplied by a number λ, the value of the determinant is multiplied by λ.
5 The value of a determinant is unaltered by adding to the elements of any row (or column) a constant multiple of the corresponding elements of any other row (or column).

Outline proofs
1 Expand the determinant in terms of the elements of the row or column of zeros.
2 to 4. These follow by induction from the fact that the results are true for a second order determinant.
5 This follows from 2 and 3.

Example 52.9

Given that

$$\Delta = \begin{vmatrix} 3 & 1 & -2 \\ 8 & -5 & 7 \\ 4 & 0 & 1 \end{vmatrix} = -35,$$

find, without using the expansion rule, the value of the following determinants:

(i) $\begin{vmatrix} 3 & -2 & -2 \\ 8 & 7 & 10 \\ 4 & 1 & 0 \end{vmatrix}$;

(ii) $\begin{vmatrix} 3 & 1 & -2 \\ 4 & -5 & 6 \\ 4 & 0 & 1 \end{vmatrix}$;

(iii) $\begin{vmatrix} 11 & 1 & -2 \\ -20 & -5 & 7 \\ 0 & 0 & 1 \end{vmatrix}$.

Solution

(i) We need to transform the determinant to relate it to the given determinant. Interchanging columns (2) and (3) gives

$$\begin{vmatrix} 3 & -2 & -2 \\ 8 & 7 & 10 \\ 4 & 1 & 0 \end{vmatrix} = (-1) \begin{vmatrix} 3 & -2 & -2 \\ 8 & 10 & 7 \\ 4 & 0 & 1 \end{vmatrix} = (-1)(-2) \begin{vmatrix} 3 & 1 & 2 \\ 8 & -5 & 7 \\ 4 & 0 & 1 \end{vmatrix}$$

interchange
column (2) and (3)

remove factor
(− 2) from column (2)

$$= 2\Delta = -70.$$

(ii) Rows (1) and (3) agree with the given determinant so they may remain unaltered. Row (2) will agree if we add to it the elements of row (3) to obtain

$$\begin{vmatrix} 3 & 1 & -2 \\ 4 & -5 & 6 \\ 4 & 0 & 1 \end{vmatrix} = \begin{vmatrix} 3 & 1 & -2 \\ 8 & -5 & 7 \\ 4 & 0 & 1 \end{vmatrix} = \Delta = -35.$$

add row (3)
to row (2)

(iii) Columns (2) and (3) agree with the given determinant and so they may remain unaltered. Column (1) will agree if we add to it four times the elements of column (3) to obtain

$$\begin{vmatrix} 11 & 1 & -2 \\ -20 & -5 & 7 \\ 0 & 0 & 1 \end{vmatrix} = \begin{vmatrix} 3 & 1 & -2 \\ 8 & -5 & 7 \\ 4 & 0 & 1 \end{vmatrix} = \Delta = -35.$$

add four times
column (3) to
column (1)

▲

Example 52.10

Make use of the rules for the manipulation of determinants to expand:

$$\Delta = \begin{vmatrix} 2 & 1 & -1 & 1 \\ 1 & 0 & 2 & 3 \\ 1 & 2 & 1 & 3 \\ -1 & 4 & 0 & -1 \end{vmatrix}.$$

Solution

To simplify Δ let us modify it to make row (2) contain three zeros as follows:

$$\Delta = \begin{vmatrix} 2 & 1 & -5 & -5 \\ 1 & 0 & 0 & 0 \\ 1 & 2 & -1 & 0 \\ -1 & 4 & 2 & 2 \end{vmatrix}$$

New column (3) = old column (3)
 − 2 × old column (1)
New column (4) = old column (4)
 − 3 × old column (1).

Expanding in terms of the elements of the first column now reduces the problem to the expansion of a third order determinant, so

$$\Delta = (-1) \begin{vmatrix} 1 & -5 & -5 \\ 2 & -1 & 0 \\ 4 & 2 & 2 \end{vmatrix}.$$

To simplify Δ still further, we now subtract column (3) from column (2) to obtain:

$$\Delta = (-1) \begin{vmatrix} 1 & 0 & -5 \\ 2 & -1 & 0 \\ 4 & 0 & 2 \end{vmatrix} \qquad \text{New column (2) = old column(2)}$$
$$\text{- old column (3).}$$

Expanding in terms of elements of the second column gives:

$$\Delta = (-1)(-1) \begin{vmatrix} 1 & -5 \\ 4 & 2 \end{vmatrix} = 22. \qquad \blacktriangle$$

In practice, the simplest way to expand an nth order determinant is to use the rules for the manipulation of a determinant to reduce it to upper-triangular form, when its value is given by the product of the elements on the leading diagonal.

Example 52.11

Find the value of the following determinant by reducing it to upper-triangular form

$$\Delta = \begin{vmatrix} 1 & 6 & -2 \\ 4 & 1 & 2 \\ 3 & 1 & 0 \end{vmatrix}.$$

Solution

$$\Delta = \begin{vmatrix} 1 & 6 & -2 \\ 4 & 1 & 2 \\ 3 & 1 & 0 \end{vmatrix} = \begin{vmatrix} 1 & 6 & -2 \\ 0 & -23 & 10 \\ 0 & -17 & 6 \end{vmatrix} \qquad \begin{array}{l} \text{New row (2) = old row (2)} \\ -4 \times \text{old row (1)} \\ \text{New row (3) = old row (3)} \\ -3 \times \text{old row (1)} \end{array}$$

$$= \begin{vmatrix} 1 & 6 & -2 \\ 0 & -23 & 10 \\ 0 & 0 & \left(6 - \dfrac{170}{23}\right) \end{vmatrix} \qquad \begin{array}{l} \text{New row (3) = old row (3)} \\ -(17/23) \times \text{old row (2)} \end{array}$$

$$= (1)(-23)(-32/23) = 32. \qquad \blacktriangle$$

Example 52.12

Prove that

$$\begin{vmatrix} 1 & 1 & 1 \\ a & b & c \\ a^2 & b^2 & c^2 \end{vmatrix} = (c-b)(c-a)(b-a).$$

A determinant of this form is called an **alternant** of order 3.

Solution

$$\begin{vmatrix} 1 & 1 & 1 \\ a & b & c \\ a^2 & b^2 & c^2 \end{vmatrix} = \begin{vmatrix} 1 & 1 & 1 \\ a & (b-a) & (c-a) \\ a^2 & (b^2-a^2) & (c^2-a^2) \end{vmatrix} \quad \begin{array}{l} \text{New column (2) = old} \\ \text{column (2) - old column (1)} \\ \text{New column (3) = old} \\ \text{column (3) - old column (1)} \end{array}$$

$$= (b-a)(c-a)\begin{vmatrix} 1 & 0 & 0 \\ a & 1 & 1 \\ a^2 & (b+a) & (c+a) \end{vmatrix} \quad \begin{array}{l} \text{Remove factor } (b-a) \text{ from} \\ \text{column (2) and factor } (c-a) \\ \text{from column (3)} \end{array}$$

$$= (b-a)(c-a)\begin{vmatrix} 1 & 0 & 0 \\ a & 1 & 0 \\ a^2 & (b+a) & (c-b) \end{vmatrix} \quad \begin{array}{l} \text{New column (3) = old} \\ \text{column (3) - old column (2)} \end{array}$$

$$= (b-a)(c-a)(c-b),$$

because this is now a lower-triangular determinant.   ▲

The system of linear simultaneous equations

$$a_{11}x_1 + a_{12}x_2 = k_1$$

$$a_{21}x_1 + a_{22}x_2 = k_2$$

is said to be **non-homogeneous (inhomogeneous)** if at least one of the numbers k_1 and k_2 is non-zero. If may be solved by elimination to yield the solution

$$x_1 = \frac{k_1 a_{22} - k_2 a_{12}}{a_{11}a_{22} - a_{12}a_{21}}$$

and

$$x_2 = \frac{k_2 a_{11} - k_1 a_{21}}{a_{11}a_{22} - a_{12}a_{21}},$$

provided $a_{11}a_{22} - a_{12}a_{21} \neq 0$.

If we set

$$\Delta = \begin{vmatrix} a_{11} & a_{12} \\ a_{21} & a_{22} \end{vmatrix}, \quad \Delta = \begin{vmatrix} k_1 & a_{12} \\ k_2 & a_{22} \end{vmatrix} \quad \text{and} \quad \Delta_2 = \begin{vmatrix} a_{11} & k_1 \\ a_{21} & k_2 \end{vmatrix},$$

we see that

$$x_1 = \frac{\Delta_1}{\Delta} \quad \text{and} \quad x_2 = \frac{\Delta_2}{\Delta}.$$

Notice that Δ_1 is obtained from Δ by replacing the first column by the non-homogeneous terms, and Δ_2 is obtained from Δ by replacing the second column by the non-homogeneous terms. Generalizing this result to a system of n non-homogeneous linear simultaneous equations leads to **Cramer's rule**.

Cramer's rule for the solution of simultaneous equations by determinants
To solve the system of n non-homogeneous linear simultaneous equations

$$a_{11} x_1 + a_{12} x_2 + \cdots + a_{1n} x_n = k_1$$
$$a_{21} x_1 + a_{22} x_2 + \cdots + a_{2n} x_n = k_2$$
$$\cdot \qquad \cdot \qquad \cdots \qquad \cdot \qquad \cdot$$
$$a_{n1} x_1 + a_{n2} x_2 + \cdots + a_{nn} x_n = k_n,$$

set

$$\Delta = \begin{vmatrix} a_{11} & a_{12} & \cdots & a_{1n} \\ a_{21} & a_{22} & \cdots & a_{2n} \\ \cdot & \cdot & \cdot & \cdot \\ a_{n1} & a_{n2} & \cdots & a_{nn} \end{vmatrix},$$

and let Δ_i be the determinant obtained when the ith column of Δ is replaced by the non-homogeneous terms $k_1, k_2, ..., k_n$. Then, provided $\Delta \neq 0$, the solution is

$$x_1 = \frac{\Delta_1}{\Delta}, \quad x_2 = \frac{\Delta_2}{\Delta}, \quad ..., \quad x_n = \frac{\Delta_n}{\Delta}.$$

The practical solution of simultaneous equations is best carried out by means of **gaussian elimination** (to be described later). This is because the task of evaluating the determinants involved when applying Cramer's rule becomes excessive if $n > 3$. The main use of the rule is in connection with theoretical investigations involving simultaneous equations. The next example illustrates the use of the rule when $n = 3$.

Example 52.13

Solve by Cramer's rule

$$x_1 + 2x_2 + 5x_3 = -9$$
$$x_1 - x_2 + 3x_3 = 2$$
$$3x_1 - 6x_2 - x_3 = 25.$$

Solution

$$\Delta = \begin{vmatrix} 1 & 2 & 5 \\ 1 & -1 & 3 \\ 3 & -6 & -1 \end{vmatrix} = 24 \qquad \Delta_1 = \begin{vmatrix} -9 & 2 & 5 \\ 2 & -1 & 3 \\ 25 & -6 & -1 \end{vmatrix} = 48$$

$$\Delta_2 = \begin{vmatrix} 1 & -9 & 5 \\ 1 & 2 & 3 \\ 3 & 25 & -1 \end{vmatrix} = -72 \qquad \Delta_3 = \begin{vmatrix} 1 & 2 & -9 \\ 1 & -1 & 3 \\ 3 & -6 & 25 \end{vmatrix} = -24.$$

Thus

$$x_1 = \frac{48}{24} = 2, \quad x_2 = \frac{-72}{24} = -3, \quad x_3 = \frac{-24}{24} = -1.$$ ▲

PROBLEMS 52

Evaluate the determinants in problems 1 to 8.

1. $\begin{vmatrix} 1 & 4 \\ -1 & 2 \end{vmatrix}.$

2. $\begin{vmatrix} 3 & -1 \\ -2 & 1 \end{vmatrix}.$

3. $\begin{vmatrix} a & 3a \\ 2 & 1 \end{vmatrix}.$

4. $\begin{vmatrix} (1+i) & i \\ -1 & (2+3i) \end{vmatrix}.$

5. $\begin{vmatrix} (3-\lambda) & 1 \\ 4 & (2-\lambda) \end{vmatrix}.$

6. $\begin{vmatrix} \sin x & -\cos x \\ \cos x & \sin x \end{vmatrix}.$

7. $\begin{vmatrix} \cosh 2x & \sinh 2x \\ \sinh 2x & \cosh 2x \end{vmatrix}.$

8. $\begin{vmatrix} e^x & 3 \\ 1 & e^{-x} \end{vmatrix}.$

In problems 9 and 10 find the minors of the elements of the determinant.

9. $\begin{vmatrix} 1 & 3 & -1 \\ 2 & 1 & 2 \\ 1 & 0 & 5 \end{vmatrix}.$

10. $\begin{vmatrix} -2 & 1 & -2 \\ 1 & 2 & 1 \\ -1 & 1 & 3 \end{vmatrix}.$

Find the cofactors of the elements in the determinants in problems 11 and 12.

11. $\begin{vmatrix} 3 & 1 & 2 \\ -1 & 2 & -1 \\ 4 & 0 & 3 \end{vmatrix}.$

12. $\begin{vmatrix} 4 & 1 & 2 \\ 0 & 1 & 2 \\ 1 & 2 & 1 \end{vmatrix}.$

13. Verify the Laplace expansion rule for determinants by (a) expanding the following determinant in terms of elements of row (2) and (b) in terms of elements of column (3):

$$\begin{vmatrix} 4 & -2 & 3 \\ 1 & 4 & -1 \\ 2 & 2 & -3 \end{vmatrix}.$$

14. Verify the Laplace expansion rule for determinants by (a) expanding the following determinant in terms of elements of column (1) and (b) in terms of elements of column (2):

$$\begin{vmatrix} 3 & 4 & -1 \\ 2 & 1 & 0 \\ -2 & -4 & 3 \end{vmatrix}.$$

15. Expand

$$\begin{vmatrix} (3-\lambda) & 1 & 0 \\ 2 & (1-\lambda) & 1 \\ 1 & 2 & (2-\lambda) \end{vmatrix}.$$

16. Expand

$$\begin{vmatrix} (2-\lambda) & 2 & 1 \\ 0 & (2-\lambda) & 3 \\ 2 & 1 & (1-\lambda) \end{vmatrix}.$$

17. Given that

$$\begin{vmatrix} 1 & 4 & 3 \\ 4 & 2 & 1 \\ 1 & 2 & 2 \end{vmatrix} = -8,$$

use the properties of determinants to find without expansion the value of the following determinants:

(a) $\begin{vmatrix} 1 & 2 & 3 \\ 4 & 2 & 1 \\ 1 & 0 & 2 \end{vmatrix}$,

(b) $\begin{vmatrix} 1 & 4 & 3 \\ 0 & 2 & 1 \\ 4 & 2 & 1 \end{vmatrix}.$

18. Use the properties of determinants to expand the fourth order alternant

$$\begin{vmatrix} 1 & 1 & 1 & 1 \\ a & b & c & d \\ a^2 & b^2 & c^2 & d^2 \\ a^3 & b^3 & c^3 & d^3 \end{vmatrix}.$$

19. Evaluate

$$\Delta = \begin{vmatrix} 1 & 1 & 1 \\ 2 & -3 & 4 \\ 4 & 9 & 16 \end{vmatrix}.$$

20. Evaluate

$$\Delta = \begin{vmatrix} 1 & 1 & 1 \\ p+q & p+r & p+s \\ (p+q)^2 & (p+r)^2 & (p+s)^2 \end{vmatrix}.$$

Solve problems 21 to 24 by Cramer's rule.

21. $x_1 - 2x_2 + x_3 = 1$
$x_1 + 3x_2 - x_3 = 2$
$2x_1 + 4x_2 - 3x_3 = 0.$

22. $2x_1 + 3x_2 - x_3 = 2$
$x_1 + 4x_2 - 2x_3 = -2$
$4x_1 - x_2 + x_3 = 1.$

23. $3x_1 - x_2 - x_3 = 4$
$2x_1 + x_2 - 3x_3 = 1$
$x_1 + x_2 + x_3 = 1.$

24. $2x_1 - 2x_2 + x_3 = 4$
$x_1 - 3x_2 + 2x_3 = 5$
$2x_1 - x_2 + x_3 = 2.$

25. An important and useful result related to the Laplace expansion rule may be stated as follows:

The sum of the products of the elements of a row (or column) with the corresponding cofactors of a different row (or column) is zero.

This is easily proved for the second order determinant

$$\Delta = \begin{vmatrix} a_{11} & a_{12} \\ a_{21} & a_{22} \end{vmatrix}.$$

Consider, for example, the sum of the products of the elements of the first row with the corresponding cofactors of the second row

$$a_{11}C_{21} + a_{12}C_{22}.$$

As $C_{21} = -a_{12}$ and $C_{22} = a_{11}$ it follows that

$$a_{11}C_{21} + a_{12}C_{22} = 0.$$

The corresponding results for the other row and for the two columns follows in similar fashion.

Construct a third order determinant with arbitrary numerical elements and verify the result using the second and third columns.

53   Matrices: equality, addition, subtraction, scaling and transposition

A rectangular array of mn **elements** arranged in m rows and n columns is called an $m \times n$ (read m by n) **matrix**. If the element in the ith row and jth column of matrix A is denoted by a_{ij} we write

$$A = \left.\begin{bmatrix} a_{11} & a_{12} & \cdots & a_{1n} \\ a_{21} & a_{22} & \cdots & a_{2n} \\ . & . & \cdots & . \\ a_{m1} & a_{m2} & \cdots & a_{mn} \end{bmatrix}\right\} \quad m \text{ rows.}$$

$$\underbrace{}_{n \text{ columns}}$$

The elements of a matrix may either be numbers (real or complex) or functions, and the numbers $m \times n$ describe the **shape** of the matrix (it has m rows and n columns).

A matrix with n rows and n columns is called a **square matrix** of **order** n. In a square matrix the order is the number of elements on the **leading diagonal**, which is the diagonal running from top left to bottom right (as in a determinant).

Thus

$$\begin{bmatrix} 1 & 2 \\ 3 & 4 \\ 1 & 1 \\ 0 & 2 \end{bmatrix}$$

is a 4×2 matrix;

$$\begin{bmatrix} 1 & 3 & 1 \\ 2 & 1 & 2 \\ 1 & 1 & 0 \end{bmatrix}$$

is a square matrix of order 3 with elements 1, 1, 0 on it is leading diagonal;

$$\begin{bmatrix} \cos\theta & \sin\theta \\ -\sin\theta & \cos\theta \end{bmatrix}$$

is a square matrix of order 2 with functions as elements and with elements $\cos\theta$, $\cos\theta$ on its leading diagonal.

A square matrix of order n in which all elements are zero apart from those on the leading diagonal, each of which equals unity, is called a **unit matrix** of order n, and it is usually denoted by I (irrespective of its order). Thus a unit matrix of order 3 is

$$I = \begin{bmatrix} 1 & 0 & 0 \\ 0 & 1 & 0 \\ 0 & 0 & 1 \end{bmatrix}.$$

If it is essential to distinguish between unit matrices of different orders this is usually done by adding the suffix n to the symbol I to indicate the order. Thus, for example, in this notation

$$I_2 = \begin{bmatrix} 1 & 0 \\ 0 & 1 \end{bmatrix} \quad \text{and} \quad I_3 = \begin{bmatrix} 1 & 0 & 0 \\ 0 & 1 & 0 \\ 0 & 0 & 1 \end{bmatrix}.$$

A matrix comprising a single row of m elements is called an m element **row vector** and one comprising a single column of n elements is called an n element **column vector**. Thus the 1×4 matrix

$$[1, -4, 3, 2]$$

is a four element row vector, and the 3×1 matrix

$$\begin{bmatrix} 1 \\ 4 \\ -2 \end{bmatrix}$$

is a three element column vector. A **null** or **zero matrix** is a matrix in which each element is zero.

Matrices A and B with the respective **general elements** a_{ij} and b_{ij} are said to be **equal** if A and B have the same shape and corresponding elements are identical.

Thus if

$$A = \begin{bmatrix} a & 3 & 1 \\ 2 & b & 4 \end{bmatrix} \quad \text{and} \quad B = \begin{bmatrix} -3 & 3 & c \\ 2 & 7 & d \end{bmatrix},$$

the equality $A = B$ means that corresponding elements are equal, so

$$a = -3, \quad b = 7, \quad c = 1 \quad \text{and} \quad d = 4$$

If matrices A and B with the respective general elements a_{ij} and b_{ij} are the same shape, their **sum** $A + B$ is defined as the matrix with the general element

$a_{ij} + b_{ij}$ and their **difference** $A - B$ is defined as the matrix with the general element $a_{ij} - b_{ij}$.

If follows from the definition of matrix addition that the order in which matrices are summed is immaterial, so that

$$A + B = B + A.$$

The following example illustrates matrix addition and subtraction. If

$$A = \begin{bmatrix} 1 & 3 & 1 \\ 2 & -1 & 0 \end{bmatrix} \quad \text{and} \quad B = \begin{bmatrix} 2 & -4 & 3 \\ 1 & 2 & 1 \end{bmatrix},$$

then

$$A + B = \begin{bmatrix} (1+2) & (3-4) & (1+3) \\ (2+1) & (-1+2) & (0+1) \end{bmatrix} = \begin{bmatrix} 3 & -1 & 4 \\ 3 & 1 & 1 \end{bmatrix},$$

and

$$A - B = \begin{bmatrix} (1-2) & (3-(-4)) & (1-3) \\ (2-1) & (-1-2) & (0-1) \end{bmatrix} = \begin{bmatrix} -1 & 7 & -2 \\ 1 & -3 & -1 \end{bmatrix}.$$

If λ is a number and matrix A has the general element a_{ij}, the matrix λA is defined as the matrix with the general element λa_{ij}. This process is called **scaling** a matrix by the number λ.

Thus if $\lambda = -2$ and

$$A = \begin{bmatrix} -2 & 4 & 3 \\ 1 & 4 & 2 \\ -1 & 2 & -1 \end{bmatrix},$$

the matrix

$$\lambda A = -2A = \begin{bmatrix} 4 & -8 & -6 \\ -2 & -8 & -4 \\ 2 & -4 & 2 \end{bmatrix}.$$

Correspondingly, if

$$A = \begin{bmatrix} 2 & 1 & 4 \\ 1 & 2 & 1 \end{bmatrix} \quad \text{and} \quad B = \begin{bmatrix} -1 & 2 & -3 \\ 2 & 1 & -1 \end{bmatrix},$$

then

$$3A - 2B = 3\begin{bmatrix} 2 & 1 & 4 \\ 1 & 2 & 1 \end{bmatrix} - 2\begin{bmatrix} -1 & 2 & -3 \\ 2 & 1 & -1 \end{bmatrix}$$

$$= \begin{bmatrix} 6 & 3 & 12 \\ 3 & 6 & 3 \end{bmatrix} + \begin{bmatrix} 2 & -4 & 6 \\ -4 & -2 & 2 \end{bmatrix}$$

$$= \begin{bmatrix} (6+2) & (3-4) & (12+6) \\ (3-4) & (6-2) & (3+2) \end{bmatrix}$$

$$= \begin{bmatrix} 8 & -1 & 18 \\ -1 & 4 & 5 \end{bmatrix}.$$

Similarly, if λ is any number and

$$A = \begin{bmatrix} 3 & 1 & -7 \\ 2 & 4 & 1 \\ -5 & 2 & 3 \end{bmatrix},$$

then

$$A - \lambda I = \begin{bmatrix} 3 & 1 & -7 \\ 2 & 4 & 1 \\ -5 & 2 & 3 \end{bmatrix} - \lambda \begin{bmatrix} 1 & 0 & 0 \\ 0 & 1 & 0 \\ 0 & 0 & 1 \end{bmatrix}$$

$$= \begin{bmatrix} 3 & 1 & -7 \\ 2 & 4 & 1 \\ -5 & 2 & 3 \end{bmatrix} + \begin{bmatrix} -\lambda & 0 & 0 \\ 0 & -\lambda & 0 \\ 0 & 0 & -\lambda \end{bmatrix}$$

$$= \begin{bmatrix} (3-\lambda) & 1 & -7 \\ 2 & (4-\lambda) & 1 \\ -5 & 2 & (3-\lambda) \end{bmatrix}.$$

The **transpose** of an $m \times n$ matrix A, denoted by A^T (sometimes also by A'), is the $n \times m$ matrix obtained from A by interchanging its rows and columns. Thus row 1 of A becomes column 1 of A^T, row 2 of A becomes column 2 of A^T ..., and row m of A becomes column m of A^T.

If

$$A = \begin{bmatrix} 3 & 1 \\ 4 & 2 \\ -2 & 6 \end{bmatrix}, \quad \text{then} \quad A^T = \begin{bmatrix} 3 & 2 & -2 \\ 1 & 2 & 6 \end{bmatrix},$$

and if

$$A = \begin{bmatrix} 1 & 3 & 7 \\ 2 & 1 & 4 \\ 1 & 2 & 1 \end{bmatrix}, \quad \text{then} \quad A^T = \begin{bmatrix} 1 & 2 & 1 \\ 3 & 1 & 2 \\ 7 & 4 & 1 \end{bmatrix}.$$

It is clear that transposing a transposed matrix yields the original matrix, so

$$(A^T)^T = A$$

If A is square and $A^T = A$ we say A is a **symmetric matrix**, and if $A^T = -A$ we say A is a **skew-symmetric matrix**. Thus

$$\begin{bmatrix} 1 & 5 & 7 \\ 5 & 2 & 6 \\ 7 & 6 & 3 \end{bmatrix}$$

is a symmetric matrix, but

$$\begin{bmatrix} 0 & -3 & 7 \\ 3 & 0 & 6 \\ -7 & -6 & 0 \end{bmatrix}$$

is a skew-symmetric matrix. It follows at once that the elements on the leading diagonal of a skew-symmetric matrix are all zero.

PROBLEMS 53

1. If

$$A = \begin{bmatrix} 2 & 1 \\ 3 & 4 \end{bmatrix}, \quad B = \begin{bmatrix} -1 & -2 \\ 2 & 1 \end{bmatrix},$$

   find

$$A + B, \quad A - B \quad \text{and} \quad 2A + 3B.$$

2. If

$$A = \begin{bmatrix} 2 & 1 & 4 \\ -2 & 1 & 0 \end{bmatrix}, \quad B = \begin{bmatrix} 4 & -2 & 1 \\ 2 & -1 & 1 \end{bmatrix},$$

   find

$$A + B, \quad A - B \quad \text{and} \quad A - 2B.$$

3. When they are defined, find the sum and difference of the following matrices:

$$A = \begin{bmatrix} 2 & 1 \\ 3 & -2 \end{bmatrix}, \quad B = \begin{bmatrix} 1 & 2 \\ 3 & 1 \\ 1 & 0 \end{bmatrix}, \quad C = \begin{bmatrix} -1 & 2 \\ 2 & -1 \end{bmatrix}, \quad D = \begin{bmatrix} -2 & 1 \\ 2 & 3 \\ 1 & -2 \end{bmatrix}.$$

4. If

$$A = \begin{bmatrix} 3 & a & 2 \\ b & -1 & c \end{bmatrix} \quad \text{and} \quad B = \begin{bmatrix} d & -1 & 2 \\ 4 & e & 7 \end{bmatrix}$$

   find the condition that $A = B$.

5. If

$$A = \begin{bmatrix} a & 2 \\ 3 & 7 \\ b & -4 \end{bmatrix} \quad \text{and} \quad B = \begin{bmatrix} 2 & c \\ 6 & d \\ 4 & e \end{bmatrix}$$

   find the condition that $2A = B$.

6. Find and simplify the matrix sum $A + B$, given that

$$A = \begin{bmatrix} \sin A \cos B & \cos A \cos B \\ \cosh A \cosh B & \sinh A \cosh B \end{bmatrix}$$

   and

$$B = \begin{bmatrix} \cos A \sin B & \sin A \sin B \\ \sinh A \sinh B & -\cosh A \sinh B \end{bmatrix}.$$

7. Given that
$$A = \begin{bmatrix} 1 & 4 & 2 \\ 7 & 6 & 1 \\ 9 & 2 & 4 \end{bmatrix} \quad \text{and} \quad B = \begin{bmatrix} 1 & 5 & -9 \\ 5 & 0 & 6 \\ -9 & 6 & 3 \end{bmatrix}$$

find A^T and B^T.

8. Given that
$$A = \begin{bmatrix} 1 & 3 & 7 & 2 \\ 0 & 2 & 5 & 3 \end{bmatrix} \quad \text{and} \quad B = \begin{bmatrix} 0 & 5 & 6 & 1 \\ -5 & 0 & -3 & -2 \\ -6 & 3 & 0 & 1 \\ -1 & 2 & -1 & 0 \end{bmatrix}$$

find A^T and B^T.

54   Matrix multiplication

The fundamental idea underlying matrix multiplication is the multiplication of an n element row vector $\mathbf{u}$ and an n element column vector $\mathbf{v}$.

If the row vector

$$\mathbf{u} = [u_1, u_2, ..., u_n]$$

and the column vector

$$\mathbf{v} = \begin{bmatrix} v_1 \\ v_2 \\ \vdots \\ v_n \end{bmatrix},$$

the **product uv** (in this order) is defined as

$$\mathbf{uv} = u_1 v_1 + u_2 v_2 + ... + u_n v_n.$$

Thus $\mathbf{uv}$ is the sum of the products of the corresponding elements in $\mathbf{u}$ and $\mathbf{v}$. It is immaterial whether or not the product $\mathbf{uv}$ is regarded as a 1×1 matrix, or simply as a number, because their properties are identical.

Example 54.1

Find $\mathbf{uv}$, given that

(i) $\mathbf{u} = [1, 2, -1]$ and $\mathbf{v} = \begin{bmatrix} 3 \\ 2 \\ 2 \end{bmatrix}$;

(ii) $\mathbf{u} = [3, -1, 2, 0]$ and $\mathbf{v} = \begin{bmatrix} 1 \\ -2 \\ 1 \\ 2 \end{bmatrix}$.

Solution

(i) $\mathbf{uv} = (1)(3) + (2)(2) + (-1)(1) = 6.$

(ii) $\mathbf{uv} = (3)(1) + (-1)(-2) + (2)(1) + (0)(2) = 7.$ ▲

If A and B are any two matrices, the **matrix product AB** is only defined if the number of columns in A equals the number of rows in B. The product matrix $C = AB$ is then a $p \times q$ matrix, where p is the number of rows in A and q is the number of columns in B. This may be shown symbolically as follows. If A is a $p \times m$ matrix, and B is an $m \times q$ matrix,

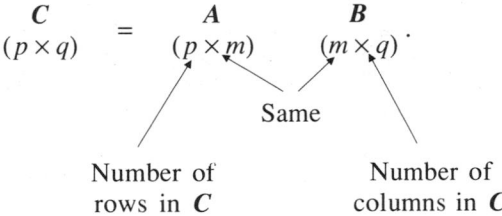

Definition of matrix multiplication
Let A be a $p \times m$ matrix and B be an $m \times q$ matrix, and let $\mathbf{a}_i$ be the row vector formed from the ith row of A and $\mathbf{b}_j$ be the column vector formed from the jth column of B. Then the element c_{ij} in the ith row and jth column of the product matrix $C = AB$ is defined as

$$c_{ij} = \mathbf{a}_i \mathbf{b}_j.$$

Example 54.2

Given

$$A = \begin{bmatrix} 1 & 2 & 3 \\ 2 & -1 & 0 \end{bmatrix}, \quad B = \begin{bmatrix} -1 & 2 \\ 2 & 3 \\ 1 & 2 \end{bmatrix} \quad \text{and} \quad I = \begin{bmatrix} 1 & 0 & 0 \\ 0 & 1 & 0 \\ 0 & 0 & 1 \end{bmatrix},$$

find
(i) AB;
(ii) BA; and
(iii) AI.

Solution
(i)   The product AB is defined and will yield a 2×2 matrix:

$$AB = \begin{bmatrix} 1 & 2 & 3 \\ 2 & -1 & 0 \end{bmatrix} \begin{bmatrix} -1 & 2 \\ 2 & 3 \\ 1 & 2 \end{bmatrix}$$

$$= \begin{bmatrix} (1)(-1)+(2)(2)+(3)(1) & (1)(2)+(2)(3)+(3)(2) \\ (2)(-1)+(-1)(2)+(0)(1) & (2)(2)+(-1)(3)+(0)(2) \end{bmatrix}$$

$$= \begin{bmatrix} 6 & 14 \\ -4 & 1 \end{bmatrix}.$$

(ii)   The product BA is defined and will yield a 3×3 matrix:

$$BA = \begin{bmatrix} -1 & 2 \\ 2 & 3 \\ 1 & 2 \end{bmatrix} \begin{bmatrix} 1 & 2 & 3 \\ 2 & -1 & 0 \end{bmatrix}$$

$$= \begin{bmatrix} (-1)(1)+(2)(2) & (-1)(2)+(2)(-1) & (-1)(3)+(2)(0) \\ (2)(1)+(3)(2) & (2)(2)+(3)(-1) & (2)(3)+(3)(0) \\ (1)(1)+(2)(2) & (1)(2)+(2)(-1) & (1)(3)+(2)(0) \end{bmatrix}$$

$$= \begin{bmatrix} 3 & -4 & -3 \\ 8 & 1 & 6 \\ 5 & 0 & 3 \end{bmatrix}.$$

(iii) The product AI is defined and will yield a 2×3 matrix.

$$AI = \begin{bmatrix} 1 & 2 & 3 \\ 2 & -1 & 0 \end{bmatrix} \begin{bmatrix} 1 & 0 & 0 \\ 0 & 1 & 0 \\ 0 & 0 & 1 \end{bmatrix}$$

$$= \begin{bmatrix} (1)(1)+(2)(0)+(3)(0) & (1)(0)+(2)(1)+(3)(0) & (1)(0)+(2)(0)+(3)(1) \\ (2)(1)+(-1)(0)+(0)(0) & (2)(0)+(-1)(1)+(0)(0) & (2)(0)+(-1)(0)+(0)(0) \end{bmatrix}$$

$$= \begin{bmatrix} 1 & 2 & 3 \\ 2 & -1 & 0 \end{bmatrix} = A. \qquad \blacktriangle$$

The last example has shown that, in general, the order in which matrices are multiplied influences the result. To make this order perfectly clear, when speaking of matrix multiplication we say that in the matrix product AB the matrix A **premultiplies** B (multiplies it from the left) and that the matrix B **postmultiplies** A (multiplies it from the right).

Example 54.3

Given that

$$A = [1, 2, 3], \quad B = \begin{bmatrix} 2 \\ -1 \\ 2 \end{bmatrix}, \quad C = [1, -4] \quad \text{and} \quad D = \begin{bmatrix} 2 & -1 \\ 0 & 3 \end{bmatrix},$$

find all possible matrix products involving pairs of matrices.

Solution

$$AB = [2, 2, 3] \begin{bmatrix} 2 \\ -1 \\ 2 \end{bmatrix} = (2)(2)+(2)(-1)+(3)(2) = 8.$$

$$BA = \begin{bmatrix} 2 \\ -1 \\ 2 \end{bmatrix} [2, 2, 3] = \begin{bmatrix} (2)(2) & (2)(2) & (2)(3) \\ (-1)(2) & (-1)(2) & (-1)(3) \\ (2)(2) & (2)(2) & (2)(3) \end{bmatrix}$$

$$= \begin{bmatrix} 4 & 4 & 6 \\ -2 & -2 & -3 \\ 4 & 4 & 6 \end{bmatrix}.$$

AC, CA, AD, DA and DC are not defined.

$$CD = [1, -4] \begin{bmatrix} 2 & -1 \\ 0 & 3 \end{bmatrix} = [(1)(2) + (-4)(0) \qquad (1)(-1) + (-4)(3)]$$

$$= [2, -13].$$ ▲

Example 54.4

Given that

$$A = \begin{bmatrix} 4 & -1 \\ 2 & 3 \end{bmatrix} \quad \text{and} \quad B = \begin{bmatrix} 3/14 & 1/14 \\ -1/7 & 2/7 \end{bmatrix},$$

show that $AB = BA = I$.

Solution

$$AB = \begin{bmatrix} 4 & -1 \\ 2 & 3 \end{bmatrix} \begin{bmatrix} 3/14 & 1/14 \\ -1/7 & 2/7 \end{bmatrix}$$

$$= \begin{bmatrix} (4)(3/14) + (-1)(-1/7) & (4)(1/14) + (-1)(2/7) \\ (2)(3/14) + 3(-1/7) & (2)(1/14) + (3)(2/7) \end{bmatrix}$$

$$= \begin{bmatrix} 1 & 0 \\ 0 & 1 \end{bmatrix}$$

$$BA = \begin{bmatrix} 3/14 & 1/14 \\ -1/7 & 2/7 \end{bmatrix} \begin{bmatrix} 4 & -1 \\ 2 & 3 \end{bmatrix}$$

$$= \begin{bmatrix} (3/14)(4) + (1/14)(2) & (3/14)(-1) + (1/14)(3) \\ (-1/7)(4) + (2/7)(2) & (-1/7)(-1) + (2/7)(3) \end{bmatrix}$$

$$= \begin{bmatrix} 1 & 0 \\ 0 & 1 \end{bmatrix}.$$ ▲

Example 54.5

Given that

$$A = \begin{bmatrix} 3 & -2 & 1 \\ 4 & 3 & 6 \\ 1 & -4 & 2 \end{bmatrix}, \quad X = \begin{bmatrix} x \\ y \\ z \end{bmatrix} \quad \text{and} \quad B = \begin{bmatrix} 2 \\ 5 \\ 6 \end{bmatrix},$$

expand and interpret the matrix equation $AX = B$.

Solution
The matrix equation $AX = B$ is

$$\begin{bmatrix} 3 & -2 & 1 \\ 4 & 3 & 6 \\ 1 & -4 & 2 \end{bmatrix} \begin{bmatrix} x \\ y \\ z \end{bmatrix} = \begin{bmatrix} 2 \\ 5 \\ 6 \end{bmatrix},$$

so carrying out the matrix product on the left this becomes

$$\begin{bmatrix} 3x - 2y + z \\ 4x + 3y + 6z \\ x - 4y + 2z \end{bmatrix} = \begin{bmatrix} 2 \\ 5 \\ 6 \end{bmatrix}.$$

However, the equality of two matrices means the equality of their corresponding elements, so the above result is equivalent to the set of three simultaneous equations:

$$3x - 2y + z = 2$$

$$4x + 3y + 6z = 5$$

$$x - 4y + 2z = 6.$$ ▲

Example 54.6

Write the simultaneous equations

$$2x + 5y - z = 6$$

$$x - 7y + 9z = -1$$

$$3x + 4y - 3z = 17$$

in the matrix form $AX = B$.

Solution
Consideration of Example 54.5 shows that the **coefficient matrix** (the matrix of multipliers of x, y and z) is

$$A = \begin{bmatrix} 2 & 5 & -1 \\ 1 & -7 & 9 \\ 3 & 4 & -3 \end{bmatrix},$$

the column vector

$$X = \begin{bmatrix} x \\ y \\ z \end{bmatrix}$$

and the column vector **B** (the vector of non-homogeneous terms) is

$$B = \begin{bmatrix} 6 \\ -1 \\ 17 \end{bmatrix}.$$

▲

GENERAL PROPERTIES OF MATRIX MULTIPLICATION

Provided the matrix products are defined it follows from the definitions of the sum, product and transpose of matrices that:

1 $A(B+C) = AB + AC$;
2 $A(BC) = (AB)C$
3 $AI = IA$ (where I is the appropriate unit matrix);
4 $A^n = \underbrace{A \cdot A \ldots A}_{n \text{ times}}$;

5 $I^n = I$.
6 $(AB)^T = B^T A^T$.

Example 54.7

Given

$$A = \begin{bmatrix} 1 & 4 \\ -1 & 3 \end{bmatrix}, \quad B = \begin{bmatrix} 2 & 1 \\ 0 & 2 \end{bmatrix} \quad \text{and} \quad C = \begin{bmatrix} 1 & -1 \\ 2 & 3 \end{bmatrix},$$

(i) verify that

$$A(B+C) = AB + AC;$$

(ii) verify that

$$A(BC) = (AB)C;$$

(iii) find A^3;
(iv) verify that

$$(AB)^T = B^T A^T.$$

Solution
Since the matrix products are straightforward we only present outline solutions.

(i) $A(B+C) = \underbrace{\begin{bmatrix} 1 & 3 \\ -1 & 3 \end{bmatrix}}_{A} \underbrace{\begin{bmatrix} 3 & 0 \\ 2 & 5 \end{bmatrix}}_{B+C} = \begin{bmatrix} 11 & 20 \\ 3 & 15 \end{bmatrix}$

$$AB + AC = \underbrace{\begin{bmatrix} 1 & 4 \\ -1 & 3 \end{bmatrix} \begin{bmatrix} 2 & 1 \\ 0 & 2 \end{bmatrix}}_{AB} + \underbrace{\begin{bmatrix} 1 & 4 \\ -1 & 3 \end{bmatrix} \begin{bmatrix} 1 & -1 \\ 2 & 3 \end{bmatrix}}_{AC}$$

$$= \begin{bmatrix} 2 & 9 \\ -2 & 5 \end{bmatrix} + \begin{bmatrix} 9 & 11 \\ 5 & 10 \end{bmatrix} = \begin{bmatrix} 11 & 20 \\ 3 & 15 \end{bmatrix},$$

and thus we have verified the property that

$$A(B + C) = AB + AC.$$

(ii) $A(BC) = \underbrace{\begin{bmatrix} 1 & 4 \\ -1 & 3 \end{bmatrix}}_{A} \underbrace{\begin{bmatrix} 4 & 1 \\ 4 & 6 \end{bmatrix}}_{B+C} = \begin{bmatrix} 20 & 25 \\ 8 & 17 \end{bmatrix}$

$$(AB)C = \underbrace{\begin{bmatrix} 2 & 9 \\ -2 & 5 \end{bmatrix}}_{AB} \underbrace{\begin{bmatrix} 1 & -1 \\ 2 & 3 \end{bmatrix}}_{C} = \begin{bmatrix} 20 & 25 \\ 8 & 17 \end{bmatrix}$$

and thus we have verified the property that

$$A(BC) = (AB)C$$

(iii) $A^3 = AA^2 = \underbrace{\begin{bmatrix} 1 & 4 \\ -1 & 3 \end{bmatrix}}_{A} \underbrace{\begin{bmatrix} -3 & 16 \\ -4 & 5 \end{bmatrix}}_{A^2} = \begin{bmatrix} -19 & 36 \\ -9 & -1 \end{bmatrix}$

and, of course,

$$A^3 = A^2 A = \underbrace{\begin{bmatrix} -3 & 16 \\ -4 & 5 \end{bmatrix}}_{A^2} \underbrace{\begin{bmatrix} 1 & 4 \\ -1 & 3 \end{bmatrix}}_{A} = \begin{bmatrix} -19 & 36 \\ 9 & -1 \end{bmatrix}.$$

(iv) $AB = \begin{bmatrix} 1 & 4 \\ -1 & 3 \end{bmatrix} \begin{bmatrix} 2 & 1 \\ 0 & 2 \end{bmatrix} = \begin{bmatrix} 2 & 9 \\ -2 & 5 \end{bmatrix}$, so

$$(AB)^T = \begin{bmatrix} 2 & -2 \\ 9 & 5 \end{bmatrix}$$

$$B^T A^T = \underbrace{\begin{bmatrix} 2 & 0 \\ 1 & 2 \end{bmatrix}}_{B^T} \underbrace{\begin{bmatrix} 1 & -1 \\ 4 & 3 \end{bmatrix}}_{A^T} = \begin{bmatrix} 2 & -2 \\ 9 & 5 \end{bmatrix},$$

▲

and thus we have verified the property

$$(AB)^T = B^T A^T.$$

PROBLEMS 54

1.   Given that

$$A = \begin{bmatrix} 1 & 4 \\ 6 & 2 \end{bmatrix} \quad \text{and} \quad B = \begin{bmatrix} 2 & 5 \\ -2 & 1 \end{bmatrix},$$

find AB and BA.

2.   Given that

$$A = \begin{bmatrix} 1 & 2 & 1 \\ -2 & 0 & 6 \\ 4 & -1 & 2 \end{bmatrix} \quad \text{and} \quad B = \begin{bmatrix} 2 & 6 \\ 1 & -1 \\ 3 & -2 \end{bmatrix},$$

find AB.

3.   Given that

$$A = [1, 4, -3, 2] \quad \text{and} \quad B = \begin{bmatrix} 2 \\ -1 \\ 2 \\ 6 \end{bmatrix},$$

find AB and BA.

4.   Given that

$$A = \begin{bmatrix} 1 & 4 & -1 & 2 \\ 2 & 0 & 1 & 3 \\ -1 & -2 & 0 & 4 \end{bmatrix} \quad \text{and} \quad B = \begin{bmatrix} 3 & 4 & 1 \\ 2 & 2 & 4 \end{bmatrix},$$

find whichever of the products AB and BA is defined.

5.   Given that

$$A = [1, -2, 1, 3], \quad B = \begin{bmatrix} 1 \\ 1 \\ 1 \\ 0 \end{bmatrix}, \quad C = \begin{bmatrix} 1 \\ 3 \\ 5 \\ 2 \end{bmatrix} \quad \text{and} \quad D = [1, 3, -2],$$

find AB, AC and BD.

6.   Given that

$$A = \begin{bmatrix} 1 & -3 \\ 2 & -7 \end{bmatrix} \quad \text{and} \quad B = \begin{bmatrix} 2 & 1 \\ -3 & 4 \end{bmatrix},$$

find AB and BA.

7.   Given that

$$A = \begin{bmatrix} 1-3i & 2i \\ 4 & 2+i \end{bmatrix} \quad \text{and} \quad B = \begin{bmatrix} 3i & -1+i \\ 1+i & 1-i \end{bmatrix},$$

find AB and BA.

8. Given that

$$A = \begin{bmatrix} 1+x & 3 \\ 2x & 1-x \end{bmatrix} \quad \text{and} \quad B = \begin{bmatrix} 1-x & -2 \\ 2 & 1+x \end{bmatrix},$$

find AB and BA.

9. Given that

$$A = \begin{bmatrix} 3 & 1 & 4 \\ 2 & -1 & 2 \end{bmatrix}, \quad B = \begin{bmatrix} 1 & 2 & 1 \\ 2 & 1 & -1 \\ 3 & 0 & 1 \\ 1 & 2 & 4 \end{bmatrix} \quad \text{and} \quad C = \begin{bmatrix} 1 & 2 \\ 4 & 2 \\ 6 & 1 \end{bmatrix},$$

find all possible matrix products.

10. Given that

$$A = \begin{bmatrix} 1 & 4 & 6 & -3 \\ 3 & -1 & 2 & 1 \\ 4 & -2 & 3 & 6 \end{bmatrix}, \quad B = \begin{bmatrix} 2 & 1 & 4 \\ 3 & -1 & 2 \\ 1 & 2 & 1 \end{bmatrix} \quad \text{and} \quad C = \begin{bmatrix} 3 \\ 2 \end{bmatrix},$$

find all possible matrix products.

11. Given that

$$A = \begin{bmatrix} 2 & 1 & 3 \\ 1 & 4 & -1 \\ 1 & -1 & 2 \end{bmatrix},$$

find A^3.

12. Given that

$$A = \begin{bmatrix} 0 & 0 & 1 \\ 0 & 1 & 0 \\ 1 & 0 & 0 \end{bmatrix},$$

find A^2 and A^3 and hence deduce A^n for $n > 3$.

13. Given that

$$A = \begin{bmatrix} 2 & 4 \\ -1 & -2 \end{bmatrix}, \quad B = \begin{bmatrix} 4 & 1 \\ 3 & -1 \end{bmatrix} \quad \text{and} \quad C = \begin{bmatrix} 1 & -1 \\ -1 & 1 \end{bmatrix},$$

verify that

$$A(B+C) = AB + AC.$$

14. Using the matrices A, B and C in problem 13 verify that

$$A(BC) = (AB)C,$$

15. Given that

$$A = \begin{bmatrix} 1 & 3 \\ -2 & 1 \end{bmatrix} \quad \text{and} \quad B = \begin{bmatrix} 2 & 4 \\ 3 & -2 \end{bmatrix},$$

find $A^T B$ and $B^T A$.

16. Given that

$$A = \begin{bmatrix} 1 & -3 & 0 \\ 2 & 1 & 4 \\ 1 & 2 & 1 \end{bmatrix} \quad \text{and} \quad B = \begin{bmatrix} -7 & 3 & -12 \\ 2 & 1 & -4 \\ 3 & -5 & 7 \end{bmatrix},$$

show that

$$AB = -13I,$$

where I is the 3×3 unit matrix.

17. Given that

$$A = \begin{bmatrix} \sin x & -\cos x \\ \cos x & \sin x \end{bmatrix},$$

find A^2 and simplify the result.

18. Given that

$$A = \begin{bmatrix} \cos x & \sin x \\ -\sin x & \cos x \end{bmatrix},$$

find A^2 and simplify the result.

19. Given that

$$A = \begin{bmatrix} 0 & 1 & 0 \\ 0 & 0 & 1 \\ 1 & 0 & 0 \end{bmatrix} \quad \text{and} \quad B = \begin{bmatrix} 1 & 2 & 3 \\ 4 & 5 & 6 \\ 7 & 8 & 9 \end{bmatrix},$$

find AB and comment on the effect on B of premultiplication by A.

20. Write down the system of equations described in matrix form by

$$AX = B,$$

when

$$A = \begin{bmatrix} 3 & 4 & 7 \\ -2 & 0 & 1 \\ 4 & 3 & -2 \end{bmatrix}, \quad X = \begin{bmatrix} x \\ y \\ z \end{bmatrix} \quad \text{and} \quad B = \begin{bmatrix} -19 \\ 6 \\ 4 \end{bmatrix}.$$

21. Find the matrices A, X and B if the system of equations

$$x + 6y - 7z + 8u = -1$$
$$3x - y + 4z - 9u = 3$$
$$x + 2z + u = -14$$
$$4y - 6z + 7u = 0$$

is written in the matrix form

$$AX = B.$$

22. Given that

$$A = \begin{bmatrix} 4 & 1 \\ 3 & 2 \end{bmatrix} \text{ and } Q = \begin{bmatrix} 2/5 & -1/5 \\ -3/5 & 4/5 \end{bmatrix},$$

show that $QA = I$, where I is the 2×2 unit matrix. Write the system of equations

$$4x + y = 1$$
$$3x + 2y = -1$$

as the matrix equation

$$AX = B,$$

and by premultiplying this result by Q find x and y.

23. Given that

$$A = \begin{bmatrix} 1 & 3 & 4 \\ 3 & -2 & 1 \\ 4 & 1 & 2 \end{bmatrix} \text{ and } X = \begin{bmatrix} x \\ y \\ z \end{bmatrix},$$

find $X^T A X$.

24. Given that

$$A = \begin{bmatrix} 2 & -1 & 3 \\ -1 & 1 & -2 \\ 3 & -2 & 5 \end{bmatrix} \text{ and } X = \begin{bmatrix} x \\ y \\ z \end{bmatrix},$$

find $X^T A X$.

The inverse matrix   55

Matrix division is not defined, but provided a square matrix A has a non-zero associated determinant $|A|$, a **multiplicative inverse** A^{-1} exists with the property that

$$A^{-1}A = AA^{-1} = I.$$

Thus A^{-1} and A are mutually inverse, in the sense that A^{-1} is the multiplicative inverse of A, and A is the multiplicative inverse of A^{-1}. To discover how to compute A^{-1} from A we need to make use of the Laplace expansion rule for determinants and a result mentioned only in Problem 25 of Problems 52 that the sum of the products of the elements in any row (or column) of a determinant with the corresponding cofactors of a different row (or column) is zero. It then follows that if C is the matrix of cofactors of A,

$$AC^T = C^TA = \begin{bmatrix} |A| & 0 & 0 & \cdots & 0 \\ 0 & |A| & 0 & \cdots & 0 \\ 0 & 0 & |A| & \cdots & 0 \\ \cdot & \cdot & \cdot & \cdots & \cdot \\ 0 & 0 & 0 & \cdots & |A| \end{bmatrix} = |A|\, I,$$

and so, provided $|A| \neq 0$,

$$A\left(\frac{C^T}{|A|}\right) = \left(\frac{C^T}{|A|}\right)A = I.$$

Thus, the inverse A^{-1} of A is given by

$$A^{-1} = \frac{C^T}{|A|}, \text{ provided } |A| \neq 0.$$

The transpose of the matrix of cofactors C^T is important in its own right and it is called the **adjoint matrix** and written adj A. Thus, provided $|A| \neq 0$,

$$A^{-1} = \frac{\text{adj } A}{|A|}.$$

A square matrix A is said to be **non-singular** if $|A| \neq 0$, and to be **singular** if $|A| = 0$. Thus only non-singular square matrices possess inverses and if A is singular,

$$A(\text{adj } A) = (\text{adj } A)A = 0,$$

where 0 denotes the null matrix.

Rule for finding an inverse matrix
Let A be a non-singular square matrix. Then the inverse matrix A^{-1} may be found as follows:
Step 1
Find $|A|$ and the matrix C of cofactors of A.
Step 2
Form the adjoint of A given by

$$\text{adj } A = C^{\text{T}}.$$

Step 3
The inverse matrix A^{-1} is then given by

$$A^{-1} = \frac{\text{adj } A}{|A|}.$$

Example 55.1

Find A^{-1} given that

$$A = \begin{bmatrix} 3 & 1 \\ 2 & 4 \end{bmatrix}.$$

Solution

Step 1
$|A| = 10$, so A is non-singular and we may proceed to find A^{-1}. The matrix of cofactors is

$$C = \begin{bmatrix} 4 & -2 \\ -1 & 3 \end{bmatrix}.$$

Step 2
The adjoint matrix adj A is

$$\text{adj } A = C^{\text{T}} = \begin{bmatrix} 4 & -1 \\ -2 & 3 \end{bmatrix}.$$

Step 3
The inverse matrix A^{-1} is thus

$$A^{-1} = \frac{\text{adj } A}{|A|} = \frac{1}{10} \begin{bmatrix} 4 & -1 \\ -2 & 3 \end{bmatrix}$$

$$= \begin{bmatrix} 2/5 & -1/10 \\ -1/5 & 3/10 \end{bmatrix}.$$

▲

Example 55.2

Find A^{-1} given that

$$A = \begin{bmatrix} 1 & 2 & 1 \\ 2 & 1 & 0 \\ 0 & 1 & 3 \end{bmatrix}.$$

Solution
Step 1
The matrix of cofactors

$$C = \begin{bmatrix} 3 & -6 & 2 \\ -5 & 3 & 1 \\ -1 & 2 & -3 \end{bmatrix},$$

so expanding $|A|$ in terms of the elements of the first row gives
$$|A| = (1)(3) + (2)(-6) + (1)(2) = -7.$$

As A is non-singular we may proceed to find A^{-1}.
Step 2
The adjoint matrix adj A is

$$\text{adj } A = C^{\mathrm{T}} = \begin{bmatrix} 3 & -5 & -1 \\ -6 & 3 & 2 \\ 2 & 1 & -3 \end{bmatrix}.$$

Step 3
The inverse matrix A^{-1} is thus

$$A^{-1} = \frac{\text{adj } A}{|A|} = \frac{1}{-7} \begin{bmatrix} 3 & -5 & -1 \\ -6 & 3 & 2 \\ 2 & 1 & -3 \end{bmatrix}$$

$$= \begin{bmatrix} -3/7 & 5/7 & 1/7 \\ 6/7 & -3/7 & -2/7 \\ -2/7 & -1/7 & 3/7 \end{bmatrix}. \qquad \blacktriangle$$

Example 55.3

Verify that

$$A = \begin{bmatrix} 4 & 3 & 1 \\ 2 & 1 & 3 \\ 2 & 2 & -2 \end{bmatrix}$$

is singular, and that

$$A(\text{adj } A) = (\text{adj } A)A = 0.$$

Solution
$|A| = 0$ because

$$\text{Row}(3) \text{ of } A = \text{Row}(1) - \text{Row}(2),$$

and so A is singular.

The matrix of cofactors

$$C = \begin{bmatrix} -8 & 10 & 2 \\ 8 & -10 & -2 \\ 8 & -10 & -2 \end{bmatrix},$$

so

$$\text{adj } A = C^{\mathrm{T}} = \begin{bmatrix} -8 & 8 & 8 \\ 10 & -10 & -10 \\ 2 & -2 & -2 \end{bmatrix}.$$

Routine calculation then shows that

$$A(\text{adj } A) = (\text{adj } A)A = \begin{bmatrix} 0 & 0 & 0 \\ 0 & 0 & 0 \\ 0 & 0 & 0 \end{bmatrix}.$$

The last matrix is the 3×3 null matrix. ▲

The interchange of rows in an $n \times n$ matrix A, and the addition of a multiple of the elements of one row of A to a multiple of the corresponding elements of another row are called **elementary row operations**. It follows from the definition of matrix multiplication that if A is an $n \times n$ matrix, pre multiplication of A by an $n \times n$ matrix R to form the matrix product RA is equivalent to performing elementary row operations on A.

Suppose, if possible, that m matrices $R_1, R_2, ..., R_m$ can be found such that

$$R_m R_{m-1} ... R_2 R_1 A = I.$$

Then post multiplication by A^{-1} (provided it exists) gives the result

$$R_m R_{m-1} ... R_2 R_1 = A^{-1},$$

which we may rewrite as

$$A^{-1} = R_m R_{m-1} ... R_2 R_1 I.$$

Thus the sequence of elementary row operations performed on a matrix A which possesses an inverse (A is non-singular), will also transform the unit matrix I into A^{-1}.

This result provides an alternative method for the computation of an inverse matrix which does not involve finding $|A|$ and the cofactors of A. The method is formulated as the following rule.

Determination of an inverse matrix by elementary row transformations
Let

$$A = \begin{bmatrix} a_{11} & a_{12} & \cdots & a_{1n} \\ a_{21} & a_{22} & \cdots & a_{2n} \\ \cdot & \cdot & \cdots & \cdot \\ a_{n1} & a_{n2} & \cdots & a_{nn} \end{bmatrix} \quad \text{and} \quad I = \begin{bmatrix} 1 & 0 & \cdots & 0 \\ 0 & 1 & \cdots & 0 \\ 0 & 0 & \cdots & 0 \\ 0 & 0 & \cdots & 1 \end{bmatrix}$$

both be $n \times n$ matrices. Then if a sequence of elementary row operations can be found which when performed on A reduces it to I, the same sequence of operations when performed on I in the same order will transform it to A^{-1}.

Example 55.4

Use row transformations to find A^{-1} given that

$$A = \begin{bmatrix} 1 & 0 & 1 \\ 1 & 3 & 0 \\ 4 & 0 & 2 \end{bmatrix}.$$

Solution
We will use the notation $R_3 = R_3 - 2R_1 + R_2$ to signify that the new row (3) is formed from the combination row $(3) - 2$ row $(1) +$ row (2) of the old rows.
   We start by writing A and I side by side as follows:

$$\begin{bmatrix} 1 & 0 & 1 \\ 1 & 3 & 0 \\ 4 & 0 & 2 \end{bmatrix} \begin{bmatrix} 1 & 0 & 0 \\ 0 & 1 & 0 \\ 0 & 0 & 1 \end{bmatrix}.$$

Now we perform elementary row operations on A and I simultaneously, so that A is reduced to I:

$$\begin{matrix} R_1 = R_1 \\ R_2 = R_2 - R_1 \\ R_3 = R_3 - 4R_1 \end{matrix} \quad \begin{bmatrix} 1 & 0 & 1 \\ 0 & 3 & -1 \\ 0 & 0 & -2 \end{bmatrix} \begin{bmatrix} 1 & 0 & 0 \\ -1 & 1 & 0 \\ -4 & 0 & 1 \end{bmatrix}$$

$$\begin{matrix} R_1 = R_1 + \frac{1}{2}R_1 \\ R_2 = R_2 - \frac{1}{2}R_3 \\ R_3 = R_3 \end{matrix} \quad \begin{bmatrix} 1 & 0 & 0 \\ 0 & 3 & 0 \\ 0 & 0 & -2 \end{bmatrix} \begin{bmatrix} -1 & 0 & 1/2 \\ 1 & 1 & -1/2 \\ -4 & 0 & 1 \end{bmatrix}$$

$$\begin{matrix} R_1 = R_1 \\ R_2 = \frac{1}{3}R_2 \\ R_3 = -\frac{1}{2}R_3 \end{matrix} \quad \begin{bmatrix} 1 & 0 & 0 \\ 0 & 1 & 0 \\ 0 & 0 & 1 \end{bmatrix} \begin{bmatrix} -1 & 0 & 1/2 \\ 1/3 & 1/3 & -1/6 \\ 2 & 0 & -1/2 \end{bmatrix}.$$

The reduction of A to the matrix I is now complete, so the transformed unit matrix on the right is A^{-1}, and thus

$$A^{-1} = \begin{bmatrix} -1 & 0 & 1/2 \\ 1/3 & 1/3 & -1/6 \\ 2 & 0 & -1/2 \end{bmatrix}.$$ ▲

PROBLEMS 55

In problems 1 to 10 find A^{-1}.

1. $A = \begin{bmatrix} 1 & 3 \\ 9 & -2 \end{bmatrix}$.

2. $A = \begin{bmatrix} 4 & 5 \\ 5 & 1 \end{bmatrix}$.

3. $A = \begin{bmatrix} 4 & -6 \\ 2 & 1 \end{bmatrix}$.

4. $A = \begin{bmatrix} -6 & 7 \\ 1 & 2 \end{bmatrix}$.

5. $A = \begin{bmatrix} i & 1+i \\ -i & 2+i \end{bmatrix}$.

6. $A = \begin{bmatrix} 1+i & 3-i \\ 2i & 1-i \end{bmatrix}$.

7. $A = \begin{bmatrix} 1 & 4 & 9 \\ 2 & 4 & 0 \\ 0 & 1 & 1 \end{bmatrix}$.

8. $A = \begin{bmatrix} 0 & 0 & 1 \\ 0 & 1 & 0 \\ 1 & 1 & 0 \end{bmatrix}$.

9. $A = \begin{bmatrix} -2 & 4 & 1 \\ 0 & 2 & 0 \\ 1 & 2 & 1 \end{bmatrix}$.

10. $A = \begin{bmatrix} 0 & -1 & 4 \\ 2 & 1 & 1 \\ -2 & 2 & 3 \end{bmatrix}$.

11. Given that

$$A = \begin{bmatrix} 2 & 4 & 1 \\ 3 & 1 & 0 \\ 2 & 2 & 1 \end{bmatrix},$$

verify the general result that $(A^{-1})^T = (A^T)^{-1}$.

12. Given that

$$A = \begin{bmatrix} 1 & 2 & 4 \\ 1 & 0 & 1 \\ 2 & 1 & 2 \end{bmatrix} \quad \text{and} \quad B = \begin{bmatrix} 3 & 1 & 2 \\ 1 & 2 & 1 \\ 0 & 1 & 2 \end{bmatrix},$$

verify the general result that

$$(AB)^{-1} = B^{-1}A^{-1}.$$

13. Given that

$$A = \begin{bmatrix} 1 & 4 \\ 2 & 1 \end{bmatrix}, \quad B = \begin{bmatrix} -1 & 3 \\ 1 & 2 \end{bmatrix} \quad \text{and} \quad C = \begin{bmatrix} 2 & 1 \\ 0 & 3 \end{bmatrix},$$

verify the general result that

$$(ABC)^{-1} = C^{-1}B^{-1}A^{-1}.$$

14. Given that

$$A = \begin{bmatrix} 4 & 3 \\ -1 & 2 \end{bmatrix} \quad \text{and} \quad B = \begin{bmatrix} 1 & 3 \\ -1 & 1 \end{bmatrix},$$

verify the general result that

$$((AB)^T)^{-1} = (A^{-1})^T(B^{-1})^T.$$

15. Given that

$$A = \begin{bmatrix} -1 & 4 & 3 \\ 2 & 0 & 1 \\ 1 & -1 & 2 \end{bmatrix},$$

find A^{-1}, and hence solve

$$-x + 4y + 3z = 1$$
$$2x + z = 3$$
$$x - y + 2z = -5.$$

16. Given that

$$A = \begin{bmatrix} 1 & 3 & -1 \\ 2 & 1 & 0 \\ 1 & 2 & 3 \end{bmatrix},$$

find A^{-1}, and hence solve

$$x + 3y - z = 2$$
$$2x + y = 1$$
$$x + 2y + 3z = 4.$$

56   Solution of a system of linear equations: Gaussian elimination

We return to the problem touched upon in the previous section, and discuss the **Gaussian elimination** method for solving the following system of n linear simultaneous equations in the n unknowns $x_1, x_2, ..., x_n$

$$a_{11}x_1 + a_{12}x_2 + \cdots + a_{1n}x_n = k_1$$
$$a_{21}x_1 + a_{22}x_2 + \cdots + a_{2n}x_n = k_2$$
$$\cdot \qquad \cdot \quad \cdot \quad \cdots \qquad \cdot \qquad \cdot$$
$$a_{n1}x_1 + a_{n2}x_2 + \cdots + a_{nn}x_n = k_n.$$

Such a system is said to be non-homogeneous (inhomogeneous) if not all of the $k_1, k_2, ..., k_n$ are zero, and homogeneous if $k_1 = k_2 = ... = k_n = 0$.

The system may be written in the matrix form

$$AX = B,$$

where

$$A = \begin{bmatrix} a_{11} & a_{12} & \cdots & a_{1n} \\ a_{21} & a_{22} & \cdots & a_{2n} \\ \cdot & \cdot & \cdots & \cdot \\ a_{n1} & a_{n2} & \cdots & a_{nn} \end{bmatrix}, \quad X = \begin{bmatrix} x_1 \\ x_2 \\ \vdots \\ x_n \end{bmatrix} \quad \text{and} \quad B = \begin{bmatrix} k_1 \\ k_2 \\ \vdots \\ k_n \end{bmatrix}.$$

For obvious reasons, the matrix A is called the **coefficient matrix**.

If A is non-singular, an inverse matrix A^{-1} exists, so premultiplying the matrix equation by A^{-1} we have

$$A^{-1}AX = A^{-1}B,$$

but $A^{-1}A = I$ and $IX = X$, so this reduces to

$$X = A^{-1}B.$$

Thus, when A is non-singular, the system has a unique solution, but when A is singular no inverse matrix A^{-1} exists so this method of approach fails. To proceed further we need to make use of the method of Gaussian elimination, which is the practical method for solving equations. The method does not require the existence of an inverse of the coefficient matrix, the system can be homogeneous or non-homogeneous, and the coefficient matrix need not even be square.

The principle of the method is simple, and it is best understood in terms of a system of three equations in the three unknowns x_1, x_2 and x_3. Consider the system

$$a_{11}x_1 + a_{12}x_2 + a_{13}x_3 = k_1$$
$$a_{21}x_1 + a_{22}x_2 + a_{23}x_3 = k_2$$
$$a_{31}x_1 + a_{32}x_2 + a_{33}x_3 = k_3.$$

Then, when using Gaussian elimination to solve for x_1, x_2 and x_3, we start by eliminating x_1 from the second and third equations by subtracting from them suitable multiples of the first equation. This leads to a new, but equivalent, system of the form

$$a_{11}x_1 + a_{12}x_2 + a_{13}x_3 = k_1$$
$$\tilde{a}_{22}x_2 + \tilde{a}_{23}x_3 = \tilde{k}_2$$
$$\tilde{a}_{32}x_2 + \tilde{a}_{33}x_3 = \tilde{k}_3.$$

Next, x_2 is eliminated from the new third equation by subtracting from it a suitable multiple of the new second equation. As a result we arrive at another equivalent system of equations of the form

$$a_{11}x_1 + a_{12}x_2 + a_{13}x_3 = k_1$$
$$\tilde{a}_{22}x_2 + \tilde{a}_{23}x_3 = \tilde{k}_2$$
$$\hat{a}_{33}x_3 = \hat{k}_3.$$

The third of these equations is solved for x_3, the result is used in the second equation to solve for x_2, and the two results are used in the first equation to solve for x_1. This last step is called **back-substitution.**

Example 56.1

Solve by Gaussian elimination the non-homogeneous system of equations:

$$x_1 + 2x_2 + 3x_3 = 4$$
$$x_1 + 3x_2 + 5x_3 = 1$$
$$x_1 + 5x_2 + 12x_3 = 2.$$

Solution
Using the first equation to eliminate x_1 from the second and third equations gives:

$$x_1 + 2x_2 + 3x_3 = 4$$
$$x_2 + 2x_3 = -3$$
$$3x_2 + 9x_3 = -2.$$

Using the new second equation to eliminate x_2 from the new third equation gives:

$$x_1 + 2x_2 + 3x_3 = 4$$
$$x_2 + 2x_3 = -3$$
$$3x_3 = 7 \quad .$$

Solving by back-substitution gives, in this order, $x_3 = 7/3, x_2 = -23/3$ and $x_1 = 37/3$. ▲

The examples which follow show how Gaussian elimination may be used in some different but typical cases to which matrix inverse methods do not apply.

Example 56.2

Solve the non-homogeneous system of three equations in the three unknowns x_1, x_2 and x_3:

$$2x_1 + 3x_2 + 4x_3 = 1$$
$$5x_1 + 6x_2 + 7x_3 = 2$$
$$8x_1 + 9x_2 + 10x_3 = 4.$$

Solution
This system cannot be solved by means of an inverse matrix since the coefficient matrix is singular, because it is easily shown that

$$\begin{vmatrix} 2 & 3 & 4 \\ 5 & 6 & 7 \\ 8 & 9 & 10 \end{vmatrix} = 0.$$

Applying Gaussian elimination to eliminate x_1 from the last two equations gives:

$$2x_1 + 3x_2 + 4x_3 = 1$$
$$-3x_2 - 6x_3 = -1$$
$$-6x_2 - 12x_3 = 0 \quad .$$

Using the second equation to eliminate x_2 from the third equation leads to an inconsistency in the third equation, for we have

$$2x_1 + 3x_2 + 4x_3 = 1$$
$$-3x_2 - 6x_3 = -1$$
$$0 = 2 \quad .$$

The inconsistency in the last result tells us that this system has no solution (the first two equations contradict the last equation). Systems such as this are said to be **inconsistent**. ▲

Example 56.3

Solve the non-homogeneous system of three equations in the three unknowns x_1, x_2 and x_3:

$$\begin{aligned} 2x_1 + 4x_2 + x_3 &= 1 \\ 3x_1 + 5x_2 &= 1 \\ 5x_1 + 13x_2 + 7x_3 &= 4. \end{aligned}$$

Solution
Here again the coefficient matrix is singular, so we must use Gaussian elimination. Eliminating x_1 from the last two equations by subtracting from them suitable multiples of the first equation gives:

$$\begin{aligned} 2x_1 + 4x_2 + x_3 &= 1 \\ -2x_2 - 3x_3 &= -1 \\ 6x_2 - 9x_3 &= 3 \quad . \end{aligned}$$

Using the second equation to eliminate x_2 from the last equation shows that:

$$\begin{aligned} 2x_1 + 4x_2 + x_3 &= 1 \\ -2x_2 - 3x_3 &= -1 \\ 0 &= 0. \quad . \end{aligned}$$

These equations are consistent, since no contradictions are involved, but in this case there are only two independent equations connecting the three variables x_1, x_2 and x_3. If we set $x_3 = k$, where k is an arbitrary number, we can solve for x_1 and x_2 in terms of k.
   The second equation gives

$$x_2 = \frac{1}{2}(1 - 3x_3) = \frac{1}{2}(1 - 3k),$$

and substituting for x_3 and x_2 in the first equation we find that

$$x_1 = \frac{1}{2}(-1 + 5k),$$

so the solution is of the form

$$x_1 = \frac{1}{2}(-1 + 5k), \quad x_2 = \frac{1}{2}(1 - 3k), \quad x_3 = k,$$

with k a parameter. Such a solution is said to be a **one-parameter family of solutions**. We have shown that in this case although a solution exists, it is not unique.

Example 56.4

Solve the non-homogeneous system of three equations in the two unknowns x_1 and x_2:

$$x + x_2 = 1$$
$$2x_1 - x_2 = 5$$
$$x_1 + px_2 = 0,$$

with p a parameter.

Solution
In this case we have more equations than unknowns, so it is to be expected that this system might be inconsistent.

Using the first equation to eliminate x_1 from the second and third equations leads to the result:

$$x_1 + x_2 = 1$$
$$-3x_2 = 3$$
$$(p-1)x_2 = 0.$$

These are seen to be inconsistent if $p \neq 1$, for then the last equation shows $x_2 = 0$, while the second equation shows that $x_2 = -1$. If $p = 1$ the last equation is satisfied by any x_2, while from the second equation we have $x_2 = -1$ and from the first equation we see that $x_1 = 2$.

Thus these equations are inconsistent, and so have no solution if $p \neq 1$, but they are consistent and have the unique solution $x_1 = 2$, $x_2 = -1$ when $p = 1$.

▲

Example 56.5

Solve the homogeneous system of three equations in the three unknowns x_1, x_2, x_3:

$$x_1 - 2x_2 + 3x_3 = 0$$
$$2x_1 + 4x_2 + 5x_3 = 0$$
$$x_1 + 2x_2 + 6x_3 = 0.$$

Solution
Using the first equation to eliminate x_1 from the last two equations gives:

$$x_1 - 2x_2 + 3x_3 = 0$$
$$8x_2 - x_3 = 0$$
$$4x_2 + 3x_3 = 0.$$

Using the second equation to eliminate x_2 from the last equation we arrive at the system:

$$x_1 - 2x_2 + 3x_2 = 0$$
$$8x_2 - x_3 = 0$$
$$\frac{7}{2}x_3 = 0.$$

Thus $x_3 = 0$, and back-substitution shows that $x_2 = x_1 = 0$, and so the equations are consistent and the solution is unique, but it is the **trivial solution** (the uninteresting solution)

$$x_1 = x_2 = x_3 = 0.$$

This could have been found by matrix methods, because the determinant of the coefficient matrix A is 28, so the matrix

$$A = \begin{bmatrix} 1 & -2 & 3 \\ 2 & 4 & 5 \\ 1 & 2 & 6 \end{bmatrix}$$

is non-singular and thus an inverse matrix A^{-1} exists. As the equations can be written in the form

$$AX = 0,$$

we have

$$A^{-1}AX = A^{-1}0$$

or

$$X = 0 = \begin{bmatrix} 0 \\ 0 \\ 0 \end{bmatrix}. \qquad\qquad \blacktriangle$$

Example 56.6

Solve the homogeneous system of three equations in the three unknowns x_1, x_2, x_3:

$$x_1 + 5x_2 + 3x_3 = 0$$
$$5x_1 + x_2 - x_3 = 0$$
$$x_1 + 2x_2 + x_3 = 0.$$

Solution
Notice first that the coefficient matrix A is singular, because

$$A = \begin{bmatrix} 1 & 5 & 3 \\ 5 & 1 & -1 \\ 1 & 2 & 1 \end{bmatrix} \quad \text{and} \quad |A| = 0.$$

Thus no inverse matrix A^{-1} exists so we must solve by using Gaussian elimination. Using the first equation to eliminate x_1 from the last two equations gives:

$$x_1 + 5x_2 + 3x_3 = 0$$
$$- 24x_2 - 16x_3 = 0$$
$$3x_2 - 2x_3 = 0.$$

Using the second of these equations to eliminate x_2 from the last equation gives:

$$x_1 + 5x_2 + 3x_3 = 0$$
$$-24x_2 - 16x_3 = 0$$
$$0 = 0,$$

so the equations are consistent, but there are only two equations connecting the three variables x_1, x_2 and x_3. Setting $x_3 = k$, with k an arbitrary parameter, and using back-substitution to solve for x_2 and x_1 gives:

$$x_1 = \frac{1}{3}k, \quad x_2 = -\frac{2}{3}k \quad \text{and} \quad x_3 = k.$$

Thus we have a one parameter family of solutions of the form

$$X = \begin{bmatrix} \frac{1}{3}k \\ -\frac{2}{3}k \\ k \end{bmatrix} = k \begin{bmatrix} 1/3 \\ -2/3 \\ 1 \end{bmatrix}.$$

The system was of the form

$$AX = 0,$$

so if X is a solution, so also is μX, with μ any number. Thus if, for example, we choose to set $\mu = 3$, we see that a solution is

$$X = \begin{bmatrix} 1 \\ -2 \\ 3 \end{bmatrix}.$$

This example has demonstrated the important fact that if a homogeneous system

$$AX = 0$$

has a singular coefficient matrix ($|A| = 0$), its solution determines the ratios between x_1, x_2 and x_3, and not their absolute values. Thus in this case, x_1, x_2 and x_3 may be taken as any three numbers such that

$$\frac{x_1}{1} = \frac{x_2}{-2} = \frac{x_3}{3}. \qquad \blacktriangle$$

We now express the result demonstrated by this last example in the form of a general property of a homogeneous system with a singular coefficient matrix.

Solution of homogeneous systems
The homogeneous system of n linear equations in the n unknowns $x_1, x_2, \ldots, x_n$

$$a_{11}x_1 + a_{12}x_2 + \ldots + a_{1n}x_n = 0$$
$$x_{21}x_1 + a_{22}x_2 + \ldots + a_{2n}x_n = 0$$
$$\cdot \qquad \cdot \qquad \ldots \qquad \cdot$$
$$a_{n1}x_1 + a_{n2}x_2 + \ldots + a_{nn}x_n = 0$$

will only have a non-trivial solution if the coefficient matrix is singular ($|A| = 0$). When $|A| = 0$, the solution can only be determined up to an arbitrary multiplicative constant, in the sense that if $\tilde{x}_1, \tilde{x}_2 \ldots, \tilde{x}_n$ is a solution, then so also is $k\tilde{x}_1, k\tilde{x}_2, \ldots, k\tilde{x}_n$ where k is an arbitrary number.

THE AUGMENTED MATRIX

Gaussian elimination is performed on the **numerical coefficients** of $x_1, x_2, \ldots,$ and x_n on the non-homogeneous terms $k_1, k_2, \ldots, k_n$. Thus the actual variables $x_1, x_2, \ldots, x_n$ may be omitted, and the operations performed instead on the coefficient matrix to which, on the right, has been adjoined a column containing the non- homogeneous terms. This new matrix is called the **augmented matrix**, and the element in the jth row and mth column, with $m = 1, 2, \ldots, n$, will be the multiplier of x_m in the jth equation. Thus in Example 56.1 the augmented matrix is

$$\begin{bmatrix} 1 & 2 & 3 & \vdots & 4 \\ 1 & 3 & 5 & \vdots & 1 \\ 1 & 5 & 12 & \vdots & 2 \end{bmatrix},$$

in which the dashed line has been inserted to indicate that the entries to its right are the non-homogeneous terms.

We will use the notation $R_1 = R_1 + 3R_2 - 2R_3$ to signify that the new row (1) is obtained as the combination row (1) + 3 row (2) – 2 row (3) of the old rows. The calculations in Example 56.1 may then be represented as follows:

$$\begin{bmatrix} 1 & 2 & 3 & \vdots & 4 \\ 1 & 3 & 5 & \vdots & 1 \\ 1 & 5 & 12 & \vdots & 2 \end{bmatrix} \quad \begin{matrix} R_1 = R_1 \\ R_2 = R_2 - R_1 \\ R_3 = R_3 - R_1 \end{matrix} \quad \begin{bmatrix} 1 & 2 & 3 & \vdots & 4 \\ 0 & 1 & 2 & \vdots & -3 \\ 0 & 3 & 9 & \vdots & -2 \end{bmatrix}$$

$$\begin{matrix} R_1 = R_1 \\ R_2 = R_2 \\ R_3 = R_3 - 3R_2 \end{matrix} \quad \begin{bmatrix} 1 & 2 & 3 & \vdots & 4 \\ 0 & 1 & 2 & \vdots & -3 \\ 0 & 0 & 3 & \vdots & 7 \end{bmatrix}.$$

This augmented matrix is seen to be equivalent to

$$x_1 + 2x_2 + 3x_3 = 4$$
$$x_2 + 2x_3 = -3$$
$$3x_3 = 7 \ ,$$

so, as before, back-substitution gives $x_3 = 7/3$, $x_2 = -23/3$ and $x_1 = 37/3$.

PROBLEMS 56

Solve problems 1 to 14 by Gaussian elimination.

1. $x - 3y = 1$
    $3x + 7y = -4.$

2. $2x - 5y = 3$
    $3x - 3y = 2.$

3. $2x - 5y = -7$
    $5x + 3y = 2.$

4. $4x - 3y = 4$
    $3x + 2y = 1.$

5. $2.1x + 7.3y = 4.6$
    $0.9x - 2.1y = 3.2.$

6. $1.2x + 3.1y = 2.5$
    $-2.5x + 1.4y = 1.5.$

7. $3x - y - 2z = 1$
    $2x + y - 3z = 2$
    $2x - 3y - z = 4.$

8. $x + 2y - z = 5$
    $2x + y + 2z = 1$
    $x + 5y + z = 4.$

9. $2x - y + 4z = 3$
    $x - 4y + 2z = 1$
    $4x + 2y + z = -4.$

10. $3x + y + z = -3$
    $6x + 2y - z = 4$.
    $2x + y + 3z = 1.$

11. $4.2x - 1.4y + 2.1z = 4.2$
    $3.1x + 2.4y - 3.6z = -2.4$
    $2.1x - 2.4y + 3.2z = 1.3.$

12. $3.2x - 1.7y - 4.1z = -0.4$
    $1.3x + 2.5y + 3.7z = 0.9$
    $2.7x - 1.3y - 2.8z = -0.6.$

13. $1.4x + 3.7y - 0.9z = 1.5$
    $0.8x - 1.9y - 3.1z = -0.4.$
    $1.9x - 2.1y + 1.4z = 0.$

14. $2.7x - 1.4y - 2.9z = -0.8$
    $2.1x + 2.5y - 1.5z = 0.7$
    $1.8x + 3.1y + 1.6z = 3.2.$

In the following problems use Gaussian elimination to find a solution when it exists.

15. $3x + y - 3z = 4$
$x + 3y - z = 3$
$5x - y - 5z = 6.$

16. $3x - y - 3z = -4$
$x - 3y + z = -3$
$5x + y - 5z = -5.$

17. $x + 3y + 2z = 1$
$2x - y - 4z = -3$
$3x - 5y - 10z = -7.$

18. $x - y + z = 4$
$3x + 2y + 3z = 1$
$7x + 8y + 7z = -5.$

19. $x - y + z = 0$
$2x + y - z = 0$
$x + 5y - 5z = 0.$

20. $x + 3y - 2z = 0$
$2x + y - 3z = 0$
$4x + 2y - 7z = 0.$

21. $3x - y - z = 0$
$2x + 4y + 6z = 0$
$5x - 11y - 15z = 0.$

22. $x - y + z = 0$
$3x - 2y + 3z = 0$
$5x - 4y + 5z = 0.$

23. $2x + y = 1$
$x - 3y = 11$
$x + py = 1,$

with p a parameter.

24. $3x + y - 2z = 0$
$2x + 4y + z = 0$
$x + py + z = 0,$

with p a parameter.

25. Repeat problem 7 using the augmented matrix approach.
26. Repeat problem 8 using the augmented matrix approach.
27. Repeat problem 9 using the augmented matrix approach.
28. Repeat problem 10 using the augmented matrix approach.

57

The Gauss–Seidel iterative method

When very large systems of simultaneous equations require a solution, iterative methods are used. These methods are particularly useful and efficient if many of the coefficients in the equations are zero, which is often the case in engineering applications. In this section we shall only describe the **Gauss–Seidel iterative method** for solving the n linear non-homogeneous equations:

$$a_{11}x_1 + a_{12}x_2 + a_{13}x_3 + \ldots + a_{1n}x_n = k_1$$
$$a_{21}x_1 + a_{22}x_2 + a_{23}x_3 + \ldots + a_{2n}x_n = k_2$$

$$\cdots$$

$$a_{n1}x_1 + a_{n2}x_2 + a_{n3}x_3 + \ldots + a_{nn}x_n = k_n,$$

in the n unknowns $x_1, x_2, \ldots, x_n$.

An **iterative method of solution** is a method of successive approximations which starts from an initial approximation that is usually chosen arbitrarily. In the case of the system of equations shown above, the rth approximation to the solution $x_1, x_2, \ldots, x_n$ will be denoted by $x_1^{(r)}, x_2^{(r)}, \ldots, x_n^{(r)}$. The calculations leading to the determination of $x_1^{(r)}, x_2^{(r)}, \ldots, x_1^{(r)}$ will be said to comprise the rth iteration, and the individual number $x_m^{(r)}$ will be called the rth iterate of x_m.

In an iterative calculation each iteration is obtained from the result of the previous iteration by means of the same method of calculation. The method will be said to converge if the numbers $x_1^{(r)}, x_2^{(r)}, \ldots, x_n^{(r)}$ all tend to limits as r increases.

When an iterative method converges, it is usual to stop the iteration process when

$$\left| x_m^{(r+1)} - x_m^{(r)} \right| < \varepsilon ,$$

for some suitably small number ε and all $m = 1, 2, \ldots, n$. Thus, if $\varepsilon = 10^{-4}$ the iterations would be terminated when the approximations to $x_1, x_2, \ldots, x_n$ had all converged to four decimal places.

If the iteration process fails to converge owing to oscillation of the iterates, when the magnitude of the difference between iterates usually increases as r increases, the process is said to diverge. Divergence of an iterative process does not mean that no solution exists, but simply that it cannot be found by that particular iterative method starting from the given initial approximation.

To arrive at the **Gauss–Seidel iterative scheme** we start by solving the first equation for x_1, the second for x_2, ..., and the last for x_n, to obtain

$$x_1 = (k_1 - a_{12}x_2 - a_{13}x_3 - a_{14}x_4 - \ldots - a_{1n}x_n)/a_{11},$$
$$x_2 = (k_2 - a_{21}x_1 - a_{23}x_3 - a_{24}x_4 - \ldots - a_{2n}x_n)/a_{22},$$
$$x_3 = (k_3 - a_{31}x_1 - a_{32}x_2 - a_{34}x_4 - \ldots - a_{3n}x_n)/a_{33}$$
$$\vdots \quad\quad \vdots \quad\quad \vdots \quad\quad\quad\quad \vdots$$
$$x_n = (k_n - a_{n1}x_1 - a_{n2}x_2 - a_{n3}x_3 - \ldots - a_{nn-1}x_{n-1})/a_{nn}.$$

To convert this to an iterative process, in each of the above equations we now make use of the *best available estimate* of the solution at that stage. Thus the $(r + 1)$th iterates are obtained from the rth iterates by means of the following scheme, which makes use of the $(r + 1)$ iterates themselves whenever possible.

Gauss–Seidel iterative scheme
Starting with the initial values $x_1^{(0)}, x_2^{(0)}, \ldots, x_n^{(0)}$, the $(r + 1)$th iterates $x_1^{(r + 1)}$, $x_2^{(r + 1)}, \ldots, x_n^{(r + 1)}$ are obtained from the rth iterates $x_1^{(r)}, x_2^{(r)}, \ldots, x_n^{(r)}$ by means of the equations

$$x_1^{(r + 1)} = (k_1 - a_{12}x_2^{(r)} - a_{13}x_3^{(r)} - a_{14}x_4^{(r)} - \ldots - a_{1n}x_n^{(r)})/a_{11}$$
$$x_2^{(r + 1)} = (k_2 - a_{21}x_1^{(r + 1)} - a_{23}x_3^{(r)} - a_{24}x_4^{(r)} - \ldots - a_{2n}x_n^{(r)})/a_{22}$$
$$x_3^{(r + 1)} = (k_3 - a_{31}x_1^{(r + 1)} - a_{32}x_2^{(r + 1)} - a_{34}x_4^{(r)} - \ldots - a_{3n}x_n^{(r)})/a_{33}$$
$$\vdots \quad\quad \vdots \quad\quad \vdots \quad\quad\quad\quad \vdots$$
$$x_n^{(r + 1)} = (k_n - a_{1n}x_1^{(r + 1)} - a_{n2}x_2^{(r + 1)} - a_{n3}x_3^{(r + 1)} - \ldots - a_{nn-1}x_{n-1}^{(r + 1)})/a_{nn}.$$

It can be shown that a sufficient condition for the convergence of the Gauss–Seidel method is that the original system of equations is in **diagonally dominant** form. The condition for diagonal dominance is as follows:

$$|a_{11}| > |a_{12}| + |a_{13}| + |a_{14}| + \ldots + |a_{1n}|$$
$$|a_{22}| > |a_{21}| + |a_{23}| + |a_{24}| + \ldots + |a_{2n}|$$
$$|a_{33}| > |a_{31}| + |a_{32}| + |a_{34}| + \ldots + |a_{3n}|$$
$$\cdot \quad\quad \cdot \quad\quad \cdot \quad\quad \cdot \quad\quad \cdot \quad\quad \cdot$$
$$|a_{nn}| > |a_{n1}| + |a_{n2}| + |a_{n3}| + \ldots + |a_{nn-1}|.$$

Thus, in words, diagonal dominance means that in the mth equation the absolute value of the coefficient a_{mm} (the coefficient on the leading diagonal) must exceed the sum of the absolute values of all the other coefficients in the mth equation; for $m = 1, 2, \ldots, n$. The non-homogeneous terms $k_1, k_2, \ldots, k_n$ do not enter into the determination of diagonal dominance.

Thus, for example, the system

$$4x_1 - 6x_2 = 5$$
$$7x_1 - 2x_2 = 1$$

is not in diagonally dominant form, because in the first equation

$$|4| \not> |-6|$$

and in the second equation

$$|-2| \not> |7|.$$

However, by interchanging the order of the equations we obtain the system in diagonally dominant form

$$7x_1 - 2x_2 = 1$$
$$4x_1 - 6x_2 = 5,$$

because in the first equation we now have

$$|7| > |-2|,$$

while in the second equation we have

$$|-6| > |4|.$$

The checking for diagonal dominance and, if necessary, the interchange of equations to bring a system into a diagonally dominant form, is a necessary preliminary to writing down the Gauss–Seidel scheme.

For simplicity, unless an approximate solution is known, the iterations are started either by taking for the initial approximation

$$x_1^{(0)} = x_2^{(0)} = \dots = x_n^{(0)} = 0,$$

or

$$x_1^{(0)} = x_2^{(0)} = \dots = x_n^{(0)} = 1.$$

This iterative process is normally performed by a computer, but we illustrate the method here using a simple example with integer solutions to show the convergence properties of the method.

Example 57.1

Perform six iterations using the Gauss–Seidel scheme working to four decimal places to determine the approximate solution of the following system, starting:
(i)   with $x_1^{(0)} = x_2^{(0)} = x_3^{(0)} = 0$; and
(ii) with $x_1^{(0)} = x_2^{(0)} = x_3^{(0)} = 1$.

$$3x_1 + 5x_2 - x_3 = -14$$
$$7x_1 - 2x_2 + 3x_3 = 19$$
$$2x_1 - x_2 + 6x_3 = 17.$$

The equations have the exact solution

$$x_1 = 1, \quad x_2 = -3 \quad \text{and} \quad x_3 = 2.$$

Solution

The equations are not in diagonally dominant form as they stand, but they can be brought into this form by interchanging the first two equations to obtain

$$7x_1 - 2x_2 + 3x_3 = 19$$
$$3x_1 + 5x_2 - x_3 = -14$$
$$2x_1 - x_2 + 6x_3 = 17.$$

To check these for diagonal dominance, we see that from the first equation

$$|7| > |-2| + |3|,$$

from the second equation

$$|5| > |3| + |-1|$$

and from the third equation

$$|6| > |2| + |-1|.$$

Thus the Gauss–Seidel scheme for the system in the rearranged form is

$$x_1^{(r+1)} = (19 + 2x_2^{(r)} - 3x_3^{(r)})/7$$
$$x_2^{(r+1)} = (-14 - 3x_1^{(r+1)} + x_3^{(r)})/5$$
$$x_3^{(r+1)} = (17 - 2x_1^{(r+1)} + x_2^{(r+1)})/6.$$

(i) Starting the iteration process with $x_1^{(0)} = x_2^{(0)} = x_3^{(0)} = 0$ gives when $r = 0$,

$$x_1^{(1)} = (19 - 2x_2^{(0)} - x_3^{(0)})/7$$
$$= 19/7 = 2.7143$$
$$x_2^{(1)} = (-14 - 3x_1^{(1)} + x_3^{(0)})/5$$
$$= [-14 - (3)(2.7143)]/5 = -4.4286$$
$$x_3^{(1)} = (17 - 2x_1^{(1)} + x_2^{(1)})/6$$
$$= [17 - (2)(2.714) + (-4.4286)]/6 = 1.1905.$$

To proceed to the next iteration we set $r = 1$, when we find that

$$x_1^{(2)} = (19 - 2x_2^{(1)} - 3x_3^{(1)})/7$$
$$= [19 + (2)(-4.4286) - (3)(1.1905)]/7 = 0.9388$$
$$x_2^{(2)} = (-14 - 3x_1^{(2)} + x_3^{(1)})/5$$
$$= [-14 - (3)(0.9388) + 1.1905]/5 = -3.1252$$
$$x_3^{(2)} = (17 - 2x_1^{(2)} - x_2^{(2)})/6$$
$$= [17 - (2)(0.9388) + (-3.1252)]/6 = 1.9995.$$

Combining these results into a table and continuing the iterations gives the results shown in Table 8. These show fairly rapid convergence to the exact solution $x_1 = 1$, $x_2 = -3$ and $x_3 = 2$, with only an error of 0.0001 in x_2 after six iterations.

Table 8

n	$x_1^{(n)}$	$x_2^{(n)}$	$x_3^{(n)}$
0	0	0	0
1	2.7143	−4.4286	1.1905
2	0.9388	−3.1252	1.9995
3	0.9644	−2.9787	2.0154
4	0.9995	−2.9966	2.0007
5	1.0007	−3.0002	1.9997
6	1	−3.0001	2

(ii)   Starting the iteration process with $x_1^{(0)} = x_2^{(0)} = x_3^{(0)} = 1$, and repeating the above calculations, gives the results shown in Table 9. Here also the convergence is rapid, and it is seen that in this case the choice of the initial approximation has had little effect on the rate of convergence. In general, if a good initial approximation is used, the convergence will be accelerated.

Table 9

n	$x_1^{(n)}$	$x_2^{(n)}$	$x_3^{(n)}$
0	1	1	1
1	2.5714	−4.1429	1.2857
2	0.9796	−3.1306	1.9850
3	0.9691	−2.9845	2.0129
4	0.9989	−2.9968	2.0009
5	1.0005	−3.0001	1.9998
6	1	−3.0001	2

▲

To see the effect of applying the Gauss–Seidel scheme to a system which is not in diagonally dominant form, we need only consider the system of equations in Example 57.1 in their original form. Table 10 shows the effect of starting with the initial approximation $x_1^{(0)} = x_2^{(0)} = x_3^{(0)} = 0$ and using the Gauss–Seidel scheme, which then becomes

$$x_1^{(r+1)} = (-14 - 5x_2^{(r)} + x_3^{(r)})/3$$
$$x_2^{(r+1)} = (-19 + 7x_1^{(r+1)} + 3x_3^{(r)})/2$$
$$x_3^{(r+1)} = (17 - 2x_1^{(r+1)} + x_2^{(r+1)})/6.$$

Table 10

n	$x_1^{(n)}$	$x_2^{(n)}$	$x_3^{(n)}$
0	0	0	0
1	−4.6667	−25.8333	0.0833
2	38.4167	125.0833	10.8750
3	−209.5139	−726.4861	−48.4097
4	1.19×10^3	4.08×10^3	286.65

The unrestricted growth of the iterates and their alternation in sign is typical of a numerically divergent scheme.

In conclusion, we remark that since diagonal dominance is only a sufficient condition for the convergence of the Gauss–Seidel scheme, the method may still converge if although a system cannot be rearranged to bring it into diagonally dominant form, the majority of its equations can be so arranged. For example, the system

$$-5x_1 + 4x_2 = 24$$
$$8x_1 - x_2 = 35$$

cannot be arranged in diagonally dominant form, and if the Gauss–Seidel scheme is applied to it as it stands the iterations will diverge. If, however, the order of the equations is reversed to produce the system

$$8x_1 - x_2 = 35$$
$$-5x_1 + 4x_2 = 24,$$

and the Gauss–Seidel scheme is applied, the iterations will converge to the exact solution $x_1 = 164/27$, $x_2 = 367/27$. Check this by performing a few iterations with each system.

The reason for the convergence in the second case is because the magnitude of the coefficient of x_1 in the first equation, namely 8, strongly dominates the first equation, and its effect is also strong enough to compensate for the lack of diagonal dominance in the second equation in which the magnitude of the coefficient of x_2, namely 4, is only slightly less than the magnitude of the coefficient of x_1, namely $|-5|$.

Often, by addition and subtraction of equations, a system which cannot be arranged in diagonally dominant form as it stands can be converted to an equivalent system which is diagonally dominant, and to which the Gauss–Seidel scheme can be applied. This happens, for example, in the case of the system above, because if the second equation is replaced by the sum of the first equation and twice the second equation it produces the system

$$8x_1 - x_2 = 35$$
$$-2x_1 + 7x_2 = 83,$$

which is equivalent to the original system and is also diagonally dominant.

PROBLEMS 57

In problems 1 to 4 arrange the system of equations in diagonally dominant form, when necessary, and then working to four decimal places perform five iterations starting (a) with $x_1^{(0)} = x_2^{(0)} = 0$ and (b) with $x_1^{(0)} = x_2^{(0)} = 1$. Compare the results in each case with the given exact solution.

1. $4.31x_1 - 2.1x_2 = 5.34$
     $2.52x_1 + 7.32x_2 = 1.92$
     Exact solution is $x_1 = 1.1705$, $x_2 = -0.1406$.

2. $2.32x_1 - 9.12x_2 = 5.14$
    $7.25x_1 + 3.12x_2 = 2.67$
    Exact solution is $x_1 = 0.5505$, $x_2 = -0.4235$.

3. $3.24x_1 + 7.76x_2 = -3.15$
    $9.19x_1 + 2.13x_2 = 7.37$
    Exact solution is $x_1 = 0.9920$, $x_2 = -0.8201$.

4. $3.72x_1 + 1.24x_2 = -2.14$
    $1.11x_1 - 5.43x_2 = 4.67$
    Exact solution is $x_1 = -0.2702$, $x_2 = -0.9153$.

5. Starting with $x_1^{(0)} = x_2^{(0)} = 0$ and working to four decimal places (a) perform five iterations with the system of equations in diagonally dominant form, and (b) perform five iterations with the system of equations not in diagonally dominant form, and compare the results.
    $2.31x_1 - 4.79x_2 = 3.67$
    $6.27x_1 + 3.42x_2 = -2.43$
    Exact solution is $x_1 = 0.0240$, $x_2 = -0.7546$.

    In problems 6 to 10 arrange the equations in diagonally dominant form, where necessary, and starting with $x_1^{(0)} = x_2^{(0)} = x_3^{(0)} = 0$, perform five iterations. Compare the results with the exact solution given to four decimal places.

6. $1.25x_1 - 3.12x_2 + 6.03x_3 = 0.46$
    $5.17x_1 + 2.26x_2 + 1.41x_3 = 2.27$
    $1.21x_1 + 4.13x_2 + 1.32x_3 = 6.71$
    Exact solution $x_1 = -0.6850$, $x_2 = 1.5065$, $x_3 = 0.9978$.

7. $2.03x_1 + 4.12x_2 - 1.12x_3 = 1.23$
    $1.05x_1 + 2.28x_2 - 6.27x_3 = 1.08$
    $5.17x_1 - 1.02x_2 + 2.18x_3 = 3.04$
    Exact solution $x_1 = 0.6160$, $x_2 = -0.0264$, $x_3 = -0.0787$.

8. $1.31x_1 + 2.17x_2 + 6.14x_3 = 2.17$
    $3.12x_1 - 1.09x_2 + 1.03x_3 = 4.12$
    $2.01x_1 + 5.27x_2 - 1.34x_3 = 1.14$
    Exact solution $x_1 = 1.1953$, $x_2 = -0.1990$, $x_3 = 0.1687$.

9. $1.27x_1 - 4.22x_2 + 1.13x_3 = 2.07$
    $4.37x_1 + 1.03x_2 + 0.97x_3 = 1.16$
    $2.01x_1 + 1.11x_2 + 3.89x_3 = 0.27$
    Exact solution $x_1 = 0.3573$, $x_2 = -0.3845$, $x_3 = -0.0055$.

10. $4.37x_1 + 1.21x_2 - 0.93x_3 = 1.26$
    $0.96x_1 + 1.13x_2 + 3.57x_3 = -1.67$
    $0.95x_1 - 5.92x_2 + 2.13x_3 = 3.12$
    Exact solution $x_1 = 0.3748$, $x_2 = -0.6028$, $x_3 = -0.3778$.

The algebraic eigenvalue problem 58

The study of many problems in engineering and science give rise to what is known as the **algebraic eigenvalue problem**. The problem involves finding for what values of the parameter λ the system of linear algebraic equations

$$a_{11}x_1 + a_{12}x_2 + a_{13}x_3 + \ldots + a_{1n}x_n = \lambda x_1$$
$$a_{21}x_1 + a_{22}x_2 + a_{23}x_3 + \ldots + a_{2n}x_n = \lambda x_2$$

$$\cdot \qquad \cdot \qquad \cdot \qquad \cdot$$
$$\cdot \qquad \cdot \qquad \cdot \qquad \cdot$$
$$\cdot \qquad \cdot \qquad \cdot \qquad \cdot$$

$$a_{n1}x_1 + a_{n2}x_2 + a_{n3}x_3 + \ldots + a_{nn}x_n = \lambda x_n,$$

has **non-trivial solutions** (not all the $x_1, x_2, \ldots, x_n$ vanish), and then finding the form of these solutions.

At first sight the system appears to be non-homogeneous, but when it is rewritten in the equivalent form

$$(a_{11} - \lambda)x_1 + a_{12}x_2 + a_{13}x_3 + \ldots + a_{1n}x_n = 0$$
$$a_{21}x_1 + (a_{22} - \lambda)x_2 + a_{23}x_3 + \ldots + a_{2n}x_n = 0$$
$$a_{31}x_1 + a_{32}x_2 + (a_{33} - \lambda)x_3 + \ldots + a_{3n}x_n = 0$$

$$\cdot \qquad \cdot \qquad \cdot \qquad \qquad \cdot$$
$$\cdot \qquad \cdot \qquad \cdot \qquad \qquad \cdot$$
$$\cdot \qquad \cdot \qquad \cdot \qquad \qquad \cdot$$

$$a_{n1}x_1 + a_{n2}x_2 + a_{n3}x_3 + \ldots + (a_{nn} - \lambda)x_n = 0,$$

it is seen to be homogeneous.

If the coefficient matrix of the original system is denoted by A, I is the $n \times n$ unit matrix and $\mathbf{X}$ is the column vector with the elements $x_1, x_2, \ldots, x_n$, the original system can be written

$$A\mathbf{X} = \lambda \mathbf{X},$$

and the rewritten equivalent system then becomes

$$(A - \lambda I)\mathbf{X} = \mathbf{0},$$

where here the $\mathbf{0}$ is the n element null column matrix (the $n \times 1$ vector whose elements are all zeros).

We see from our previous consideration of homogeneous equations that this matrix system will only have a non-trivial solution if the determinant of its coefficient matrix is zero, so we must require that

$$|A - \lambda I| = 0.$$

As λ occurs once on each element of the leading diagonal of this nth order determinant, when expanded this will give rise to a polynomial equation in λ of degree n of the form

$$\lambda^n + c_1 \lambda^{n-1} c_2 \lambda^{n-2} + \dots + c_{n-1} \lambda + c_n = 0$$

This is called the **characteristic equation** of A, and its roots, the numbers $\lambda_1, \lambda_2, \dots, \lambda_n$ are called the **eigenvalues** of A. The eigenvalues may be real or complex, but we will only consider the case in which they are all **real** and **distinct** (no two eigenvalues are equal).

To each of the n eigenvalues λ_r, with $r = 1, 2, \dots, n$, there will correspond a matrix vector $\mathbf{X}_r$ satisfying

$$(A - \lambda_r I)\mathbf{X}_r = 0, \quad \text{for} \quad r = 1, 2, \dots, n.$$

The vector $\mathbf{X}_r$ is called the **eigenvector** corresponding to the eigenvalue λ_r.

As the system is homogeneous, if $\mathbf{X}_r$ is a solution, so also is $k\mathbf{X}_r$ with k an arbitrary constant which may be either positive or negative. This is because the solution of a homogeneous system only determines the **ratios** of the components $x_1, x_2, \dots, x_n$, and not their absolute values.

This property of $\mathbf{X}_r$ is used to normalize eigenvectors so that the magnitudes of their elements remain within reasonable bounds. Such a normalization is usually necessary in matrix calculations where repeated multiplication by eigenvectors is involved.

If the eigenvector $\mathbf{X}_r$ is of the form

$$\mathbf{X}_r = \begin{bmatrix} c_1 \\ c_2 \\ \vdots \\ c_n \end{bmatrix},$$

we set

$$k = (\pm 1)/(c^2 + c_2^2 + \dots + c_n^2)^{1/2}$$

and define the **normalized eigenvector** $\hat{\mathbf{X}}_r$ to be

$$\hat{\mathbf{X}}_r = \frac{(\pm 1)}{(c_1^2 + c_2^2 + \dots + c_n^2)^{1/2}} \begin{bmatrix} c_1 \\ c_2 \\ \vdots \\ c_n \end{bmatrix}.$$

The choice of sign in the factor (± 1) is arbitrary, and it reflects the fact that when solving for $n - 1$ variables in terms of the nth variable, the sign of that variable may be either positive or negative.

THE ALGEBRAIC EIGENVALUE PROBLEM

Let A be an $n \times n$ matrix. Then to find the eigenvalues, eigenvectors and normalized eigenvectors of A the following steps are involved.

1 The eigenvalues of A are the roots $\lambda_1, \lambda_2, ..., \lambda_n$ of the characteristic equation

$$|A - \lambda I| = 0.$$

2 The eigenvectors of A are the solutions X_r, with $r = 1, 2, .., n$, corresponding to the solutions of

$$(A - \lambda_r I) X_r = 0.$$

3 If required, the normalized eigenvector $\hat{X}_r$ corresponding to an eigenvector X_r of the form

$$X_r = \begin{bmatrix} c_1 \\ c_2 \\ \vdots \\ c_n \end{bmatrix},$$

is

$$\hat{X}_r = \frac{(\pm 1)}{(c_1^2 + c_2^2 + ... + c_n^2)^{1/2}} \begin{bmatrix} c_1 \\ c_2 \\ \vdots \\ c_n \end{bmatrix}.$$

Example 58.1

Find the eigenvalues, eigenvectors and normalized eigenvectors of

$$A = \begin{bmatrix} 3 & 2 \\ 1 & 2 \end{bmatrix}.$$

Solution
Step 1
The eigenvalues are the roots of the characteristic equation

$$|A - \lambda I| = 0,$$

which in this case becomes

$$\begin{vmatrix} 3 - \lambda & 2 \\ 1 & 2 - \lambda \end{vmatrix} = 0.$$

Expanding this determinant shows the characteristic equation to be

$$(3 - \lambda)(2 - \lambda) - 2 = 0,$$

or, equivalently,

$$\lambda^2 - 5\lambda + 4 = 0.$$

This has the roots $\lambda = 1$ and $\lambda = 4$, which are thus the eigenvalues of A. It is convenient to arrange these eigenvalues in numerical order and to number them

$$\lambda_1 = 1 \quad \text{and} \quad \lambda_2 = 4.$$

Steps 2 and 3
To find the eigenvector $\mathbf{X}_1$ corresponding to $\lambda = \lambda_1$ we must solve the system of equations

$$\begin{bmatrix} 3 - \lambda_1 & 2 \\ 1 & 2 - \lambda_1 \end{bmatrix} \begin{bmatrix} x_1 \\ x_2 \end{bmatrix} = \begin{bmatrix} 0 \\ 0 \end{bmatrix}.$$

After setting $\lambda_1 = 1$ this is seen to be equivalent to

$$\begin{bmatrix} 2 & 2 \\ 1 & 1 \end{bmatrix} \begin{bmatrix} x_1 \\ x_2 \end{bmatrix} = \begin{bmatrix} 0 \\ 0 \end{bmatrix}$$

or, when expanded, to the pair of equations

$$2x_1 + 2x_2 = 0$$
$$x_1 + x_2 = 0.$$

These equations are equivalent, so we have only the one equation $x_2 = -x_1$ relating the two variables x_1 and x_2, in which we make take x_1 to be arbitrary. Setting $x_1 = 1$ shows that the eigenvector

$$\mathbf{X}_1 = \begin{bmatrix} 1 \\ -1 \end{bmatrix},$$

and when normalized this becomes

$$\hat{\mathbf{X}}_1 = \frac{(\pm 1)}{\sqrt{2}} \begin{bmatrix} 1 \\ -1 \end{bmatrix}.$$

To find the second eigenvector $\mathbf{X}_2$ we must solve the system of equations

$$\begin{bmatrix} 3 - \lambda_2 & 2 \\ 1 & 2 - \lambda_2 \end{bmatrix} \begin{bmatrix} x_1 \\ x_2 \end{bmatrix} = \begin{bmatrix} 0 \\ 0 \end{bmatrix}.$$

After setting $\lambda_2 = 4$ this matrix equation is seen to be equivalent to the pair of equations

$$-x_1 + 2x_2 = 0$$
$$x_1 - 2x_2 = 0.$$

The equations are equivalent and we again have only the one equation $x_1 = 2x_2$ relating the two variables x_1 and x_2, in which we may take x_2 to be arbitrary. Setting $x_2 = 1$ shows the second eigenvector to be

$$\mathbf{X}_2 = \begin{bmatrix} 2 \\ 1 \end{bmatrix}.$$

After normalization the normalized eigenvector $\hat{\mathbf{X}}_2$ is seen to be

$$\hat{\mathbf{X}}_2 = \frac{(\pm 1)}{\sqrt{5}} \begin{bmatrix} 2 \\ 1 \end{bmatrix}.$$

In summary, the eigenvalues of

$$A = \begin{bmatrix} 3 & 2 \\ 1 & 2 \end{bmatrix}$$

are $\lambda_1 = 1$ and $\lambda_2 = 4$, the corresponding eigenvectors are

$$\mathbf{X}_1 = \begin{bmatrix} 1 \\ -1 \end{bmatrix} \quad \text{and} \quad \mathbf{X}_2 = \begin{bmatrix} 2 \\ 1 \end{bmatrix},$$

and the corresponding normalized eigenvectors are

$$\hat{\mathbf{X}}_1 = \frac{(\pm 1)}{\sqrt{2}} \begin{bmatrix} 1 \\ -1 \end{bmatrix} \quad \text{and} \quad \hat{\mathbf{X}}_2 = \frac{(\pm 1)}{\sqrt{5}} \begin{bmatrix} 2 \\ 1 \end{bmatrix}. \qquad \blacktriangle$$

Example 58.2

Find the eigenvalues, eigenvectors and normalized eigenvectors of

$$A = \begin{bmatrix} 3 & 2 & 2 \\ 2 & 2 & 0 \\ 2 & 0 & 4 \end{bmatrix}.$$

Solution
Step 1
The eigenvalues of A are the roots of the characteristic equation

$$|A - \lambda I| = 0,$$

which in this case reduces to

$$\begin{vmatrix} 3 - \lambda & 2 & 2 \\ 2 & 2 - \lambda & 0 \\ 2 & 0 & 4 - \lambda \end{vmatrix} = 0.$$

Expanding this in terms of the elements of the first row gives

$$(3 - \lambda)[(2 - \lambda)(4 - \lambda)] - 2[2(4 - \lambda)] + 2[-2(2 - \lambda)] = 0,$$

or

$$\lambda^3 - 9\lambda^2 + 18\lambda = 0.$$

Writing the characteristic equation as

$$\lambda(\lambda^2 - 9\lambda + 18) = 0,$$

shows the eigenvalues to be $\lambda = 0$ and the two roots of

$$\lambda^2 - 9\lambda + 18 = 0,$$

which are $\lambda = 3$ and $\lambda = 6$. Thus numbering the eigenvalues in their numerical order (for convenience) we see that the eigenvalues of A are

$$\lambda_1 = 0, \quad \lambda_2 = 3 \quad \text{and} \quad \lambda_3 = 6.$$

Steps 2 and 3

We must find the three eigenvectors and normalized eigenvectors corresponding to the three eigenvalues.

Case $\lambda = \lambda_1$: to find $\mathbf{X}_1$ we must solve

$$\begin{bmatrix} 3 - \lambda_1 & 2 & 2 \\ 2 & 2 - \lambda_1 & 0 \\ 2 & 0 & 4 - \lambda_1 \end{bmatrix} \begin{bmatrix} x_1 \\ x_2 \\ x_3 \end{bmatrix} = \begin{bmatrix} 0 \\ 0 \\ 0 \end{bmatrix},$$

which after setting $\lambda_1 = 0$ is seen to yield the three equations

$$3x_1 + 2x_2 + 2x_3 = 0$$
$$2x_1 + 2x_2 \qquad = 0$$
$$2x_1 \qquad + 4x_3 = 0.$$

These may be solved in terms of x_3 to give

$$x_1 = -2x_3, \quad x_2 = 2x_3,$$

where x_3 is arbitrary. Setting $x_3 = 1$ gives for the eigenvector $\mathbf{X}_1$ corresponding
to λ_1

$$\mathbf{X}_1 = \begin{bmatrix} -2 \\ 2 \\ 1 \end{bmatrix}.$$

The normalized eigenvector $\hat{\mathbf{X}}_1$ is thus

$$\hat{\mathbf{X}} = \frac{(\pm 1)}{3} \begin{bmatrix} -2 \\ 2 \\ 1 \end{bmatrix}.$$

Case $\lambda = \lambda_2$: to find $\mathbf{X}_3$ we must solve

$$\begin{bmatrix} 3 - \lambda_2 & 2 & 2 \\ 2 & 2 - \lambda_2 & 0 \\ 2 & 0 & 4 - \lambda_2 \end{bmatrix} \begin{bmatrix} x_1 \\ x_2 \\ x_3 \end{bmatrix} = \begin{bmatrix} 0 \\ 0 \\ 0 \end{bmatrix}.$$

Setting $\lambda_2 = 3$ in this matrix equation yields the three equations

$$2x_2 + 2x_3 = 0$$
$$2x_1 - x_2 = 0$$
$$2x_1 + x_3 = 0.$$

These may be solved in terms of x_1 to give

$$x_2 = 2x_1, \quad x_3 = -2x_1,$$

where x_1 is arbitrary. Setting $x_1 = 1$ gives for the eigenvector $\mathbf{X}_2$ corresponding
to λ_2

$$\mathbf{X}_2 = \begin{bmatrix} 1 \\ 2 \\ -2 \end{bmatrix}.$$

The normalized eigenvector $\hat{\mathbf{X}}_2$ is thus

$$\hat{\mathbf{X}}_2 = \frac{(\pm 1)}{3} \begin{bmatrix} 1 \\ 2 \\ -2 \end{bmatrix}.$$

Case $\lambda = \lambda_3$: to find $\mathbf{X}_3$ we must solve

$$\begin{bmatrix} 3 - \lambda_3 & 2 & 2 \\ 2 & 2 - \lambda_3 & 0 \\ 2 & 0 & 4 - \lambda_3 \end{bmatrix} \begin{bmatrix} x_1 \\ x_2 \\ x_3 \end{bmatrix} = \begin{bmatrix} 0 \\ 0 \\ 0 \end{bmatrix}.$$

Setting $\lambda_3 = 6$ and proceeding as before yields the three equations

$$-3x_1 + 2x_2 + 2x_3 = 0$$
$$2x_1 - 4x_2 \qquad = 0$$
$$2x_1 \qquad - 2x_3 = 0.$$

These may be solved in terms of x_2 to give

$$x_1 = 2x_2, \quad x_3 = 2x_2,$$

where x_2 is arbitrary. Setting $x_2 = 1$ gives for the eigenvector $\mathbf{X}_3$ corresponding to λ_3

$$\mathbf{X}_3 = \begin{bmatrix} 2 \\ 1 \\ 2 \end{bmatrix}.$$

The normalized eigenvector $\hat{\mathbf{X}}_3$ is thus

$$\hat{\mathbf{X}}_3 = \frac{(\pm 1)}{3} \begin{bmatrix} 2 \\ 1 \\ 2 \end{bmatrix}.$$

In summary, the eigenvalues of

$$A = \begin{bmatrix} 3 & 2 & 2 \\ 2 & 2 & 0 \\ 2 & 0 & 4 \end{bmatrix}$$

are $\lambda_1 = 0$, $\lambda_2 = 3$ and $\lambda_3 = 6$, the corresponding eigenvectors are

$$\mathbf{X}_1 = \begin{bmatrix} -2 \\ 2 \\ 1 \end{bmatrix}, \quad \mathbf{X}_2 = \begin{bmatrix} 1 \\ 2 \\ -2 \end{bmatrix} \quad \text{and} \quad \mathbf{X}_3 = \begin{bmatrix} 2 \\ 1 \\ 2 \end{bmatrix},$$

while the corresponding normalized eigenvectors are

$$\hat{X}_1 = \frac{(\pm 1)}{3}\begin{bmatrix} -2 \\ 2 \\ 1 \end{bmatrix}, \quad X_2 = \frac{(\pm 1)}{3}\begin{bmatrix} 1 \\ 2 \\ -2 \end{bmatrix} \text{ and } X_3 = \frac{(\pm 1)}{3}\begin{bmatrix} 2 \\ 1 \\ 2 \end{bmatrix}. \qquad \blacktriangle$$

PROBLEMS 58

In the following problems find the characteristic equation, the eigenvalues, the eigenvectors and normalized eigenvectors of the matrix A.

1. $A = \begin{bmatrix} 5 & 4 \\ 1 & 2 \end{bmatrix}$.

2. $A = \begin{bmatrix} 1 & 2 \\ 3 & 2 \end{bmatrix}$.

3. $A = \begin{bmatrix} 1 & 2 \\ 4 & 3 \end{bmatrix}$.

4. $A = \begin{bmatrix} 4 & 1 \\ 2 & 3 \end{bmatrix}$.

5. $A = \begin{bmatrix} 3 & 2 & -1 \\ 3 & 4 & 1 \\ 1 & 1 & 3 \end{bmatrix}$,

   given that $\lambda = 3$ is a root of the characteristic equation.

6. $A = \begin{bmatrix} 3 & 0 & 1 \\ 2 & 2 & 2 \\ 4 & 2 & 5 \end{bmatrix}$,

   given that $\lambda = 1$ is a root of the characteristic equation.

7. $A = \begin{bmatrix} 0 & 2 & 4 \\ 1 & 1 & -2 \\ -2 & 0 & 5 \end{bmatrix}$,

   given that $\lambda = 1$ is a root of the characteristic equation.

8. $A = \begin{bmatrix} 0 & 1 & 0 \\ 0 & 0 & 1 \\ 2 & 1 & -2 \end{bmatrix}$,

given that $\lambda = -1$ is a root of the characteristic equation.

9. $A = \begin{bmatrix} 2 & 0 & 1 \\ 1 & -2 & 1 \\ -1 & -2 & 0 \end{bmatrix}.$

10. $A = \begin{bmatrix} 1 & -9 & 5 \\ -9 & 15 & -9 \\ 5 & -9 & 1 \end{bmatrix},$

given that $\lambda = -3$ is a root of the characteristic equation.

11. $A = \begin{bmatrix} -1 & 2 & 2 \\ 2 & 2 & 2 \\ -3 & -6 & -6 \end{bmatrix}.$

12. $A = \begin{bmatrix} -1 & 6 & -12 \\ 0 & -13 & 30 \\ 0 & -9 & 20 \end{bmatrix},$

given that $\lambda = 5$ is a root of the characteristic equation.

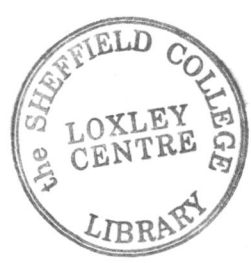

SHEFFIELD COLLEGE
the LOXLEY CENTRE
LIBRARY

59   Scalars, vectors and vector addition

When describing physical situations, many quantities can be completely specified by means of a single number which measures their **magnitude** in appropriate units. Such quantities are called **scalars**, and typical examples are mass, density, time, work done, temperature, speed and electric charge, to name but a few.

Other physical quantities are more complicated, and in order to specify them it is necessary to give both their **magnitude** and their **direction**. These are called **vectors**, and they have a convenient geometrical representation in terms of a straight line segment to which has been added an arrow. The length of the line segment is proportional to the magnitude of the vector which is always considered to be non-negative, and the orientation of the line in space together with the arrow indicates the direction of the vector. A reversal of the arrow leaves the magnitude of the vector unchanged but reverses its direction.

It is understood that two vectors are **equal** if they have the same magnitude and direction. Expressed differently, two vectors are equal if their magnitudes are equal, the line segments representing their magnitudes are parallel and the arrows indicating the sense along each of the line segments both point in the same direction. Thus a vector remains unchanged if it is moved parallel to itself without change of length or direction. Such a shift of a vector is called a **translation**.

Typical vector quantities are velocity (speed in a given direction), force, momentum, heat flux, displacement, acceleration and electric field intensity.

Sometimes it is convenient to represent the vector directed from A, called the **initial point**, or **base**, of the vector, to B, called the **terminal point**, or **tip**, of the vector, by $\underline{AB}$, but more frequently it is simply denoted by a single bold face symbol like **a**. Thus
Thus

$$\underline{AB} = \mathbf{a},$$

and the two representations of this vector are illustrated in Fig. 118, in which the two lines are parallel, of equal length and have arrows in the same direction. The choice of the proportionality constant is arbitrary, but it is often chosen such that a line segment of length 1 represents a vector of magnitude 1 (in appropriate units).

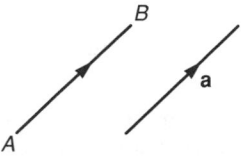

Fig. 118

The essential property underlying vectors is the definition of **vector addition**. The **sum** of the two vectors **a** and **b** is defined to be a third vector **a** + **b** determined by the **parallelogram** or **triangle law for addition**.

Parallelogram and triangle laws for vector addition
The parallelogram law for the vector sum **a** + **b** is illustrated in Fig. 119(a), and the equivalent triangle law is illustrated in Fig. 119(b). Vector summation of **a** and **b** by means of the parallelogram law involves bringing the initial points of vectors **a** and **b** into coincidence, completing the parallelogram as shown, and equating the sum **a** + **b** to the diagonal of the parallelogram drawn from the common initial point of **a** and **b** as shown, with the arrow directed away from O. Vector summation by means of the triangle law is equivalent, and it involves translating **b** so that its initial point is at the terminal point of **a**, and then equating the sum **a** + **b** to the third side of the triangle, with the arrow directed from the initial point of **a** to the terminal point of **b**, as shown in Fig. 119(b).

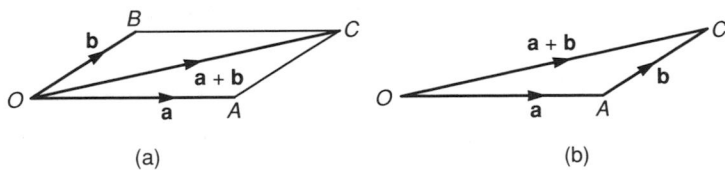

Fig. 119

The **magnitude**, or **modulus**, of a vector $\mathbf{a} = \underline{AB}$ is the length of the line AB, and it is convenient to denote the magnitude of a vector denoted by the bold face symbol **a** by $|\mathbf{a}|$ and to write this simply as a, so that if $\mathbf{a} = \underline{AB}$, then

$$AB = |\mathbf{a}| = a.$$

A vector of unit length in the direction of **a** is called a **unit vector**, and it is written $\hat{\mathbf{a}}$, so that

$$|\hat{\mathbf{a}}| = 1.$$

A number of important properties of vectors follow directly from the law for vector addition.

Commutative law

$$\mathbf{a} + \mathbf{b} = \mathbf{b} + \mathbf{a}$$

This follows from the parallelogram law which is seen to comprise two triangle laws, one of which gives $\mathbf{a} + \mathbf{b}$ and the other which gives $\mathbf{b} + \mathbf{a}$, both represented by the same diagonal. Thus the **order** in which vectors are added is immaterial.

Associative law

$$\mathbf{a} + (\mathbf{b} + \mathbf{c}) = (\mathbf{a} + \mathbf{b}) + \mathbf{c}$$

The proof of this follows by considering Fig. 120. We see from this that

$$\mathbf{b} + \mathbf{c} = \underline{AC},$$

so

$$\mathbf{a} + (\mathbf{b} + \mathbf{c}) = \underline{OC},$$

but

$$\mathbf{a} + \mathbf{b} = \underline{AB},$$

so

$$(\mathbf{a} + \mathbf{b}) + \mathbf{c} = \underline{OC},$$

and thus

$$\mathbf{a} + (\mathbf{b} + \mathbf{c}) = (\mathbf{a} + \mathbf{b}) + \mathbf{c}.$$

This last result means that a sum such as $\mathbf{a} + \mathbf{b} + \dots + \mathbf{c}$ is unique (the order in which the vectors are added does not influence their sum).

Thus $\mathbf{a} + \mathbf{a}$ is a vector with magnitude $2\,|\mathbf{a}|$ and the direction of $\mathbf{a}$, so we write this as $2\mathbf{a}$. In general, if k, l are scalars, we have

$$k\mathbf{a} + l\mathbf{a} = (k + l)\,\mathbf{a},$$

$$k\mathbf{a} + k\mathbf{b} = k(\mathbf{a} + \mathbf{b}),$$

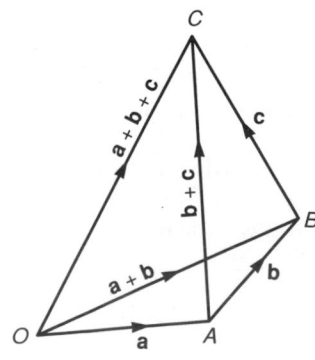

Fig. 120

and

$$k(l\mathbf{a}) = l(k\mathbf{a}) = kl\mathbf{a}.$$

If we now set $k = |\mathbf{a}|$ and $l = 1/|\mathbf{a}|$, we see from this last result that

$$|\mathbf{a}| \left(\frac{1}{|\mathbf{a}|} \mathbf{a} \right) = \mathbf{a},$$

but

$$\frac{1}{|\mathbf{a}|} \mathbf{a} = \hat{\mathbf{a}} \qquad \text{(the unit vector in the direction of a),}$$

so we have arrived at the general result that

$$\mathbf{a} = |\mathbf{a}| \, \hat{\mathbf{a}}.$$

In words, this expresses the fact that any vector **a** may be expressed as the product of the unit vector $\hat{\mathbf{a}}$ in the direction of **a** scaled by the magnitude of **a**.

SUBTRACTION OF VECTORS

The vector $- \mathbf{b}$ is defined to be the vector with the same magnitude as **b**, but with the opposite direction. Thus the vector **difference** $\mathbf{c} = \mathbf{a} - \mathbf{b}$ is defined to be the vector sum

$$\mathbf{c} = \mathbf{a} + (- \mathbf{b}).$$

This is illustrated in Fig. 121 in which first the bases of **a** and **b** are brought into coincidence. Then the direction of **b** is reversed to form $- \mathbf{b}$, after which **a** and $- \mathbf{b}$ are added by the parallelogram law to form the difference $\mathbf{a} - \mathbf{b}$.

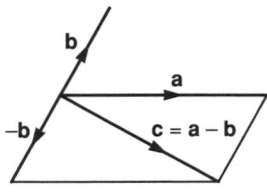

Fig. 121

If $\mathbf{b} = \mathbf{a}$ then $\mathbf{a} - \mathbf{a} = \mathbf{0}$ is the **zero** or **null vector**. All null vectors are regarded as equal and they have magnitude zero but no direction.

SCALING VECTORS

Scaling vectors means multiplying them by a number (a scalar). It follows from the arguments given above that when a vector **a** is scaled (multiplied) by a

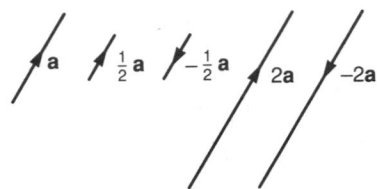

Fig. 122

number μ, its magnitude becomes $|\mu|\,|\mathbf{a}|$ (here $|\mu|$ is the absolute value of μ) and its direction is unchanged if $\mu > 0$ but its direction is reversed if $\mu < 0$. Figure 122 shows the effect of scaling the vector $\mathbf{a}$ by various factors μ.

The position of a point in space is a vector quantity when referred to a fixed origin O. Such vectors, called **position vectors**, are of considerable importance in the study of vectors. If, for example, the point O in Fig. 120 is taken to be the origin, then the position vectors of points A, B and C are, respectively, $\mathbf{a}$, $\mathbf{a} + \mathbf{b}$ and $\mathbf{a} + \mathbf{b} + \mathbf{c}$.

PROBLEMS 59

1. Draw diagrams to illustrate the commutative property

$$\mathbf{a} + \mathbf{b} = \mathbf{b} + \mathbf{a}.$$

2. A vehicle is moved 3 miles due east and 3 miles due south of its initial position. Find the position vector of its final location relative to its starting point.

3. Find the vector $\mathbf{x}$ in terms of $\mathbf{a}$ and $\mathbf{b}$, where $\mathbf{a}$, $\mathbf{b}$ and $\mathbf{x}$ are as shown in Fig. 123.

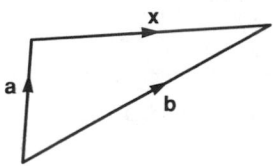

Fig. 123

4. Find the vector $\mathbf{x}$ in terms of $\mathbf{a}$, $\mathbf{b}$ and $\mathbf{c}$, where $\mathbf{a}$, $\mathbf{b}$, $\mathbf{c}$ and $\mathbf{x}$ are as shown in Fig. 124.

5. Find the position vector $\mathbf{r}$ of the point R shown in Fig. 125 which divides the line AB in the ratio $m : n$, given that the position vectors of A and B are, respectively, $\mathbf{a}$ and $\mathbf{b}$.

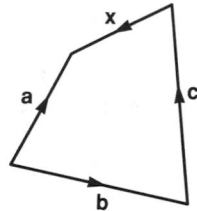

Fig. 124

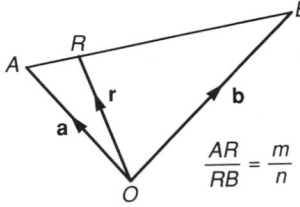

Fig. 125

6. If A and B have the respective position vectors **a** and **b**, find the vector **x** which is oppositely directed to the position vector **r** of the mid-point P of AB and twice its magnitude.

7. Find the position vector **x** of the mid-point M of the median BP, in terms of the position vectors **a**, **b** and **c** of the respective vertices A, B and C of the triangle in Fig. 126.

8. Let a unit vector represent a force of unit magnitude acting in its direction. What is the magnitude of the sum of forces of magnitudes 1, 2 and 3 which are mutually perpendicular, and how can the direction of this resultant force be found?

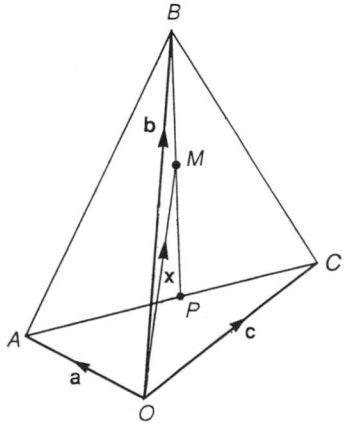

Fig. 126

Vectors in component form

60

The rule for vector addition may be used to express an arbitrary vector as the sum of multiples of three mutually perpendicular unit vectors. When working with Cartesian coordinates these unit vectors are denoted by **i**, **j** and **k**. We will take them to be directed in the positive sense along the three Cartesian axes Ox, Oy and Oz, respectively, as shown in Fig. 127. Notice that the axes are arranged so that the z-axis points in the direction in which a right-handed screw will advance if turned from x to y. This is called a **right-handed set of axes**, and we will always work with such a set. The set of vectors **i**, **j**, **k** is called a **right-handed set of unit vectors** or, sometimes, an **orthogonal triad of unit vectors**, where by orthogonal vectors we mean mutually perpendicular vectors.

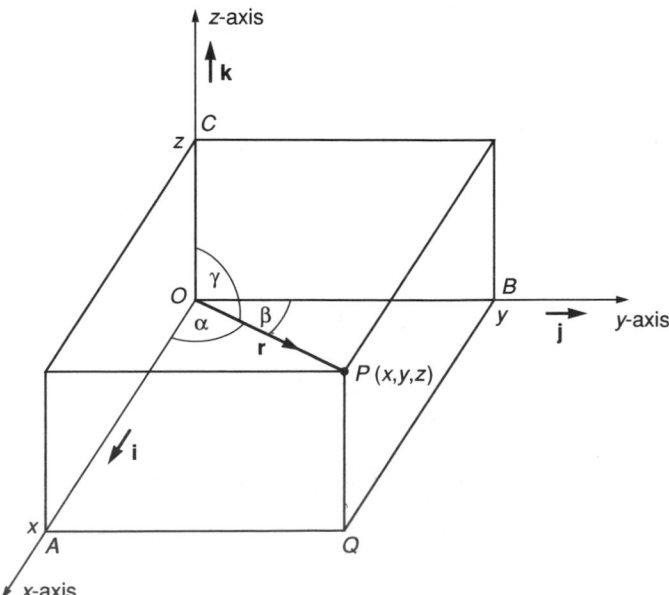

Fig. 127

If a point P has the Cartesian coordinates $P(x, y, z)$ it follows that $OA = x$ $OB = y$ and $OC = z$. Thus $\underline{OA} = x\mathbf{i}$, $\underline{OB} = y\mathbf{j}$ and $\underline{OC} = z\mathbf{k}$, and by vector addition we see that the position vector of P relative to O is

$$\mathbf{r} = \underline{OP} = x\mathbf{i} + y\mathbf{j} + z\mathbf{k}.$$

The numbers x, y and z are called the **components** of vector $\mathbf{r}$, and the representation $\mathbf{r} = x\mathbf{i} + y\mathbf{j} + z\mathbf{k}$ is called the **Cartesian form** of vector $\mathbf{r}$.

It follows from Pythagoras' theorem that the **modulus**

$$r = |\mathbf{r}| = (x^2 + y^2 + z^2)^{1/2}.$$

This can be seen from Fig. 127, because

$$OP^2 = OQ^2 + QP^2 = OQ^2 + z^2,$$

but

$$OQ^2 = x^2 + y^2,$$

so

$$OP^2 = x^2 + y^2 + z^2,$$

and thus

$$r = |\mathbf{r}| = (x^2 + y^2 + z^2)^{1/2}.$$

If α, β and γ are the angles between OP and the x, y and z-axes, respectively, we see from Fig. 127 that if we set

$$l = \cos \alpha, \quad m = \cos \beta, \quad n = \cos \gamma$$

it follows that

$$x = r \cos \alpha = rl$$
$$y = r \cos \beta = rm$$
$$z = r \cos \gamma = rn.$$

Consequently

$$\mathbf{r} = rl\mathbf{i} + rm\mathbf{j} + rn\mathbf{k}$$
$$= r(l\mathbf{i} + m\mathbf{j} + n\mathbf{k}),$$

and thus

$$\frac{\mathbf{r}}{r} = \hat{\mathbf{r}} = l\mathbf{i} + m\mathbf{j} + n\mathbf{k}.$$

The numbers (l, m, n), in this order, are called the **direction cosines** of $\mathbf{r}$ and since

$$\hat{\mathbf{r}} = l\mathbf{i} + m\mathbf{j} + n\mathbf{k}$$

it follows that l, m and n are related by the expression

$$l^2 + m^2 + n^2 = 1.$$

In terms of r and the components of $\mathbf{r}$, it is seen that

$$l = x/r, \quad m = y/r, \quad \text{and} \quad n = z/r.$$

Any set of numbers (a, b, c) which are proportional to the direction cosines (l, m, n) are called **direction ratios**. Thus if

$$\mathbf{r} = x\mathbf{i} + y\mathbf{j} + z\mathbf{k},$$

as well as x, y and z being the components of $\mathbf{r}$ they are also its **direction ratios**, as would be the numbers λx, λy and λz with $\lambda > 0$ any scalar.

Example 60.1

If $\mathbf{r} = 8\mathbf{i} + 4\mathbf{j} - \mathbf{k}$, find $r, \hat{\mathbf{r}}$ and the direction cosines of $\mathbf{r}$.

Solution

$$r = |\mathbf{r}| = [8^2 + 4^2 + (-1)^2]^{1/2} = 9.$$

$$\hat{\mathbf{r}} = \frac{\mathbf{r}}{r} = \frac{1}{9}(8\mathbf{i} + 4\mathbf{j} - \mathbf{k})$$

$$= \frac{8}{9}\mathbf{i} + \frac{4}{9}\mathbf{j} - \frac{1}{9}\mathbf{k}.$$

The direction cosines follow from this last result, since l, m and n are the coefficients of $\mathbf{i}$, $\mathbf{j}$ and $\mathbf{k}$, in the representation of the unit vector $\hat{\mathbf{r}}$. Thus we see that

$$l = 8/9, \quad m = 4/9 \quad \text{and} \quad n = -1/9. \qquad \blacktriangle$$

It is an immediate consequence of the laws for the addition and scaling of vectors that if

$$\mathbf{a} = a_1\mathbf{i} + a_2\mathbf{j} + a_3\mathbf{k} \quad \text{and} \quad \mathbf{b} = b_1\mathbf{i} + b_2\mathbf{j} + b_3\mathbf{k},$$

$$\mathbf{a} + \mathbf{b} = (a_1 + b_1)\mathbf{i} + (a_2 + b_2)\mathbf{j} + (a_3 + b_3)\mathbf{k},$$

$$\mathbf{a} - \mathbf{b} = (a_1 - b_1)\mathbf{i} + (a_2 - b_2)\mathbf{j} + (a_3 - b_3)\mathbf{k},$$

and if λ, μ are scalars,

$$\lambda\mathbf{a} + \mu\mathbf{b} = (\lambda a_1 + \mu b_1)\mathbf{i} + (\lambda a_2 + \mu b_2)\mathbf{j} + (\lambda a_3 + \mu b_3)\mathbf{k}.$$

Thus when adding vectors in component form the corresponding components must be added, and when scaling a vector by λ, each component must be scaled by λ.

Example 60.2

If

$$\mathbf{a} = 2\mathbf{i} - 7\mathbf{j} + \mathbf{k} \quad \text{and} \quad \mathbf{b} = 3\mathbf{i} + 2\mathbf{j} - 5\mathbf{k},$$

find
(i) $2\mathbf{a}$;
(ii) $-3\mathbf{b}$;
(iii) $3\mathbf{a} - \mathbf{b}$; and
(iv) a unit vector in the direction of $\mathbf{a}$.

Solution
(i) $2\mathbf{a} = 4\mathbf{i} - 14\mathbf{j} + 2\mathbf{k}.$
(ii) $-3\mathbf{b} = -9\mathbf{i} - 6\mathbf{j} + 15\mathbf{k}.$
(iii) $3\mathbf{a} - \mathbf{b} = 6\mathbf{i} - 21\mathbf{j} + 3\mathbf{k} - (3\mathbf{i} + 2\mathbf{j} - 5\mathbf{k})$
$$= 6\mathbf{i} - 21\mathbf{j} + 3\mathbf{k} - 3\mathbf{i} - 2\mathbf{j} + 5\mathbf{k}$$
$$= 3\mathbf{i} - 23\mathbf{j} + 8\mathbf{k}.$$

(iv) $\hat{\mathbf{a}} = \dfrac{\mathbf{a}}{|\mathbf{a}|} = \dfrac{2\mathbf{i} - 7\mathbf{j} + \mathbf{k}}{[(2)^2 + (-7)^2 + (1)^2]^{1/2}}$

$$= \frac{1}{\sqrt{54}}(2\mathbf{i} - 7\mathbf{j} + \mathbf{k}). \qquad \blacktriangle$$

Example 60.3

Given that A is the point $(5, -2, 3)$ and B is the point $(2, 1, -2)$ find
(i)   the position vectors of A and B relative to the origin;
(ii)   the vector $\underline{AB}$; and
(iii) the position of the mid-point P of AB.

Solution
(i) $\mathbf{a} = \underline{OA} = 5\mathbf{i} - 2\mathbf{j} + 3\mathbf{k}$ and $\mathbf{b} = \underline{OB} = 2\mathbf{i} + \mathbf{j} - 2\mathbf{k}.$
(ii)   The configuration is illustrated in Fig. 128. We have

$$\underline{OA} + \underline{AB} = \underline{OB},$$

or

$$\mathbf{a} + \underline{AB} = \mathbf{b},$$

and so

$$\underline{AB} = \mathbf{b} - \mathbf{a}$$
$$= (2\mathbf{i} + \mathbf{j} - 2\mathbf{k}) - (5\mathbf{i} - 2\mathbf{j} + 3\mathbf{k})$$
$$= -3\mathbf{i} + 3\mathbf{j} - 5\mathbf{k}.$$

(iii) $\mathbf{r} = \underline{OP} = \underline{OA} + \underline{AP}$
$$= \mathbf{a} + \tfrac{1}{2}\underline{AB}$$
$$= \mathbf{a} + \tfrac{1}{2}(\mathbf{b} - \mathbf{a})$$
$$= \tfrac{1}{2}(\mathbf{a} + \mathbf{b}).$$

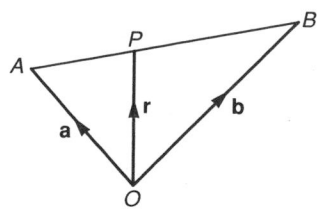

Fig. 128 $\blacktriangle$

Velocity is a vector quantity, since it is a speed in a given direction. Sometimes the velocity of a point P of interest is observed from an observation point Q which is itself moving. If the velocities of P and Q are $\mathbf{v}_P$ and $\mathbf{v}_Q$, respectively, the velocity

$$\mathbf{v}_R = \mathbf{v}_P - \mathbf{v}_Q$$

is called the **relative velocity** of P with respect to Q. The notion of relative velocity is illustrated in the next example.

Example 60.4

A man travelling due east at 24 km/h finds the wind appears to blow from the north. If he doubles his speed he finds it appears to blow from the north east. Find the velocity of the wind.

Solution
Take a unit vector $\mathbf{i}$ pointing east and a unit vector $\mathbf{k}$ pointing north, and let a unit vector represent a velocity of 1 km/h. Then the man's velocity is $24\mathbf{i}$, and the relative velocity $\mathbf{u}$ of the wind with respect to the man is $-u\mathbf{k}$, where $u = |\mathbf{u}|$. The situation is illustrated in Fig. 129(a), in which the true velocity of the wind $\mathbf{V}$ (relative to a fixed observer on the east) blows as shown with the angle θ as yet undetermined.

On doubling his speed, the man's velocity becomes $48\mathbf{i}$, the true velocity of the wind $\mathbf{V}$ remains unchanged, but relative to the man the wind now blows along CD in Fig. 129(b), with the angle BCD equal to $\pi/4$. Comparison of Figs. 129(a) and (b) shows that $AB = BC = 24$, and as angle BCD is equal to $\pi/4$ and BD is perpendicular to AC, the angle BAD must also equal $\pi/4$. Thus the wind velocity is

$$\mathbf{V} = \underline{AB} + \underline{BD}$$
$$= 24\mathbf{i} + (-24\mathbf{k})$$

so

$$\mathbf{V} = 24(\mathbf{i} - \mathbf{k}),$$

and thus the true wind speed

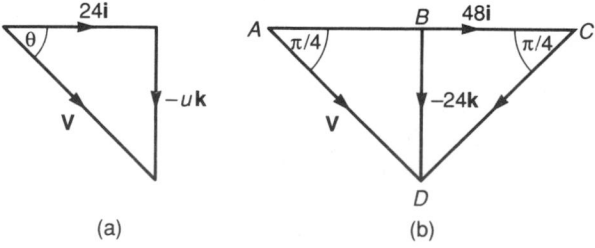

(a)   (b)

Fig. 129

$$V = |\mathbf{V}| = [24^2 + 24^2]^{1/2} = 24\sqrt{2} \text{ km/h.} \qquad \blacktriangle$$

If two forces F_1 and F_2 act on a point, the **resultant force R** is defined as

$$\mathbf{R} = \mathbf{F}_1 + \mathbf{F}_2.$$

The next example illustrates the determination of the resultant force in a simple case.

Example 60.5

A force **F** of magnitude 3 newtons acts along the line of the vector $-2\mathbf{i} + 3\mathbf{j} + \mathbf{k}$ and another force **G** of magnitude 2 newtons acts along the line of the vector $-3\mathbf{i} + \mathbf{j} + 2\mathbf{k}$. Find
(i) unit vectors $\hat{\mathbf{f}}$ and $\hat{\mathbf{g}}$ in the direction of **F** and **G**, and
(ii) the resultant **R** of **F** and **G** and $|\mathbf{R}|$.

Solution
(i) $\hat{\mathbf{f}} = \dfrac{-2\mathbf{i} + 3\mathbf{j} + \mathbf{k}}{[(-2)^2 + 3^2 + 1^2]^{1/2}} = \dfrac{1}{\sqrt{14}} (-2\mathbf{i} + 3\mathbf{j} + 2\mathbf{k})$

and

$\hat{\mathbf{g}} = \dfrac{-3\mathbf{i} + \mathbf{j} + 2\mathbf{k}}{[(-3)^2 + 1^2 + 2^2]^{1/2}} = \dfrac{1}{\sqrt{14}} (-3\mathbf{i} + \mathbf{j} + 2\mathbf{k}).$

(ii) Letting a force of 1 newton be represented by a unit vector we see that

$$\mathbf{F} = 3\hat{\mathbf{f}} \quad \text{and} \quad \mathbf{G} = 2\hat{\mathbf{g}},$$

so that the resultant force

$$\mathbf{R} = \mathbf{F} + \mathbf{G} = 3\hat{\mathbf{f}} + 2\hat{\mathbf{g}}$$

$$= \frac{3}{\sqrt{14}} (-2\mathbf{i} + 3\mathbf{j} + \mathbf{k}) + \frac{2}{\sqrt{14}} (-3\mathbf{i} + \mathbf{j} + 2\mathbf{k})$$

$$= \frac{1}{\sqrt{14}} (-12\mathbf{i} + 11\mathbf{j} + 7\mathbf{k})$$

The magnitude $R = |\mathbf{R}|$ of the resultant force is thus

$$R = [(-12/\sqrt{14})^2 + (11/\sqrt{14})^2 + (7/\sqrt{14})^2]^{1/2}$$

$$= \sqrt{(157/7)} \text{ newton.} \qquad \blacktriangle$$

Finally, we give the definition of the **centroid** of a system of point masses. If point masses $m_1, m_2, ..., m_n$ have position vectors $\mathbf{r}_1, \mathbf{r}_2, ..., \mathbf{r}_n$, the centroid (centre of mass) of the system has the position vector

$$\mathbf{r} = \frac{m_1\mathbf{r}_1 + m_2\mathbf{r}_2 + ... + m_n\mathbf{r}_n}{m_1 + m_2 + ... + m_n}.$$

PROBLEMS 60

1. Given

    $$a = 4i - 2j + 3k, \quad b = -2i + 3j + k,$$

    find $|a|$, $|b|$, $\hat{a}$, $\hat{b}$ and $3a - 2b$.

2. Given

    $$a = 6i + 2j + k, \quad b = -i - 4j + 2k,$$

    find $|a|$, $|b|$, $\hat{a}$, $\hat{b}$ and $2a + b$.

3. Given

    $$a = 3i + 4j - 2k,$$

    find the direction cosines of a.

4. Given

    $$a = i + 2j - k, \quad b = 2i - 3j + 2k,$$

    find the direction cosines of $2a - b$.

5. Given

    $$a = 3i + 7j - 4k, \quad b = 6i - 2j + 12k,$$

    find $|a|$, $|b|$ and the direction cosines of $a + b$.

6. Express the following vectors in the form $ai + bj + ck$:
    (a) $\underline{AB}$ if A is the point $(1, 3, 2)$ and B the point $(2, 1, 1)$;
    (b) the vector from the point $C(1, -1, -2)$ to the origin.

7. The position vectors of four points A, B, C and D are given by $2i + 3j - k$, k and $4i + 4j - k$, respectively. Express $\underline{AB}$ and $\underline{CD}$ in terms of i, j and k. Calculate the vector $\underline{AB} + \underline{CD}$ and determine its length.

8. Let a unit vector represent a force of 1 kg acting in its direction. Find the resultant of the forces $3i + 4j$, $2j - 5k$, $-3k$ and $6i + 7j$ kg and its inclination to the x, y and z-axes, respectively.

9. Forces of 1, 2 and 3 kg parallel to the sides BC, CA and AB of a triangle ABC act through a point. The forces act from B to C, from C to A and from A to B, where the vertices A, B and C are located at the points $(1, 1, 1)$, $(0, 2, 3)$ and $(2, 3, 0)$. Find their resultant R and the direction cosines of its line of action.

10. If the position vectors of two points P and Q are $3i + 2j - 7k$ and $5i - 2j + 4k$, respectively, find PQ and determine its direction cosines.

11. If i, j denote displacements of 1 mile to the east and north, respectively, express the following displacements in terms of them:
    (a) 4 miles N30°E;   (b) 3 miles SE;   (c) 5 miles at 240°.

12. If i, j denote displacements of 5 miles to the east and north, respectively, express in terms of their lengths and directions (a) $i + j$;   (b) $-(1/2)i + \sqrt{3}/2 j$.

13. A particle is given in succession three displacements, 1 mile SW., $2\frac{1}{2}$ miles 60°E and 3 miles E. Find the magnitude and direction of the equivalent single displacement.

14. The position vectors of the four points A, B, C and D, respectively, are **a**, **b**, $2\mathbf{a} + 3\mathbf{b}$ and $\mathbf{a} - 2\mathbf{b}$. Express $\underline{AC}$, $\underline{DB}$, $\underline{BC}$ and $\underline{CA}$ in terms of **a** and **b**.

15. A particle describes a circle uniformly in the (x, y)-plane taking 12 seconds to complete one revolution, with the centre of the circle located at the origin. If its initial position vector is **i**, and the rotation is from **i** to **j**, find the position vectors at 1, 3, 5 and 7 seconds. Also express as vectors the velocity of the particle at 3/2 and 5 seconds.

16. The velocity of a boat relative to water is represented by $3\mathbf{i} + 4\mathbf{j}$, and that of the water relative to the earth by $\mathbf{i} - 3\mathbf{j}$. What is the velocity of the boat relative to the earth if **i** and **j** represent velocities of 1 km/h to the east and north, respectively?

17. Forces of 1, 2 and 3 kg act at one corner of a cube along the diagonals of the faces meeting at that corner. Find the magnitude of the resultant force **R** and its inclination to the edges of the cube.

18. Find the position vector of the centroid of masses 3, 4 and 5 located at the points $(2, -3, 3)$, $(5, -3, -4)$ and $(2, -3, -1)$, respectively.

19. Express in the form $a\mathbf{i} + b\mathbf{j} + c\mathbf{k}$ the vector $\underline{OC}$, where O is the origin and C is the mid-point of the line AB, where A and B are the points $(2, -1, -2)$ and $(-4, 3, 2)$, respectively.

20. Prove by vectors that the centroid of three particles of identical mass located at the vertices of triangle ABC lies on a median of the triangle 2/3 of the distance from the vertex from which the median is drawn.

61 The straight line

Consider a straight line L which passes through a point A with position vector **a** and is parallel to a vector **b**, as shown in Fig. 130, and let P be any point on L with position vector **r**.

Then from the vector triangle OAP we see that

$$\underline{OA} + \underline{AP} = \underline{OP},$$

or

$$\mathbf{r} = \mathbf{a} + \underline{AP}.$$

Now $\underline{AP}$ is parallel to **b**, so we may always find a scalar multiplier λ, which may be either positive or negative, such that

$$\underline{AP} = \lambda\,\mathbf{b}.$$

Notice that λ will be positive if P lies to the side of A towards which **b** is directed, otherwise it will be negative.

Thus the vector equation of L is seen to be

$$\mathbf{r} = \mathbf{a} + \lambda\,\mathbf{b}.$$

If $\mathbf{r} = x\mathbf{i} + y\mathbf{j} + z\mathbf{k}$, $\mathbf{a} = a_1\mathbf{i} + a_2\mathbf{j} + a_3\mathbf{k}$ and $\mathbf{b} = b_1\mathbf{i} + b_2\mathbf{j} + b_3\mathbf{k}$, the equation of L becomes

$$x\mathbf{i} + y\mathbf{j} + z\mathbf{k} = a_1\mathbf{i} + a_2\mathbf{j} + a_3\mathbf{k} + \lambda\,(b_1\mathbf{i} + b_2\mathbf{j} + b_3\mathbf{k}).$$

A **vector equation** is, in fact, **three scalar equations**, for it implies the equality of the **i**, **j** and **k** components on either side of the equation. Thus the ordinary Cartesian equations of the straight line L are

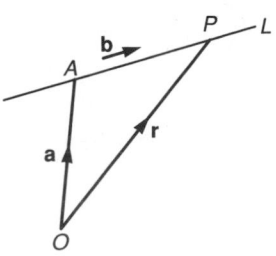

Fig. 130

$$x = a_1 + \lambda b_1$$

$$y = a_2 + \lambda b_2$$

$$z = a_3 + \lambda b_3,$$

in which λ is a parameter such that $-\infty < \lambda < \infty$. Giving different values to λ determines different points (x, y, z) on L.

Eliminating λ between these three equations we find that the Cartesian equations of L are

$$\frac{x - a_1}{b_1} = \frac{y - a_2}{b_2} = \frac{z - a_3}{b_3} \; (= \lambda).$$

When expressed in this form the Cartesian equations of L are said to be in **standard** (or **canonical**) **form**. Notice the important fact that when the equations are in standard form, the coefficients of x, y and z are all equal to **unity**.

When the Cartesian equations of a line L are in standard form, equating the numerator of each of the three expressions to zero determines the coordinates of a point on L, while the denominators of the expressions are the direction ratios of L.

Example 61.1

Write down the Cartesian equations of the straight line L passing through the point with position vector $\mathbf{a} = -3\mathbf{i} + 2\mathbf{j} + 7\mathbf{k}$ in the direction of the vector $\mathbf{b} = 2\mathbf{i} + 3\mathbf{j} + 5\mathbf{k}$.

Solution
As the vector equation of L is

$$\mathbf{r} = \mathbf{a} + \lambda \mathbf{b},$$

it follows at once that the Cartesian equations of L are

$$\frac{x + 3}{2} = \frac{y - 2}{3} = \frac{z - 7}{5}. \qquad\qquad \blacktriangle$$

Example 61.2

Find the position vector of a point on the line L and a vector along L given that its Cartesian equations are

$$\frac{3x + 1}{2} = \frac{y - 7}{3} = \frac{-2z + 1}{4}.$$

Solution
First we express the equations in standard form (we make the coefficients of x, y and z equal to 1), when they become

$$\frac{x + (1/3)}{2/3} = \frac{y - 7}{3} = \frac{z - (1/2)}{(-2)}.$$

Then equating each numerator to zero shows that the x, y and z coordinates of a point on L are $(-1/3, 7, 1/2)$. The denominators of each expression now determine the direction ratios of a vector parallel to L, which are seen to be $(2/3, 3, -2)$. Thus the position vector of a point on L is

$$\mathbf{a} = -\frac{1}{3}\mathbf{i} + 7\mathbf{j} + \frac{1}{2}\mathbf{k},$$

and a vector $\mathbf{b}$ along L is

$$\mathbf{b} = \frac{2}{3}\mathbf{i} + 3\mathbf{j} - 2\mathbf{k}. \qquad \blacktriangle$$

Example 61.3

Write down the vector equation of the straight line L with the Cartesian equations

$$\frac{-3x+1}{2} = \frac{z+7}{5}.$$

Solution
When expressed in standard form, the equations become

$$\frac{x-(1/3)}{(-2/3)} = \frac{z+7}{5}.$$

Thus, by inspection, as y is absent we see that a point on L has the coordinates $(1/3, 0, -7)$ and the direction ratios of a vector along the line are $(-2/3, 0, 5)$. Thus the position vector of a point on L is

$$\mathbf{a} = (1/3)\mathbf{i} - 7\mathbf{k}$$

and a vector along L is

$$\mathbf{b} = (-2/3)\mathbf{i} + 5\mathbf{k}.$$

Thus the vector equation of the line is

$$\mathbf{r} = (1/3)\mathbf{i} - 7\mathbf{k} + \lambda[(-2/3)\mathbf{i} + 5\mathbf{k}].$$

The component of the unit vector $\mathbf{j}$ is identically zero, so the line lies in the (x, z)-plane. $\qquad \blacktriangle$

Example 61.4

Find the Cartesian equations of the line L through the point $\mathbf{a} = \mathbf{i} - 2\mathbf{j} + \mathbf{k}$ in the direction of the vector $\mathbf{b} = -2\mathbf{j} + 3\mathbf{k}$.

Solution

$$\mathbf{r} = (\mathbf{i} - 2\mathbf{j} + \mathbf{k}) + \lambda(-2\mathbf{j} + 3\mathbf{k}),$$

so

$$\frac{x-1}{0} = \frac{y+2}{-2} = \frac{z-1}{3} \ (= \lambda).$$

The first quotient is only possible if $x \equiv 1$, so the Cartesian equations of the line L are

$$x \equiv 1, \quad 3y + 2z + 4 = 0,$$

showing that the line lies in the plane $x \equiv 1$. ▲

PROBLEMS 61

In problems 1 to 4 write the Cartesian equations of the line in standard form, and hence find the position vector **a** of a point on the line and a vector **b** parallel to the line.

1. $\dfrac{-4x + 1}{-3} = \dfrac{y + 3}{2} = \dfrac{z - 4}{1}$.

2. $\dfrac{3x + 7}{-9} = \dfrac{2y - 3}{4} = \dfrac{3z + 5}{-1}$.

3. $\dfrac{2x + 3}{2} = \dfrac{4z - 9}{-3}$.

4. $\dfrac{x + 9}{4} = \dfrac{y + 6}{2} = \dfrac{z - 16}{5}$.

5. Find the vector and Cartesian equations of the line L passing through the points $(1, 1, 1)$ and $(-2, -1, 3)$.

6. Given that the vector equation of a straight line L is

$$\mathbf{r} = \mathbf{a} + \lambda \mathbf{b}$$

where $\mathbf{a} = 2\mathbf{i} - \mathbf{j} + \mathbf{k}$ and $\mathbf{b} = 3\mathbf{i} + 2\mathbf{j} - 3\mathbf{k}$, find the points on L corresponding to $\lambda = -1$, $\lambda = 1$ and $\lambda = 2$.

7. Find the Cartesian equations of the straight line L which passes through the point $(1, 2, 3)$ and is parallel to the line joining the points $(2, 3, 1)$ and $(5, 4, 2)$.

8. Find the Cartesian equations of the straight line L which passes through the point $(3, -1, 2)$ and has the direction ratios $3 : 2 : -6$.

62   The scalar product (dot product)

The **scalar product** of two vectors **a** and **b** is a form of multiplication of two **vectors** which yields a **scalar** quantity.

Let **a** and **b** be any two vectors, and let θ be the angle between them when their initial points are brought into coincidence, with $0 \leqslant \theta \leqslant \pi$, as shown in Fig. 131. The **scalar product**, or **dot product** as it is also called, of **a** and **b** is written **a·b** and defined as

$$\mathbf{a \cdot b} = |\mathbf{a}|\,|\mathbf{b}|\,\cos\theta.$$

The definition shows that the scalar product is **commutative**, because

$$\mathbf{a \cdot b} = \mathbf{b \cdot a}.$$

It follows directly from the above definition that if **a** and **b** are **orthogonal** (perpendicular), $\theta = \pi/2$ and so

$$\mathbf{a \cdot b} = 0.$$

If, however, **a** and **b** are parallel ($\theta = 0$), then

$$\mathbf{a \cdot b} = |\mathbf{a}|\,|\mathbf{b}|$$

and, in particular,

$$\mathbf{a \cdot a} = \mathbf{a}^2 = |\mathbf{a}|^2.$$

If the line segments of two vectors **a** and **b** are parallel, but the senses (directions of the arrows) are opposite, the vectors are sometimes said to be **anti-parallel**. In this case $\theta = \pi$ and it follows that then

$$\mathbf{a \cdot b} = -|\mathbf{a}|\,|\mathbf{b}|.$$

It follows from these results that

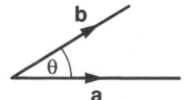

Fig. 131

$$\mathbf{i} \cdot \mathbf{i} = \mathbf{j} \cdot \mathbf{j} = \mathbf{k} \cdot \mathbf{k} = 1.$$

while

$$\mathbf{i} \cdot \mathbf{j} = \mathbf{j} \cdot \mathbf{i} = \mathbf{i} \cdot \mathbf{k} = \mathbf{k} \cdot \mathbf{i} = \mathbf{j} \cdot \mathbf{k} = \mathbf{k} \cdot \mathbf{j} = 0.$$

The scalar product also obeys the **distributive law**

$$\mathbf{a} \cdot (\mathbf{b} + \mathbf{c}) = \mathbf{a} \cdot \mathbf{b} + \mathbf{a} \cdot \mathbf{c}.$$

This last result is used to evaluate scalar products when **a** and **b** are given in their Cartesian form. If $\mathbf{a} = a_1\mathbf{i} + a_2\mathbf{j} + a_3\mathbf{k}$ and $\mathbf{b} = b_1\mathbf{i} + b_2\mathbf{j} + b_3\mathbf{k}$, we have

$$\mathbf{a} \cdot \mathbf{b} = (a_1\mathbf{i} + a_2\mathbf{j} + a_3\mathbf{k}) \cdot (b_1\mathbf{i} + b_2\mathbf{j} + b_3\mathbf{k}),$$

and an application of the distributive law coupled with the results for scalar products involving **i**, **j** and **k** gives the fundamental result

$$\mathbf{a} \cdot \mathbf{b} = a_1 b_1 + a_2 b_2 + a_3 b_3.$$

Equating the two definitions of $\mathbf{a} \cdot \mathbf{b}$ gives

$$|\mathbf{a}|\,|\mathbf{b}| \cos \theta = \mathbf{a} \cdot \mathbf{b},$$

so the angle θ between **a** and **b** follows from

$$\cos \theta = \frac{\mathbf{a} \cdot \mathbf{b}}{|\mathbf{a}|\,|\mathbf{b}|}.$$

This last result is seen to be equivalent to

$$\cos \theta = \hat{\mathbf{a}} \cdot \hat{\mathbf{b}},$$

so the cosine of the angle between **a** and **b** equals the scalar product of the unit vectors $\hat{\mathbf{a}}$ and $\hat{\mathbf{b}}$ along **a** and **b**, respectively.

Example 62.1

If $\mathbf{a} = \mathbf{i} + 2\mathbf{j} - \mathbf{k}$ and $\mathbf{b} = 3\mathbf{i} + \mathbf{j} + 2\mathbf{k}$ find $\mathbf{a} \cdot \mathbf{b}$ and the angle between **a** and **b**.

Solution
The scalar product

$$\mathbf{a} \cdot \mathbf{b} = (1)(3) + (2)(1) + (-1)(2) = 3.$$

As $|\mathbf{a}| = \sqrt{6}$ and $|\mathbf{b}| = \sqrt{14}$ if θ is the angle between **a** and **b**, then

$$\cos \theta = \frac{\mathbf{a} \cdot \mathbf{b}}{|\mathbf{a}|\,|\mathbf{b}|} = \frac{3}{\sqrt{6}\sqrt{14}} = \frac{3}{\sqrt{84}},$$

and so $\theta = 70.89°$ ▲

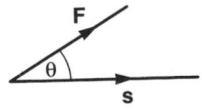

Fig. 132

The scalar product may be used to express the work W done when a force $\mathbf{F}$ moves its point of application a distance $|\mathbf{s}|$ in the direction of the unit vector $\hat{\mathbf{s}}$ along $\mathbf{s}$. We see from Fig. 132 that the work W is the product of the component of $\mathbf{F}$ along $\mathbf{s}$ with the actual displacement $|\mathbf{s}|$. Thus

$$W = |\mathbf{F}|\,|\mathbf{s}|\,\cos\theta = \mathbf{F}\cdot\mathbf{s}.$$

Example 62.2

Find the work done when a force of magnitude six force units in the direction $\mathbf{i}+\mathbf{j}+3\mathbf{k}$ moves its point of application a distance two length units parallel to $2\mathbf{i}-\mathbf{j}+\mathbf{k}$.

Solution
A unit vector $\hat{\mathbf{f}}$ parallel to $\mathbf{i}+\mathbf{j}+3\mathbf{k}$ is

$$\hat{\mathbf{f}} = \frac{1}{\sqrt{11}}\,(\mathbf{i}+\mathbf{j}+3\mathbf{k}),$$

while a unit vector $\hat{\mathbf{d}}$ parallel to $2\mathbf{i}-\mathbf{j}+\mathbf{k}$ is

$$\hat{\mathbf{d}} = \frac{1}{\sqrt{6}}\,(2\mathbf{i}-\mathbf{j}+\mathbf{k}).$$

If we let the unit vector $\hat{\mathbf{f}}$ represent a force of one unit, then a force $\mathbf{F}$ of six units is

$$\mathbf{F} = \frac{6}{\sqrt{11}}\,(\mathbf{i}+\mathbf{j}+3\mathbf{k}).$$

If $\hat{\mathbf{d}}$ represents a displacement of one unit in the direction $2\mathbf{i}-\mathbf{j}+\mathbf{k}$, a displacement $\mathbf{s}$ of two units in this direction is

$$\mathbf{s} = \frac{2}{\sqrt{6}}\,(2\mathbf{i}-\mathbf{j}+\mathbf{k}).$$

Thus the work W done by the force is

$$W = \mathbf{F}\cdot\mathbf{s} = \frac{6}{\sqrt{11}}\,(\mathbf{i}+\mathbf{j}+3\mathbf{k})\cdot\frac{2}{\sqrt{6}}\,(2\mathbf{i}-\mathbf{j}+\mathbf{k})$$

$$= \frac{12}{\sqrt{66}}\,[(1)(2)+(1)(-1)+(3)(1)] = \frac{48}{\sqrt{66}}\ \text{work units.} \qquad \blacktriangle$$

The effect of forming the scalar product of a vector $\mathbf{a}$ and an arbitrary unit vector $\hat{\mathbf{n}}$ is to give the projection of $\mathbf{a}$ in the direction of $\hat{\mathbf{n}}$, with the projection being non-negative if $0 \leqslant \theta < \pi/2$ and negative if $\pi/2 < \theta \leqslant \pi$. This follows from the fact that

$$\mathbf{a}\cdot\hat{\mathbf{n}} = |\mathbf{a}|\,|\hat{\mathbf{n}}|\,\cos\theta = |\mathbf{a}|\,\cos\theta.$$

The result is illustrated in Fig. 133, both for the case $0 \leqslant \theta \leqslant \pi/2$ and for $\pi/2 < \theta \leqslant \pi$. Notice that the projection is positive when $0 \leqslant \theta \leqslant \pi/2$ and negative when $\pi/2 < \theta < \pi$. If the length of the projection is required, then

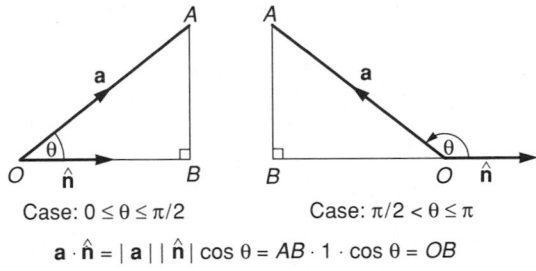

Case: $0 \le \theta \le \pi/2$ Case: $\pi/2 < \theta \le \pi$

$$\mathbf{a} \cdot \hat{\mathbf{n}} = |\mathbf{a}| |\hat{\mathbf{n}}| \cos \theta = AB \cdot 1 \cdot \cos \theta = OB$$

Fig. 133

since length is non-negative, it is necessary to take the absolute value of the scalar product.

Example 62.3

Given that $\mathbf{a} = \mathbf{i} + 4\mathbf{j} - \mathbf{k}$ and $\mathbf{b} = 2\mathbf{i} - 3\mathbf{j} + \mathbf{k}$ find
(i) the projection of $\mathbf{a}$ in the direction of $\mathbf{b}$; and
(ii) the projection of $\mathbf{b}$ in the direction of $\mathbf{a}$.

Solution
(i) To find the projection of $\mathbf{a}$ in the direction of $\mathbf{b}$ we must form the scalar product $\mathbf{a} \cdot \hat{\mathbf{b}}$. We have

$$\mathbf{a} \cdot \hat{\mathbf{b}} = (\mathbf{i} + 4\mathbf{j} - \mathbf{k}) \cdot \frac{1}{\sqrt{14}} (2\mathbf{i} - 3\mathbf{j} + \mathbf{k})$$

$$= \frac{-11}{\sqrt{14}}.$$

(ii) To find the projection of $\mathbf{b}$ in the direction of $\mathbf{a}$ we must form the scalar product $\hat{\mathbf{a}} \cdot \mathbf{b}$. We have

$$\hat{\mathbf{a}} \cdot \mathbf{b} = \frac{1}{\sqrt{18}} (\mathbf{i} + 4\mathbf{j} - \mathbf{k}) \cdot (2\mathbf{i} - 3\mathbf{j} + \mathbf{k}).$$

$$= \frac{-11}{\sqrt{18}}. \qquad\qquad \blacktriangle$$

PROBLEMS 62

1. Given $\mathbf{a} = \mathbf{i} + 3\mathbf{j} - \mathbf{k}$ and $\mathbf{b} = 2\mathbf{i} + \mathbf{j} - \mathbf{k}$ find $\mathbf{a} \cdot \mathbf{b}$ and the angle between the vectors.
2. Given $\mathbf{a} = 2\mathbf{i} - 2\mathbf{j} + \mathbf{k}$ and $\mathbf{b} = \mathbf{i} + 4\mathbf{j} - 3\mathbf{k}$ find $\mathbf{a} \cdot \mathbf{b}$ and the angle between the vectors.
3. Given $\mathbf{a} = 3\mathbf{i} + \mathbf{j} + 2\mathbf{k}$ and $\mathbf{b} = -6\mathbf{i} - 2\mathbf{j} + 4\mathbf{k}$ find $\mathbf{a} \cdot \mathbf{b}$ and the angle between the vectors.

4. Given $a = 3i - j + 2k$ and $b = 2i - 4j - k$ find $a \cdot b$ and the angle between the vectors.

5. Which pairs of the vectors **a**, **b**, **c** and **d** are orthogonal, given that

$$a = i - 3j - k, \quad b = 4i + 3j + k, \quad c = 2i + j - k, \quad d = 5i + 2j - k?$$

6. Given that $a = 5i + 3j - 4k$, $b = 2i + j - k$ and $c = i + 2j + 3k$, verify that

$$a \cdot (b + c) = a \cdot b + a \cdot c.$$

7. For what value of α will the vectors $a = 5i + 2j + 3k$ and $b = 2i + \alpha j + \alpha k$ be orthogonal?

8. Find the work done when a force of magnitude eight force units in the direction $i + j + k$ moves its point of application a distance five length units in the direction $2i - j + 3k$.

9. Given that $a = i + j + k$ and $b = 3i - 2j + 4k$, find (a) the projection of **a** in the direction of **b** and (b) the projection of **b** in the direction of **a**.

10. Given that $a = -4i + 2j + 2k$ and $b = 3i - 2j + k$, find (a) the length of the projection of **a** in the direction of **b** and (b) the length of the projection of **b** in the direction of **a**.

11. Find numbers n_1, n_2 and n_3 such that the vector $n = n_1 i + n_2 j + n_3 k$ is orthogonal to both $a = i - j + k$ and $b = 3i + 2j - 2k$.

The plane

A geometrical **plane** is characterized by the fact that a vector **N** which is perpendicular to it at any point is perpendicular to it at every other point. Such a vector **N** is called a **normal** to the plane, and apart from the arbitrariness of $|\mathbf{N}|$ it is unique apart from its sign (the normal can point to either side of the plane). A plane Π is completely determined once a point on the plane is specified together with a normal vector **N**.

To derive the vector and Cartesian equations of a plane let us consider Fig. 134 in which the plane Π contains the point A with position vector **a** and has a vector **N** as its normal.

If **r** is the position vector of an arbitrary point P on the plane Π, the vector $\underline{AP} = \mathbf{r} - \mathbf{a}$ is a vector in the plane. As **N** is normal to the plane Π, it must be orthogonal to any line in the plane, and hence orthogonal to $\underline{AP}$. Thus

$$(\mathbf{r} - \mathbf{a}) \cdot \mathbf{N} = 0,$$

which is the **vector equation** of the plane Π. If required, this can be rewritten in the form

$$\mathbf{r} \cdot \mathbf{N} = \mathbf{a} \cdot \mathbf{N}.$$

If $\mathbf{r} = x\mathbf{i} + y\mathbf{j} + z\mathbf{k}$, $\mathbf{a} = a_1\mathbf{i} + a_2\mathbf{j} + a_3\mathbf{k}$, and $\mathbf{N} = N_1\mathbf{i} + N_2\mathbf{j} + N_3\mathbf{k}$, the **Cartesian equation** of the plane Π is seen to be

$$N_1 x + N_2 y + N_3 z = N_1 a_1 + N_2 a_2 + N_3 a_3.$$

Inspection of this general expression shows that the coefficients N_1, N_2, N_3 are the **direction ratios** of a normal to the plane.

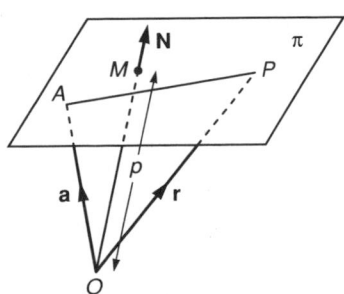

Fig. 134

Let us define a unit normal

$$\hat{\mathbf{n}} = \frac{\mathbf{N}}{|\mathbf{N}|},$$

then if the vector equation of the plane is divided by $|\mathbf{N}|$ it becomes

$$\mathbf{r} \cdot \hat{\mathbf{n}} = \mathbf{a} \cdot \hat{\mathbf{n}}.$$

Now $\mathbf{a} \cdot \hat{\mathbf{n}}$ is the **projection** of $\mathbf{a}$ in the direction of $\hat{\mathbf{n}}$, and from Fig. 134 this is seen to be OM, where M is the point on Π at which the normal from O cuts the plane. If we set $\mathbf{a} \cdot \hat{\mathbf{n}} = p$, it follows that p will be positive if M lies on the side of O towards which $\hat{\mathbf{n}}$ is directed, and it will be negative if it is on the opposite side. The perpendicular distance of the plane from O is the length OM (regarded as non-negative), so

$$OM = |\mathbf{a} \cdot \hat{\mathbf{n}}| = |p|.$$

Example 63.1

Find the Cartesian form of the equation of the plane through the point $(3, -2, 1)$ with a normal $\mathbf{N} = 4\mathbf{i} + 7\mathbf{j} - 4\mathbf{k}$. Determine the perpendicular distance of the plane from the origin.

Solution
In terms of the previous notation, $\mathbf{a} = 3\mathbf{i} - 2\mathbf{j} + \mathbf{k}$ and $\mathbf{N} = 4\mathbf{i} + 7\mathbf{j} - 4\mathbf{k}$, so the vector equation of the plane

$$\mathbf{r} \cdot \mathbf{N} = \mathbf{a} \cdot \mathbf{N}$$

becomes

$$(x\mathbf{i} + y\mathbf{j} + z\mathbf{k}) \cdot (4\mathbf{i} + 7\mathbf{j} - 4\mathbf{k}) = (3\mathbf{i} - 2\mathbf{j} + \mathbf{k}) \cdot (4\mathbf{i} + 7\mathbf{j} - 4\mathbf{k}).$$

When expanded this gives the Cartesian equation of the plane

$$4x + 7y - 4z = -6.$$

The perpendicular distance $\mathbf{d}$ of the plane from the origin is

$$d = \left| \mathbf{a} \cdot \frac{\mathbf{N}}{|\mathbf{N}|} \right|$$

$$= \left| (3\mathbf{i} - 2\mathbf{j} + \mathbf{k}) \cdot \frac{1}{9} (4\mathbf{i} + 7\mathbf{j} - 4\mathbf{k}) \right|$$

$$= \left| \frac{-6}{9} \right| = \frac{2}{3}. \qquad \blacktriangle$$

The **angle between two planes** is the angle between their normals. Thus if the planes have the vector equations

$$\mathbf{r} \cdot \mathbf{N}_1 = \mathbf{a}_1 \cdot \mathbf{N}_1 \quad \text{and} \quad \mathbf{r} \cdot \mathbf{N}_2 = \mathbf{a}_2 \cdot \mathbf{N}_2,$$

the angle θ between them is given by finding θ from the result

$$\cos \theta = \frac{\mathbf{N}_1 \cdot \mathbf{N}_2}{|\mathbf{N}_1| \, |\mathbf{N}_2|}.$$

Example 63.2

Find the angle between the planes

$$2x - 3y - 6z = 5 \quad \text{and} \quad 6x + 2y - 9z = 4.$$

Solution
The direction ratios of the normal $\mathbf{N}_1$ to the first plane are $2, -3, -6$, so

$$\mathbf{N}_1 = 2\mathbf{i} - 3\mathbf{j} - 6\mathbf{k}.$$

The direction ratios of the normal N_2 to the second plane are $6, 2, -9$, so

$$\mathbf{N}_2 = 6\mathbf{i} + 2\mathbf{j} - 9\mathbf{k}.$$

Thus the angle θ between the planes is such that

$$\cos \theta = \frac{\mathbf{N}_1 \cdot \mathbf{N}_2}{|\mathbf{N}_1| \, |\mathbf{N}_2|} = \frac{60}{\sqrt{49}\,\sqrt{121}} = \frac{60}{77},$$

so $\theta = 38.81°$.   ▲

The perpendicular distance between a point B in space with position vector $\mathbf{b}$ and the plane

$$\mathbf{r} \cdot \mathbf{N} = \mathbf{a} \cdot \mathbf{N}$$

is the perpendicular distance between this plane and a parallel plane through B (it will have the same normal $\mathbf{N}$).

In terms of the notation already introduced, after division by $|\mathbf{N}|$ to make $\mathbf{N}/|\mathbf{N}|$ a unit vector, the first plane becomes

$$\mathbf{r} \cdot \frac{\mathbf{N}}{|\mathbf{N}|} = p_1, \quad \text{with} \quad p_1 = \mathbf{a} \cdot \frac{\mathbf{N}}{|\mathbf{N}|},$$

correspondingly, the second parallel plane through B has the equation

$$\mathbf{r} \cdot \frac{\mathbf{N}}{|\mathbf{N}|} = p_2, \quad \text{with} \quad p_2 = \mathbf{b} \cdot \frac{\mathbf{N}}{|\mathbf{N}|},$$

where p_1 and p_2 are the projections of $\mathbf{a}$ and $\mathbf{b}$ in the direction of the unit vector $\mathbf{N}/|\mathbf{N}|$.
Thus the vector formula for the perpendicular distance d of point B from the plane is

$$d = |p_1 - p_2| = \frac{|\mathbf{a} \cdot \mathbf{N} - \mathbf{b} \cdot \mathbf{N}|}{|\mathbf{N}|}.$$

This result takes on a particularly simple form if the equation of the plane is expressed in Cartesian form. For if the plane has the equation

$$px + qy + rz = s,$$

and B is the point (x_0, y_0, z_0) so its position vector $\mathbf{b} = x_0\mathbf{i} + y_0\mathbf{j} + z_0\mathbf{k}$, we see that

$$\mathbf{N} = p\mathbf{i} + q\mathbf{j} + r\mathbf{k},$$

$$|\mathbf{N}| = (p^2 + q^2 + r^2)^{1/2},$$

$$\mathbf{a} \cdot \mathbf{N} = s$$

and

$$\mathbf{b} \cdot \mathbf{N} = px_0 + qy_0 + rz_0,$$

so the Cartesian formula for d is

$$d = \frac{|s - px_0 - qy_0 - rz_0|}{(p^2 + q^2 + r^2)^{1/2}} = \frac{|px_0 + qy_0 + rz_0 - s|}{(p^2 + q^2 + r^2)^{1/2}}.$$

Example 63.3

Find the distance d of the point $(2, -1, -4)$ from the plane

$$4x - 12y - 3z = 7$$

(i) using the vector formula for d; and
(ii) using the Cartesian formula.

Solution
(i) Inspection shows that

$$\mathbf{N} = 4\mathbf{i} - 12\mathbf{j} - 3\mathbf{k}, \quad |\mathbf{N}| = 13 \quad \text{and} \quad \mathbf{a} \cdot \mathbf{N} = 7.$$

Setting $\mathbf{b} = 2\mathbf{i} - \mathbf{j} - 4\mathbf{k}$ we find that $\mathbf{b} \cdot \mathbf{N} = 32$, so from the vector formula for d we have

$$d = \frac{|\mathbf{a} \cdot \mathbf{N} - \mathbf{b} \cdot \mathbf{N}|}{|\mathbf{N}|} = \frac{|7 - 32|}{13} = \frac{25}{13}.$$

(ii) Making the identifications $x_0 = 2, y_0 = -1, z_0 = -4, p = 4, q = -12, r = -3$ and $s = 7$ and substituting into the Cartesian formula for d gives

$$d = \frac{|7 - 32|}{13} = \frac{25}{13}. \qquad\qquad \blacktriangle$$

PROBLEMS 63

1. Find the Cartesian equation of the plane with normal $3\mathbf{i} + \mathbf{j} + 2\mathbf{k}$ which contains the point $(1, 1, 1)$.
2. Find the Cartesian equation of the plane with normal $7\mathbf{i} - \mathbf{j} + 3\mathbf{k}$ which contains the point $(1, 2, -1)$.
3. Find the Cartesian equation of the plane with normal $3\mathbf{i} + 6\mathbf{j} - 4\mathbf{k}$ which contains the point at the origin.

4. Find the angle between the two planes with the equations $2x - y + x = 4$ and $x + 4y + 3z = 1$.
5. Find a vector $\mathbf{N}$ which is normal to the plane

$$4x - 2y + 5z = 4.$$

What is the perpendicular distance d of this plane from the origin?
6. Find a unit vector $\hat{\mathbf{n}}$ which is normal to the plane

$$3x + 4y - 2z = 0.$$

What is the perpendicular distance d of this plane from the origin?
7. Find the perpendicular distance d of the point $(2, 1, -3)$ from the plane with normal $\mathbf{i} + 2\mathbf{j} + \mathbf{k}$ which passes through the point $(1, 1, -1)$.
8. Find the equation of the plane through the point $(2, 3, -1)$ normal to the line joining this point to the origin.
9. Find the distances of the point $(2, 3, -5)$ and the origin from the plane

$$x + 2y - 2z = 9.$$

Are these two points on the same side of the plane?

64 The vector product (cross product)

The **vector product**, or **cross product**, is a form of multiplication of two vectors which yields a vector. The vector product of the two vectors **a** and **b**, written **a** $\times$ **b** is defined as the vector

$$\mathbf{a} \times \mathbf{b} = |\mathbf{a}| \ |\mathbf{b}| \sin\theta \ \hat{\mathbf{n}},$$

where θ is the angle between **a** and **b** when their initial points are brought into coincidence, and $\hat{\mathbf{n}}$ is a unit vector perpendicular to both **a** and **b** pointing in the direction in which a right-handed screw would advance if rotated from **a** to **b**. The situation is illustrated in Fig. 135.

Notice that the definition of a vector product implies that

$$\mathbf{a} \times \mathbf{b} = -\mathbf{b} \times \mathbf{a},$$

so the vector product is not commutative.

Inspection of Fig. 135 shows that the area of the parallelogram $OAPB$ (the product of the base of length $|\mathbf{a}|$ and the height $|\mathbf{b}| \sin\theta$) is $S = |\mathbf{a}| \ |\mathbf{b}| \sin\theta$, so $S = |\mathbf{a} \times \mathbf{b}|$.

If the vectors **a** and **b** are parallel, $\theta = 0$ and $\mathbf{a} \times \mathbf{b} = 0$ so that, in particular,

$$\mathbf{a} \times \mathbf{a} = \mathbf{0}.$$

If, however, **a** and **b** are orthogonal, $\theta = \pi/2$ and then

$$|\mathbf{a} \times \mathbf{b}| = |\mathbf{a}| \ |\mathbf{b}|.$$

Important particular cases of these last results are

$$\mathbf{i} \times \mathbf{j} = \mathbf{k} \quad \text{and} \quad \mathbf{j} \times \mathbf{i} = -\mathbf{k}$$
$$\mathbf{j} \times \mathbf{k} = \mathbf{i} \quad \text{and} \quad \mathbf{k} \times \mathbf{j} = -\mathbf{i}$$

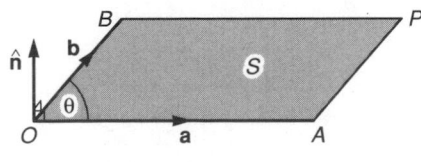

Fig. 135

$$\mathbf{k} \times \mathbf{i} = \mathbf{j} \quad \text{and} \quad \mathbf{i} \times \mathbf{k} = -\mathbf{j},$$

while

$$\mathbf{i} \times \mathbf{i} = \mathbf{j} \times \mathbf{j} = \mathbf{k} \times \mathbf{k} = \mathbf{0}.$$

It is easily shown that the **distributive law** applies to the vector product, so that

$$\mathbf{a} \times (\mathbf{b} + \mathbf{c}) = \mathbf{a} \times \mathbf{b} + \mathbf{a} \times \mathbf{c},$$

from which we can deduce the result of a vector product in Cartesian form. If $\mathbf{a} = a_1\mathbf{i} + a_2\mathbf{j} + a_3\mathbf{k}$ and $\mathbf{b} = b_1\mathbf{i} + b_2\mathbf{j} + b_3\mathbf{k}$, then after applying the above results and collecting terms we have

$$\mathbf{a} \times \mathbf{b} = (a_1\mathbf{i} + a_2\mathbf{j} + a_3\mathbf{k}) \times (b_1\mathbf{i} + b_2\mathbf{j} + b_3\mathbf{k})$$

$$= (a_2 b_3 - a_3 a_2)\mathbf{i} + (a_3 b_1 - a_1 b_3)\mathbf{j} + (a_1 b_2 - a_2 b_1)\mathbf{k}.$$

This last result is seen to be equivalent to the easily remembered result

$$\mathbf{a} \times \mathbf{b} = \begin{vmatrix} \mathbf{i} & \mathbf{j} & \mathbf{k} \\ a_1 & a_2 & a_3 \\ b_1 & b_2 & b_3 \end{vmatrix},$$

where the determinant is to be expanded in terms of the elements $\mathbf{i}$, $\mathbf{j}$ and $\mathbf{k}$ of its first row. Notice that in this form the components of the first vector in the vector product form the first row to follow $\mathbf{i}$, $\mathbf{j}$ and $\mathbf{k}$, while the components of the second vector in the vector product form the last row.

Example 64.1

Find $\mathbf{a} \times \mathbf{b}$ given that $\mathbf{a} = \mathbf{i} + 2\mathbf{j} - \mathbf{k}$ and $\mathbf{b} = 2\mathbf{i} - \mathbf{j} + \mathbf{k}$.

Solution

$$\mathbf{a} \times \mathbf{b} = \begin{vmatrix} \mathbf{i} & \mathbf{j} & \mathbf{k} \\ 1 & 2 & -1 \\ 2 & -1 & 1 \end{vmatrix}$$

$$= \begin{vmatrix} 2 & -1 \\ -2 & 1 \end{vmatrix}\mathbf{i} + \begin{vmatrix} 1 & -1 \\ 2 & 1 \end{vmatrix}\mathbf{j} + \begin{vmatrix} 1 & 2 \\ 2 & -1 \end{vmatrix}\mathbf{k}$$

$$= \mathbf{i} - 3\mathbf{j} - 5\mathbf{k}. \qquad \blacktriangle$$

Example 64.2

Find a unit vector $\hat{\mathbf{n}}$ perpendicular to both $\mathbf{a} = 3\mathbf{i} + \mathbf{j} - \mathbf{k}$ and $\mathbf{b} = 2\mathbf{i} - 2\mathbf{k}$.

Solution
By definition, a vector (not necessarily a unit vector) perpendicular to both $\mathbf{a}$ and $\mathbf{b}$ is the vector $\mathbf{n} = \mathbf{a} \times \mathbf{b}$. Thus a unit vector perpendicular to both $\mathbf{a}$ and $\mathbf{b}$ is

$$\hat{\mathbf{n}} = \frac{\mathbf{a} \times \mathbf{b}}{|\mathbf{a} \times \mathbf{b}|} \, .$$

In this case $\mathbf{a} = 3\mathbf{i} + \mathbf{j} - \mathbf{k}$ and $\mathbf{b} = 2\mathbf{i} - 2\mathbf{k}$, so

$$\mathbf{a} \times \mathbf{b} = \begin{vmatrix} \mathbf{i} & \mathbf{j} & \mathbf{k} \\ 3 & 1 & -1 \\ 2 & 0 & -2 \end{vmatrix}$$

$$= \begin{vmatrix} 1 & -1 \\ 0 & -2 \end{vmatrix} \mathbf{i} + \begin{vmatrix} 3 & -1 \\ 2 & -2 \end{vmatrix} \mathbf{j} + \begin{vmatrix} 3 & 1 \\ 2 & 0 \end{vmatrix} \mathbf{k}$$

$$= -2\mathbf{i} + 4\mathbf{j} - 2\mathbf{k}.$$

Thus

$$|\mathbf{a} \times \mathbf{b}| = [(-2)^2 + 4^2 + (-2)^2]^{1/2} = \sqrt{24},$$

and so

$$\hat{\mathbf{n}} = \frac{1}{\sqrt{24}} (-2\mathbf{i} + 4\mathbf{j} - 2\mathbf{k})$$

$$= \frac{1}{\sqrt{6}} (-\mathbf{i} + 2\mathbf{j} - \mathbf{k}). \qquad \blacktriangle$$

The scalar and vector products can be combined in certain ways to form **triple products** of different types. As $\mathbf{a} \cdot \mathbf{b}$ is a scalar, no further vector operations can be performed on it, but $\mathbf{a} \times \mathbf{b}$ is a vector, so it may either be combined with a third vector $\mathbf{c}$ to form a scalar product or a vector product.

The **triple scalar product** $(\mathbf{a} \times \mathbf{b}) \cdot \mathbf{c}$ is a scalar which has a simple geometrical interpretation, as may be seen from Fig. 136.

The parallelepiped shown is formed from the vectors $\mathbf{a}$, $\mathbf{b}$ and $\mathbf{c}$ involved in a triple scalar product. We have already seen that the area S of the parallelogram $OAFB$ is given by

$$S = |\mathbf{a} \times \mathbf{b}|.$$

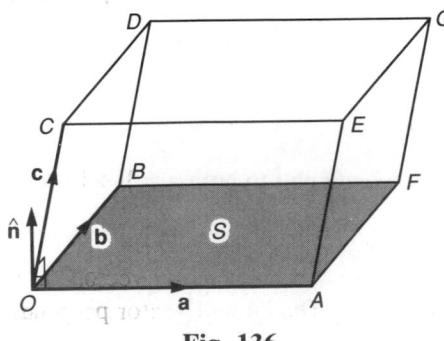

Fig. 136

The scalar product $\hat{\mathbf{n}} \cdot \mathbf{c}$ is the projection of $\mathbf{c}$ in the direction of $\hat{\mathbf{n}}$, so that $|\hat{\mathbf{n}} \cdot \mathbf{c}|$ is the height of the parallelepiped. Thus if we consider the triple scalar product $(\mathbf{a} \times \mathbf{b}) \cdot \mathbf{c}$ we see that

$$|(\mathbf{a} \times \mathbf{b}) \cdot \mathbf{c}| = V$$

is the volume of the parallelepiped. This result provides a useful test by which to establish if the vectors $\mathbf{a}$, $\mathbf{b}$ and $\mathbf{c}$ are coplanar (all in the same plane). If they are coplanar then $V = 0$, otherwise $V \neq 0$.

The volume V is independent of the manner in which it is calculated, so by using different faces of the parallelepiped as base we see that

$$\mathbf{a} \cdot (\mathbf{b} \times \mathbf{c}) = \mathbf{b} \cdot (\mathbf{c} \times \mathbf{a}) = \mathbf{c} \cdot (\mathbf{a} \times \mathbf{b}).$$

Furthermore, since the scalar product is commutative it follows that

$$(\mathbf{b} \times \mathbf{c}) \cdot \mathbf{a} = (\mathbf{c} \times \mathbf{a}) \cdot \mathbf{b} = (\mathbf{a} \times \mathbf{b}) \cdot \mathbf{c},$$

but interchanging the order of the vectors in the vector product will change the sign of the triple scalar product.

When expressed in component form, since

$$\mathbf{a} \times \mathbf{b} = (a_2 b_3 - a_3 b_2)\mathbf{i} + (a_3 b_1 - a_1 b_3)\mathbf{j} + (a_1 b_2 - a_2 b_1)\mathbf{k},$$

the triple scalar product $(\mathbf{a} \times \mathbf{b}) \cdot \mathbf{c}$ with $\mathbf{c} = c_1 \mathbf{i} + c_2 \mathbf{j} + c_3 \mathbf{k}$ is

$$(\mathbf{a} \times \mathbf{b}) \cdot \mathbf{c} = (a_2 b_3 - a_3 b_2) c_1 + (a_3 b_1 - a_1 b_3) c_2 + (a_1 b_2 - a_2 b_1) c_3,$$

which is simply

$$(\mathbf{a} \times \mathbf{b}) \cdot \mathbf{c} = \begin{vmatrix} a_1 & a_2 & a_3 \\ b_1 & b_2 & b_3 \\ c_1 & c_2 & c_3 \end{vmatrix}.$$

Notice that the order of the rows of the determinant is the same as the order of the vectors $\mathbf{a}$, $\mathbf{b}$ and $\mathbf{c}$ in the triple scalar product. In a triple scalar product the $\cdot$ and $\times$ may be interchanged without altering the result, but the order of the vectors must not be changed.

Example 64.3

Find $(\mathbf{a} \times \mathbf{b}) \cdot \mathbf{c}$, given that $\mathbf{a} = \mathbf{i} - 2\mathbf{j}$, $\mathbf{b} = 3\mathbf{j} + \mathbf{k}$ and $\mathbf{c} = \mathbf{i} + \mathbf{j} - \mathbf{k}$.

Solution

$$(\mathbf{a} \times \mathbf{b}) \cdot \mathbf{c} = \begin{vmatrix} 1 & -2 & 0 \\ 0 & 3 & 1 \\ 1 & 1 & -1 \end{vmatrix} = -6. \qquad \blacktriangle$$

Example 64.4

Prove that the vectors $\mathbf{a} = \mathbf{i} - 2\mathbf{j} + \mathbf{k}$, $\mathbf{b} = 2\mathbf{i} + 5\mathbf{j} - 3\mathbf{k}$ and $\mathbf{c} = 4\mathbf{i} + \mathbf{j} - \mathbf{k}$ are coplanar.

Solution

$$(\mathbf{a} \times \mathbf{b}) \cdot \mathbf{c} = \begin{vmatrix} 1 & -2 & 1 \\ 2 & 5 & -3 \\ 4 & 1 & -1 \end{vmatrix} = 0,$$

so **a**, **b** and **c** are coplanar. ▲

The **triple vector product** $(\mathbf{a} \times \mathbf{b}) \times \mathbf{c}$ is a vector perpendicular to both **c** and $\mathbf{a} \times \mathbf{b}$, and so lies in the plane of **a** and **b**. A routine calculation establishes the basic result that

$$(\mathbf{a} \times \mathbf{b}) \times \mathbf{c} = (\mathbf{a} \cdot \mathbf{c})\mathbf{b} - (\mathbf{b} \cdot \mathbf{c})\mathbf{a}.$$

The order and the brackets in a triple vector product must not be changed, for to do so will alter the result.

If **c** is normal to the plane of **a** and **b** then $(\mathbf{a} \times \mathbf{b}) \times \mathbf{c} = 0$. This result may be used as a test to determine whether **c** is perpendicular to the vectors **a** and **b**.

Example 64.5

Find $(\mathbf{a} \times \mathbf{b}) \times \mathbf{c}$ and $\mathbf{a} \times (\mathbf{b} \times \mathbf{c})$, given that $\mathbf{a} = \mathbf{i} + 2\mathbf{j} - \mathbf{k}, \mathbf{b} = 2\mathbf{i} - \mathbf{j} - \mathbf{k}$ and $\mathbf{c} = \mathbf{i} + 3\mathbf{j} + 2\mathbf{k}$.

Solution

$$(\mathbf{a} \times \mathbf{b}) \times \mathbf{c} = (\mathbf{a} \cdot \mathbf{c})\mathbf{b} - (\mathbf{b} \cdot \mathbf{c})\mathbf{a}.$$
$$= 5\mathbf{b} + 3\mathbf{a}$$
$$= 13\mathbf{i} + \mathbf{j} - 8\mathbf{k}.$$
$$\mathbf{a} \times (\mathbf{b} \times \mathbf{c}) = -(\mathbf{b} \times \mathbf{c}) \times \mathbf{a}$$
$$= -[(\mathbf{b} \cdot \mathbf{a})\mathbf{c} - (\mathbf{c} \cdot \mathbf{a})\mathbf{b}]$$
$$= -\mathbf{c} + 5\mathbf{b}$$
$$= 9\mathbf{i} - 8\mathbf{j} - 7\mathbf{k}. \qquad ▲$$

Example 64.6

Which of the vectors **c** and **d** is orthogonal to both of the vectors **a** and **b**, given that

$$\mathbf{a} = \mathbf{i} + \mathbf{j} + \mathbf{k}, \quad \mathbf{b} = -\mathbf{i} + 2\mathbf{j} - \mathbf{k},$$
$$\mathbf{c} = \mathbf{j}, \quad \text{and} \quad \mathbf{d} = \mathbf{i} - \mathbf{k} ?$$

Solution

We may use the triple vector product as a test, because if **r** is orthogonal to both **p** and **q**, then $(\mathbf{p} \times \mathbf{q}) \times \mathbf{r} = 0$.

$$(\mathbf{a} \times \mathbf{b}) \times \mathbf{c} = (\mathbf{a} \cdot \mathbf{c})\mathbf{b} - (\mathbf{b} \cdot \mathbf{c})\mathbf{a}$$

$$= \mathbf{b} - 2\mathbf{a} = -3\mathbf{i} + 3\mathbf{k} \neq \mathbf{0},$$

so **c** is not orthogonal to both **a** and **b**.

$$(\mathbf{a} \times \mathbf{b}) \times \mathbf{d} = (\mathbf{a} \cdot \mathbf{d})\mathbf{b} - (\mathbf{b} \cdot \mathbf{d})\mathbf{a}$$

$$= 0\mathbf{b} - 0\mathbf{a} = \mathbf{0},$$

so **d** is orthogonal to both **a** and **b**.   ▲

PROBLEMS 64

1. Find $\mathbf{a} \times \mathbf{b}$, $\mathbf{a} \times \mathbf{c}$ and $\mathbf{b} \times \mathbf{c}$ given that $\mathbf{a} = 2\mathbf{i} - \mathbf{j} - \mathbf{k}$, $\mathbf{b} = 3\mathbf{i} + 2\mathbf{j} + 2\mathbf{k}$ and $\mathbf{c} = \mathbf{i} + \mathbf{j} - \mathbf{k}$.
2. Find $\mathbf{u} = \mathbf{a} \times \mathbf{b}$, $\mathbf{v} = \mathbf{b} \times \mathbf{c}$ and $\mathbf{u} \times \mathbf{v}$ given that $\mathbf{a} = 3\mathbf{i} + \mathbf{j} + \mathbf{k}$, $\mathbf{b} = \mathbf{i} + 2\mathbf{j} + 2\mathbf{k}$ and $\mathbf{c} = -\mathbf{i} + 3\mathbf{j} - \mathbf{k}$.
3. Find the area of the parallelogram with two adjacent sides $\mathbf{a} = 4\mathbf{i} - \mathbf{j} + 2\mathbf{k}$ and $\mathbf{b} = 3\mathbf{i} + \mathbf{j} + 4\mathbf{k}$.
4. Find the area of the parallelogram with two adjacent sides $\mathbf{a} = \mathbf{i} + \mathbf{j} + 4\mathbf{k}$ and $\mathbf{b} = -6\mathbf{i} + 2\mathbf{j} - 4\mathbf{k}$.
5. Verify the distributive law

$$\mathbf{a} \times (\mathbf{b} + \mathbf{c}) = \mathbf{a} \times \mathbf{b} + \mathbf{a} \times \mathbf{c},$$

given that $\mathbf{a} = 3\mathbf{i} + 2\mathbf{j} - \mathbf{k}$, $\mathbf{b} = \mathbf{i} + 2\mathbf{j} - 3\mathbf{k}$ and $\mathbf{c} = \mathbf{i} - 7\mathbf{j} + 3\mathbf{k}$.
6. Find a unit vector normal to $\mathbf{a} = 2\mathbf{i} - \mathbf{j} + 4\mathbf{k}$ and $\mathbf{b} = \mathbf{i} + 3\mathbf{j} + 2\mathbf{k}$.
7. Find $\mathbf{a} \cdot (\mathbf{b} \times \mathbf{c})$ given that $\mathbf{a} = \mathbf{i} + 3\mathbf{j} + 4\mathbf{k}$, $\mathbf{b} = 2\mathbf{i} - \mathbf{j} - 4\mathbf{k}$ and $\mathbf{c} = 3\mathbf{i} + 2\mathbf{j} + 3\mathbf{k}$.
8. Find $\mathbf{b} \cdot (\mathbf{c} \times \mathbf{a})$ given that $\mathbf{a} = 2\mathbf{i} + 2\mathbf{j} - \mathbf{k}$, $\mathbf{b} = \mathbf{i} - 2\mathbf{j} + 3\mathbf{k}$ and $\mathbf{c} = 3\mathbf{i} - \mathbf{k}$.
9. Given that $\mathbf{a} = 2\mathbf{i} - 2\mathbf{j} + 3\mathbf{k}$ and $\mathbf{b} = \mathbf{i} + \mathbf{j} + 4\mathbf{k}$, find the number α such that $\mathbf{c} = \mathbf{i} - \mathbf{j} + \alpha\mathbf{k}$ is coplanar with **a** and **b**.
10. Find $(\mathbf{a} \times \mathbf{b}) \times \mathbf{c}$ and $\mathbf{a} \times (\mathbf{b} \times \mathbf{c})$ given that $\mathbf{a} = \mathbf{i} + 2\mathbf{j} + 4\mathbf{k}$, and $\mathbf{b} = \mathbf{i} - 6\mathbf{k}$ and $\mathbf{c} = 2\mathbf{i} + 3\mathbf{j} + \mathbf{k}$.
11. Find $(\mathbf{a} \times \mathbf{b}) \times \mathbf{c}$ and $\mathbf{a} \times (\mathbf{b} \times \mathbf{c})$, given that $\mathbf{a} = \mathbf{i} + \mathbf{j} + \mathbf{k}$, $\mathbf{b} = \mathbf{i} - \mathbf{j} - 2\mathbf{k}$ and $\mathbf{c} = \mathbf{i} - \mathbf{j} + \mathbf{k}$.
12. Find α such that the vector $\mathbf{c} = -8\mathbf{i} + \alpha\mathbf{j} + 6\mathbf{k}$ is orthogonal to both $\mathbf{a} = \mathbf{i} + \mathbf{j} + \mathbf{k}$ and $\mathbf{b} = \mathbf{i} - 2\mathbf{j} + 2\mathbf{k}$.
13. Consider Fig. 137, and justify the result that

$$\mathbf{a} + \mathbf{b} + \mathbf{c} = \mathbf{0}.$$

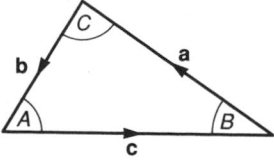

Fig 137

By forming the vector product of this result first with **a** and then with **b**, prove the **sine rule**

$$\frac{\sin A}{a} = \frac{\sin B}{b} = \frac{\sin C}{c},$$

where $a = |\mathbf{a}|$, $b = |\mathbf{b}|$ and $c = |\mathbf{c}|$.

14. If vectors **a**, **b** and **c** are such that

$$\mathbf{a} + \mathbf{b} + \mathbf{c} = \mathbf{0},$$

form the triple scalar product $(\mathbf{a} \times \mathbf{b}) \cdot \mathbf{c}$ and hence show that **c** is orthogonal to both **a** and **b**.

Applications of the vector product   **65**

THE ANGLE BETWEEN TWO VECTORS

If θ is the angle between vectors **a** and **b**, as shown in Fig. 135, it follows from the definition of the vector product that

$$\sin \theta = \frac{|\mathbf{a} \times \mathbf{b}|}{|\mathbf{a}| \, |\mathbf{b}|}.$$

This result is less convenient to use than the one used so far, namely,

$$\cos \theta = \frac{\mathbf{a} \cdot \mathbf{b}}{|\mathbf{a}| \, |\mathbf{b}|},$$

since the scalar product $\mathbf{a} \cdot \mathbf{b}$ is easier to evaluate than the vector product $\mathbf{a} \times \mathbf{b}$.

Example 65.1

Use the vector product to find the angle between $\mathbf{a} = \mathbf{i} + 2\mathbf{j} - 2\mathbf{k}$ and $\mathbf{b} = 2\mathbf{i} - 2\mathbf{j} + \mathbf{k}$.

Solution

$|\mathbf{a}| = 3, |\mathbf{b}| = 3$ and $\mathbf{a} \times \mathbf{b} = \begin{vmatrix} \mathbf{i} & \mathbf{j} & \mathbf{k} \\ 1 & 2 & -2 \\ 2 & -2 & 1 \end{vmatrix} = -2\mathbf{i} - 5\mathbf{j} - 6\mathbf{k}$, so $|\mathbf{a} \times \mathbf{b}| = \sqrt{65}$. Thus we have

$$\sin \theta = \frac{|\mathbf{a} \times \mathbf{b}|}{|\mathbf{a}| \, |\mathbf{b}|} = \frac{\sqrt{65}}{9},$$

and thus

$$\theta = 0.4606 \, \text{rad} \ (26.39°). \qquad \blacktriangle$$

A PLANE THROUGH THREE POINTS

Instead of specifying a plane as in Section 63, by giving a point in the plane and a vector **m** normal to the plane, it may equally well be specified by giving three points in the plane which are not collinear (not in a straight line). Let **a**, **b** and **c** be the position vectors of three such points A, B and C. Then $\mathbf{a} - \mathbf{b}$ and $\mathbf{a} - \mathbf{c}$ are vectors in the plane containing A, B and C. Thus the vector

$$\mathbf{m} = (\mathbf{a} - \mathbf{b}) \times (\mathbf{a} - \mathbf{c})$$

is normal to the plane, and as **a** is the position vector of a point in the plane it follows from Section 63 that the vector equation of the plane is

$$(\mathbf{r} - \mathbf{a}) \cdot \mathbf{m} = 0.$$

Example 65.2

Find the vector and Cartesian equations of the plane through the points $A(2, 4, 7)$, $B(1, 1, 2)$ and $C(1, 0, -1)$.

Solution
Set $\mathbf{a} = 2\mathbf{i} + 4\mathbf{j} + 7\mathbf{k}$, $\mathbf{b} = \mathbf{i} + \mathbf{j} + 2\mathbf{k}$ and $\mathbf{c} = \mathbf{i} - \mathbf{k}$. Then $\mathbf{a} - \mathbf{b} = \mathbf{i} + 3\mathbf{j} + 5\mathbf{k}$, $\mathbf{a} - \mathbf{c} = \mathbf{i} + 4\mathbf{j} + 8\mathbf{k}$ and

$$\mathbf{m} = (\mathbf{a} - \mathbf{b}) \times (\mathbf{a} - \mathbf{c}) = \begin{vmatrix} \mathbf{i} & \mathbf{j} & \mathbf{k} \\ 1 & 3 & 5 \\ 1 & 4 & 8 \end{vmatrix} = 4\mathbf{i} - 3\mathbf{j} + \mathbf{k}.$$

Thus the vector equation of the plane is

$$(\mathbf{r} - \mathbf{a}) \cdot \mathbf{m} = 0,$$

with $\mathbf{a} = 2\mathbf{i} + 4\mathbf{j} + 7\mathbf{k}$ and $\mathbf{m} = 4\mathbf{i} - 3\mathbf{j} + \mathbf{k}$. When expanded, this shows the Cartesian equation to be

$$4x - 3y + z = 3.$$

We could equally well have chosen **b** or **c** to be the given point on the plane, when we would have obtained the respective vector equations

$$(\mathbf{r} - \mathbf{b}) \cdot \mathbf{m} = 0 \quad \text{and} \quad (\mathbf{r} - \mathbf{c}) \cdot \mathbf{m} = 0.$$

Both of these results are equivalent to $(\mathbf{r} - \mathbf{a}) \cdot \mathbf{m} = 0$, and they yield the same Cartesian equation (check this)

$$4x - 3y + z = 3. \qquad \blacktriangle$$

THE LINE OF INTERSECTION OF TWO PLANES

Let the two planes be

$$\mathbf{n}_1 \cdot \mathbf{r} = p_1 \quad \text{and} \quad \mathbf{n}_2 \cdot \mathbf{r} = p_2.$$

Then the **line of intersection** L of the two planes will be perpendicular to both $\mathbf{n}_1$ and $\mathbf{n}_2$, and so will be in the direction $\mathbf{n}_1 \times \mathbf{n}_2$.

If the position vector of a point on the line is $\mathbf{a}$, the vector equation of the line will be

$$\mathbf{r} = \mathbf{a} + \lambda\, \mathbf{n}_1 \times \mathbf{n}_2.$$

As L lies on both planes it follows that

$$\mathbf{n}_1 \cdot (\mathbf{a} + \lambda\, \mathbf{n}_1 \times \mathbf{n}_2) = p_1$$

and

$$\mathbf{n}_2 \cdot (\mathbf{a} + \lambda\, \mathbf{n}_1 \times \mathbf{n}_2) = p_2,$$

but

$$\mathbf{n}_1 \cdot (\mathbf{n}_1 \times \mathbf{n}_2) = \mathbf{n}_2 \cdot (\mathbf{n}_1 \times \mathbf{n}_2) = 0,$$

and so

$$\mathbf{n}_1 \cdot \mathbf{a} = p_1 \quad \text{and} \quad \mathbf{n}_2 \cdot \mathbf{a} = p_2.$$

Setting $\mathbf{n}_1 = n_1^{(1)}\mathbf{i} + n_2^{(1)}\mathbf{j} + n_3^{(1)}\mathbf{k}$, $\mathbf{n}_2 = n_1^{(2)}\mathbf{i} + n_2^{(2)}\mathbf{j} + n_3^{(2)}\mathbf{k}$ and $\mathbf{a} = a_1\mathbf{i} + a_2\mathbf{j} + a_3\mathbf{k}$, the above two equations reduce to

$$n_1^{(1)}a_1 + n_2^{(1)}a_2 + n_3^{(1)}a_3 = p_1$$

and

$$n_1^{(2)}a_1 + n_2^{(2)}a_2 + n_3^{(2)}a_3 = p_2.$$

These are two equations for the three coordinates a_1, a_2 and a_3 of the point on line L with position vector $\mathbf{a}$. If one of the three coordinates is allocated an arbitrary numerical value, the two equations may then be solved for the other two coordinates, and the position vector $\mathbf{a}$ is then known. It is simplest to set $a_3 = 0$ and to solve for a_1 and a_2 using the equations

$$n_1^{(1)}a_1 + n_2^{(1)}a_2 = p_1$$
$$n_1^{(2)}a_1 + n_2^{(2)}a_2 = p_2.$$

The equation of the line of intersection L then becomes

$$\mathbf{r} = a_1\mathbf{i} + a_2\mathbf{j} + \lambda\, (\mathbf{n}_1 \times \mathbf{n}_2).$$

Example 65.3

Find the line of intersection of the planes

$$x + 2y - z = 3 \quad \text{and} \quad 2x + y + 2z = 0,$$

and the angle between the two planes.

Solution
The normal $\mathbf{n}_1$ to the first plane is

$$\mathbf{n}_1 = \mathbf{i} + 2\mathbf{j} - \mathbf{k},$$

and the normal $\mathbf{n}_2$ to the second plane is

$$\mathbf{n}_2 = 2\mathbf{i} + \mathbf{j} + 2\mathbf{k},$$

while $p_1 = 3$ and $p_2 = 0$.

Thus, setting $a_3 = 0$, it follows that a_1 and a_2 must satisfy

$$a_1 + 2a_2 = 3$$

$$2a_1 + a_2 = 0,$$

and so $a_1 = -1$ and $a_2 = 2$.

$$\mathbf{n}_1 \times \mathbf{n}_2 = \begin{vmatrix} \mathbf{i} & \mathbf{j} & \mathbf{k} \\ 1 & 2 & -1 \\ 2 & 1 & 2 \end{vmatrix} = 5\mathbf{i} - 4\mathbf{j} - 3\mathbf{k}.$$

Thus the vector equation of the line of intersection is

$$\mathbf{r} = -\mathbf{i} + 2\mathbf{j} + \lambda(5\mathbf{i} - 4\mathbf{j} - 3\mathbf{k}),$$

so the Cartesian equations of the line are

$$\frac{x+1}{5} = \frac{y-2}{-4} = \frac{z}{-3} \, (= \lambda).$$

The angle θ between the planes is the angle between their normals $\mathbf{n}_1$ and $\mathbf{n}_2$, so θ is determined by solving

$$\cos \theta = \frac{\mathbf{n}_1 \cdot \mathbf{n}_2}{|\mathbf{n}_2| \, |\mathbf{n}_2|} = \frac{2}{3\sqrt{6}},$$

so $\theta = 74.21°$. ▲

THE PERPENDICULAR DISTANCE FROM A POINT TO A STRAIGHT LINE

Consider a straight line L through point A with position vector $\mathbf{a}$ and parallel to the vector $\mathbf{b}$, as shown in Fig. 138. Let a point C in space have the position vector $\mathbf{c}$, and let d be the perpendicular distance from C to L.

We see from Fig. 138 that $\underline{AC} = \mathbf{c} - \mathbf{a}$, and

$$|\mathbf{b} \times (\mathbf{c} - \mathbf{a})| = |\mathbf{b}| \, |\mathbf{c} - \mathbf{a}| \sin \theta$$

$$= |\mathbf{b}| \, AC \sin \theta$$

$$= |\mathbf{b}| \, d,$$

and so

$$d = \frac{|\mathbf{b} \times (\mathbf{c} - \mathbf{a})|}{|\mathbf{b}|}.$$

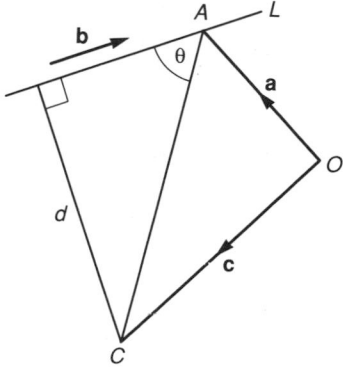

Fig. 138

Example 65.4

Find the perpendicular distance d from the point $(1, 2, 3)$ to the straight line

$$\frac{x-2}{1} = \frac{y+4}{2} = \frac{z-1}{-2}.$$

Solution

The equation of the straight line is in standard form, so the position vector of a point on the line is $\mathbf{a} = 2\mathbf{i} - 4\mathbf{j} + \mathbf{k}$, while the vector $\mathbf{b}$ along the line is $\mathbf{b} = \mathbf{i} + 2\mathbf{j} - 2\mathbf{k}$.

The point whose perpendicular distance d from the line is required has the position vector $\mathbf{c} = \mathbf{i} + 2\mathbf{j} + 3\mathbf{k}$.

Thus

$$d = \frac{|\mathbf{b} \times (\mathbf{c} - \mathbf{a})|}{|\mathbf{b}|},$$

but $\mathbf{c} - \mathbf{a} = -\mathbf{i} + 6\mathbf{j} + 2\mathbf{k}$, so

$$\mathbf{b} \times (\mathbf{c} - \mathbf{a}) = \begin{vmatrix} \mathbf{i} & \mathbf{j} & \mathbf{k} \\ 1 & 2 & -2 \\ -1 & 6 & 2 \end{vmatrix} = 16\mathbf{i} + 8\mathbf{k},$$

$|\mathbf{b} \times (\mathbf{c} - \mathbf{a})| = 8\sqrt{5}$ and $|\mathbf{b}| = 3$, so that

$$d = \frac{8\sqrt{5}}{3}. \qquad\qquad \blacktriangle$$

ANGULAR VELOCITY

Consider a rigid body pivoted about a point O and rotating about an axis OC, as shown in Fig. 139. Let its angular speed about OC be ω rad/s, and let $\hat{\mathbf{n}}$ be a unit vector in the direction of OC. Then the **angular velocity** is defined as

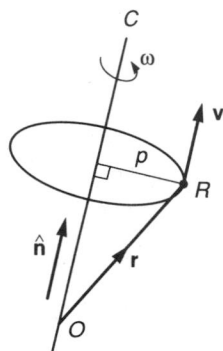

Fig. 139

$$\omega = \omega \hat{n}.$$

Let the perpendicular distance of R from the line OC be p. Then the velocity of a point R in the body with position vector $\mathbf{r}$ relative to O has magnitude $p\omega$, and is in a direction perpendicular to the plane containing the line OC and the point R, and is such that

$$\mathbf{v} = \omega \times \mathbf{r}.$$

Example 65.5

A rigid body spins about an axis OC in the direction $\mathbf{i} + \mathbf{j} + \mathbf{k}$ at the uniform rate of 5 rad/s. The point O has the position vector $\mathbf{a} = 2\mathbf{i} + \mathbf{j} + 3\mathbf{k}$ relative to an origin O', with a unit vector representing a displacement of 1 cm. Find the instantaneous velocity of a point R with the position vector $\mathbf{b} = 4\mathbf{i} + 3\mathbf{j} + 2\mathbf{k}$ relative to O'.

Solution
The configuration is illustrated in Fig. 140. The position vector of R relative to O is $\mathbf{r} = \mathbf{b} - \mathbf{a}$, $\omega = 5$ and $\hat{n} = (\mathbf{i} + \mathbf{j} + \mathbf{k})/\sqrt{3}$, so

$$\omega = \frac{5}{\sqrt{3}} (\mathbf{i} + \mathbf{j} + \mathbf{k})$$

and thus

$$\mathbf{v} = \frac{5}{\sqrt{3}} (\mathbf{i} + \mathbf{j} + \mathbf{k}) \times (\mathbf{b} - \mathbf{a}),$$

but $\mathbf{b} - \mathbf{a} = 2\mathbf{i} + 2\mathbf{j} - \mathbf{k}$, so

$$\mathbf{v} = \frac{5}{\sqrt{3}} (\mathbf{i} + \mathbf{j} + \mathbf{k}) \times (2\mathbf{i} + 2\mathbf{j} - \mathbf{k})$$

$$= 5\sqrt{3}(-\mathbf{i} + \mathbf{j}) \, \text{cm/s}. \qquad \blacktriangle$$

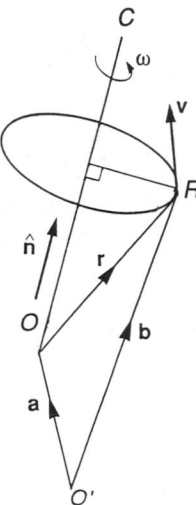

Fig. 140

MOMENTS

Consider a system of forces F_1, F_2, ..., F_n acting on a rigid body. If the resultant is $F = F_1 + F_2 + ... + F_n$, it is **necessary** that $F = 0$ for equilibrium, but this is not a sufficient condition. The additional condition necessary to ensure equilibrium concerns the turning effect the resultant force has on the body.

Let a force F act on a body, and r be the position vector of any point P on the line of application of the force, as shown in Fig. 141. The **moment** of the force about O is defined as

$$M = r \times F.$$

Thus from Fig. 141 and the definition of M we see that $d = OP \sin \theta$ and $|M| = |r|\,|F|\sin \theta = d\,|F|\sin \theta$. To see that M is independent of the choice of the point P on the line of action of F, let r' be the position vector of another point Q on the line of action of F. Then, by writing

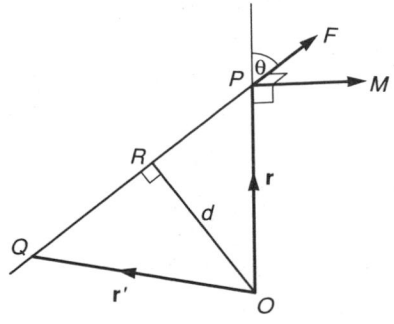

Fig. 141

$$\mathbf{r}' = \mathbf{r} + (\mathbf{r}' - \mathbf{r}),$$

we see that

$$\mathbf{M}' = \mathbf{r}' \times \mathbf{F} = [\mathbf{r} + (\mathbf{r}' - \mathbf{r})] \times \mathbf{F}$$
$$= \mathbf{r} \times \mathbf{F},$$

because $\mathbf{r}' - \mathbf{r}$ and $\mathbf{F}$ are parallel vectors, so $(\mathbf{r}' - \mathbf{r}) \times \mathbf{F} = \mathbf{0}$.

Example 65.6

A force $\mathbf{F} = 2\mathbf{i} - 3\mathbf{j} + 4\mathbf{k}$ acts at the point $(1, 2, 1)$. Find its moment
(i) about the origin; and
(ii) about the point $(4, 1, -1)$.

Solution
(i)   The position vector $\mathbf{r}$ of the point $(1, 2, 1)$ relative to the origin is
      $\mathbf{r} = \mathbf{i} + 2\mathbf{j} + \mathbf{k}$, so the moment about the origin is

$$\mathbf{M} = (\mathbf{i} + 2\mathbf{j} + k) \times (2\mathbf{i} + 3\mathbf{j} + 4\mathbf{k})$$
$$= 11\mathbf{i} - 2\mathbf{j} - 7\mathbf{k} \text{ torque units.}$$

(ii) The position vector $\mathbf{r}$ of the point $(1, 2, 1)$ relative to the point $(4, 1, -1)$
     is

$$\mathbf{r} - (\mathbf{i} + 2\mathbf{j} + \mathbf{k}) - (4\mathbf{i} + \mathbf{j} - \mathbf{k}) = -3\mathbf{i} + \mathbf{j} + 2\mathbf{k},$$

so the moment about the point $(4, 1, -1)$ is

$$\mathbf{M} = (-3\mathbf{i} + \mathbf{j} + 2\mathbf{k}) \times (2\mathbf{i} - 3\mathbf{j} + 4\mathbf{k})$$
$$= 10\mathbf{i} + 16\mathbf{j} + 7\mathbf{k} \text{ torque units.} \qquad \blacktriangle$$

For a system of forces $\mathbf{F}_1, \mathbf{F}_2, ..., \mathbf{F}_n$ acting at points with position vectors
$\mathbf{r}_1, \mathbf{r}_2, ..., \mathbf{r}_n$, the moment of the system about the origin is

$$\mathbf{G} = \mathbf{r}_1 \times \mathbf{F}_1 + \mathbf{r}_2 \times \mathbf{F}_2 + ... + \mathbf{r}_n \times \mathbf{F}_n.$$

For a rigid body $\mathbf{F} = \mathbf{G} = \mathbf{0}$ is sufficient to ensure equilibrium. If $\mathbf{F} = \mathbf{0}$ but
$\mathbf{G} \neq \mathbf{0}$ it can be shown that the moment is the same about any point and the
system reduces to a **couple** (a simple turning effect).

In component form, if $\mathbf{F} = X\mathbf{i} + Y\mathbf{j} + Z\mathbf{k}$ and $\mathbf{r} = x\mathbf{i} + y\mathbf{j} + z\mathbf{k}$, then

$$\mathbf{r} \times \mathbf{F} = (yZ - zY)\mathbf{i} + (zX - xZ)\mathbf{j} + (xY - yX)\mathbf{k}.$$

For a system in the (x, y)-plane $z = 0$ and $Z = 0$, and

$$\mathbf{M} = \mathbf{r} \times \mathbf{F} = (xY - yX)\mathbf{k}.$$

Now $xY - yX$ is the usual counterclockwise moment about the origin. We
can interpret this scalar quantity as the moment about a line, which in this case
is the z-axis. In general the moment about a line through the origin O in the
direction of the unit vector $\hat{\mathbf{n}}$ is

$$\hat{\mathbf{n}} \cdot (\mathbf{r} \times \mathbf{F}).$$

Thus for the above two-dimensional system the moment about the z-axis is

$$\mathbf{k} \cdot (xY - yX)\mathbf{k} = xY - yX.$$

Example 65.7

The force $\mathbf{F} = 3\mathbf{i} - 2\mathbf{j} + 4\mathbf{k}$ acts at the point $(1, 3, -2)$. Find the moment

(i) about the origin; and
(ii) about the line through O in the direction $\mathbf{i} + 2\mathbf{j} - 3\mathbf{k}$.

Solution
(i) The moment about the origin is

$$\mathbf{M} = \mathbf{r} \times \mathbf{F} = (\mathbf{i} + 3\mathbf{j} - 2\mathbf{k}) \times (3\mathbf{i} - 2\mathbf{j} + 4\mathbf{k})$$

$$= 8\mathbf{i} - 10\mathbf{j} - 11\mathbf{k} \text{ torque units.}$$

(ii) The unit vector $\hat{\mathbf{n}}$ in the direction of $\mathbf{i} + 2\mathbf{j} + 3\mathbf{k}$ is

$$\hat{\mathbf{n}} = (\mathbf{i} + 2\mathbf{j} + 3\mathbf{k})/\sqrt{14},$$

so the moment about this line is

$$\hat{\mathbf{n}} \cdot \mathbf{M} = \frac{1}{\sqrt{14}} (\mathbf{i} + 2\mathbf{j} = 3\mathbf{k}) \cdot (8\mathbf{i} - 10\mathbf{j} - 11\mathbf{k})$$

$$= 21 \text{ torque units.} \qquad \blacktriangle$$

The notion of a moment may be applied to any vector quantity that has a line of application (a vector which acts in a given direction through a specific point, and so cannot be translated).

PROBLEMS 65

1. Find a unit vector $\hat{\mathbf{n}}$ perpendicular to each of the vectors $2\mathbf{j} - \mathbf{j} + \mathbf{k}$ and $3\mathbf{i} + 4\mathbf{j} - \mathbf{k}$. Determine the sine of the angle, and hence the angle, between these two vectors. Also find unit vectors in the plane of these vectors, one perpendicular to each vector.
2. Obtain the equation of the line passing through the points $(1, 1, 1)$ and $(-2, -1, 3)$. Determine the equation of the plane with the vector along this line as its normal and passing through the point $(2, 1, 1)$.
3. Find the equation of the plane through the origin and the points $(1, 1, 1)$ and $(1, 2, 3)$. Find the perpendicular distance d from the point $(3, -2, -4)$ to the plane.
4. Find a unit vector normal $\hat{\mathbf{n}}$ to the plane through the points $A(1, 1, 1)$, $B(1, 2, 3)$ and $C(2, -2, -1)$. By projecting OA in the direction of this unit vector, find the distance d of the plane from the origin O.
5. Find the equation of the line of intersection of the two planes with the equations

$$4x + 20y + 20z + 11 = 0$$

$$4x - 5y + 10z - 9 = 0.$$

Find the equation of the plane containing the origin which has the vector along this line as its normal. Determine the angle between the two planes.

6.   Show that the lines

$$\frac{x-2}{1} = \frac{y+1}{2} = \frac{z-2}{2} \quad \text{and} \quad \frac{x-1}{3} = \frac{y-1}{4} = \frac{z-2}{5}$$

intersect and find the angle between the lines. Find the equation of the plane containing both lines.

7.   Show that the four points $(0, -1, 0)$ and $(2, 1, -1)$, $(1, 1, 1)$ and $(3, 3, 0)$ are coplanar.

8.   Show that the four points $(1, 1, 0)$, $(2, 0, -1)$, $(-2, 1, 2)$ and $(4, 4, -1)$ are coplanar and find the equation of the plane containing them.

9.   Find the distance p, measured parallel to the line

$$\frac{x}{2} = \frac{y}{3} = \frac{z}{-6},$$

from the point $(1, -2, 3)$ to the plane

$$x - y + z = 5.$$

10.   A rigid body spins about an axis OC in the direction $2\mathbf{i} + \mathbf{j} + 2\mathbf{k}$ at the uniform rate of 9 rad/s. The point O has the position vector $\mathbf{a} = \mathbf{i} + 2\mathbf{j} + \mathbf{k}$ relative to an origin O', with a unit vector representing a displacement of 1 cm. Find the instantaneous velocity of a point R with the position vector $\mathbf{b} = 3\mathbf{i} + \mathbf{j} - 3\mathbf{k}$ relative to O'.

11.   A force $\mathbf{F} = \mathbf{i} - \mathbf{j} + 3\mathbf{k}$ acts at the point $(1, 1, 1)$. Find its moment about the origin and about the point $(2, 0, -1)$.

Differentiation and integration of vectors 66

A vector function of the single scalar variable t has the form

$$\mathbf{r} = x(t)\mathbf{i} + y(t)\mathbf{j} + z(t)\mathbf{k},$$

with $x(t)$, $y(t)$ and $z(t)$ scalar functions of t. Relative to the origin O of Cartesian coordinates $\mathbf{r}$ may be considered as the position vector of a point P in space whose position depends on the parameter t (often the time). Then, as t increases, so the point P moves in space and traces out a space curve Γ.

Thus, for example, the position vector

$$\mathbf{r} = R\cos t\mathbf{i} + R\sin t\mathbf{j} + a\mathbf{k}$$

traces out a circle of radius R with its centre at $(0, 0, a)$ in the plane $z = a$. To see this, notice that

$$\mathbf{r} - a\mathbf{k} = R(\cos t\mathbf{i} + \sin t\mathbf{j}),$$

and so

$$|\mathbf{r} - a\mathbf{k}| = [R^2(\cos^2 t + \sin^2 t)]^{1/2} = R.$$

Hence in the plane $z = a$ the curve traced out by the vector $\mathbf{r} - a\mathbf{k}$ has a constant modulus R relative to the z-axis, and so must be a circle.

DIFFERENTIATION

Consider Fig. 142 which shows the curve Γ traced out by the position vector $\mathbf{r}(t)$ as t increases. Let $\underline{OP}$ be the vector $\mathbf{r}$ at some value of t and $\underline{OP'} = \mathbf{r} + \delta\mathbf{r}$ be the vector at some subsequent value $t + \delta t$. Then Fig. 142 shows that

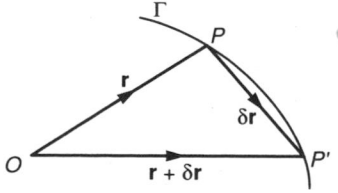

Fig. 142

$$PP' = \delta \mathbf{r}.$$

The quantity $\delta \mathbf{r}/\delta t$ is a vector along $\underline{PP'}$, and as $\delta t \to 0$, so the chord PP' approaches the tangent at P. We define the **derivative** of $\mathbf{r}$ with respect to t by

$$\frac{d\mathbf{r}}{dt} = \lim_{\delta t \to 0}\left(\frac{\delta \mathbf{r}}{\delta t}\right) = \lim_{h \to 0}\left[\frac{\mathbf{r}(t+h) - \mathbf{r}(t)}{h}\right],$$

which is a vector in the direction of the tangent vector at P.

A repetition of this argument shows that higher order derivatives may be defined in similar fashion, with

$$\frac{d}{dt}\left(\frac{d\mathbf{r}}{dt}\right) = \frac{d^2\mathbf{r}}{dt^2}, \quad \frac{d}{dt}\left(\frac{d^2\mathbf{r}}{dt^2}\right) = \frac{d^3\mathbf{r}}{dt^3}, \quad \dots .$$

The following results are easily shown to be true. Let $\mathbf{c}$ be a constant vector, A be a scalar constant and $\mathbf{r}, \mathbf{s}$ differentiable vectors. Then

1 $\dfrac{d}{dt}[\mathbf{c}] = \mathbf{0}$;

2 $\dfrac{d}{dt}[A\mathbf{r}] = A\dfrac{d\mathbf{r}}{dt}$;

3 $\dfrac{d}{dt}[\mathbf{r} + \mathbf{s}] = \dfrac{d\mathbf{r}}{dt} + \dfrac{d\mathbf{s}}{dt}$;

4 $\dfrac{d\mathbf{r}}{dt} = \dfrac{d\mathbf{r}}{d\alpha}\dfrac{d\alpha}{dt}$, where $\mathbf{r} = \mathbf{r}(\alpha)$ and $\alpha = \alpha(t)$.

We shall only prove rule 4. Let us set

$$\mathbf{r}(\alpha) = x(\alpha)\mathbf{i} + y(\alpha)\mathbf{j} + z(\alpha)\mathbf{k},$$

where $\alpha = \alpha(t)$. Then letting t change to $t + \delta t$, and setting $\alpha(t + \delta t) = \alpha + \delta\alpha$, we can write

$$\frac{d\mathbf{r}}{dt} = \lim_{\delta t \to 0}\left[\frac{\mathbf{r}(\alpha + \delta\alpha) - \mathbf{r}(\alpha)}{\delta t}\right]$$

$$= \lim_{\delta t \to 0}\left[\frac{\mathbf{r}(\alpha + \delta\alpha) - \mathbf{r}(\alpha)}{\delta\alpha} \cdot \frac{\delta\alpha}{\delta t}\right].$$

However, $\delta\alpha \to 0$ as $\delta t \to 0$, so in the limit this result becomes

$$\frac{d\mathbf{r}}{dt} = \frac{d\mathbf{r}}{d\alpha}\frac{d\alpha}{dt},$$

as was to be proved.

DERIVATIVES OF PRODUCTS

Let $u = u(t)$ be a differentiable scalar function of t and $\mathbf{r}(t), \mathbf{s}(t)$, be differentiable vector functions of t. Then the derivatives of $u\mathbf{r}$, $\mathbf{r} \cdot \mathbf{s}$ and $\mathbf{r} \times \mathbf{s}$ obey the following rules

1 $\dfrac{d}{dt}[u\mathbf{r}] = \dfrac{du}{dt}\mathbf{r} + u\dfrac{d\mathbf{r}}{dt}$,

2 $\dfrac{d}{dt}[\mathbf{r}\cdot\mathbf{s}] = \dfrac{d\mathbf{r}}{dt}\cdot\mathbf{s} + \mathbf{r}\cdot\dfrac{d\mathbf{s}}{dt}$,

3 $\dfrac{d}{dt}[\mathbf{r}\times\mathbf{s}] = \dfrac{d\mathbf{r}}{dt}\times\mathbf{s} + \mathbf{r}\times\dfrac{d\mathbf{s}}{dt}$.

We shall only prove rule 1 since the others follow in similar fashion. Let u change by δu and $\mathbf{r}$ by $\delta\mathbf{r}$ when t changes by δt. Then we can write

$$\delta(u\mathbf{r}) = (u + \delta u)(\mathbf{r} + \delta\mathbf{r}) - u\mathbf{r}$$
$$= \delta u\mathbf{r} + u\delta\mathbf{r} + \delta u\delta\mathbf{r},$$

and so

$$\frac{\delta(u\mathbf{r})}{\delta t} = \frac{\delta u}{\delta t}\mathbf{r} + u\frac{\delta\mathbf{r}}{\delta t} + \frac{\delta u}{\delta t}\delta\mathbf{r}.$$

Proceeding to the limit as $\delta t \to 0$ this becomes

$$\frac{d}{dt}[u\mathbf{r}] = \frac{du}{dt}\mathbf{r} + u\frac{d\mathbf{r}}{dt},$$

since the last term $(du/dt)\delta\mathbf{r} \to 0$, because $\delta\mathbf{r} \to 0$ as $\delta t \to 0$, so the result is proved.

As a special case of this last result let us set

$$\mathbf{r} = x\mathbf{i} + y\mathbf{j} + z\mathbf{k},$$

then

$$\frac{d\mathbf{r}}{dt} = \frac{dx}{dt}\mathbf{i} + \frac{dy}{dt}\mathbf{j} + \frac{dz}{dt}\mathbf{k},$$

because

$$\frac{d\mathbf{i}}{dt} = \frac{d\mathbf{j}}{dt} = \frac{d\mathbf{k}}{dt} = 0.$$

Consider the curve Γ in Fig. 143(a) traced out by

$$\mathbf{r} = x(t)\mathbf{i} + y(t)\mathbf{j} + z(t)\mathbf{k},$$

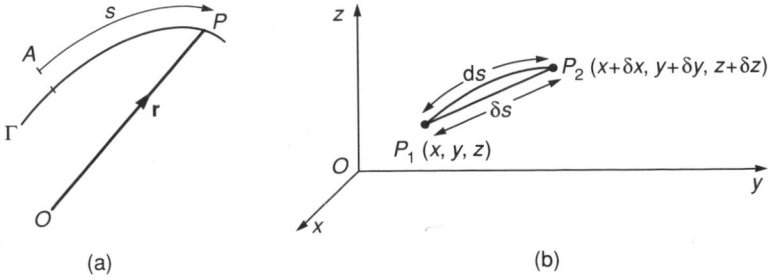

(a)   (b)

Fig. 143

and suppose that s is the distance along Γ measured from some fixed point A on Γ. Then considering adjacent points $P_1(x, y, z)$ and $P_2(x + \delta x, y + \delta y, z + \delta z)$ on Γ corresponding, respectively, to t and $t + \delta t$ we see from Pythagoras' theorem and Fig. 143(b) that

$$(\delta s)^2 = (\delta x)^2 + (\delta y)^2 + (\delta z)^2,$$

and thus, after division by δt, this becomes

$$\left(\frac{\delta s}{\delta t}\right)^2 = \left(\frac{\delta x}{\delta t}\right)^2 + \left(\frac{\delta y}{\delta t}\right)^2 + \left(\frac{\delta z}{\delta t}\right)^2.$$

Proceeding to the limit as $\delta t \to 0$ this reduces to

$$\frac{ds}{dt} = \left[\left(\frac{dx}{dt}\right)^2 + \left(\frac{dy}{dt}\right)^2 + \left(\frac{dz}{dt}\right)^2\right]^{1/2}.$$

Comparing this result with

$$\frac{ds}{dt} = \frac{dx}{dt}\mathbf{i} + \frac{dy}{dt}\mathbf{j} + \frac{dz}{dt}\mathbf{k}$$

shows that

$$\frac{ds}{dt} = \left|\frac{d\mathbf{r}}{dt}\right|.$$

Thus if $\hat{\mathbf{T}}$ is a unit vector in the direction of the tangent to Γ at P we have

$$\frac{d\mathbf{r}}{dt} = \frac{ds}{dt}\hat{\mathbf{T}}.$$

Expressed differently, this gives the basic result that the unit tangent $\hat{\mathbf{T}}$ to Γ is

$$\hat{\mathbf{T}} = \left(\frac{d\mathbf{r}}{dt}\right)\Big/\left|\frac{d\mathbf{r}}{dt}\right|.$$

Example 66.1

Find $d\mathbf{r}/dt$ and the tangent vector $\hat{\mathbf{T}}$ to the curve traced out by

$$\mathbf{r} = R\cos t\,\mathbf{i} + R\sin t\,\mathbf{j} + a\mathbf{k}.$$

Solution
We have

$$\frac{d\mathbf{r}}{dt} = -R\sin t\,\mathbf{i} + R\cos t\,\mathbf{j},$$

so that

$$\left|\frac{d\mathbf{r}}{dt}\right| = [(-R\sin t)^2 + (R\cos t)^2]^{1/2} = R,$$

and thus

$$\hat{\mathbf{T}} = \left(\frac{d\mathbf{r}}{dt}\right) \bigg/ \left|\frac{d\mathbf{r}}{dt}\right| = -\sin t\mathbf{i} + \cos t\mathbf{j}.$$ ▲

Example 66.2

Given that a curve $\varGamma$ is traced out by the position vector

$$\mathbf{r} = t\cos t\mathbf{i} + t^2\mathbf{j} + \cos t\mathbf{k},$$

find $\mathbf{r}$, $d\mathbf{r}/dt$ and a unit vector $\hat{\mathbf{T}}$ tangent to $\varGamma$ at $t = \pi/2$.

Solution
Setting $t = \pi/2$ in $\mathbf{r}$ gives

$$\mathbf{r}(\pi/2) = \frac{\pi^2}{4}\mathbf{j}.$$

Differentiation of $\mathbf{r}$ gives

$$\frac{d\mathbf{r}}{dt} = \frac{d}{dt}[t\cos t]\mathbf{i} + \frac{d}{dt}[t^2]\mathbf{j} + \frac{d}{dt}[\cos t]\mathbf{k}$$

$$= (\cos t - t\sin t)\mathbf{i} + 2t\mathbf{j} - \sin t\mathbf{k},$$

so setting $t = \pi/2$ gives

$$\left(\frac{d\mathbf{r}}{dt}\right)_{t=\pi/2} = -\frac{\pi}{2}\mathbf{i} + \pi\mathbf{j} - \mathbf{k}.$$

Thus when $t = \pi/2$,

$$\left|\frac{d\mathbf{r}}{dt}\right| = [(-\pi/2)^2 + \pi^2 + (-1)^2]^{1/2}$$

$$= \frac{1}{2}(4 + 5\pi^2)^{1/2},$$

and hence

$$\hat{\mathbf{T}} = \left(\frac{d\mathbf{r}}{dt}\right) \bigg/ \left|\frac{d\mathbf{r}}{dt}\right|$$

$$= \frac{-\pi\mathbf{i} + 2\pi\mathbf{j} - 2\mathbf{k}}{4 + 5\pi^2}.$$ ▲

Example 66.3

Find $d^2\mathbf{r}/dt^2$ given that

$$\mathbf{r} = t^3\mathbf{i} + \left(t^2 + \frac{1}{t^2}\right)\mathbf{j} + (3t^2 + 1)\mathbf{k}.$$

Solution

Differentiating **r** with respect to t gives

$$\frac{d\mathbf{r}}{dt} = 3t^2\mathbf{i} + \left(2t - \frac{2}{t^3}\right)\mathbf{j} + 6t\mathbf{k}.$$

A further differentiation then yields

$$\frac{d^2\mathbf{r}}{dt^2} = 6t\mathbf{i} + \left(2 + \frac{6}{t^4}\right)\mathbf{j} + 6\mathbf{k}. \qquad \blacktriangle$$

Example 66.4

Given that s in the arc length along the curve Γ traced out by the position vector

$$\mathbf{r} = \sin^2 t\mathbf{i} + \cos^2 t\mathbf{j} + t\mathbf{k},$$

find ds/dt.

Solution

We must calculate $d\mathbf{r}/dt$, because $ds/dt = |d\mathbf{r}/dt|$. Differentiation of **r** with respect to t gives

$$\frac{d\mathbf{r}}{dt} = 2 \sin t \cos t\mathbf{i} - 2 \cos t \sin t\mathbf{j} + \mathbf{k},$$

so

$$\frac{ds}{dt} = \left|\frac{d\mathbf{r}}{dt}\right| [(2 \sin t \cos t)^2 + (-2 \cos t \sin t)^2 + 1^2]^{1/2}$$

$$= [8 \sin^2 t \cos^2 t + 1]^{1/2}.$$

INTEGRATION

Given a vector function $\mathbf{r}(t)$, the process of determining a vector function $\mathbf{F}(t)$ whose derivative with respect to t is $\mathbf{r}(t)$ is called **integration**. Thus, using the usual notation, we have

$$\mathbf{F} = \int \mathbf{r} \, dt, \text{ and, equivalently, } \frac{d\mathbf{F}}{dt} = \mathbf{r}.$$

If

$$\mathbf{r} = x(t)\mathbf{i} + y(t)\mathbf{j} + z(t)\mathbf{k},$$

then

$$\mathbf{F} = F_1\mathbf{i} + F_2\mathbf{j} + F_3\mathbf{k},$$

where

$$F_1 = \int x(t) \, dt, \quad F_2 = \int y(t) \, dt \quad \text{and} \quad F_3 = \int z(t) \, dt.$$

The **antiderivative F** (or **indefinite integral**) will have an arbitrary additive **constant vector** of integration, since a scalar arbitrary constant will be introduced when each component of **r** is integrated.

Example 66.5

Find

$$\mathbf{F} = \int (t^2 \mathbf{i} + \cos 2t \mathbf{j} + e^{-t} \mathbf{k}) \, dt.$$

Solution

$$\mathbf{F} = \left[\int t^2 \, dt \right] \mathbf{i} + \left[\int \cos 2t \, dt \right] \mathbf{j} + \left[\int e^{-t} \, dt \right] \mathbf{k}$$

$$= \frac{t^3}{3} \mathbf{i} + \frac{1}{2} \sin 2t \mathbf{j} - e^{-t} \mathbf{k} + \mathbf{c},$$

where **c** is an arbitrary constant vector.   ▲

VELOCITY AND ACCELERATION

Let P be a moving point and $\mathbf{r}(t)$ its position vector at time t. Then the **velocity** **v** of P at time t is

$$\mathbf{v} = \frac{d\mathbf{r}}{dt},$$

and its **acceleration**

$$\mathbf{a} = \frac{d\mathbf{v}}{dt} = \frac{d^2\mathbf{r}}{dt^2},$$

and so

$$\mathbf{v} = \int \mathbf{a} \, dt \quad \text{and} \quad \mathbf{r} = \int \mathbf{v} \, dt.$$

If s is the arc length along the curve traced out by P, then

$$\mathbf{v} = \frac{ds}{dt} \hat{\mathbf{T}},$$

so the point P has **speed** ds/dt in the direction of the unit tangent vector $\hat{\mathbf{T}}$ to the curve traced out by P.

Example 66.6

Given that the position vector of a point at time t is given by

$$\mathbf{r} = R \cos t\mathbf{i} + R \sin t\mathbf{j} + t\mathbf{k},$$

find its velocity and acceleration when $t = \pi/4$.

Solution
Differentiation with respect to t gives

$$\mathbf{v} = \frac{\mathrm{d}\mathbf{r}}{\mathrm{d}t} = -R \sin t\mathbf{i} + R \cos t\mathbf{j} + \mathbf{k},$$

so when $t = \pi/4$ the velocity is

$$\mathbf{v} = -\frac{R}{\sqrt{2}}(-\mathbf{i} + \mathbf{j}) + \mathbf{k}.$$

A further differentiation of $\mathbf{v}$ yields

$$\mathbf{a} = \frac{\mathrm{d}\mathbf{v}}{\mathrm{d}t} = -R \cos t\mathbf{i} - R \sin t\mathbf{j},$$

so when $t = \pi/4$ the acceleration is

$$\mathbf{a} = -\frac{R}{\sqrt{2}}(\mathbf{i} + \mathbf{j}). \qquad\qquad \blacktriangle$$

Example 66.7

Given that the acceleration of a moving point P is given by

$$\mathbf{a} = t\mathbf{i} + 2 \cos 3t\mathbf{j} + \mathbf{k},$$

find its velocity and position vector at time t if $\mathbf{v} = \mathbf{v}_0$ and $\mathbf{r} = \mathbf{r}_0$ when $t = 0$.

Solution
We have $\mathbf{a} = \mathrm{d}\mathbf{v}/\mathrm{d}t$, so

$$\frac{\mathrm{d}\mathbf{v}}{\mathrm{d}t} = t\mathbf{i} + 2 \cos 3t\mathbf{j} + \mathbf{k},$$

and hence

$$\int \left(\frac{\mathrm{d}\mathbf{v}}{\mathrm{d}t}\right) \mathrm{d}t = \left[\int t \, \mathrm{d}t\right]\mathbf{i} + \left[\int 2 \cos 3t \, \mathrm{d}t\right]\mathbf{j} + \left[\int \mathrm{d}t\right]\mathbf{k}$$

but $(\mathrm{d}\mathbf{v}/\mathrm{d}t)\,\mathrm{d}t = \mathrm{d}\mathbf{v}$, so it follows that

$$\int \mathrm{d}\mathbf{v} = \left[\int t \, \mathrm{d}t\right]\mathbf{i} + \left[\int 2 \cos 3t \, \mathrm{d}t\right]\mathbf{j} + \left[\int \mathrm{d}t\right]\mathbf{k}$$

or

$$\mathbf{v} = \frac{t^2}{2}\mathbf{i} + \frac{2}{3} \sin 3t\mathbf{j} + t\mathbf{k} + \mathbf{c},$$

where $\mathbf{c}$ is an arbitrary additive constant vector of integration.

Now we are told that $\mathbf{v} = \mathbf{v}_0$ when $t = 0$, so setting $\mathbf{v} = \mathbf{v}_0$ and $t = 0$ in the vector equation for $\mathbf{v}$ gives

$$\mathbf{v}_0 = \mathbf{c},$$

and so the velocity at time t is

$$\mathbf{v} = \mathbf{v}_0 + \frac{t^2}{2}\mathbf{i} + \frac{2}{3}\sin 3t\,\mathbf{j} + t\mathbf{k}.$$

To find the position at time t we use the fact that

$$\mathbf{v} = \frac{d\mathbf{r}}{dt},$$

so

$$\frac{d\mathbf{r}}{dt} = \mathbf{v}_0 + \frac{t^2}{2}\mathbf{i} + \frac{2}{3}\sin 3t\,\mathbf{j} + t\mathbf{k},$$

and thus

$$\int\left(\frac{d\mathbf{r}}{dt}\right)dt = \int \mathbf{v}_0\,dt + \left[\int \frac{t^2}{2}\,dt\right]\mathbf{i} + \frac{2}{3}\left[\int \sin 3t\,dt\right]\mathbf{j} + \left[\int t\,dt\right]\mathbf{k}.$$

Using the fact that $(d\mathbf{r}/dt)\,dt = d\mathbf{r}$ this becomes

$$\int d\mathbf{r} = \int \mathbf{v}_0\,dt + \left[\int \frac{t^2}{2}\,dt\right]\mathbf{i} + \frac{2}{3}\left[\int \sin 3t\,dt\right]\mathbf{j} + \left[\int t\,dt\right]\mathbf{k},$$

and so

$$\mathbf{r} = \mathbf{v}_0 t + \frac{t^3}{6}\mathbf{i} - \frac{2}{9}\cos 3t\,\mathbf{j} + \frac{t^2}{2}\mathbf{k} + \mathbf{d},$$

where $\mathbf{d}$ is an arbitrary additive constant vector of integration. However, we know that $\mathbf{r} = \mathbf{r}_0$ when $t = 0$, so substituting into the vector equation for $\mathbf{r}$ gives

$$\mathbf{r}_0 = -\frac{2}{9}\mathbf{j} + \mathbf{d} \quad \text{so} \quad \mathbf{d} = \mathbf{r}_0 + \frac{2}{9}\mathbf{j}.$$

Thus the position vector of the point P at time t is

$$\mathbf{r} = \mathbf{r}_0 + \mathbf{v}_0 t + \frac{t^3}{6}\mathbf{i} + \frac{2}{9}(1 - \cos 3t)\mathbf{j} + \frac{t^2}{2}\mathbf{k}. \qquad \blacktriangle$$

PROBLEMS 66

1. Describe the curve traced out by the position vector

$$\mathbf{r} = R\cos t\,\mathbf{i} + R\sin t\,\mathbf{j} + t\mathbf{k}.$$

2. Describe the curve traced out by the position vector

$$\mathbf{r} = t \cos t\mathbf{i} + t \sin t\mathbf{j} + t\mathbf{k}.$$

3. Find $d\mathbf{r}/dt$ and $d^2\mathbf{r}/dt^2$, given that
   (a) $\mathbf{r} = (1 - 3t^2)\mathbf{i} + 2t\mathbf{j} - \cos 2t\mathbf{k};$

   (b) $\mathbf{r} = t\mathbf{a} - \dfrac{1}{t^2}\mathbf{b}$ (**a**, **b** constant vectors).

4. Find $d\mathbf{r}/dt$ at $t = 0$, given that
   (a) $\mathbf{r} = \sinh 2t\mathbf{i} + e^{3t}\mathbf{j} + t \cos t\mathbf{k},$

   (b) $\mathbf{r} = (t^3 + t^2 + 1)\mathbf{i} + \left(\dfrac{1}{1+t^2}\right)\mathbf{j} + \ln(1 + 3t^2)\mathbf{k}.$

5. If ω is a scalar constant, **a**, **b** are constant vectors and

   $$\mathbf{r} = \cos \omega t\mathbf{a} - \sin \omega t\mathbf{b},$$

   find $d\mathbf{r}/dt$ and $d^2\mathbf{r}/dt^2$ and prove that

   $$\frac{d^2\mathbf{r}}{dt^2} + \omega^2\mathbf{r} = 0.$$

6. If ω is a scalar constant, **a**, **b** are constant vectors and

   $$\mathbf{r} = e^{\omega t}\mathbf{a} + e^{-\omega t}\mathbf{b},$$

   find $d\mathbf{r}/dt$ and $d^2\mathbf{r}/dt^2$, and prove that

   $$\frac{d^2\mathbf{r}}{dt^2} - \omega^2\mathbf{r} = 0.$$

7. Find $d[\mathbf{r} \cdot \mathbf{s}]/dt$, given that
   (a) $\mathbf{r} = \sinh t\mathbf{i} - \cosh t\mathbf{j} + t\mathbf{k}$ and $\mathbf{s} = 2 \sinh t\mathbf{i} + 2 \cosh t\mathbf{j} + e^t\mathbf{k};$
   (b) $\mathbf{r} = \sin 2t\mathbf{i} + \cos 2t\mathbf{j} + e^{-t}\mathbf{k}$ and $\mathbf{s} = 4 \sin 2t\mathbf{i} + 4 \cos 2t\mathbf{j} + e^t\mathbf{k}.$

8. Find $d\mathbf{r}/dt$ given that
   (a) $\mathbf{r} = (t\mathbf{i} + e^{-t}\mathbf{j} + \sin t\mathbf{k}) \times (\mathbf{i} + t^2\mathbf{j} - \mathbf{k});$
   (b) $\mathbf{r} = (1 + t^2 + \cos t)(\mathbf{i} + 4\mathbf{j} - 6\mathbf{k});$
   (c) $\mathbf{r} = 2\mathbf{i} - \mathbf{j} + \mathbf{k}.$

9. Find $d\mathbf{r}/dt$, given that
   (a) $\mathbf{r} = (t^2\mathbf{i} + \mathbf{j} - e^{-t}\mathbf{k}) \cdot (\mathbf{i} + t\mathbf{j} + \mathbf{k});$
   (b) $\mathbf{r} = (\sin t\mathbf{i} + \cos t\mathbf{j} + \mathbf{k}) \cdot (\sin t\mathbf{i} + \cos t\mathbf{j} + \mathbf{k});$
   (c) $\mathbf{r} = [(t\mathbf{i} + t^2\mathbf{j}) \times (\mathbf{i} + 3\mathbf{j})] \cdot t\mathbf{k}.$

10. Find $d\mathbf{r}/dt$ given that
   (a) $\mathbf{r}(u) = \ln(1 + u^2)\mathbf{i} + u\mathbf{j} + \tan u^3\mathbf{k}$ and $u = \sin t;$
   (b) $\mathbf{r}(u) = (1 + u^2)^{1/2}\mathbf{i} + u^2\mathbf{j} + \cosh(2u + 1)\mathbf{k}$ and $u = \ln(1 + t).$

11. Find $d[\mathbf{r} \times \mathbf{s}]/dt$, given that
   (a) $\mathbf{r} = (1 + t^2)\mathbf{i} + t\mathbf{j} + \sin t\mathbf{k}$ and $\mathbf{s} = 2\mathbf{i} - t^2\mathbf{j} + \mathbf{k};$
   (b) $\mathbf{r} = \sin t\mathbf{i} + \cos t\mathbf{j} + e^t\mathbf{k}$ and $\mathbf{s} = \cos t\mathbf{i} - \sin t\mathbf{j} + \mathbf{k}.$

12. Find

   $$\frac{d}{dt}\left[\mathbf{r} \times \frac{d\mathbf{r}}{dt}\right].$$

13. The **curvature** κ of a curve traced out by the position vector **r** is defined as

$$\kappa = \frac{|d\mathbf{r}/dt \times d^2\mathbf{r}/dt^2|}{|d\mathbf{r}/dt^3|}.$$

Find κ, given that

$$\mathbf{r} = t \sin t\mathbf{i} + t \cos t\mathbf{j}.$$

14. Find

(a) $\displaystyle\int \left(\frac{\mathbf{i} + t\mathbf{j} + t^2\mathbf{k}}{t^4}\right) dt$; and

(b) $\displaystyle\int_0^\pi (\sin kt\mathbf{a} + \cos kt\mathbf{b}) \, dt.$

15. Find

$$\int (\sinh t\mathbf{i} + e^{-2t}\mathbf{j} + t\mathbf{k}) \times (\mathbf{i} - \mathbf{j} + \mathbf{k}) \, dt.$$

16. Find **r**, given that

$$\frac{d^2\mathbf{r}}{dt^2} = \mathbf{a},$$

where **a** is a constant vector and $\mathbf{r} = \mathbf{r}_0$, $d\mathbf{r}/dt = \mathbf{u}$ when $t = 0$.

17. Given that a point P has the position vector

$$\mathbf{r} = \cos t\mathbf{i} + \sin t\mathbf{j} + t^2\mathbf{k},$$

find the tangent vector **T** to the curve traced out by P when $t = t_1$, and the equation of the plane with **T** as its normal which contains the point $(1, 2, 3)$.

18. A particle, whose velocity is given by

$$\mathbf{v} = -t\mathbf{i} + (1 - 2k)\mathbf{k}$$

was at the origin at time $t = 0$. Find the position and acceleration of the particle for $t \geq 0$, and find the times for which the position and acceleration vectors are orthogonal.

19. The velocity of a particle at time t is given by

$$\mathbf{v} = \sin 2t\mathbf{i} + 2 \cos 2t\mathbf{j} + t\mathbf{k}.$$

Find its position as a function of time, given that at time $t = 0$ it was located at the point $(3, 1, -3)$. Show the velocity and acceleration vectors can never be orthogonal if $t > 3$.

20. A particle has the position vector

$$\mathbf{r} = -\cos 3t\mathbf{i} + \sin 3t\mathbf{j} + \left(t^2 - 4t - \frac{1}{2}\right)\mathbf{k}.$$

Find its velocity **v** and acceleration **a** at time t. If the motion starts at time $t = 0$, find the subsequent time at which the acceleration vector is orthogonal to **r**.

Dynamics of a particle and the motion of a particle in a plane

DYNAMICS OF A PARTICLE

Consider a particle of mass m and position vector $\mathbf{r}(t)$ at time t. Its velocity $\mathbf{v} = d\mathbf{r}/dt$ and its **linear momentum** is defined as

$$\mathbf{M} = m\mathbf{v},$$

so by Newton's second law of motion the force $\mathbf{F}$ on the particle is

$$\mathbf{F} = \frac{d\mathbf{M}}{dt}.$$

When the mass m is constant,

$$\mathbf{F} = m\frac{d\mathbf{v}}{dt} = m\frac{d^2\mathbf{r}}{dt^2} = m\mathbf{a},$$

where $\mathbf{a}$ is the acceleration.

The **moment of momentum (angular momentum)** of the particle about the origin is

$$\mathbf{H} = \mathbf{r} \times (m\mathbf{v}) = m(\mathbf{r} \times \mathbf{v}),$$

so

$$\frac{d\mathbf{H}}{dt} = m\left(\frac{d\mathbf{r}}{dt} \times \mathbf{v} + \mathbf{r} \times \frac{d\mathbf{v}}{dt}\right)$$

$$= m\left(\mathbf{v} \times \mathbf{v} + \mathbf{r} \times \frac{d\mathbf{v}}{dt}\right),$$

and as $\mathbf{v} \times \mathbf{v} = \mathbf{0}$ this reduces to

$$\frac{d\mathbf{H}}{dt} = \mathbf{r} \times \mathbf{F}.$$

This result is called the **principle of angular momentum**.

If $\mathbf{F}$ has a zero moment about the origin, it follows from the principle of angular momentum that $\mathbf{H} = $ constant. This last result is called the **principle**

of conservation of angular momentum, and in words it asserts that the angular momentum remains constant when no external moment acts on the particle.

Example 67.1

A particle of constant mass m on a rough horizontal plane is projected horizontally from the origin at time $t = 0$ with velocity $\mathbf{v}_0$ and is resisted by a frictional force $km\mathbf{v}$. Determine the velocity $\mathbf{v}$ of the particle and its position vector $\mathbf{r}$ as functions of the time t.

Solution

To arrive at the equation of motion we must equate the rate of change of momentum of the particle to the external force acting upon it, both of which act horizontally. This leads to the result

$$m \frac{d\mathbf{v}}{dt} = -km\mathbf{v},$$

where the negative sign is necessary because the resistance opposes the motion. Cancelling the factor m and rearranging terms shows that the motion of the particle is governed by the linear homogeneous first order differential equation

$$\frac{d\mathbf{v}}{dt} + k\mathbf{v} = 0,$$

for the vector $\mathbf{v}$.

This equation has an integrating factor μ (see Section 74) given by

$$\mu = \exp\left(\int k\,dt \right) = e^{kt},$$

and multiplying the vector differential equation by μ gives

$$e^{kt} \frac{d\mathbf{v}}{dt} + ke^{kt}\mathbf{v} = \mathbf{0}.$$

This can be rewritten as

$$\frac{d}{dt}(e^{kt}\mathbf{v}) = \mathbf{0},$$

and after integration it shows that

$$e^{kt}\mathbf{v} = \mathbf{c},$$

where $\mathbf{c}$ is an arbitrary constant vector. Thus we arrive at the general result

$$\mathbf{v} = \mathbf{c}e^{-kt}.$$

The initial condition requires that $\mathbf{v} = \mathbf{v}_0$ when $t = 0$, so $\mathbf{c} = \mathbf{v}_0$ and the velocity as a function of time is seen to be given by

$$\mathbf{v} = \mathbf{v}_0 e^{-kt}.$$

Using the fact that $\mathbf{v} = d\mathbf{r}/dt$ this last result may be written

$$\frac{d\mathbf{r}}{dt} = \mathbf{v}_0 e^{-kt},$$

so

$$\mathbf{r} = \int \mathbf{v}_0 e^{-kt} dt$$

$$= -\frac{\mathbf{v}_0}{k} e^{-kt} + \mathbf{a},$$

where $\mathbf{a}$ is an arbitrary constant vector.

The particle starts from the origin at time $t = 0$, so

$$\mathbf{0} = -\frac{\mathbf{v}_0}{k} + \mathbf{a},$$

showing that $\mathbf{a} = \mathbf{v}_0/k$, and hence that

$$\mathbf{r} = \frac{1}{k}(1 - e^{-kt})\mathbf{v}_0.$$

As $t \to \infty$, so $\mathbf{r} \to \mathbf{v}_0/k$ which is the total displacement of the particle before it comes to rest. ▲

MOTION OF A PARTICLE IN A PLANE

When considering the motion of a particle in a plane as, for example, when studying orbits, it is often convenient to use the polar coordinates (r, θ). The path of a particle P in the (x, y)-plane is shown in Fig. 144, where the radius $OP = r$ and the angle between OP and the x-axis is θ. The **radial unit vector** $\hat{\mathbf{e}}$ is in the direction in which r increases, and the **transverse unit vector** $\hat{\mathbf{s}}$ is perpendicular to $\hat{\mathbf{e}}$ and in the direction in which θ increases. In terms of the

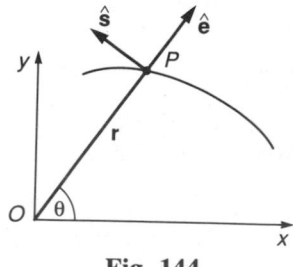

Fig. 144

usual unit vectors **i**, **j** and **k** along the x, y and z-axes, we see that $\hat{s} = \mathbf{k} \times \hat{e}$. Thus as

$$\hat{e} = \cos \theta \, \mathbf{i} + \sin \theta \, \mathbf{j},$$

it follows that

$$\hat{s} = -\sin \theta \, \mathbf{i} + \cos \theta \, \mathbf{j}.$$

By definition, $\mathbf{r} = r\hat{e}$, so the particle velocity

$$\mathbf{v} = \frac{d}{dt} [r\hat{e}]$$

$$= \frac{dr}{dt} \hat{e} + r \frac{d}{dt} [\hat{e}].$$

However,

$$\frac{d}{dt} [\hat{e}] = (-\sin \theta \, \mathbf{i} + \cos \theta \, \mathbf{j}) \frac{d\theta}{dt} = \hat{s} \frac{d\theta}{dt},$$

so denoting differentiation with respect to t by a dot we arrive at the result

$$\mathbf{v} = \dot{r}\hat{e} + r\dot{\theta}\hat{s}.$$

The acceleration of particle P is

$$\mathbf{a} = \frac{d\mathbf{v}}{dt} = \frac{d}{dt} [\dot{r}\hat{e} + r\dot{\theta}\hat{s}]$$

$$= \ddot{r}\hat{e} + \dot{r} \frac{d}{dt} [\hat{e}] + \dot{r}\dot{\theta}\hat{s} + r\ddot{\theta}\,\hat{s} + r\dot{\theta}\,\hat{s} + r\dot{\theta} \frac{d}{dt} [\hat{s}].$$

Using the fact that

$$\frac{d}{dt} [\hat{e}] = \dot{\theta}\hat{s} \quad \text{and} \quad \frac{d}{dt} [\hat{s}] = -\dot{\theta}\hat{e}$$

the above result simplifies to

$$\mathbf{a} = (\ddot{r} - r\dot{\theta}^2)\hat{e} + (r\ddot{\theta} + 2\dot{r}\dot{\theta})\hat{s}.$$

An alternative form of this last result which is often useful, and is easily verified, is

$$\mathbf{a} = (\ddot{r} - r\dot{\theta}^2)\hat{e} + \frac{1}{r} \frac{d}{dt} [r^2\dot{\theta}]\hat{s}.$$

Thus, summarizing results, we have established that

$$\hat{e} = \cos \theta \, \mathbf{i} + \sin \theta \, \mathbf{j}$$

$$\hat{s} = -\sin \theta \, \mathbf{i} + \cos \theta \, \mathbf{j}$$

$$\dot{\hat{e}} = \dot{\theta}\hat{s}$$

$$\dot{\hat{s}} = -\dot{\theta}\hat{e}$$

$$\mathbf{r} = r\hat{\mathbf{e}}$$

$$\mathbf{v} = \dot{r}\hat{\mathbf{e}} + r\dot{\theta}\hat{\mathbf{s}}$$

$$\mathbf{a} = (\ddot{r} - r\dot{\theta}^2)\hat{\mathbf{e}} + (r\ddot{\theta} + 2\dot{r}\dot{\theta})\hat{\mathbf{s}}$$

or, equivalently,

$$\mathbf{a} = (\ddot{r} - r\dot{\theta}^2)\,\hat{\mathbf{e}} + \frac{1}{r}\frac{\mathrm{d}}{\mathrm{d}t}[r^2\dot{\theta}]\hat{\mathbf{s}}.$$

Two special cases
1 Motion in a circle: in this case $r = \text{const.}$, so $\dot{r} = \ddot{r} = 0$, and as a result

$$\mathbf{v} = r\dot{\theta}\hat{\mathbf{s}} \quad \text{and} \quad \mathbf{a} = -r\dot{\theta}^2\hat{\mathbf{e}} + r\ddot{\theta}\,\hat{\mathbf{s}}.$$

2 Constant angular velocity: in this case $\dot{\theta} = \omega = \text{const.}$, so $\ddot{\theta} = 0$, and as a result

$$\mathbf{v} = \dot{r}\hat{\mathbf{e}} + r\omega\hat{\mathbf{s}} \quad \text{and} \quad \mathbf{a} = (\ddot{r} - r\omega^2)\hat{\mathbf{e}} + 2\dot{r}\omega\hat{\mathbf{s}}.$$

Example 67.2

A particle P moves in a plane with constant angular velocity ω in such a way that the rate of increase of the acceleration is parallel to the radius vector OP. Prove that

$$\dddot{r} = \frac{1}{3}r\omega^2.$$

Solution
The acceleration is determined by case 2 above, and so is given by

$$\mathbf{a} = (\ddot{r} - r\omega^2)\hat{\mathbf{e}} + 2\dot{r}\omega\hat{\mathbf{s}}.$$

Differentiating with respect to time gives

$$\dot{\mathbf{a}} = \dddot{r}\,\hat{\mathbf{e}} + \ddot{r}\,\dot{\hat{\mathbf{e}}} - \dot{r}\omega^2\hat{\mathbf{e}} - r\omega^2\dot{\hat{\mathbf{e}}} + 2\ddot{r}\,\omega\hat{\mathbf{s}} + 2\dot{r}\omega\dot{\hat{\mathbf{s}}}$$

$$= (\dddot{r} - 3\dot{r}\omega^2)\,\hat{\mathbf{e}} + (3\ddot{r} - r\omega^2)\,\omega\hat{\mathbf{s}}.$$

As the rate of change of acceleration is parallel to the radius vector OP, the transverse component along $\hat{\mathbf{s}}$ must vanish, so that

$$3\ddot{r} - r\omega^2 = 0, \quad \text{or} \quad \ddot{r} = \frac{1}{3}r\omega^2. \qquad\blacktriangle$$

PROBLEMS 67

1. A particle of constant mass m acting under the influence of gravity is projected from a point on a horizontal plane at time $t = 0$ with a velocity $\mathbf{u}$ in the vertical plane. Find the velocity $\mathbf{v}$ and position vector $\mathbf{r}$ of the

particle as a function of time. If $\mathbf{u} = u(\cos \alpha \mathbf{i} + \sin \alpha \mathbf{j})$, with y measured vertically and x horizontally from the origin, show that

$$x = ut \cos \alpha \quad \text{and} \quad y = ut \sin \alpha - \frac{1}{2} gt^2.$$

Find the distance from the origin at which the particle hits the ground.

2. A particle of constant mass m moving in the vertical plane under gravity is projected from the origin at time $t = 0$ with velocity $\mathbf{v}_0$. Determine its velocity $\mathbf{v}$ and position vector $\mathbf{r}$ at time t if it experiences a force $km\mathbf{v}$ due to air resistance.

3. A particle P moves in a plane with constant angular velocity ω in such a way that the rate of increase of the acceleration is perpendicular to the· radius vector OP. Prove that

$$\dddot{r} - 3r\omega^2 = \text{const.}$$

4. A particle moves around the cardioid $r = a(1 - \cos \theta)$ in such a manner that the radius vector rotates about the origin with the constant angular velocity ω. Show that the radial and transverse components of the acceleration are, respectively,

$$\omega^2(a - 2r) \quad \text{and} \quad 2a\omega^2 \sin \theta.$$

5. A point P moves on the curve

$$r = a \exp(\theta \cot \alpha)$$

in such a way that its radius vector OP rotates about the origin with the constant angular velocity ω. Find the radial and transverse components of its velocity, and show that the resultant velocity makes a constant angle with the radius vector (it is an **equiangular spiral**).

68 Scalar and vector fields and the gradient of a scalar function

SCALAR AND VECTOR FIELDS

A scalar function φ is a single-valued function which is defined in some domain D of space, and whose value at any point P of D is a real number. The value of φ depends only on the position of P, and not on the coordinate system used to specify it. The domain of definition D of φ may be a curve, a surface or a region in space. We say φ defines a **scalar field** in D, since it associates a scalar $\varphi(P)$ with each point P in D.

When using Cartesian coordinates (x, y, z) to specify the point P with position vector $\mathbf{r} = x\mathbf{i} + z\mathbf{j} + z\mathbf{k}$ at which φ is to be evaluated, we write

$$\varphi(x, y, z), \quad \varphi(\mathbf{r}) \quad \text{or} \quad \varphi(P).$$

The following are typical examples of scalar fields:

1 The distance $\varphi(P)$ of a point $P(x, y, z)$ from some fixed point $P_0(x_0, y_0, z_0)$. This defines a scalar field determined by the function

$$\varphi(x, y, z) = [(x - x_0)^2 + (y - y_0)^2 + (z - z_0)^2]^{1/2},$$

which is defined throughout all space.

2 The temperature $T(P)$ at a point P inside a body. This defines a scalar field throughout the body.

3 The pressure p at a point on the wall of a container filled with fluid. This defines a scalar field over a finite surface.

4 The density $\rho(P)$ of the metal in a thin twisted wire of non-homogeneous composition. This defines a scalar field over a curve in space.

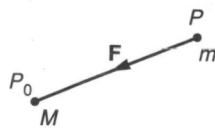

Fig. 145

5 The electrostatic potential $\varphi(x, y, z)$ inside a dielectric. This defines a scalar
field throughout the dielectric.

Suppose it is possible to assign a unique vector $\mathbf{v}(P)$ to each point P in a
region D in space, and that $\mathbf{v}(P)$ depends only on the position of P, and not
on the coordinate system used to specify it. Then $\mathbf{v}(P)$ is said to specify a
vector field throughout the region D.

In terms of Cartesian coordinates we write

$$\mathbf{v}(x, y, z) = v_1(x, y, z)\,\mathbf{i} + v_2(x, y, z)\,\mathbf{j} + v_3(x, y, z)\,\mathbf{k},$$

where v_1, v_2 and v_3 are scalar fields in D.

The following are typical examples of vector fields:

1 The **velocity field** $\mathbf{v}$ inside a rigid body rotating with angular velocity $\boldsymbol{\omega}$
about an axis through the origin. This vector field is defined by the vector ·
equation

$$\mathbf{v} = \boldsymbol{\omega} \times \mathbf{r},$$

where $\mathbf{r}$ is the position vector of a point in the body. If the axis coincides
with the z-axis, so that $\boldsymbol{\omega} = \omega\mathbf{k}$, then

$$\mathbf{v} = \omega\mathbf{k} \times (x\mathbf{i} + y\mathbf{j} + z\mathbf{k})$$
$$= \omega(-y\mathbf{i} + x\mathbf{j}).$$

2 A **gravitational force field** $\mathbf{F}$. Let a particle of mass M be at a point P_0, and
suppose that a particle of mass m is located at a general point P, as shown
in Fig. 145. Then by **Newton's law of gravitation** mass M attracts mass m
(and conversely) with a force along PP_0 which is inversely proportional to
$r^2 = (PP_0)^2$. The magnitude of the force is given by

$$|\mathbf{F}| = \frac{k}{r^2},$$

where $k = GMm$, with G the universal gravitational constant.

If $P_0 P = \mathbf{r}$, then the unit vector along PP_0 is $-\mathbf{r}/r$, so

$$\mathbf{F} = -\frac{GMm\,\mathbf{r}}{r^3}$$

$$= -\frac{GMm}{r^3}[(x - x_0)\mathbf{i} + (y - y_0)\mathbf{j} + (z - z_0)\mathbf{k}].$$

3. The **electric field** $\mathbf{E}$ at a point in a dielectric medium between two electri-
cally charged plates.

4 The **heat flux vector** $\mathbf{Q}$ at a point in a solid in which there is an uneven
temperature distribution. The vector $\mathbf{Q}$ determines the direction in which
heat is conducted at any given point in the solid, and $|\mathbf{Q}|$ is the energy per
unit area per unit time transferred in the direction of $\mathbf{Q}$.

The surfaces $\varphi = \text{const.}$ associated with a scalar field are called **level surfaces** and, by definition, two different level surfaces do not intersect. Typical
examples of level surfaces are **isotherms**, which are level surfaces of temperature (surfaces of constant temperature) and **isobars**, which are level surfaces
of pressure (surfaces of constant pressure).

Thus, for example, the level surfaces of the function

$$\varphi = (x - x_0)^2 + (y - y_0)^2, \quad \text{for all} \quad z,$$

are the surfaces determined by setting $\varphi = $ constant, which in this case must be a non-negative constant because φ is the sum of two squared quantities. If we set $\varphi = k^2$, say, the level surfaces become

$$(x - x_0)^2 + (y - y_0)^2 = k^2, \quad \text{for all} \quad z.$$

The equation describes a circle of radius k centred on the point (x_0, y_0), and as this is true for all z, the level surfaces are concentric cylinders with their common axis parallel to the z-axis and passing through the point (x_0, y_0) in the (x, y)-plane.

If $\mathbf{F}(x, y, z)$ is a vector function, a **field line** at a point P is a line in space such that the direction of the tangent to the line at P is that of $\mathbf{F}$. In a velocity field in a moving body (solid or fluid) such lines are called **streamlines**, while in a force field they are called **lines of force**. If the vector $\mathbf{F}$ is given by

$$\mathbf{F} = F_1 \mathbf{i} + F_2 \mathbf{j} + F_3 \mathbf{k},$$

the field lines are determined by

$$d\mathbf{r} = k\mathbf{F},$$

where $d\mathbf{r} = dx \mathbf{i} + dy \mathbf{j} \, dz \mathbf{k}$ is an increment along the field line from the point with position vector $\mathbf{r}$. Equivalently, the field lines are determined by the scalar equations

$$\frac{dx}{F_1} = \frac{dy}{F_2} = \frac{dz}{F_3} \, (= k).$$

An example of a velocity field was given earlier for the case of a rigid body rotating about the z-axis with constant angular velocity $\boldsymbol{\omega}$, where it was seen that

$$\mathbf{v} = \omega(-y\mathbf{i} + x\mathbf{j}).$$

In this case the streamlines are given by

$$\frac{dx}{-\omega y} = \frac{dy}{\omega x}$$

or, equivalently, by

$$x dx = - y dy.$$

Integration then shows that the streamlines have the equation

$$x^2 + y^2 = k^2,$$

so they are circles centred on the z-axis (as would be expected from the nature of the problem).

THE GRADIENT OF A SCALAR FUNCTION

Consider a scalar field $\varphi(x, y, z)$ defined in some region of space D. Construct the level surfaces through two adjacent point P and P' of D, and let these level

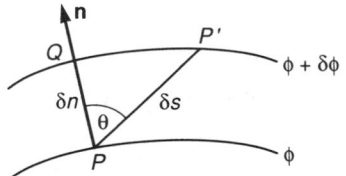

Fig. 146

surfaces have the respective values φ and $\varphi + \delta\varphi$, as shown in Fig. 146. Setting the length $PP' = \delta s$ we define the expression

$$\lim_{\delta s \to 0} \frac{\delta\varphi}{\delta s} = \frac{\partial\varphi}{\partial s}$$

to be the **directional derivative** of φ in the direction PP'. Let Q be the point at which the normal to the level surface through P cuts the level surface through P', and let $PQ = \delta n$. The directional derivative along the normal at P is then

$$\lim_{\delta n \to 0} \frac{\delta\varphi}{\delta n} = \frac{\partial\varphi}{\partial n} .$$

However, $\delta n / \delta s = \cos\theta$, where θ is the angle between PQ and PP', so as

$$\frac{\delta\varphi}{\delta s} = \frac{\delta\varphi}{\delta n} \frac{\delta n}{\delta s} ,$$

by proceeding to the limit, as $\delta s \to 0$ this becomes

$$\frac{\partial\varphi}{\partial s} = \frac{\partial\varphi}{\partial n} \cos\theta .$$

This last result shows that the **maximum rate of change** of φ occurs along the normal to the level surface. The **gradient** of the scalar field φ at any given point, written grad φ (and also $\nabla\varphi$), is defined as the maximum rate of change of φ in magnitude and direction, and thus

$$\text{grad } \varphi = \frac{\partial\varphi}{\partial n} \hat{\mathbf{n}},$$

where $\hat{\mathbf{n}}$ is the unit normal to the level surface at any given point.

Forming the scalar product of this result with the unit vector $\hat{\mathbf{s}}$ in the direction PP' shows that the directional derivative in this direction is

$$\frac{\partial\varphi}{\partial s} = \frac{\partial\varphi}{\partial n} \cos\theta = \hat{\mathbf{s}} \cdot \text{grad } \varphi .$$

In component form, $\partial\varphi/\partial x$, $\partial\varphi/\partial y$ and $\partial\varphi/\partial z$ are seen to be the directional derivatives of φ along the x, y and z-axes, respectively. As the unit vectors along these axes are $\mathbf{i}, \mathbf{j}$ and $\mathbf{k}$, it follows directly that

$$\frac{\partial\varphi}{\partial x} = \mathbf{i} \cdot \text{grad } \varphi$$

$$\frac{\partial \varphi}{\partial y} = \mathbf{j} \cdot \text{grad } \varphi$$

$$\frac{\partial \varphi}{\partial z} = \mathbf{k} \cdot \text{grad } \varphi .$$

The vector function grad φ is a vector, so it can be written as

$$\text{grad } \varphi = A\mathbf{i} + B\mathbf{j} + C\mathbf{k}.$$

Forming the scalar product of this expression with $\mathbf{i}$, $\mathbf{j}$ and $\mathbf{k}$, and using the previous result, shows that

$$A = \frac{\partial \varphi}{\partial x} , \quad B = \frac{\partial \varphi}{\partial y} \quad \text{and} \quad C = \frac{\partial \varphi}{\partial z} ,$$

so we may write

$$\text{grad } \varphi = \frac{\partial \varphi}{\partial x} \mathbf{i} + \frac{\partial \varphi}{\partial y} \mathbf{j} + \frac{\partial \varphi}{\partial z} \mathbf{k} .$$

This is the result we use to determine grad φ when φ is specified in terms of the Cartesian coordinates x, y and z. The **vector differential operator** grad is defined as

$$\text{grad} \equiv \mathbf{i} \frac{\partial}{\partial x} + \mathbf{j} \frac{\partial}{\partial y} + \mathbf{k} \frac{\partial}{\partial z} .$$

Properties of grad φ

1 grad $\varphi = \dfrac{\partial \varphi}{\partial x} \mathbf{i} + \dfrac{\partial \varphi}{\partial y} \mathbf{j} + \dfrac{\partial \varphi}{\partial z} \mathbf{k}.$

2 If $\hat{\mathbf{s}}$ is a unit vector, then

$$\hat{\mathbf{s}} \cdot \text{grad } \varphi$$

is the directional derivative of φ in the direction of $\hat{\mathbf{s}}$.

3 grad φ is directed in the direction of the maximum rate of increase of φ.

4 $|\text{grad } \varphi|$ is the maximum rate of increase of φ per unit displacement.

5 If $P_0(x_0, y_0, z_0)$ is a point at which grad $\varphi \neq \mathbf{0}$, then $(\text{grad } \varphi)_{P_0}$ is normal to the level surface through P_0.

6 If a, b are constants and φ, ψ, are scalar fields, then

$$\text{grad}(a\varphi + b\psi) = a \text{ grad } \varphi + b \text{ grad } \psi.$$

Example 68.1

Find grad φ and $(\text{grad } \varphi)_{(1, 0, -1)}$ given that

(i) $\varphi = 3x - 4y + 7z;$

(ii) $\varphi = \dfrac{x^2}{4} + \dfrac{y^2}{9} + \dfrac{z^2}{16} ;$

(iii) $\varphi = \dfrac{1}{x^2 + y^2} - z^2.$

Solution

(i) grad $\varphi = \dfrac{\partial \varphi}{\partial x} \mathbf{i} + \dfrac{\partial \varphi}{\partial y} \mathbf{j} + \dfrac{\partial \varphi}{\partial z} \mathbf{k}$,

$= 3\mathbf{i} - 4\mathbf{j} + 7\mathbf{k}.$

As in this case grad φ is a constant vector, and so is the same at all points in space, it follows that

$$(\text{grad } \varphi)_{(1, 0, -1)} = 3\mathbf{i} - 4\mathbf{j} + 7\mathbf{k}.$$

(ii) grad $\varphi = \dfrac{\partial \varphi}{\partial x} \mathbf{i} + \dfrac{\partial \varphi}{\partial y} \mathbf{j} + \dfrac{\partial \varphi}{\partial z} \mathbf{k}$

$= \dfrac{1}{2} x\mathbf{i} + \dfrac{2}{9} y\mathbf{j} + \dfrac{1}{8} z\mathbf{k},$

and thus

$$(\text{grad } \varphi)_{(1, 0, -1)} = \dfrac{1}{2} \mathbf{i} - \dfrac{1}{8} \mathbf{k}.$$

(iii) grad $\varphi = \dfrac{\partial \varphi}{\partial x} \mathbf{i} + \dfrac{\partial \varphi}{\partial y} \mathbf{j} + \dfrac{\partial \varphi}{\partial z} \mathbf{k}$

$= \dfrac{-2x}{(x^2 + y^2)^2} \mathbf{i} - \dfrac{2y}{(x^2 + y^2)^2} \mathbf{j} - 2z\mathbf{k},$

and thus

$$(\text{grad } \varphi)_{(1, 0, -1)} = -2\mathbf{i} + 2\mathbf{k}. \qquad \blacktriangle$$

Example 68.2

Given that

$$\varphi = 3x^2 + xy^2 + yz,$$

find grad φ and the directional derivative of φ in the direction of the vector $\mathbf{s} = \mathbf{i} + 2\mathbf{j} - 2\mathbf{k}$. Find the value of this directional derivative at the point $(1, -2, -1)$.

Solution

$$\text{grad } \varphi = \dfrac{\partial \varphi}{\partial x} \mathbf{i} + \dfrac{\partial \varphi}{\partial y} \mathbf{j} + \dfrac{\partial \varphi}{\partial z} \mathbf{k}$$

$$= (6x + y^2)\mathbf{i} + (2xy + z)\mathbf{j} + y\mathbf{k}.$$

The unit vector $\hat{\mathbf{s}}$ in the direction of $\mathbf{s} = \mathbf{i} + 2\mathbf{j} - 2\mathbf{k}$ is

$$\hat{\mathbf{s}} = \dfrac{1}{3} (\mathbf{i} + 2\mathbf{j} - 2\mathbf{k}),$$

so the directional derivative of φ in the direction of $\mathbf{s}$ is

$$\hat{\mathbf{s}} \cdot \text{grad } \varphi = \dfrac{1}{3} (\mathbf{i} + 2\mathbf{j} - 2\mathbf{k}) \cdot [(6x + y^2)\mathbf{i} + (2xy + z)\mathbf{j} + y\mathbf{k}]$$

$$= \frac{1}{3} [6x + y^2 + 4xy + 2x - 2y].$$

At the point $(1, -2, -1)$, the directional derivative has the value

$$\hat{s} \cdot \text{grad}\, \varphi = 4/3.$$

▲

Example 68.3

Find grad φ, given that

$$\varphi = r^n \quad \text{and} \quad r^2 = x^2 + y^2 + z^2.$$

Solution
By definition,

$$\text{grad}(r^n) = \frac{\partial}{\partial x}(r^n)\mathbf{i} + \frac{\partial}{\partial y}(r^n)\mathbf{j} + \frac{\partial}{\partial z}(r^n)\mathbf{k},$$

but

$$\frac{\partial}{\partial x}(r^n) = nr^{n-1}\frac{\partial r}{\partial x}, \quad \frac{\partial}{\partial y}(r^n) = nr^{n-1}\frac{\partial r}{\partial y} \quad \text{and} \quad \frac{\partial}{\partial z}(r^n) = nr^{n-1}\frac{\partial r}{\partial z},$$

so

$$\text{grad}(r^n) = nr^{n-1}\left(\frac{\partial r}{\partial x}\mathbf{i} + \frac{\partial r}{\partial y}\mathbf{j} + \frac{\partial r}{\partial z}\mathbf{k}\right) = nr^{n-1}\,\text{grad}\, r.$$

Differentiating $r^2 = x^2 + y^2 + z^2$ partially with respect to x gives

$$2r\frac{\partial r}{\partial x} = 2x,$$

showing that

$$\frac{\partial r}{\partial x} = \frac{x}{r}.$$

Similar arguments show that

$$\frac{\partial r}{\partial y} = \frac{y}{r} \quad \text{and} \quad \frac{\partial r}{\partial z} = \frac{z}{r},$$

and thus

$$\text{grad}\, r = \frac{\partial r}{\partial x}\mathbf{i} + \frac{\partial r}{\partial y}\mathbf{j} + \frac{\partial r}{\partial z}\mathbf{k}$$

$$= \frac{1}{r}(x\mathbf{i} + y\mathbf{j} + z\mathbf{k}) = \frac{\mathbf{r}}{r}.$$

Combining this with the previous result then shows that

$$\text{grad}\, \varphi = nr^{n-1}\frac{\mathbf{r}}{r} = nr^{n-2}\mathbf{r}.$$

▲

From the definition of grad φ, we see that at any point P on the level surface $\varphi = $ constant, the vector $(\text{grad}\,\varphi)_P$ is **normal** to the surface at P. Thus, if required, the tangent plane at any point on the level surface may be found, since the normal to the tangent plane at a given point is known together with the point P itself which lies on the plane.

Example 68.4

Find the normal and a unit normal to the surface

$$x^2 + 2y^2 - z^2 - 8 = 0$$

at the point $(1, 2, 1)$, and the equation of the tangent plane at this point.

Solution
If we set

$$\varphi = x^2 + 2y^2 - z^2 - 8,$$

the level surface $\varphi = 0$ is the surface to which the tangent plane is required at the point $(1, 2, 1)$. We have

$$\text{grad}\,\varphi = 2x\mathbf{i} + 4y\mathbf{j} - 2z\mathbf{k},$$

and at the point $(1, 2, 1)$ it follows that

$$\mathbf{n} = (\text{grad}\,\varphi)_{(1, 2, 1)} = 2\mathbf{i} + 8\mathbf{j} - 2\mathbf{k}.$$

A unit normal at this same point is

$$\hat{\mathbf{n}} = \frac{\mathbf{n}}{|\mathbf{n}|} = \frac{1}{3\sqrt{2}}(\mathbf{i} + 4\mathbf{j} - \mathbf{k}).$$

The tangent plane through the point with position vector $\mathbf{a}$ and normal $\mathbf{n}$ is

$$(\mathbf{r} - \mathbf{a}) \cdot \mathbf{n} = 0, \quad \text{or} \quad \mathbf{r} \cdot \mathbf{n} = \mathbf{a} \cdot \mathbf{n}.$$

Setting $\mathbf{r} = x\mathbf{i} + y\mathbf{j} + z\mathbf{k}$, $\mathbf{n} = 2\mathbf{i} + 8\mathbf{j} - 2\mathbf{k}$ and $\mathbf{a} = \mathbf{i} + 2\mathbf{j} + \mathbf{k}$ in the equation of the plane gives

$$(x\mathbf{i} + y\mathbf{j} + z\mathbf{k}) \cdot (2\mathbf{i} + 8\mathbf{j} - 2\mathbf{k}) = (\mathbf{i} + 2\mathbf{j} + \mathbf{k}) \cdot (2\mathbf{i} + 8\mathbf{j} + 2\mathbf{k}),$$

and after the cancellation of a numerical factor this reduces to

$$x + 4y - z = 8. \qquad \blacktriangle$$

Example 68.5

Given that

$$f(x, y, z) = \cosh 2x \sinh 3y \sin z$$

find grad f, and setting $\mathbf{u} = \text{grad}\,f$ with $\mathbf{u} = u_1\mathbf{i} + u_2\mathbf{j} + u_3\mathbf{k}$ show that

$$\frac{\partial u_1}{\partial x} + \frac{\partial u_2}{\partial y} + \frac{\partial u_3}{\partial z} = 12f.$$

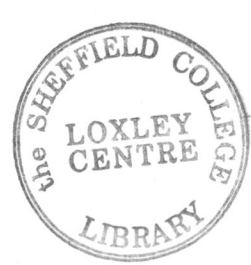
SHEFFIELD COLLEGE
the LOXLEY CENTRE LIBRARY

Solution
We have

$$\operatorname{grad} f = 2 \sinh 2x \sinh 3y \sin z\mathbf{i} + 3 \cosh 2x \cosh 3y \sin z\mathbf{j}$$
$$+ \cosh 2x \sinh 3y \cos z\mathbf{k},$$

and thus

$$u_1 = 2 \sinh 2x \sinh 3y \sin z,$$

$$u_2 = 3 \cosh 2x \cosh 3y \sin z,$$

$$u_3 = \cosh 2x \sinh 3y \cos z.$$

Differentiation then gives

$$\frac{\partial u_1}{\partial x} = 4 \cosh 2x \sinh 3y \sin z = 4f$$

$$\frac{\partial u_2}{\partial y} = 9 \cosh 2x \sinh 3y \sin z = 9f$$

$$\frac{\partial u_3}{\partial z} = - \cos 2x \sinh 3y \sin z = -f,$$

and so

$$\frac{\partial u_1}{\partial x} + \frac{\partial u_2}{\partial y} + \frac{\partial u_3}{\partial z} = 12f. \qquad\blacktriangle$$

PROBLEMS 68

1. Show that the level surfaces of the function

$$\varphi = \frac{x^2}{4} + \frac{y^2}{9}$$

   in three dimensions are elliptic cylinders.
2. Show that the level surfaces of the function

$$\varphi = x^2 - y^2$$

   in three dimensions are hyperbolic cylinders.
3. Show that the level surfaces of

$$\varphi = x^2 + y^2 + z^2$$

   are concentric spheres.
4. Show that the level surfaces of

$$\varphi = x + y + z$$

   are parallel planes.

In problems 5 to 10 find grad φ and a unit vector $\hat{\mathbf{n}}$ in the direction of grad φ at the stated point.

5. $\varphi = x^2 + 2y^2 - 3z^2$; $(1, 2, -1)$.
6. $\varphi = xy^2 z^3$; $(1, 1, -1)$.
7. $\varphi = \sin(xyz)$; $(-1, \pi/4, -1)$.
8. $\varphi = \ln(x^2 + y^2 + z^2)$; $(1, 1, 1)$.
9. $\varphi = x \sin y + y \cos z$; $(\pi/4, \pi/4, \pi/4)$.

10. $\varphi = \dfrac{1}{x^2 + 3y^2 + z^2}$; $(1, 0, -1)$.

11. Find the equation of the plane tangent to the surface

$$x^2 + 2xyz + yz^2 + 1 = 0$$

at the point $(-1, 0, 1)$.

12. Find the equation of the plane tangent to the surface

$$x^2 + 3y^2 + 2z^2 - 15 = 0$$

at the point $(1, 2, 1)$.

13. A force $\mathbf{F}$ is given by

$$\mathbf{F} = \text{grad}(x^2 + 2xyz + z^3).$$

Find $\mathbf{F}$ and $|\mathbf{F}|$ at the point $(1, -1, 1)$ and the component of $\mathbf{F}$ at this point in the direction of the vector $\mathbf{i} + \mathbf{j} - \mathbf{k}$.

14. Find the angle between the tangent planes to the surface

$$x^2 + 4y^2 + z^2 = 6$$

at the point $(1, 1, 1)$ and $(1, -1, -1)$.

15. Find the equation of the line normal to the surface

$$\varphi = x^3 + 2x^2 y^2 z + y^2 z^2 - 4$$

at the point $(1, 1, 1)$.

16. Find the equation of the plane tangent to the surface

$$\varphi = x^3 + 2y^2 - 2z^2 + 1$$

at the point $(-1, -1, -1)$, and determine its distance from the origin.

17. Find the directional derivative of

$$\varphi = \dfrac{x}{x^2 + 2y^2 + 3z^2 + 1}$$

at the point $(1, -1, -1)$ in the direction of the vector $\mathbf{i} - 3\mathbf{j} + 3\mathbf{k}$.

18. Given that $\mathbf{u} = u_1 \mathbf{i} + u_2 \mathbf{j}$ satisfies the vector equation

$$\mathbf{a} \times \mathbf{u} = \text{grad}\,\varphi,$$

find $\mathbf{u}$ given that $\mathbf{a} = \mathbf{k}$ and

$$\varphi = \sin x \sin y.$$

19. Find the equation of the normal to the surface

$$x^2 + 2y^2 + a^2 z^2 = 18$$

at the point $(1, 2, 3/\alpha)$. For what values of α does the normal pass through the point $(0, -2, 8)$?

20.   The equation of a surface is

$$3x^2 - y^2 + 2xyz = 4.$$

Show that the tangent planes to the surface at the points $(1, 1, 1)$ and $(-1, -1, 1)$ are both parallel to the y-axis and obtain their equations. Show that each plane is at a perpendicular distance $5/\sqrt{17}$ from the origin, but on opposite sides.

Ordinary differential equations: order and degree, initial and boundary conditions 69

An **ordinary differential equation** for the function $y(x)$ is an equation relating x, y and one or more derivatives of y with respect to x. It is called an ordinary differential equation because y only depends on x, and so only ordinary derivatives of y with respect to x are involved.

The following are examples of different types of ordinary differential equations.

1 The differential equation describing the free fall of a unit mass under the influence of gravity, neglecting air resistance, is

$$\frac{d^2 x}{dt^2} = g,$$

where x is the distance fallen in time t and g is the acceleration due to gravity.

2 The differential equation describing the current I flowing at time t in the RL circuit shown in Fig. 147 is

$$L\frac{dI}{dt} + RI = E,$$

where R is the resistance, L the inductance and E is the applied voltage.

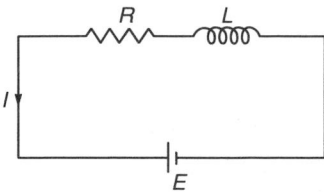

Fig. 147

3 The differential equation describing the vertical displacement from equilibrium x at time t of a mass m suspended by a spring and subject to air resistance proportional to the speed is

$$m\frac{\mathrm{d}^2x}{\mathrm{d}t^2} + D\frac{\mathrm{d}x}{\mathrm{d}t} + kx = 0,$$

where $D > 0$ is the resistance coefficient and $k > 0$ is the spring constant.

4 The differential equation describing **Newton's law of cooling**, which asserts that the rate of decrease of the temperature of a hot body is proportional to the excess of the temperature T over the ambient temperature T_0 is

$$\frac{\mathrm{d}T}{\mathrm{d}t} = -k(T - T_0),$$

where T is the temperature at time t and T_0 is the ambient temperature.

5 The differential equation determining the vertical deflection y of a uniform beam of length L and weight W/unit length supported at each end, as shown in Fig. 148

$$EI\frac{\mathrm{d}^2y}{\mathrm{d}x^2} = \frac{1}{2}W(x^2 - Lx^2),$$

where E is Young's modulus of elasticity for the material of the beam, I is the moment of inertia of the cross-section of the beam and x is the distance along the beam.

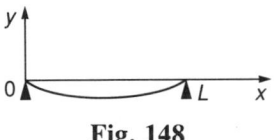

Fig. 148

It is necessary to have a simple classification of differential equations which gives some indication of their complexity. This is accomplished by specifying their **order** and **degree**. If the highest derivative to occur in a differential equation involving y as a function of x is $\mathrm{d}^ny/\mathrm{d}x^n$ the equation is said to be of order n. The degree of the equation is the power to which the highest derivative is raised. The typical examples which follow illustrate this classification:

1 $\dfrac{\mathrm{d}y}{\mathrm{d}x} = kx$, order 1, degree 1;

2 $x^2(1 + y)\dfrac{\mathrm{d}y}{\mathrm{d}x} - (1 + x)y^2 = 0$, order 1, degree 1;

3 $\dfrac{\mathrm{d}^3y}{\mathrm{d}x^2} + \dfrac{2\mathrm{d}^2y}{\mathrm{d}x^2} - \dfrac{\mathrm{d}y}{\mathrm{d}x} + 4y = 0$, order 3, degree 1;

4 $x\left(\dfrac{\mathrm{d}^3y}{\mathrm{d}x^3}\right)^2 + \dfrac{3\mathrm{d}^2y}{\mathrm{d}x} + x^2\left(\dfrac{\mathrm{d}y}{\mathrm{d}x}\right)^5 = 0$, order 3, degree 2.

In general, although the complexity of a differential equation increases as the order increases, the degree is more important, and equations of degree 1 are significantly simpler than those of higher degree.

One of the most important types of ordinary differential equation is one in which y and its derivatives only occur with degree 1, and derivatives of y are never multiplied by y or any function of y. Such equations are called **linear differential equations**. Differential equations which are not linear are said to be **non-linear**. Here are some illustrative examples:

1 $\dfrac{dy}{dx} + ky = 0$, first order and linear;

2 $(1+x)^2 \dfrac{dy}{dx} + (\sin x)y = 0$, first order and linear;

3 $\dfrac{dy}{dx} + x \sin y = 0$, first order and non-linear;

4 $(1+x)\dfrac{d^2 y}{dx^2} + x \dfrac{dy}{dx} + 6y = 0$, second order and linear;

5 $(1+x^2)\dfrac{d^3 y}{dx^2} + \dfrac{3d^2 y}{dx^2} + \left(\dfrac{dy}{dx}\right)^2 + y = 0$, third order and non-linear;

6 $x\dfrac{d^4 y}{dx^4} + (1+x^2)\dfrac{d^2 y}{dx^2} + (\sin x)y = 0$, fourth order and linear.

Given a differential equation, the object is to find a function $y = Y(x)$ which when substituted into the equation satisfies it identically. Such a function is called a **solution** of the differential equation. In general, special techniques are needed to find solutions of differential equations, but the simplest differential equations can be solved by means of direct integration.

Consider, for example, the equation

$$\frac{dy}{dx} = kx \quad (k = \text{const.}).$$

Direct integration with respect to x gives

$$\int \left(\frac{dy}{dx}\right) dx = \int kx\, dx,$$

or

$$\int dy = \int kx\, dx,$$

so that

$$y = \frac{1}{2} kx^2 + A,$$

where A is an arbitrary constant of integration.

Arguing in similar fashion shows that the equation

$$\frac{d^2 y}{dx^2} = x$$

has the solution

$$y = \frac{1}{6}x^3 + Ax + B,$$

where A is the arbitrary constant of integration introduced as a result of the first integration, and B is another arbitrary constant of integration introduced as a result of the second integration needed to arrive at y from dy/dx.

An extension of this argument establishes the fundamental property that the **general solution** (the most general solution possible) of an nth order differential equation will contain n arbitrary constants.

In physical problems a unique solution is expected, so if an nth order differential equation is involved, n conditions to be satisfied by the solution must be specified if the values of these n arbitrary constants are to be determined. If these conditions are all specified at a **single** value of x they are called **initial conditions**. When the conditions are specified at **two different** values of x they are called **boundary conditions**. Solutions satisfying initial or boundary conditions are called **particular solutions**, and they contain no arbitrary constants.

In the RL circuit in Fig. 147 an initial condition is appropriate, and it involves the specification of the current I when $t = 0$. Thus an initial condition for this equation would be $I = I_0$ when $t = 0$, where I_0 is the given value of I when $t = 0$. Since I is a function of t it follows that $I = I(t)$, and this result is often used to state the initial condition more concisely as

$$I(0) = I_0.$$

In the beam problem in Fig. 148 boundary conditions are appropriate, and they involve the specification of the fact that $y = 0$ when $x = 0$ and also when $x = L$, because the beam is supported at these points so there can be no deflection at the ends of the beam. As $y = y(x)$, these boundary conditions can also be written

$$y(0) = 0 \quad \text{and} \quad y(L) = 0.$$

A simple initial value problem involves solving the equation in illustration 1 describing the free fall of a particle under the influence of gravity when air resistance is neglected.
The differential equation is

$$\frac{d^2x}{dt^2} = g,$$

where x is measured vertically downwards from the position of the particle at time $t = 0$. Thus when the particle starts to fall, $x = 0$, which is one of the two initial conditions necessary to identify a particular solution. The other initial condition which needs to be specified is whether or not the particle starts from rest. Let us suppose it starts by being projected downwards with an initial speed u. Then we are required to solve

$$\frac{d^2x}{dt^2} = g,$$

subject to the initial conditions

$$x = 0 \quad \text{and} \quad \frac{\mathrm{d}x}{\mathrm{d}t} = u, \quad \text{when} \quad t = 0,$$

or, using the more concise notation, and a prime to denote differentiation with respect to t,

$$x(0) = 0 \quad \text{and} \quad x'(0) = u.$$

Integrating once with respect to t gives

$$\frac{\mathrm{d}x}{\mathrm{d}t} = gt + A,$$

where A is an arbitrary constant. However, from the initial conditions we know that $\mathrm{d}x/\mathrm{d}t = u$ when $t = 0$ (equivalently, $x'(0) = u$), so that $A = u$, and thus

$$\frac{\mathrm{d}x}{\mathrm{d}t} = u + gt.$$

This, then, is the equation determining the **speed** of the particle at a time $t > 0$.

A further integration with respect to t gives

$$x = ut + \frac{1}{2}gt^2 + B,$$

where B is an arbitrary constant. The so far unused initial condition is $x = 0$ when $t = 0$ (equivalently, $x(0) = 0$) which shows that $B = 0$, so the required particular solution determining the distance fallen in a time $t > 0$ is

$$x = ut + \frac{1}{2}gt^2.$$

Had the particle started from the position $x = x_0$ with speed u at $t = 0$ we would have found that $B = x_0$ and the particular solution would then have been

$$x = x_0 + ut + \frac{1}{2}gt^2.$$

As an example of a simple boundary value problem let us solve

$$\frac{\mathrm{d}^2 y}{\mathrm{d}x^2} = 2x^2 + 3$$

subject to the boundary conditions

$$y(0) = 1 \quad \text{and} \quad y(1) = -2.$$

Integrating once gives

$$\frac{\mathrm{d}^2 y}{\mathrm{d}x^2} = \frac{2}{3}x^3 + 3x + A,$$

where A is an arbitrary constant. A further integration gives

$$y = \frac{1}{6}x^4 + \frac{3}{2}x^2 + Ax + B,$$

where B is a second arbitrary constant.

Substituting the boundary condition $y(0) = 1$ gives

$$1 = B,$$

so

$$y = \frac{1}{6}x^4 + \frac{3}{2}x^2 + Ax + 1.$$

Substituting the boundary condition $y(1) = -2$ gives

$$-2 = \frac{8}{3} + A, \quad \text{so} \quad A = -\frac{14}{3},$$

and thus the required solution is

$$y = \frac{1}{6}x^4 + \frac{3}{2}x^2 - \frac{14}{3}x + 1.$$

The general solution of an nth order ordinary differential equation contains n arbitrary constants. Thus, if such a general solution is known, differentiating it n times and eliminating the arbitrary constants will yield the original differential equation.

Thus if the general solution of an equation is

$$y = Ae^t + 2Be^{2t},$$

it follows that it must be a second order equation because there are two arbitrary constants. Differentiation yields

$$\frac{dy}{dx} = Ae^t + 2Be^{2t}$$

and

$$\frac{d^2y}{dx^2} = Ae^t + 4Be^{2t}.$$

Thus

$$\frac{dy}{dt} - y = Be^{2t} \quad \text{and} \quad \frac{d^2y}{dt^2} - \frac{dy}{dt} = 2Be^{2t},$$

and so

$$\frac{d^2y}{dt^2} - \frac{dy}{dt} = 2\left(\frac{dy}{dt} - y\right),$$

which yields the governing differential equation

$$\frac{d^2y}{dt^2} - 3\frac{dy}{dt} + 2y = 0.$$

PROBLEMS 69

1. Determine the order and degree of each of the following differential equations:

(a) $\left(\dfrac{d^4y}{dx^4}\right)^3 + \dfrac{d^3y}{dx^3} - 6\left(\dfrac{dy}{dx}\right)^2 + y = 0;$

(b) $\dfrac{d^3y}{dx^3} + 9\dfrac{d^2y}{dx^2} + 4\dfrac{dy}{dx} + 7y = 0;$

(c) $\left(\dfrac{dy}{dx}\right)^2 + x\sin y = 0;$

(d) $x\dfrac{dy}{dx} + (1 + x^2 + x^3)y = 0;$

(e) $\sin x\dfrac{d^2y}{dx^2} + (1 + x^2)\dfrac{dy}{dx} + xy = 0;$

(f) $x^2\dfrac{d^2y}{dx^2} + 5\dfrac{dy}{dx} + (x^2 - 9)y = 0.$

2.   Determine the order of each of the following differential equations, and whether or not they are linear.

(a) $(1 + x)\dfrac{dy}{dx} + (1 + 2x + 4x^3)y = 0;$

(b) $x^2\dfrac{d^2y}{dx^2} + (2x + 1)\dfrac{dy}{dx} + 3y^2 = 0;$

(c) $(1 + x^2)y\dfrac{d^2y}{dx^2} + x\dfrac{dy}{dx} + 2y = 0;$

(d) $x^2\dfrac{d^2y}{dx^2} + x\dfrac{dy}{dx} + (x^2 - 1)y = 0;$

(e) $\dfrac{d^3y}{dx^3} + (1 + 4x)\dfrac{d^2y}{dx^2} + \sin x\dfrac{dy}{dx} + 4y = 0;$

(f) $\dfrac{d^4y}{dx^4} + 3\dfrac{d^2y}{dx^2} + \sqrt{(1 - y^2)} = 0.$

3.   Find the general solution of
$$\dfrac{d^3y}{dx^3} = 1.$$

4.   Find the general solution of
$$\dfrac{d^3y}{dx^3} = 1 + x.$$

5.   Solve the initial value problem
$$\dfrac{d^2y}{dx^3} = x^2,$$
subject to the initial conditions
$$y(1) = 2 \quad \text{and} \quad y'(1) = 3.$$

6.   Solve the initial value problem
$$\dfrac{d^2y}{dx^3} = \sin x,$$

subject to the initial conditions

$$y(0) = 1 \quad \text{and} \quad y'(0) = 2.$$

7.   Solve the boundary value problem

$$\frac{d^2y}{dx^3} = \sinh 2x,$$

subject to the boundary conditions

$$y(0) = 1 \quad \text{and} \quad y(1) = 4.$$

8.   Solve the boundary value problem

$$\frac{d^2y}{dx^3} = \cos x$$

subject to the boundary conditions

$$y(0) = 0 \quad \text{and} \quad y(\pi) = 0.$$

In problems 9 to 14 find the differential equation with the given form of general solution.

9. $y = A \cos 3x + B \sin 3x.$

10. $y = A \cosh 4x + B \sinh 4x.$

11. $y = Ae^{3x} + Bxe^{3x}.$

12. $y = Ae^{3x} + Bxe^{3x} + Ce^{-2x}.$

13. $y = Ae^{3x} \cos 4x + Be^{3x} \sin 4x.$

14. $y = Ae^{x} + B \cos x + C \sin x.$

First order differential equations solvable by separation of variables 70

Any first order ordinary differential equation can be written as

$$F(x, y, y') = 0,$$

where $y' = dy/dx$ and F is a function of x, y and y'. In many cases this can be solved explicitly for y' and rewritten as

$$\frac{dy}{dx} = f(x, y),$$

where f is a function of x and y. A further simplification occurs if the function f is of the form

$$f(x, y) = g(x)h(y),$$

for then the differential equation becomes

$$\frac{dy}{dx} = g(x)h(y),$$

A differential equation of this type is said to have **separable variables**, because in terms of differentials it can be written

$$\frac{1}{h(y)}\, dy = g(x)\, dx,$$

so after integration it becomes

$$\int \frac{1}{h(y)}\, dy = \int g(x)\, dx.$$

When a solution is found in this manner it is said to have been obtained by means of **separation of variables**.

The single arbitrary constant associated with this general solution appears as the sum of the arbitrary constants arising when the integrals on the left and right are evaluated. This follows because the sum of two arbitrary constants is simply a single arbitrary constant.

An alternative way of representing a separable first order differential equation which is often used is by writing it as

$$p(y)\,dy + q(x)\,dx = 0.$$

Example 70.1

Find the general solution of

$$\frac{dy}{dx} + ky = 0,$$

and use it to solve the initial value problem for this equation in which $y(1) = 3$.

Solution
The differential equation can be written in the form

$$\frac{dy}{y} = -\,k\,dx,$$

in which the variables have been separated. Thus

$$\int \frac{dy}{y} = -\,k \int dx,$$

so after evaluating the integrals this becomes

$$\ln |y| = C - kx,$$

where C is an arbitrary constant. Taking exponentials we arrive at the result

$$y = \exp[C - kx] = e^{C}e^{-kx}.$$

As C is an arbitrary constant, so also is e^{C}, so we now denote it by A. The general solution is thus

$$y = A\mathrm{e}^{-kx}.$$

To solve the initial value problem, A must be chosen such that $y = 3$ when $x = 1$. Substituting this condition into the general solution gives

$$3 = A\mathrm{e}^{-k}, \quad \text{or} \quad A = 3\mathrm{e}^{k}.$$

Thus the required particular solution becomes

$$y = 3\mathrm{e}^{k} \cdot \mathrm{e}^{-kx} = 3 \exp[k(1 - x)]. \qquad \blacktriangle$$

Example 70.2

Find the general solution of

$$\frac{dy}{dx} = 2(x^2 + 1)(y^2 + 1).$$

Solution
Separating variables and integrating, the differential equation becomes

$$\int \frac{dy}{y^2 + 1} = 2 \int (x^2 + 1)\,dx,$$

so after evaluating the integrals we find that

$$\arctan y = 2\left(\frac{x^3}{3} + x\right) + A,$$

where A is an arbitrary constant. Thus the general solution is seen to be

$$y = \tan\left[\frac{2x^3}{3} + 2x + A\right]. \qquad \blacktriangle$$

Example 70.3

Find the general solution of
$$(x^3 y^2 - x^3 y)\,dy - xy^2\,dx = 0, \quad x \neq 0, \quad y \neq 0.$$

Solution
At first sight this differential equation does not have separable variables, but
it can be written as
$$x^3 y(y - 1)\,dy = xy^2\,dx,$$
and after rearrangement it becomes
$$\left(\frac{y-1}{y}\right)dy = \left(\frac{1}{x^2}\right)dx.$$

Thus

$$\int \left(1 - \frac{1}{y}\right)dy = \int \frac{dx}{x^2},$$

and so the general solution is seen to be

$$y - \ln|y| = -\frac{1}{x} + C,$$

where C is an arbitrary constant. $\qquad \blacktriangle$

Example 70.4

Find the general solution of
$$(y + xy)\frac{dy}{dx} + x + xy = 0.$$

Solution
First we rewrite the differential equation as

$$y(1 + x)\frac{dy}{dx} + x(1 + y) = 0.$$

Separating variables this becomes

$$\left(\frac{y}{1+y}\right)dy = -\left(\frac{x}{1+x}\right)dx,$$

and so

$$\int \frac{y}{1+y}\,dy = -\int \frac{x}{1+x}\,dx$$

or, equivalently,

$$\int \left(1 - \frac{1}{1+y}\right)dy = -\int \left(1 - \frac{1}{1+x}\right)dx.$$

Thus the general solution is

$$y - \ln|1+y| = C_1 - (x - \ln|1+x|),$$

where C_1 is an arbitrary constant. It is convenient to set $C_1 = \ln C$, where C is an arbitrary constant, for then after rearrangement the general solution becomes

$$x + y = \ln|C(1+x)(1+y)|. \qquad\qquad \blacktriangle$$

Sometimes a simple substitution will transform a differential equation in which the variables are not separable into one in which they are.

Example 70.5

Find the general solution of

$$\frac{dy}{dx} = \cos(x+y).$$

Solution
The variables x and y are not separable in this differential equation. However, setting

$$z = x + y,$$

differentiation shows that

$$\frac{dz}{dx} = 1 + \frac{dy}{dx}.$$

After changing the variables from x and y to x and z the original differential equation becomes

$$\frac{dz}{dx} = 1 + \cos z,$$

in which the variables are now separable. Thus

$$\int \frac{dz}{1+\cos z} = \int dx$$

and so as $1 + \cos z = 2 \cos^2(z/2)$,

$$\int \frac{dz}{2 + \cos^2(z/2)} = \int dx,$$

which is equivalent to

$$\frac{1}{2} \int \cot^2(z/2) \, dz = \int dx.$$

Integration then gives

$$\tan(z/2) = x + C,$$

or

$$z = 2 \arctan(x + C),$$

where C is an arbitrary constant.

Returning to the original variables x and y we arrive at the general solution

$$y = 2 \arctan(x + C) - x. \qquad \blacktriangle$$

PROBLEMS 70

Find the general solution for each of the differential equations in problems 1 to 14 and, where necessary, use it to solve the associated initial value problem.

1. $x \dfrac{dy}{dx} = y; \quad y(-1) = 3.$

2. $y \dfrac{dy}{dx} + x = 0; \quad y(-2) = 4.$

3. $x^2 \dfrac{dy}{dx} + y = 0; \quad y(1) = 2e.$

4. $2 \dfrac{dy}{dx} \sqrt{x} = y; \quad y(9) = 1.$

5. $\dfrac{dy}{dx} = (2y + 1) \cot x; \quad y(\pi/4) = 1/2.$

6. $(x^2 + x) \dfrac{dy}{dx} = 2y + 1; \quad y(1) = 0.$

7. $\tan x \sin^2 y \, dx + \cos^2 x \cot y \, dy = 0.$

8. $3e^x \tan y \, dx + (1 - e^x) \sec^2 y \, dy = 0.$

9. $e^x(1 + e^y) \, dy + e^y(1 + e^x) \, dy = 0.$

10. $x \dfrac{dy}{dx} = \ln |x|.$

11. $(1 + x) y \, dx + (1 - y) x \, dy = 0.$

12. $(x^2 - yx^2) \dfrac{dy}{dx} + y^2 + xy^2 = 0.$

13. $\dfrac{dy}{dx} \cot x + y = 4; \quad y(0) = -1.$

14. $x^2 \dfrac{dy}{dx} - \cos 4y = 1; \quad y(+\infty) = \pi/8.$

15. Find the general solution of

$$\frac{dy}{dx} + y = 2x + 1$$

by means of the substitution $z = y - 2x - 1$.

16. Find the general solution of

$$\frac{dy}{dx} = \cos(x - y - 1)$$

by means of the substitution $z = x - y - 1$.

The method of isoclines and Euler's methods   71

The general solution of the ordinary differential equation

$$\frac{dy}{dx} = f(x, y)$$

can be represented graphically in the form of a family of curves in the (x, y)-plane. The solution corresponding to the initial condition $y(a) = b$ will be a curve starting from the point (a, b). Collectively, these solution curves are called the **integral curves** of the differential equation.

The general behaviour of the integral curves of a first order ordinary differential equation can be deduced by using a graphical approach called the **method of isoclines**.

An **isocline** is a curve in the (x, y)-plane along which the derivative of the solution dy/dx of every integral curve has a constant value k. Geometrically, dy/dx determines the slope (gradient) of an integral curve, so it follows from this that the tangents to all integral curves passing through a given isocline will have the same slope. It is this property which has given rise to the name **isocline**, which means a curve of constant slope (of dy/dx). An isocline is not an integral curve, but a curve characterizing a property possessed by all integral curves when they cross it.

To derive the equation of the isoclines we must set $dy/dx = k$ (a constant) in the original differential equation. This shows the equation of the isoclines to be

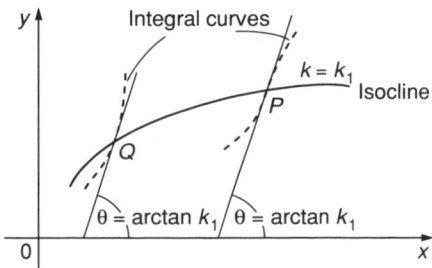

Fig. 149

$$f(x, y) = k,$$

and each different isocline is associated with a different value of k. When an integral curve intersects the isocline corresponding to $k = k_1$ its tangent at the point of intersection will make an angle $\theta = \arctan k_1$ with the positive x-axis, as shown in Fig. 149 in which integral curves pass through points P and Q.

Example 71.1

Sketch some representative isoclines of

$$\frac{dy}{dx} = y.$$

Use them to deduce the general behaviour of the solutions of this differential equation, and sketch the approximate integral curves corresponding to the initial conditions
(i) $y(0) = 0.5$; and
(ii) $y(-0.5) = -1$.

Solution
The equation of the isoclines is given by setting $dy/dx = k$ in the differential equation which gives rise to the equation

$$y = k.$$

These are lines parallel to the x-axis, as shown in Fig. 150. To each isocline has been added several short lines inclined to the positive x-axis at the angle $\theta = \arctan k$, and their purpose is to indicate the direction of the tangent to an integral curve when it crosses the isocline.

Inspection of Fig. 150 shows how if an integral curve starts at a point in the upper half-plane it will increase with increasing rapidity as x increases. The

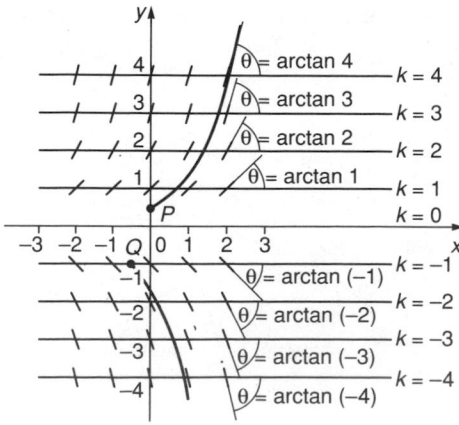

Fig. 150

converse situation arises if the integral curve starts at a point in the lower half-plane, for then it decreases with increasing rapidity as x increases. Taking into account these general properties of the integral curves, and the fact that the x-axis corresponds to the isocline on which $dy/dx = 0$, it follows that no integral curve can cross the x-axis. Thus if an integral curve starts on one side of the x-axis, it must remain on that same side for all x.

The curve starting from point P is the approximate integral curve corresponding to initial condition (i) in which $y(0) = 0.5$, and the curve starting from point Q is the approximate integral curve corresponding to initial condition (ii) in which $y(-0.5) = -1$. The general solution of this simple differential equation is, of course

$$y = Ce^x,$$

so the exact solution through P is

$$y = \frac{1}{2}e^x$$

and the exact solution through Q is

$$y = -\exp\left(x + \frac{1}{2}\right). \qquad \blacktriangle$$

Example 71.2

Sketch some representative isoclines of

$$\frac{dy}{dx} = x^2 + y^2,$$

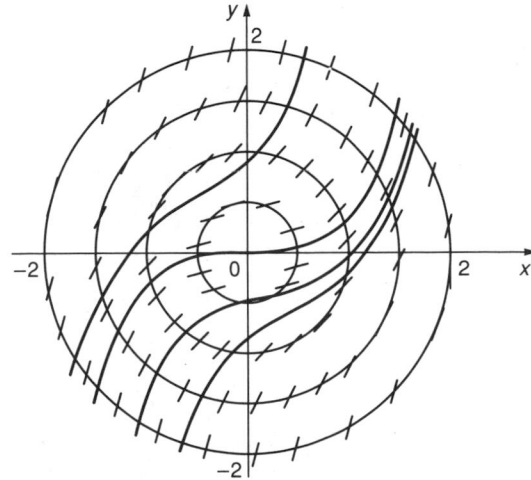

Fig. 151

and use them to construct some approximate integral curves.

Solution
The isoclines are determined by setting $dy/dx = k$, in the differential equation, and so they are the curves with the equation

$$x^2 + y^2 = k.$$

Since the left-hand side of this equation is non-negative, we must restrict k to be such that $k \geq 0$. The isocline for any given value of k is thus a circle of radius $k^{1/2}$ centred on the origin.

Some typical isoclines, together with lines showing the associated slope, are given in Fig. 151 to which has also been added four approximate integral curves.

Example 71.3

Sketch some representative isoclines and integral curves for

$$\frac{dy}{dx} = x - y^2.$$

Solution
The equation of the isoclines is given by setting $dy/dx = k$ in the differential equation which gives rise to the equation

$$k = x - y^2.$$

Thus the isoclines are the parabolas

$$y = \pm \sqrt{(x - k)}, \quad \text{with} \quad x \geq k,$$

and the integral curves intersect these at an angle $\theta = \arctan k$. These isoclines are shown as the dotted curves in Fig. 152, and representative integral curves are shown as the solid curves. ▲

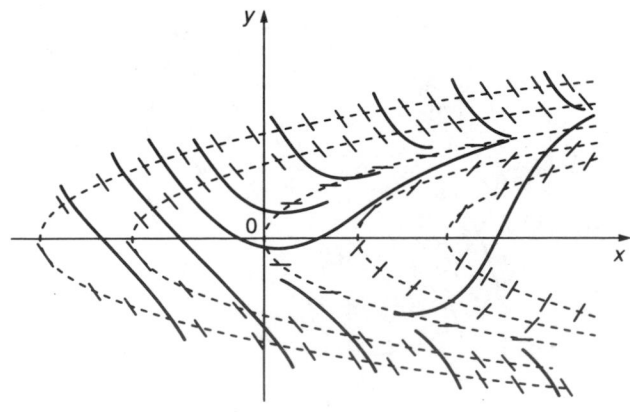

Fig. 152

EULER'S METHOD

When the solution of the initial value problem

$$\frac{dy}{dx} = f(x, y), \quad \text{with} \quad y(x_0) = y_0$$

cannot be found analytically it becomes necessary to use numerical methods. The simplest of these is **Euler's method** which uses a tangent line approximation to the integral curve through the point (x_0, y_0) in order to determine the value of y, say y_1, when x increases from x_0 to x_1. The idea is illustrated in Fig. 153, in which the tangent to the integral curve at $P(x_0, y_0)$ is used to approximate the arc PQ of the integral curve. Thus the point Q on the integral curve corresponding to $x = x_1$ is approximated by the point R. If the point R is located at (x_1, y_1) then as $SR = PS \tan \theta = (x_1 - x_0) \tan \theta$,

$$y_1 = y_0 + (x_1 - x_0) \tan \theta,$$

but

$$\tan \theta = f(x_0, y_0),$$

so **Euler's formula** for y_1 is

$$y_1 = y_0 + (x_1 - x_0) f(x_0, y_0).$$

It is customary to set $h = x_1 - x_0$ and to call this the integration **step length**, so the above result then becomes

$$y_1 = y_0 + hf(x_0, y_0).$$

Having obtained an approximation (x_1, y_1) to the point Q on the integral curve, the process can be repeated as often as necessary, and the approximate solution found at intervals h apart starting from $x = x_0$. This is Euler's method which is simple to apply, but subject to error owing to the fact that the tangent approximation at P does not take account of the curvature of the integral curve through P. The accuracy can be improved by reducing the step length.

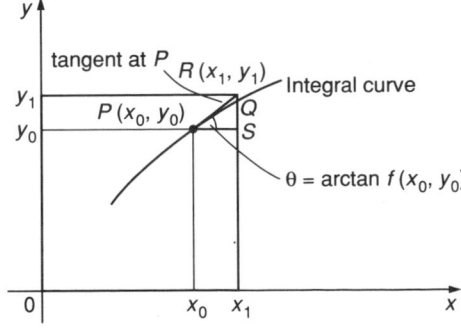

Fig. 153

The numerical algorithm for Euler's method

1 It is required to solve numerically

$$\frac{dy}{dx} = f(x, y)$$

subject to the initial condition $y(x_0) = y_0$, and to find the solution at the points

$$x_n = x_0 + nh, \quad \text{with} \quad n = 0, 1, 2, ..., N,$$

where h is a specified step length and N is the number of steps to be taken. That is, the solution is to be determined from $x = x_0$ to $x = x_0 + Nh$ at intervals h apart.

2 Euler's method involves starting from the given initial values x_0 and y_0 and applying the numerical algorithm (computational rule)

$$y_{n+1} = y_n + hf(x_n, y_n),$$

to find the approximate values of y_n when $x_n = x_0 + nh$ for $n = 0, 1, 2, ..., N$.

Example 71.4

Given the initial value problem

$$\frac{dy}{dx} = -\left(\frac{x + 2y}{x}\right) \quad \text{with} \quad y(1) = 0.5,$$

use Euler's method with ten steps of equal length to determine the solution in the interval $1 \leq x \leq 3.5$.

Solution

The function $f(x, y)$ is

$$f(x, y) = -\left(\frac{x + 2y}{x}\right),$$

and as ten steps of equal length are to be used to cover the interval $1 \leq x \leq 3.5$ it follows that the step length $h = (3.5 - 1)/10 = 0.25$. Thus in this case the Euler algorithm becomes

$$x_{n+1} = x_n + nh,$$

and

$$y_{n+1} = y_n - h\left(\frac{x_n + 2y_n}{x_n}\right),$$

with $n = 0, 1, 2, ..., 10$. The calculation uses the step length $h = 0.25$ and starts from the initial condition

$$x_0 = 1, \quad y_0 = 0.5.$$

Setting $n = 0$ we have

$$y_1 = y_0 - h\left(\frac{x_0 + 2y_0}{x_0}\right)$$

$$= 0.5 - 0.25\left(\frac{1 + 2 \times 0.5}{1}\right) = 0,$$

so $y_1 = 0$.

Setting $n = 1$ we have $x_1 = x_0 + h = 1.25$

$$y_2 = y_1 - h\left(\frac{x_1 + 2y_1}{x_1}\right)$$

$$= 0 - 0.25\left(\frac{1.25 + 2 \times 0}{1.25}\right) = -0.25,$$

so $y_2 = -0.25$.

Setting $n = 2$ we have $x_2 = x_1 + h = 1.5$

$$y_3 = y_2 - h\left(\frac{x_2 + 2y_2}{x_2}\right)$$

$$= -0.25 - 0.25\left(\frac{1.5 + 2 \times (-0.25)}{1.5}\right) = -0.4167,$$

so $y_3 = -0.4167$.

Continuing this process leads to the results given in Table 11.   ▲

Table 11

n	x_n	y_n
0	1.0	0.5
1	1.25	0
2	1.5	-0.25
3	1.75	-0.4167
4	2.0	-0.5476
5	2.25	-0.6607
6	2.5	-0.7639
7	2.75	-0.8611
8	3.0	-0.9545
9	3.25	-1.0455
10	3.5	-1.1346

MODIFIED EULER METHOD

A simple modification can be made to Euler's method which takes some account of the curvature of the integral curve and leads to improved accuracy.

The nature of the modification is best understood by considering Fig. 153. In Euler's method, instead of extrapolating to find the approximate value of y at Q using the slope at P, the slope at P is replaced by the **average** of the slopes at P and R. In terms of Fig. 153 this leads to the modified Euler result

$$y_1 = y_0 + \frac{1}{2} h[f(P) + f(R)],$$

where $f(P)$ and $f(R)$ are the values of $f(x, y)$ at P and R, respectively. Now $F(P) = f(x_0, y_0)$, and from the Euler method R is the point $[x_0 + h, y_0 + hf(x_0, y_0)]$, so

$$f(R) = f[x_0 + h, y_0 + hf(x_0, y_0)]$$

and thus the modified Euler result becomes

$$y_1 = y_0 + \frac{1}{2} h \{ f(x_0, y_0) + f[x_0 + h, y_0 + hf(x_0, y_0)] \}.$$

As with the original method, the modified Euler method may be used to advance the solution step by step as far as is required and its accuracy will be improved if smaller steps are taken.

The numerical algorithm for the modified Euler method
1 It is required to solve numerically

$$\frac{dy}{dx} = f(x, y)$$

subject to the initial condition $y(x_0) = y_0$, where x_0 and y_0 are specified, and to find the solution at the points

$$x_n = x_0 + nh, \quad \text{with} \quad n = 0, 1, 2, ..., N,$$

where h is a specified step length and N is the number of steps to be taken. That is, the solution is to be determined from $x = x_0$ to $x = x_0 + Nh$ at intervals h apart.
2 The modified Euler method involves starting from the given initial values x_0 and y_0 and applying the numerical algorithm

$$y_{n+1} = y_n + \frac{1}{2} h \{ f(x_n, y_n) + f[x_n + h, y_n + hf(x_n, y_n)] \},$$

to find the approximate values of y_n when $x_n = x_0 + nh$ for $n = 0, 1, 2, ..., N$.

Example 71.5

Repeat the calculation in Example 71.3 using the modified Euler method. Compare the results with those obtained in the previous calculation and with the exact solution

$$y = \frac{5 - 2x^3}{6x^2}.$$

Solution
The function $f(x, y)$ is again

$$f(x, y) = -\left(\frac{x + 2y}{x}\right),$$

so

$$f(x_n, y_n) = -\left(\frac{x_n + 2y_n}{x_n}\right).$$

The modified Euler algorithm

$$y_{n+1} = y_n + \frac{1}{2} h \{ f(x_n + y_n) + f[x_n + h, y_n + hf(x_n, y_n)]\}$$

is to be applied with $x_0 = 1$, $y_0 = 0.5$, $h = 0.25$ and $N = 10$.
    Setting $n = 0$ we have

$$f(x_0, y_0) = -2, \; f[x_0 + h, y_0 + hf(x_0, y_0)] = -1,$$

so

$$y_1 = 0.5 + \frac{1}{2} \times 0.25 \, [(-2) + (-1)] = 0.125$$

and $x_1 = x_0 + h = 1.25$.
    Setting $n = 1$ we have

$$f(x_1, y_1) = -1.2, \; f[x_1 + h, y_1 + hf(x_1, y_1)] = -0.7667,$$

so

$$y_2 = 0.125 + \frac{1}{2} \times 0.25 \, [(-1.2) + (-0.7667)] = -0.1208,$$

and $x_3 = x_2 + h = 1.5$.
    Setting $n = 2$ we have

$$f(x_2, y_2) = -0.8389, \; f[x_2 + h, y_2 + hf(x_2, y_2)] = -0.6272,$$

so

$$y_3 = -0.1208 + \frac{1}{2} \times 0.25 \, [-0.8389 - 0.6222] = -0.3034,$$

and $x_3 = x_2 + h = 1.75$.
    Repetition of these calculations leads to the results set out in Table 12. For the purpose of comparison we have listed the results obtained using the simple Euler method in Example 71.3, the results obtained using the modified Euler method and the exact solution given by

$$y = \frac{5 - 2x^3}{6x^2}.$$

Table 12

n	x_n	Euler's method y_n	Modified Euler method y_n	Exact y_n
0	1.0	0.5	0.5	0.5
1	1.25	0	0.125	0.1167
2	1.5	− 0.25	− 0.1208	− 0.1296
3	1.75	− 0.4167	− 0.3034	− 0.3112
4	2.0	− 0.5476	− 0.4517	− 0.4583
5	2.25	− 0.6607	− 0.5798	− 0.5354
6	2.5	− 0.7639	− 0.6953	− 0.7000
7	2.75	− 0.8611	− 0.8025	− 0.8065
8	3.0	− 0.9545	− 0.9040	− 0.9074
9	3.25	− 1.0455	− 1.0015	− 1.0044
10	3.5	− 1.1346	− 1.0961	− 1.0986

The improvement in accuracy resulting from the use of the modified Euler method is seen to be significant, and in good agreement with the exact results.

▲

PROBLEMS 71

In each of the following problems (a) find the equation of the isoclines, (b) sketch some representative isoclines together with lines showing the slope at which integral curves intersect the isoclines, and (c) use the modified Euler method to solve the associated initial value problem using the specified step length h and number of integration steps N.

1. $\dfrac{dy}{dx} = 4 - x^2 + y$; initial condition $y(1)$, $h = 0.5$ and $N = 4$.

2. $\dfrac{dy}{dx} = \dfrac{3x}{x}$; initial condition $y(1) = 1$, $h = 0.5$ and $N = 6$.

3. $\dfrac{dy}{dx} = \dfrac{x^2 + y^2}{x^2}$; initial condition $y(1) = 1$, $h = 0.5$ and $N = 4$.

4. $\dfrac{dy}{dx} = 4 - x + y$; initial condition $y(0) = 0$, $h = 0.5$ and $N = 6$.

5. $\dfrac{dy}{dx} = \dfrac{2y}{x^2}$; initial condition $y(1) = 1$, $h = 0.5$ and $N = 4$.

6. $\dfrac{dy}{dx} = \dfrac{1}{x(y+2)}$; initial condition $y(1) = 0$, $h = 0.5$ and $N = 4$.

Homogeneous and near homogeneous equations

72

A function $F(x, y)$ is said to be **algebraically homogeneous of degree** n if the sum of the powers of x and y in each term of F is equal to n. Expressed differently, $F(x, y)$ is homogeneous of degree n if

$$F(tx, ty) = t^n F(x, y).$$

Thus the function

$$xy^2 - 3x^2y + 9x^3$$

is homogeneous of degree 3, while the function

$$\sqrt{\left(4 + \frac{x^2}{2y^2}\right)}$$

is homogeneous of degree zero. However, the function

$$x + \sqrt{\left[3y^2 + \left(\frac{x^3}{2y^2}\right)\right]}$$

is not homogeneous, because the expression under the square root sign is not homogeneous of degree 2, and hence homogeneous of degree 1 after the square root operation has been performed.

If a first order ordinary differential can be written as

$$\frac{dy}{dx} = \frac{M(x, y)}{N(x, y)},$$

where M and N are algebraically homogeneous functions of the same degree, the differential equation is said to be **algebraically homogeneous** or, more simply, **homogeneous**.

If $M(x, y)$, $N(x, y)$ are homogeneous of degree n, then dividing M and N in the differential equation

$$\frac{dy}{dx} = \frac{M(x, y)}{N(x, y)}$$

by x^n enables it to be written in the form

$$\frac{dy}{dx} = f\left(\frac{y}{x}\right),$$

where f is a function of the single variable y/x. Setting $u = y/x$, so that $y = xu(x)$, it follows that

$$\frac{dy}{dx} = u + x\frac{du}{dx}.$$

Substituting into the differential equation and changing to the variable u gives

$$u + x\frac{du}{dx} = f(u),$$

or

$$x\frac{du}{dx} = f(u) - u,$$

which may now be solved by separation of variables.

Example 72.1

Find the general solution of

$$\frac{dy}{dx} = \frac{xy}{x^2 + y^2},$$

and the solution satisfying the initial condition $y(1) = 3$.

Solution
This is a homogeneous differential equation, since both the numerator and denominator of the right-hand side are homogeneous of degree 2. Dividing the numerator and denominator by x^2 the equation becomes

$$\frac{dy}{dx} = \frac{(y/x)}{1 + (y/x)^2},$$

so setting $u = y/x$ and changing to the variable u we obtain the variable separable equation

$$u + x\frac{du}{dx} = \frac{u}{1 + u^2}.$$

Thus

$$\int\left(\frac{1 + u^2}{u^3}\right)du = -\int\frac{du}{x},$$

so

$$-\frac{1}{2u^2} + \ln|u| = -\ln|x| + \ln A,$$

where $\ln A$ is an arbitrary constant (written in this form for convenience).

Hence

$$\ln\left|\frac{xu}{A}\right| = \frac{1}{2u^2},$$

and so as $u = y/x$ the general solution is seen to be

$$y = A \exp[x^2/(2y^2)].$$

To match this general solution to the initial condition, A must be chosen such that $y(2) = 1$. Substitution into the general solution gives

$$1 = Ae^2, \quad \text{or} \quad A = e^{-2},$$

and so the solution of the initial value problem is

$$y = \exp\left(\frac{x^2}{2y^2} - 2\right),$$

or

$$\dot{y} = \exp\left(\frac{x^2 - 4y^2}{2y^2}\right).$$

Notice that this solution is an implicit solution since y cannot be found explicitly from this result. The solution can, however, be solved explicitly for x in the form

$$x^2 = 2y^2(2 + e^y). \qquad\qquad\qquad \blacktriangle$$

A differential equation of the form

$$\frac{dy}{dx} = \frac{ax + by + c}{px + qy + r}$$

is said to be **near-homogeneous**, because although it is not homogeneous, it can be made so by shifting the origin to the point of intersection of the two straight lines

$$ax + by + c = 0$$

and

$$px + qy + r = 0.$$

This is accomplished by making the change of variable

$$x = X + \alpha, \quad y = Y + \beta,$$

where α and β are solutions of

$$a\alpha + b\beta + c = 0$$

$$p\alpha + q\beta + r = 0.$$

The resulting differential equation is homogeneous in X and Y and so may be solved in the usual manner. The transformation

$$X = x - \alpha, \quad Y = y - \beta$$

then gives the solution in terms of the original variables x and y.

Example 72.2

Find the general solution of

$$\frac{dy}{dx} = \frac{2x - 5y + 3}{2x + 4y - 6}.$$

Solution
This differential equation is near homogeneous. We solve for α and β using the equations

$$2\alpha - 5\beta + 3 = 0$$
$$2\alpha + 4\beta - 6 = 0,$$

which have the solution $\alpha = \beta = 1$. Thus we make the substitutions

$$x = X + 1, \quad y = Y + 1$$

in the original differential equation which becomes

$$\frac{dY}{dx} = \frac{2X - 5Y}{2X + 4Y}.$$

The further substitution

$$\frac{Y}{X} = V$$

leads to the result

$$X\frac{dV}{dX} = \frac{-4V^2 - 7V + 2}{2 + 4V},$$

and so

$$\int \frac{(4V + 2)}{(4V - 1)(V + 2)} dV = -\int \frac{dX}{X}.$$

Simplifying the first integral by means of partial fractions reduces it to

$$\frac{4}{3} \int \frac{dV}{4V - 1} + \frac{2}{3} \int \frac{dV}{V + 2} = -\int \frac{dX}{X},$$

and after integration this becomes

$$\frac{1}{3} \ln|4V - 1| + \frac{2}{3} \ln|V + 2| = -\ln|X| + \ln A,$$

where $\ln A$ is an arbitrary constant. This result simplifies to

$$(4V - 1)(V + 2)^2 X^3 = A^3 = B \quad \text{(say)},$$

so returning to the original variables by writing

$$V = Y/X, \quad X = x - 1 \quad \text{and} \quad Y = y - 1$$

we arrive at the general solution

$$(4y - x - 3)(2x + y - 3)^2 = B$$

which, as is usual in such problems, is an implicit solution.   ▲

If

$$ax + by = k(px + qy), \quad \text{with} \quad k = \text{constant},$$

the lines

$$ax + by + c = 0$$
$$px + qy + r = 0$$

will be parallel, and so will not intersect. In such a case either of the following two changes of variable

$$u = ax + by \quad \text{or} \quad u = px + qy$$

will reduce the differential equation to one of homogeneous type.

Example 72.3

Find the general solution of

$$\frac{dy}{dx} = \frac{2x - 2y + 3}{x - y + 1}.$$

Solution
The lines

$$2x - 2y + 3 = 0$$

and

$$x - y + 1 = 0$$

are parallel (because $2x - 2y = 2(x - y)$), so we have an example of the type just discussed.

Setting $u = x - y$ and differentiating with respect to x gives

$$\frac{du}{dx} = 1 - \frac{dy}{dx},$$

after which substituting into the differential equation gives

$$1 - \frac{du}{dx} = \frac{2u + 3}{u + 1}$$

or

$$\frac{du}{dx} = -\left(\frac{u + 2}{u + 1}\right).$$

Thus

$$\int \left(\frac{u + 1}{u + 2}\right) du = -\int dx,$$

but

$$\frac{u + 1}{u + 2} = 1 - \frac{1}{u + 2},$$

so

$$\int du - \int \frac{du}{u+2} = -\int dx,$$

and hence

$$u - \ln|u+2| = -x + A,$$

where A is an arbitrary constant. Returning to the original variables by setting $u = x - y$ we see that the general solution is

$$2x - y - \ln|x - y + 2| = A. \qquad \blacktriangle$$

PROBLEMS 72

1. State which of the following functions are homogeneous and, when they are, give their degree:
   (a) $(x^2 + 3xy + y^2)/xy$; (b) $x^3 + \sqrt{(x^6 + x^3 y^3)}$; (c) $3x^2 y + y^4/x$;
   (d) $(1 + x/y)/(x + y)$; (e) $x + 2y - \sqrt{(x^2 + 4y^2)}$; (f) $\exp[x^2 + y^2\sqrt{(x^2 + y^2)}/x]$.

In problems 2 to 10 find the general solution of the differential equation and, where specified, the solution satisfying the given initial condition.

2. $\dfrac{dy}{dx} = \dfrac{2y^2 - x^2}{2xy}$.

3. $\dfrac{dy}{dx} = \dfrac{x^2 + y^2}{2xy}$; initial condition $y(1) = 2$.

4. $\dfrac{dy}{dx} = \dfrac{2x + y}{2x}$; initial condition $y(1) = 0$.

5. $\dfrac{dy}{dx} = \dfrac{(x - y)y}{x^2}$.

6. $\dfrac{dy}{dx} = \dfrac{y}{x - 2\sqrt{(xy)}}$.

7. $\dfrac{dy}{dx} = -\left(\dfrac{4x^2 + 3xy + y^2}{4y^2 + 3xy + x^2}\right)$.

8. $\dfrac{dy}{dx} = \dfrac{xy - y^2}{x^2 - 2xy}$.

9. $\dfrac{dy}{dx} = \dfrac{2y^2 - x^2}{2xy}$.

10. $\dfrac{dy}{dx} = \dfrac{xy}{x^2 - y^2}$.

Find the general solution in problems 11 to 16.

11. $\dfrac{dy}{dx} = \left(\dfrac{x - 2y + 5}{2x - y + 4} \right).$

12. $\dfrac{dy}{dx} = \dfrac{1 - 3x - 3y}{1 + x + y}.$

13. $\dfrac{dy}{dx} = \dfrac{x + 2y + 1}{2x + 4y + 3}.$

14. $\dfrac{dy}{dx} = 2 \left(\dfrac{y + 1}{x + y - 2} \right)^{2}.$

15. $\dfrac{dy}{dx} = \dfrac{2x + y - 1}{4x + 2y + 5}.$

16. $\dfrac{dy}{dx} = \dfrac{x^{3} + y^{3}}{xy^{2}}.$

73

Exact differential equations

Implicit differentiation of the function $F(x, y) = C$, with C, a constant, gives

$$\frac{\partial F}{\partial x} \, \mathrm{d}x + \frac{\partial F}{\partial y} \, \mathrm{d}y = 0.$$

This is simply an ordinary differential equation written in differential form with the general solution $F(x, y) = C$. The equation can, of course, also be written in the more familiar form

$$\frac{\mathrm{d}y}{\mathrm{d}x} = -\left(\frac{\partial F}{\partial x}\right) \Big/ \left(\frac{\partial F}{\partial y}\right).$$

When a differential equation

$$M(x, y) \, \mathrm{d}x + N(x, y) \, \mathrm{d}y = 0$$

has the property that a function $F(x, y)$ exists such that

$$M(x, y) = \frac{\partial F}{\partial x} \quad \text{and} \quad N(x, y) = \frac{\partial F}{\partial y}$$

it is said to be **exact**, and its general solution is $F(x, y) = C$.

To test to see if an equation of this type is exact we use the fact that when the second order partial derivatives of $F(x, y)$ exist and are continuous, they must be such that

$$\frac{\partial^2 F}{\partial x \partial y} = \frac{\partial^2 F}{\partial y \partial x}.$$

When expressed in terms of M and N, it follows from this that the differential equation

$$M(x, y) \, \mathrm{d}x + N(x, y) \, \mathrm{d}y = 0$$

is exact if

$$\frac{\partial M}{\partial y} = \frac{\partial N}{\partial x}.$$

To find the general solution of an exact equation we start from the fact that

$$\frac{\partial F}{\partial x} = M(x, y) \quad \text{and} \quad \frac{\partial F}{\partial y} = N(x, y).$$

Integrating the first equation with respect to x, while regarding y as a constant because M was obtained by partial differentiation with respect to x, we find that

$$\int \frac{\partial F}{\partial x}\, dx = \int M(x,\, y)\, dx$$

or

$$F(x,\, y) = \int M(x,\, y)\, dx + g(y) + A.$$

In this result $g(y)$ is an **arbitrary function** of y and A is an arbitrary constant. The introduction of the arbitrary function $g(y)$ is necessary because under partial differentiation with respect to x, $f(y)$ will look like a constant.

Similarly, if we integrate the second equation with respect to y, while regarding x as a constant, we obtain

$$F(x,\, y) = \int N(x,\, y)\, dy + h(x) + B,$$

where $h(x)$ is an arbitrary function of x and B is an arbitrary constant.

These two expressions for $F(x, y)$ must be identical, so $A = B$ and the functions $g(y)$ and $h(x)$ follow by equating the two results and identifying $g(y)$ with any function solely of y and $h(x)$ with any function solely of x.

Example 73.1

Verify that

$$[2x + 3y \cos(xy)]\, dx + [2e^{2y} + 3x \cos(xy)]\, dy = 0$$

is an exact differential equation and find its general solution.

Solution
First we test this equation to check that it is in fact exact. Setting

$$M = 2x + 3y \cos(xy) \quad \text{and} \quad N = 2e^{2y} + 3x \cos(xy),$$

partial differentiation shows that

$$\frac{\partial M}{\partial y} = 3 \cos(xy) - 3xy \sin(xy)$$

and

$$\frac{\partial N}{\partial x} = 3 \cos(xy) - 3xy \sin(xy).$$

Thus

$$\frac{\partial M}{\partial y} = \frac{\partial N}{\partial x}$$

so the equation is indeed exact.

Setting

$$\frac{\partial F}{\partial x} = M(x, y) = 2x + 3y \cos(xy)$$

and integrating with respect to x, while keeping y constant, gives

$$\int \frac{\partial F}{\partial x} \, dx = \int [2x + 3y \cos(xy)] \, dx$$

or

$$F(x, y) = x^2 + 3 \sin(xy) + g(y) + A.$$

Similarly,

$$\int \frac{\partial F}{\partial x} \, dy = \int [2e^{2y} + 3x \cos(xy)] \, dy,$$

or

$$F(x, y) = e^{2y} + 3 \sin(xy) + h(x) + B.$$

These two expressions for $F(x, y)$ must be identical, so

$$x^2 + 3 \sin(xy) + g(y) + A \equiv e^{2y} + 3 \sin(xy) + h(x) + B.$$

This can only be an identity in x and y (the same for all x and y) if $h(x) = x^2$, $g(y) = e^{2y}$ and $B = A$, so the general solution is:

$$x^2 + e^{2y} + 3 \sin(xy) + A = 0. \qquad \blacktriangle$$

In some simple cases the differential equation

$$P(x, y) \, dx + Q(x, y) \, dy = 0$$

is not exact as it stands, but it can be made exact by multiplication by a factor $\mu(x, y)$, often of the form $\mu = x^m y^n$ for some m and n. Such a factor μ is called an **integrating factor**. Once found, the integration of the differential equation

$$\mu P(x, y) \, dx + \mu Q(x, y) \, dy = 0,$$

which is now exact, proceeds as before.

Example 73.2

Find an integrating factor of the form $\mu = x^m y^n$ for

$$(4xy + y^2) \, dx + (4x^2 + 3xy) \, dy = 0,$$

and hence find the general solution.

Solution
This equation is not exact, because setting

$$P = 4xy + y^2 \quad \text{and} \quad Q = 4x^2 + 3xy$$

we see that

$$\frac{\partial P}{\partial y} \neq \frac{\partial Q}{\partial x}$$

We are told that it will become exact if numbers m and n can be found such that

$$x^m y^n (4xy + y^2) \, dx + x^m y^n (4x^2 + 3xy) \, dy = 0$$

is an exact equation.

To find m and n we set

$$M = x^m y^n P \quad \text{and} \quad N = x^m y^n Q,$$

so

$$M = 4x^{m+1} y^{n+1} + x^m y^{n+2}$$

and

$$N = 4x^{m+2} y^n + 3x^{m+1} y^{n+1}.$$

The differential equation

$$M(x, y) \, dx + N(x, y) \, dy = 0$$

will be exact if

$$\frac{\partial M}{\partial y} = \frac{\partial N}{\partial x}.$$

This leads to the condition

$$4(n+1) x^{m+1} y^n + (n+2) x^m y^{n+1} = 4(m+2) x^{m+1} y^n + 3(m+1) x^m y^{n+1},$$

which can only be satisfied if

$$4(n+1) = 4(m+2) \quad \text{and} \quad n+2 = 3(m+1)$$

or, equivalently,

$$n = m+1 \quad \text{and} \quad n = 3m + 1.$$

These conditions are only true if $m = 0$ and $n = 1$, so the equation has the integrating factor $\mu = y$. The exact differential equation is thus

$$\mu P \, dx + \mu Q \, dy = 0,$$

or

$$(4xy^2 + y^3) \, dx + (4x^2 y + 3xy^2) \, dy = 0.$$

Proceeding as in Example 73.1 we have

$$\int \frac{\partial F}{\partial x} \, dx = \int (4xy^2 + y^3) \, dx$$

so

$$F(x, y) = 2x^2 y^2 + xy^3 + g(y) + A,$$

and

$$\int \frac{\partial F}{\partial y} \, dy = \int (4x^2 y + 3xy^2) \, dy$$

so

$$F(x, y) = 2x^2y^2 + xy^3 + h(x) + B.$$

For the two results to be identical we must set $h(x) \equiv 0$, $g(y) \equiv 0$ and $B = A$, so the general solution is seen to be

$$2x^2y^2 + xy^3 + A = 0. \qquad\qquad \blacktriangle$$

PROBLEMS 73

In problems 1 to 8 show the differential equations are exact and find their general solutions.

1. $(3x^2 + 2y^2)\,dx + (4xy + 2y)\,dy = 0.$

2. $(2x + y - \sin x)\,dx + (4y + x + \cos y)\,dy = 0.$

3. $\left(y + \dfrac{x}{\sqrt{(x^2 + y^2)}}\right)dx + \left(x + \dfrac{y}{\sqrt{(x^2 + y^2)}}\right)dy = 0.$

4. $(ye^x + xye^x)\,dx + (xe^x + 2y)\,dy = 0.$

5. $(x^3 - 3xy^2 + 2)\,dx - (3x^2y - y^2)\,dy = 0.$

6. $(x^2 + y^2 + 2x)\,dx + 2xy\,dy = 0.$

7. $[y + 2 + \cosh(x + 3y)]\,dx + [x + 1 + 3\cosh(x + 3y)]\,dy = 0.$

8. $\dfrac{2x}{y^3}\,dx + \left(\dfrac{y^2 - 3x^2}{y^4}\right)dy = 0.$

In problems 9 and 10 find integrating factors of the form $\mu = x^m x^n$ and hence find the general solutions.

9. $(3xy^2 + 6y^3)\,dx + (2x^2y + 9xy^2)\,dy = 0.$

10. $(4xy + 18y^3)\,dx + (3x^2 + 30xy^2)\,dy = 0.$

The first order linear differential equation

74

The **general first order linear differential equation** has the form

$$a(x)\frac{dy}{dx} + b(x)\,y = c(x),$$

and to solve it we first write it in the **standard form**

$$\frac{dy}{dx} + p(x)\,y = q(x),$$

where

$$p(x) = b(x)/a(x) \quad \text{and} \quad q(x) = c(x)/a(x).$$

Working with the equation in standard form, we now seek a factor $\mu(x)$ with the property that when the differential equation is multiplied by μ to give

$$\mu\frac{dy}{dx} + \mu p(x)\,y = \mu q(x),$$

the left-hand side can be written as

$$\frac{d}{dx}(\mu y),$$

thus reducing the equation to the simple form

$$\frac{d}{dx}(\mu y) = \mu q(x).$$

This result can be integrated to give

$$\int \frac{d}{dx}(\mu y)\,dx = \int \mu q(x)\,dx,$$

so

$$\mu y = A + \int \mu q(x)\,dx,$$

where A is an arbitrary constant. Division by μ then gives the general solution in the form

$$y = \frac{A}{\mu} + \frac{1}{\mu} \int \mu q(x)\,\mathrm{d}x.$$

It now remains for us to determine the factor μ. The function μ was required to be such that

$$\frac{\mathrm{d}}{\mathrm{d}x}(\mu y) = \mu \frac{\mathrm{d}y}{\mathrm{d}x} + \mu p(x)\,y,$$

so performing the differentiation on the left-hand side gives

$$\mu \frac{\mathrm{d}y}{\mathrm{d}x} + y \frac{\mathrm{d}y}{\mathrm{d}x} = \mu \frac{\mathrm{d}y}{\mathrm{d}x} + \mu p(x)\,y,$$

and after simplification this becomes

$$\frac{\mathrm{d}\mu}{\mathrm{d}x} = \mu p(x).$$

This is a simple differential equation for μ with separable variables, so

$$\int \frac{\mathrm{d}\mu}{\mu} = \int p(x)\,\mathrm{d}x$$

and thus

$$\ln|\mu| + \ln C = \int p(x)\,\mathrm{d}x,$$

where $\ln C$ is an arbitrary constant. It follows from this that

$$C\mu = \exp\left[\int p(x)\,\mathrm{d}x \right].$$

For convenience we set $C = 1$. This is permissible because the factor μ multiplies the entire equation so the value of C is immaterial. The factor $\mu(x)$, called the **integrating factor** for the first order linear differential equation in standard form, is thus

$$\mu = \exp\left[\int p(x)\,\mathrm{d}x \right].$$

Integration of a first order linear differential equation
To find the general solution of the first order linear differential equation

$$a(x) \frac{\mathrm{d}y}{\mathrm{d}x} + b(x)\,y = c(x)$$

the following steps are required.

1 Divide the equation by $a(x)$ to bring it into the standard form

$$\frac{dy}{dx} + p(x)y = q(x),$$

with $p(x) = b(x)/a(x)$ and $q(x) = c(x)/a(x)$.

2 Find the integrating factor

$$\mu = \exp\left[\int p(x)\,dx\right].$$

3 Replace the differential equation in standard form by the equivalent differential equation

$$\frac{d}{dx}(\mu y) = \mu q(x).$$

4 Integrate the result in step 3 to obtain

$$\mu y = A + \int \mu q(x)\,dx,$$

where A is an arbitrary constant.

5 Divide the result of step 4 by μ to obtain the general solution

$$y = \frac{A}{\mu} + \frac{1}{\mu}\int \mu q(x)\,dx.$$

Example 74.1

Find the general solution of

$$x(x-1)\frac{dy}{dx} + 2xy = 1,$$

and hence solve the initial value problem for this equation in which $y(2) = 2$.

Solution
Step 1
When written in standard form the equation becomes

$$\frac{dy}{dx} + \left(\frac{2}{x-1}\right)y = \frac{1}{x(x-1)}.$$

Step 2
The integrating factor

$$\mu = \exp\left[\int\left(\frac{2}{x-1}\right)dx\right] = \exp\left[2\ln|x-1|\right] = (x-1)^2.$$

Step 3

We replace the original differential equation in standard form by the equivalent differential equation

$$\frac{d}{dx}[(x-1)^2 y] = (x-1)^2 \cdot \frac{1}{x(x-1)},$$

which becomes

$$\frac{d}{dx}[(x-1)^2 y] = \frac{x-1}{x}.$$

Step 4

Integration of the result in step 3 gives

$$(x-1)^2 y = A + \int \left(\frac{x-1}{x}\right) dx,$$

or

$$(x-1)^2 y = A + x - \ln|x|.$$

Step 5

Dividing the result of step 4 by $(x-1)^2$ (the integrating factor) gives the general solution

$$y = \frac{A + x - \ln|x|}{(x-1)^2}.$$

To solve the initial value problem we must choose the arbitrary constant A such that $y(2) = 2$. Substituting $y = 2$ when $x = 2$ into the general solution gives

$$2 = A + 2 - \ln 2,$$

so $A = \ln 2$, and thus

$$y = \frac{\ln 2 + x - \ln|x|}{(x-1)^2}. \qquad \blacktriangle$$

Example 74.2

Find the general solution of

$$(1 + x^2)\frac{dy}{dx} - xy = 2x,$$

and hence find the solution of the initial value problem for this equation for which $y(1) = 2$.

Solution

Step 1

When written in standard form the equation becomes

$$\frac{dy}{dx} - \left(\frac{1}{1+x^2}\right)y = \frac{2x}{1+x^2}.$$

Step 2
The integrating factor

$$\mu = \exp\left[-\int\left(\frac{x}{1+x^2}\right)dx\right] = \exp\left[-\frac{1}{2}\ln(1+x^2)\right],$$

so

$$\mu = (1+x^2)^{-1/2}.$$

Step 3
Replace the original differential equation in standard form by the equivalent differential equation

$$\frac{d}{dx}\left(\frac{y}{\sqrt{(1+x^2)}}\right) = \frac{2x}{1+x^2} \cdot \frac{1}{\sqrt{(1+x^2)}},$$

or

$$\frac{d}{dx}\left(\frac{y}{\sqrt{(1+x^2)}}\right) = \frac{2x}{(1+x^2)^{3/2}}.$$

Step 4
Integrating the result of step 3 gives

$$\frac{y}{\sqrt{(1+x^2)}} = A + \int \frac{2x}{(1+x^2)^{3/2}}\,dx,$$

or

$$\frac{y}{\sqrt{(1+x^2)}} = A - \frac{2}{\sqrt{(1+x^2)}}.$$

Step 5
The general solution is thus

$$y = \sqrt{(1+x^2)}\left(A - \frac{2}{\sqrt{(1+x^2)}}\right).$$

To solve the initial value problem we must choose A such that $y = 2$ when $x = 1$, so substituting the values into the general solution gives

$$2 = \sqrt{2}(A - \sqrt{2}),$$

so $A = 2\sqrt{2}$ and thus

$$y = 2\sqrt{2}\sqrt{(1+x^2)} - 2. \qquad \blacktriangle$$

PROBLEMS 74

In Problems 1 to 8 find the general solution of the given first order linear differential equations.

1. $x\dfrac{dy}{dx} - y = -x.$

2. $x\dfrac{dy}{dx} + y = \sin x.$

3. $(x+1)\dfrac{dy}{dx} - 2y = (x+1)^4.$

4. $x\dfrac{dy}{dx} - xy = (1+x^2)e^x.$

5. $\dfrac{dy}{dx} - y\sin x = \sin x \cos x.$

6. $(1+x^2)\dfrac{dy}{dx} - 2xy = (1+x^2)^2.$

7. $x\dfrac{dy}{dx} - 2y = x^3 e^x.$

8. $(x+1)\dfrac{dy}{dx} - 2y = (x+1)^3.$

In problems 9 to 16 find the solutions to the given initial value problems.

9. $x\dfrac{dy}{dx} + y = 3,$ with $y(1) = 1.$

10. $(1+x^2)\dfrac{dy}{dx} - xy = 3x - 1,$ with $y(1) = 0.$

11. $\sin x\dfrac{dy}{dx} - y\cos x = 1,$ with $y(\pi/2) = 2.$

12. $x\dfrac{dy}{dx} - 3y = x^4 e^x,$ with $y(1) = 3e.$

13. $x^3\dfrac{dy}{dx} + 3x^2 y = 2,$ with $y(1) = 4.$

14. $x\dfrac{dy}{dx} + y = x^2 + 1,$ with $y(1) = 1.$

15. $\sin x\dfrac{dy}{dx} + y\cos x = 3,$ with $y(\pi/2) = 1.$

16. $\dfrac{dy}{dx} - y\tan x = \dfrac{1}{\cos x},$ with $y(0) = 1.$

The **Bernoulli equation**, which has the general form

$$\frac{dy}{dx} + p(x)\,y = q(x)\,y^n,$$

is a first order **non-linear** differential equation provided $n \neq 0$ or $n \neq 1$. The equation, which arises in various applications, can be transformed into a first order linear differential equation by making the change of variable

$$z = y^{1-n}.$$

To transform the equation we first differentiate the above result to obtain

$$\frac{dz}{dx} = (1-n)\,y^{-n}\,\frac{dy}{dx},$$

and then after changing the independent variable from y to z in the differential equation we obtain

$$\frac{dz}{dx} + (1-n)\,p(x)\,z = (1-n)\,q(x).$$

This is now a first order linear differential equation for z, and so may be solved by the method discussed in Section 74. Once z is known, the required solution is found by transforming back from z to y.

Example 75.1

Find the general solution of

$$x^2 y\,\frac{dy}{dx} - xy^2 = 1.$$

Solution
At first sight this differential equation does not look like a Bernoulli equation, but after division by $x^2 y$ it becomes

$$\frac{dy}{dx} - \left(\frac{1}{x}\right)y = \frac{1}{x^2}\,y^{-1}$$

which is a Bernoulli equation with $p(x) = -1/x$, $q(x) = 1/x^2$ and $n = -1$.
Thus we make the change of variable

$$z = y^2,$$

from which it follows that

$$\frac{dz}{dx} = 2y \frac{dy}{dx},$$

so changing from the dependent variable y to the new dependent variable z in the differential equation we find that it becomes

$$\frac{dz}{dx} - \frac{2z}{x} = \frac{2}{x^2}.$$

This first order linear differential equation has the integrating factor

$$\mu = \exp\left[-\int \frac{2}{x} dx\right] = 1/x^2.$$

Proceeding as in Section 74 we have

$$\frac{d}{dx}(z/x^2) = \left(\frac{2}{x^2}\right)\left(\frac{1}{x^2}\right),$$

or

$$\frac{d}{dx}(z/x^2) = \frac{2}{x^4}.$$

Integration then shows that

$$\frac{z}{x^2} = A - \frac{2}{3x^3},$$

and thus as $z = y^2$, the general solution is seen to be

$$y^2 = Ax^2 - \frac{2}{3x}.$$

PROBLEMS 75

Find the general solution for each of the following problems.

1. $\dfrac{dy}{dx} + \dfrac{y}{x} = -y^2.$

2. $x^2 \dfrac{dy}{dx} = y^2 + xy.$

3. $\dfrac{dy}{dx} - \dfrac{4y}{x} = x\sqrt{y}.$

4. $\dfrac{dy}{dx} + \dfrac{y}{x} = -xy^2.$

5. $2xy \dfrac{dy}{dx} - y^2 + x = 0.$

6. $x \dfrac{dy}{dx} + y = \dfrac{1}{2} xy^3.$

The structure of solutions of linear differential equations of any order

76

The **general linear differential equation of order** n may be written as

$$\frac{\mathrm{d}^n y}{\mathrm{d}x^n} + a_1(x)\frac{\mathrm{d}^{n-1}y}{\mathrm{d}x^{n-1}} + \ldots + a_{n-1}(x)\frac{\mathrm{d}y}{\mathrm{d}x} + a_n(x)y = f(x).$$

This becomes a **constant coefficient** linear differential equation of order n if $a_1(x), a_2(x), \ldots, a_n(x)$ are all constants. We will only consider constant coefficient linear higher order differential equations in what follows.

The above differential equation will be said to be **homogeneous** if $f(x) \equiv 0$; otherwise it will be said to be **non-homogeneous**. Thus, for example, the second order equation

$$\frac{\mathrm{d}^2 y}{\mathrm{d}x^2} + 3\frac{\mathrm{d}y}{\mathrm{d}x} - 4y = 0$$

is homogeneous, whereas the third order equation

$$2\frac{\mathrm{d}^3 y}{\mathrm{d}x^3} - 4\frac{\mathrm{d}^2 y}{\mathrm{d}x^2} + 3\frac{\mathrm{d}y}{\mathrm{d}x} + 7y = \mathrm{e}^x$$

is non-homogeneous.

Do not confuse this use of the term 'homogeneous' with the term 'algebraically homogeneous' introduced in Section 72, where it was used to refer to a property possessed by certain functions of two variables.

The concept of linearly independent functions is of fundamental importance in the theory of higher order linear differential equations. A set of functions $\varphi_1(x), \varphi_2(x), \ldots, \varphi_n(x)$ will be said to be **linearly independent** if the expression

$$C_1\varphi_1(x) + C_2\varphi_2(x) + \ldots + C_n\varphi_n(x) = 0$$

is true for all x only when the constants $C_1 = C_2 = \ldots = C_n = 0$. If this expression is true for all x when not all of the constants are zero, the functions will be said to be **linearly dependent**.

For example, the three functions $1, x, x^2$ are linearly independent, because setting $\varphi_1(x) = 1, \varphi_2(x) = x$ and $\varphi_3(x) = x^2$ we see that

$$C_1 + C_2 x + C_3 x^2 = 0$$

can only be true for all x if $C_1 = C_2 = C_3 = 0$. However, the four functions 1, x, x^2, $(1+x)^2$ are linearly dependent, because $(1+x)^2 = 1 + 2x + x^2$ so setting $\varphi_1(x) = 1$, $\varphi_2(x) = x$, $\varphi_3(x) = x^2$ and $\varphi_4(x) = (1+x)^2$, we see that

$$\varphi_4(x) = \varphi_1(x) + 2\varphi_2(x) + \varphi_3(x),$$

so $\varphi_4(x)$ is a **linear combination** (a sum of multiples) of the three functions $\varphi_1(x)$, $\varphi_2(x)$ and $\varphi_3(x)$. Thus the expression

$$\varphi_1(x) + 2\varphi_2(x) + \varphi_3(x) - \varphi_4(x) = 0$$

for all x, and the constants multiplying the functions $\varphi_1(x)$ to $\varphi_4(x)$ are not all zero. Consequently, this set of four functions is linearly dependent.

A simple but important test for the linear independence of a set of n functions $\varphi_1(x)$, $\varphi_2(x)$, ..., $\varphi_n(x)$ is provided by evaluating the following determinant

$$W = \begin{vmatrix} \varphi_1(x) & \varphi_2(x) & \cdots & \varphi_n(x) \\ \varphi_1^{(1)}(x) & \varphi_2^{(1)}(x) & \cdots & \varphi_n^{(1)}(x) \\ \varphi_1^{(2)}(x) & \varphi_2^{(2)}(x) & \cdots & \varphi_n^{(2)}(x) \\ \vdots & \vdots & \cdots & \vdots \\ \varphi_1^{(n-1)}(x) & \varphi_2^{(n-1)}(x) & \cdots & \varphi_n^{(n-1)}(x) \end{vmatrix},$$

in which

$$\varphi_m^{(r)}(x) = \frac{d^r}{dx^r}[\varphi_m(x)].$$

This determinant is called the **Wronskian** of the functions $\varphi_1(x)$, $\varphi_2(x)$, ..., $\varphi_n(x)$, and the functions will be linearly independent if $W \neq 0$. This test, called the **Wronskian test**, follows by differentiating

$$C_1 \varphi_1(x) + C_2 \varphi_2(x) + \ldots + C_n \varphi_n(x) = 0$$

successively up to $n - 1$ times and requiring the resulting system of equations

$$\begin{aligned} C_1 \varphi_1 &+ C_2 \varphi_2 &+ \ldots + C_n \varphi_n^{(1)} = 0 \\ C_1 \varphi_1^{(1)} &+ C_2 \varphi_2^{(1)} &+ \ldots + C_n \varphi_n^{(1)} = 0 \\ \vdots \qquad &\quad \vdots & \vdots \\ C_1 \varphi_1^{(n-1)} &+ C_2 \varphi_2^{(n-1)} &+ \ldots + C_n \varphi_n^{(n-1)} = 0 \end{aligned}$$

to have the solution $C_1 = C_2 = \ldots = C_n = 0$. It then follows from Section 56 that this can only be true if the determinant of the coefficients of $C_1, C_2, \ldots, C_n$ is non-vanishing, but this is simply the condition $W \neq 0$.

Example 76.1

Prove that the functions $1, e^x, e^{2x}$ are linearly independent.

Solution
We apply the Wronskian test. We have

$$W = \begin{vmatrix} 1 & e^x & e^{2x} \\ 0 & e^x & 2e^{2x} \\ 0 & e^x & 4e^{2x} \end{vmatrix} = 2e^{3x} \neq 0,$$

so the functions are linearly independent.   ▲

When seeking the general solution of the non-homogeneous linear nth order differential equation

$$\frac{d^n y}{dx^n} + a_1(x) \frac{d^{n-1} y}{dx^{n-1}} + \ldots + a_n y = f(x)$$

we first associate with it the homogeneous equation

$$\frac{d^n y}{dx^n} + a_1(x) \frac{d^{n-1} y}{dx^{n-1}} + \ldots + a_n y = 0,$$

obtained by setting $f(x) \equiv 0$.

Then it can be shown that for every such equation there exists a set of n linearly independent solutions $\varphi_1(x), \varphi_2(x), \ldots, \varphi_n(x)$. These are said to form a **fundamental set** of solutions, and we will see later how to find such a set for any constant coefficient equation. The general solution $y_c(x)$ of the homogeneous equation is called the **complementary function** of the non-homogeneous equation, and it is the arbitrary linear combination of the fundamental set of solutions

$$y_c(x) = C_1 \varphi_1(x) + C_2 \varphi_2(x) + \ldots + C_n \varphi_n(x),$$

with $C_1, C_2 \ldots, C_n$ arbitrary constants.

This result is a consequence of the fact that the operation of differentiation is linear with respect to the linear combination $\lambda g(x) + \mu h(x)$, because

$$\frac{d^r}{dx^r} [\lambda g(x) + \mu h(x)] = \lambda \frac{d^r g}{dx^r} + \mu \frac{d^r h}{dx^r},$$

with λ, μ constants. This means that if $y_1(x), y_2(x), \ldots, y_k(x)$ are any solutions of the homogeneous equation, then so also is

$$y(x) = C_1 y_1(x) + C_2 y_2(x) + \ldots + C_k y(x),$$

with $C_1, C_2, \ldots, C_k$ arbitrary constants. This result is called the **superposition property** of solutions.

Returning to the non-homogeneous equation

$$\frac{d^n y}{dx^n} + a_1(x) \frac{d^{n-1} y}{dx^{n-1}} + \ldots + a_n(x) y = f(x),$$

we call any solution of this equation which does not contain arbitrary constants a **particular solution**. In general, such particular solutions $y_p(x)$ are called **particular integrals**.

Thus $y_c(x)$ and $y_p(x)$ are such that

$$\frac{d^n y_c}{dx^n} + a_1(x)\frac{d^{n-1} y_c}{dx^{n-1}} + \ldots + a_n(x) y_c(x) = 0$$

and

$$\frac{d^n y_p}{dx^n} + a_1(x)\frac{d^{n-1} y_p}{dx^{n-1}} + \ldots + a_n(x) y_p(x) = f(x),$$

so the general solution of

$$\frac{d^n y}{dx^n} + a_1(x)\frac{d^{n-1} y}{dx^{n-1}} + \ldots + a_n(x) y(x) = f(x)$$

has the form

$$y(x) = y_c(x) + y_p(x).$$

To find the general solution of a linear differential equation of any order it is thus necessary to find both the complementary function $y_c(x)$, and a particular integral $y_p(x)$. The solution of an initial value problem then involves matching the general solution

$$y(x) = y_c(x) + y_p(x)$$

to the initial conditions, which will determine the values of the arbitrary constants in $y_c(x)$.

A special case of this general structure of a solution has already been established in Section 74 when solving the first order linear differential equation

$$\frac{dy}{dx} + p(x) y = q(x).$$

The general solution was shown to be of the form

$$y = \frac{A}{\mu} + \frac{1}{\mu} \int \mu q(x)\, dx,$$

where $\mu = \exp\left[\int p(x)\, dx\right]$ was the integrating factor. Thus, in this case,

$$y_c(x) = \frac{A}{\mu}$$

is the complementary function (it contains the arbitrary constant), and

$$y_p(x) = \frac{1}{\mu} \int \mu q(x)\, dx$$

is a particular integral (it is a solution which does not contain an arbitrary constant).

In Example 74.2, which is of this type, the general solution of

$$(1 + x^2) \frac{dy}{dx} - xy = 2x$$

was shown to be

$$y = A\sqrt{(1 + x^2)} - 2.$$

Thus in this case the complementary function is

$$y_c(x) = A\sqrt{(1 + x^2)},$$

which is the general solution of the homogeneous equation

$$(1 + x^2) \frac{dy_c}{dx} - xy_c = 0.$$

A particular integral is

$$y_p(x) = -2,$$

which is a particular solution of

$$(1 + x^2) \frac{dy_p}{dx} - xy_p = 2x,$$

so the general solution can be written as

$$y(x) = y_c(x) + y_p(x).$$

PROBLEMS 76

Prove the linear independence of the functions given in problems 1 to 6.

1. $1, x, x^2, x^3$.
2. $\sin x, \cos x$.
3. $1, e^{\lambda x}, e^{\mu x} (\lambda \neq \mu)$.
4. $e^{\lambda x} \cos \mu x, e^{\lambda x} \sin \mu x$.
5. $1, e^x, x e^x$.
6. $x \cos \mu x, x \sin \mu x$.
7. Verify that the constant coefficient second order linear differential equation

$$\frac{d^2 y}{dx^2} + 9y = 9x^2 + 11$$

has the complementary function

$$y_c(x) = A \cos 3x + B \sin 3x,$$

and that a particular integral is

$$y_p(x) = x^2 + 1.$$

8. Verify that the second order linear differential equation

$$x^2 \frac{d^2 y}{dx^2} - 3x \frac{dy}{dx} + 3y = x^4 e^x$$

has the complementary function

$$y_c(x) = C_1 x + C_2 x^3,$$

and that a particular integral is

$$y_p(x) = x(x - 1) e^x.$$

Would the function

$$y(x) = 4x - 5x^3 + x(x - 1) e^x$$

also be a particular integral?

Determining the complementary function for constant coefficient equations

77

We will discuss in detail the determination of the complementary function for the linear constant coefficient second order equation

$$\frac{d^2y}{dx^2} + a\frac{dy}{dx} + by = 0,$$

since this is the most important case. The extension of the argument to linear higher order constant coefficient equations of order $n > 2$ will then be almost immediate.

The solution of the homogeneous first order constant coefficient equation

$$\frac{dy}{dx} + ay = 0$$

can be found by separation of variables and is easily seen to be

$$y = Ae^{-ax}.$$

This suggests that we should seek solutions of the second order equation of the form

$$y = Ce^{\lambda x}.$$

When y is of this form

$$\frac{dy}{dx} = \lambda C e^{\lambda x} \quad \text{and} \quad \frac{d^2y}{dx^2} = \lambda^2 C e^{\lambda x},$$

so substituting into the second order equation gives

$$\lambda^2 C e^{\lambda x} + a\lambda C e^{\lambda x} + bCe^{\lambda x} = 0.$$

Cancelling the factor $Ce^{\lambda x}$ then shows that λ must be a solution of the quadratic equation

$$\lambda^2 + a\lambda + b = 0.$$

This is called the **characteristic equation** or **auxiliary equation** for the second order differential equation.

The roots of the equation are

$$\lambda = \frac{1}{2}[a \pm \sqrt{(a^2 - 4b)}],$$

and we will set

$$\lambda_1 = \frac{1}{2}[a - \sqrt{(a^2 - 4b)}] \quad \text{and} \quad \lambda_2 = \frac{1}{2}[a + \sqrt{(a^2 - 4b)}].$$

Three possibilities now arise:

1 the roots λ_1 and λ_2 are real with $\lambda_1 \neq \lambda_2$, which is the case if $a^2 > 4b$;
2 the roots λ_1 and λ_2 are real with $\lambda_1 = \lambda_2$, which is the case if $a^2 = 4b$;
3 the roots λ_1 and λ_2 are complex conjugates, which is the case if $a^2 < 4b$.

REAL AND DISTINCT ROOTS ($a^2 > 4b$)

In this case the roots λ_1 and λ_2 are real, with $\lambda_1 \neq \lambda_2$, so two possible solutions of the second order equation are seen to be $\exp(\lambda_1 x)$ and $\exp(\lambda_2 x)$. These two solutions are linearly independent because the Wronskian (see Section 76)

$$W = \begin{vmatrix} \exp(\lambda_1 x) & \exp(\lambda_2 x) \\ \lambda_1 \exp(\lambda_1 x) & \lambda_2 \exp(\lambda_2 x) \end{vmatrix} = (\lambda_2 - \lambda_1)\exp[(\lambda_1 + \lambda_2)x] \neq 0.$$

Thus they form a fundamental set of solutions for the second order equation, and in this case its general solution is of the form

$$y = A \exp(\lambda_1 x) + B \exp(\lambda_2 x),$$

where A and B are the two arbitrary constants we expect to find in the general solution of a second order differential equation.

Example 77.1

Find the general solution of

$$\frac{d^2 y}{dx^2} - \frac{dy}{dx} - 2y = 0$$

and hence the solution of the initial value problem for which $y(0) = 0$ and $y'(0) = 1$.

Solution
The differential equation is homogeneous, so its general solution is, in fact, the complementary function. The characteristic equation is

$$\lambda^2 - \lambda - 2 = 0, \quad \text{or} \quad (\lambda + 1)(\lambda - 2) = 0$$

and so its roots are

$$\lambda_1 = -1 \quad \text{and} \quad \lambda_2 = 2.$$

The general solution (complementary function in this case) is thus

$$y = Ae^{-x} + Be^{2x}.$$

To satisfy the initial conditions, the arbitrary constants A and B must be chosen such that $y(0) = 0$ and $y'(0) = 1$. Using the first of these conditions in the expression for y gives

$$0 = A + B.$$

Differentiation of the general solution shows that

$$\frac{dy}{dx} = -Ae^{-x} + 2Be^{2x},$$

so substituting the second initial condition into the above result gives

$$1 = -A + 2B.$$

Solving the pair of equations

$$A + B = 0$$

$$-A + 2B = 1$$

we find that

$$A = -1/3, \quad B = 1/3$$

so the solution of the initial value problem (a particular solution of the differential equation) is

$$y = \frac{1}{3}(e^{2x} - e^{-x}). \qquad \blacktriangle$$

EQUAL ROOTS ($a^2 = 4b$)

In this case the second order differential equation can be rewritten in the form

$$\frac{d^2y}{dx} - 2a\frac{dy}{dx} + a^2y = 0,$$

and its characteristic equation is

$$\lambda^2 - 2a\lambda + a^2 = 0, \quad \text{or} \quad (\lambda - a)^2 = 0.$$

Thus $\lambda_1 = \lambda_2 = a$ and there is a repeated root with multiplicity 2 (the root $\lambda = a$ occurs twice). Clearly e^{ax} is a solution of the second order equation, but we require a second linearly independent solution in order to construct the general solution.

Let us seek a second solution of the form

$$y = u(x)e^{ax},$$

and try to find the form of the function $u(x)$. We have

$$\frac{dy}{dx} = \left(au + \frac{du}{dx}\right)e^{ax}$$

and

$$\frac{d^2y}{dx^2} = \left(a^2u + 2a\frac{du}{dx} + \frac{d^2u}{dx^2}\right)e^{ax},$$

so substituting into the original second order equation

$$\frac{d^2y}{dx^2} - 2a\frac{dy}{dx} + a^2y = 0$$

leads to the result

$$a^2u + 2a\frac{du}{dx} + \frac{d^2u}{dx^2} - 2a\left(au + \frac{du}{dx}\right) + a^2u = 0.$$

After cancellation of terms this reduces to

$$\frac{d^2u}{dx^2} = 0,$$

so

$$u = A + \tilde{B}x,$$

where A and $\tilde{B}$ are arbitrary constants.

Thus the second linearly independent solution $y = ue^{ax}$ we are seeking is

$$y = (Ax + \tilde{B})e^{ax}.$$

It is a simple matter to check that the solutions e^{ax} and $(Ax + \tilde{B})e^{ax}$ are, indeed, linearly independent.

The general solution of the second order equation is an arbitrary linear combination of the two linearly independent solutions e^{ax} and $(Ax + \tilde{B})e^{ax}$, and so is the form

$$y = (Ax + \tilde{B})e^{ax} + Ce^{ax}.$$

The coefficients A, $\tilde{B}$ and C are arbitrary, so we may combine $\tilde{B}e^{ax}$ and Ce^{ax} and write the general solution in the form

$$y = (Ax + B)e^{ax},$$

where A and B are arbitrary constants.

Example 77.2

Find the general solution of

$$\frac{d^2y}{dx^2} - 6\frac{dy}{dx} + 9y = 0,$$

and hence the solution of the initial value problem for which $y(0) = 1$ and $y'(0) = 2$.

Solution
The general solution (complementary function in this case) has the characteristic equation

$$\lambda^2 - 6\lambda + 9 = 0, \quad \text{or} \quad (\lambda - 3)^2 = 0.$$

Thus the equation has the twice repeated root $\lambda = 3$ ($\lambda = 3$ occurs with multiplicity 2).

The general solution (complementary function) is thus

$$y = (Ax + B)e^{3x}.$$

To solve the initial value problem we first use the initial condition $y(0) = 1$ in the above general solution to obtain the condition

$$1 = B.$$

Then, since

$$\frac{dy}{dx} = Ae^{3x} + 3(Ax + B)e^{3x},$$

the second initial condition $y'(0) = 1$ gives

$$1 = A + 3B,$$

so $A = -2$, $B = 1$ and thus the solution of the initial value problem is

$$y = (1 - 2x)e^{3x}. \qquad \blacktriangle$$

COMPLEX CONJUGATE ROOTS ($a^2 < 4b$)

In this case we have

$$\lambda_1 = \alpha + i\beta \quad \text{and} \quad \alpha_2 = \alpha - i\beta,$$

so the general solution may be written

$$y = A_1 e^{(\alpha + i\beta)x} + B_1 e^{(\alpha - i\beta)x},$$

where A_1 and B_1 are now arbitrary **complex constants**. Thus

$$y = e^{\alpha x}(A_1 e^{i\beta x} + B_1 e^{-i\beta x})$$

$$= e^{\alpha x}(A_1 \cos \beta x + iA_1 \sin \beta x + B_1 \cos \beta x - iB_1 \sin \beta x),$$

and so we may write

$$y = e^{\alpha x}(A \cos \beta x + B \sin \beta x),$$

where if y is to be purely real

$$A = A_1 + B_1 \quad \text{and} \quad B = i(A_1 - B_1)$$

are now arbitrary **real** constants.

It is a simple matter to check that $e^{\alpha x} \cos \beta x$ and $e^{\alpha x} \sin \beta x$ are, indeed, linearly independent functions. The general solution in the case of complex conjugate roots is thus

$$y = e^{\alpha x} (A \cos \beta x + B \sin \beta x),$$

with A and B arbitrary real constants.

Example 77.3

Find the general solution of

$$\frac{d^2 y}{dx^2} + 4 \frac{dy}{dx} + 13y = 0,$$

and hence solve the initial value problem for which $y(0) = 1$ and $y'(0) = 4$.

Solution
The characteristic equation is

$$\lambda^2 + 4\lambda + 13 = 0,$$

so

$$\lambda = \frac{1}{2} [-4 \pm \sqrt{(16 - 52)}] = -2 \pm 3i.$$

Thus the general solution (complementary function in this case) is

$$y = e^{-2x} (A \cos 3x + B \sin 3x).$$

To solve the initial value problem we first substitute the initial condition $y(0) = 1$ into the above result to obtain

$$A = 1.$$

Then, as

$$\frac{dy}{dx} = e^{-2x} (-2A \cos 3x - 2B \sin 3x - 3A \sin 3x + 3B \cos 3x),$$

the second initial condition gives

$$-2 + 3B = 4, \quad \text{so} \quad B = 2.$$

The required solution of the initial value problem is thus

$$y = e^{-2x} (\cos 3x + 2 \sin 3x). \qquad \blacktriangle$$

The same form of approach can be used for the determination of complementary functions of higher order equations.

Example 77.4

Find the general solution of

$$\frac{d^3 y}{dx^3} - 3 \frac{dy}{dx} + 2y = 0.$$

Solution
The characteristic equation is

$$\lambda^3 - 3\lambda + 2 = 0.$$

This may be factorized as

$$(\lambda - 1)^2(\lambda + 2) = 0,$$

showing that the root $\lambda = 1$ has multiplicity 2 (is repeated twice) while the root $\lambda = -2$ occurs with multiplicity 1 (occurs only once). Thus the contribution to the general solution of the repeated root will be terms of the form

$$(Ax + B)e^x,$$

while the contribution from the single root will be

$$Ce^{-2x},$$

so the required general solution is

$$y = (Ax + B)e^x + Ce^{-2x}. \qquad \blacktriangle$$

Example 77.5

Find the general solution of

$$\frac{d^4y}{dx^4} + 2\frac{d^2y}{dx^2} - 8\frac{dy}{dx} + 5y = 0.$$

Solution
The characteristic equation is

$$\lambda^4 + 2\lambda^2 - 8\lambda + 5 = 0,$$

and this can be factorized to give

$$(\lambda - 1)^2(\lambda^2 + 2\lambda + 5) = 0.$$

Thus the roots are

$$\lambda = 1 \ \ \text{(twice)(multiplicity 2)}$$

$$\lambda = -1 \pm 2i \ \text{(complex conjugates)}.$$

The contribution to the general solution (complementary function in this case) from the repeated real root is

$$(ax + B)e^x,$$

while the contribution from the complex conjugate roots is

$$e^{-x}(C \cos 2x + D \sin 2x),$$

so the required general solution is

$$y = (Ax + B)e^x + e^{-x}(C \cos 2x + D \sin 2x). \qquad \blacktriangle$$

The method of arriving at the complementary function for a second order constant coefficient equation extends in an obvious manner to constant coefficient equations of any order. The general rules for constructing the complementary function can be summarized as follows.

Rules for determining the complementary function

It is required to find the general solution of the nth order linear homogeneous equation

$$\frac{d^n y}{dx^n} + a_1 \frac{d^{n-1}y}{dx^{n-1}} + \ldots + a_n y = 0,$$

with real constant coefficients $a_1\, a_2, \ldots, a_n$. The solution is called the complementary function and its form is determined as follows.

1 Find the roots of the characteristic equation

$$\lambda^n + a_1 \lambda^{n-1} + \ldots + a_n = 0.$$

2 For every simple root $\lambda = a$ (multiplicity 1) include in the solution a term

$$A e^{ax},$$

where A is an arbitrary real constant.

3 For every real root $\lambda = b$ of multiplicity r include in the solution the terms

$$B_1 e^{bx} + B_2 x e^{bx} + \ldots + B_r x^{r-1} e^{bx},$$

where $B_1, B_2, \ldots, B_r$ are arbitrary real constants.

4 For every pair of complex conjugate roots

$$\lambda = \alpha + i\beta \quad \text{and} \quad \lambda = \alpha - i\beta$$

include in the solution the terms

$$e^{\alpha x}(C \cos \beta x + D\,\sin \beta x)$$

where C and D are arbitrary real constants.

5 For every pair of complex conjugate roots $\lambda = \gamma + i\omega$ and $\lambda = \gamma - i\omega$, each with multiplicity s, include in the solution the terms

$$e^{\gamma x}(E_1 \cos \omega x + F_1 \sin \omega x + E_2 x \cos \omega x$$

$$+ F_2 x \sin \omega x + \ldots + E_s x^{s-1} \cos \omega x + F_x x^{s-1} \sin \omega x)$$

where $E_1, F_1, \ldots, E_s, F_s$ are arbitrary real constants.

6 The general solution is then the sum of all the terms generated in steps 2 to 5.

PROBLEMS 77

In problems 1 to 12 find the complementary function of the given differential equation.

1. $y'' + 3y' - 4y = 0.$
2. $y'' + 16y = 0.$
3. $y'' - 9y = 0.$
4. $y'' + 6y' + 8y = 0.$
5. $y'' + 2y' = 0.$
6. $y'' - 14y' + 49y = 0.$
7. $y'' + 8y' + 16y = 0.$

8. $y'' + 4y' + 8y = 0.$
9. $y'' - 6y' + 45y = 0.$
10. $y'' - 2y' + 5y = 0.$
11. $y'' + 2y' + 5y = 0.$
12. $y'' - 4y' + 13y = 0.$

Solve the given initial value problems in problems 13 to 18.

13. $y'' - 9y = 0,$ with $y(0) = 2$ and $y'(0) = 6.$
14. $y'' + 2y' + 5y = 0,$ with $y(0) = 1$ and $y'(0) = 1.$
15. $y'' - 10y' + 25y = 0,$ with $y(0) = 2$ and $y'(0) = 8.$
16. $y'' + 6y' + 9y = 0,$ with $y(0) = 2$ and $y'(0) = 1.$
17. $y'' - 2y' + 2y = 0,$ with $y(0) = 1$ and $y'(0) = 3.$
18. $y'' + 3y' + 2y = 0,$ with $y(0) = -1$ and $y'(0) = 3.$

Find the general solution for problems 19 to 24.

19. $\dfrac{d^4y}{dx^4} - 5\dfrac{d^2y}{dx^2} + 4y = 0.$

20. $\dfrac{d^3y}{dx^3} - 2\dfrac{d^2y}{dx^2} - \dfrac{dy}{dx} + 2y = 0.$

21. $\dfrac{d^3y}{dx^3} - 9\dfrac{d^2y}{dx^2} + 27\dfrac{dy}{dx} - 27y = 0.$

22. $\dfrac{d^4y}{dx^4} + 2\dfrac{d^2y}{dx^2} + 9y = 0.$

23. $\dfrac{d^4y}{dx^4} - 8\dfrac{d^2y}{dx^2} + 16y = 0.$

24. $\dfrac{d^4y}{dx^4} + 16y = 0.$

78

Determining particular integrals of constant coefficient equations

We will discuss in detail the determination of particular integrals for the non-homogeneous linear constant coefficient second order equation

$$\frac{d^2y}{dx^2} + a\frac{dy}{dx} + by = f(x),$$

for the case in which $f(x)$ is a polynomial, an exponential function, a sine or cosine function or a combination of such functions. The methods generalize immediately to higher order constant coefficient equations.

The method we will develop is called the **method of undetermined co-efficients**. It is based on the fact that when functions of the type just described are differentiated they give rise to functions of similar type. We shall describe the approach by means of examples.

POLYNOMIALS

A typical second order equation with a non-homogeneous term in the form of a polynomial is

$$\frac{d^2y}{dx^2} - 4y = x^2 - 3x - 4.$$

The only way in which a particular integral y_p when inserted into the left-hand side of this equation can give rise to the polynomial $x^2 - 3x - 4$ on the right-hand side is if it is of the form

$$y_p = Ax^2 + Bx + C.$$

To determine the as yet undetermined coefficients A, B and C we substitute this expression into the equation and require the result to be an identity.
We have

$$y_p = Ax^2 + Bx + C,$$

$$\frac{dy_p}{dx} = 2Ax + B,$$

$$\frac{d^2y_p}{dx^2} = 2A,$$

so substituting into the left-hand side of the differential equation gives

$$2A - 4(Ax^2 + Bx + C) = x^2 - 3x - 4.$$

For y_p to be a particular integral, this result must be an identity (true for all x), and this can only be so if the coefficients of corresponding powers of x on either side of this result are equal. Thus equating the coefficients of corresponding powers of x gives:

1 Coefficients of x^2: $-4A = 1$, so $A = -1/4$.
2 Coefficients of x: $-4B = -3$ so $B = 3/4$.
3 Coefficients of x^0: the constant terms: $2A - 4C = -4$, so $C = 7/8$.
   Thus the **particular integral** is

$$y_p = -\frac{1}{4}x^2 + \frac{3}{4}x + \frac{7}{8}.$$

The complementary function follows by finding the solution of the homogeneous equation

$$\frac{d^2y}{dx^2} - 4y = 0.$$

The characteristic equation is

$$\lambda^2 - 4 = 0, \quad \text{or} \quad (\lambda - 2)(\lambda + 2) = 0,$$

so the complementary function is

$$y_c = Ae^{2x} + Be^{-2x}.$$

The general solution $y = y_c + y_p$ is thus

$$y = Ae^{2x} + Be^{-2x} - \frac{1}{4}x^2 + \frac{3}{4}x + \frac{7}{8}.$$

EXPONENTIALS

If $f(x)$ is of the form Ke^{mx} we seek a particular integral of the form

$$y_p = Ae^{mx},$$

and if $f(x)$ contains a sum of exponentials we generalize y_p accordingly. To see how the approach works let us find the particular integral of

$$\frac{d^2y}{dx^2} + 2\frac{dy}{dx} + 5y = 4e^x + e^{-2x}.$$

We seek a particular integral of the form

$$y_p = Ae^x + Be^{-2x},$$

since the right-hand side of the equation (the non-homogeneous part) can only be produced by differentiating such a combination of exponentials. Then

$$y_p = Ae^x + Be^{-2x},$$

$$\frac{dy_p}{dx} = Ae^x - 2Be^{-2x},$$

$$\frac{d^2y_p}{dx^2} = Ae^x + 4Be^{-2x},$$

so substituting these results into the differential equation gives

$$(Ae^x + 4Be^{-2x}) + 2(Ae^x - 2Be^{-2x}) + 5(Ae^x + Be^{-2x}) = 4e^x + e^{-2x}.$$

For y_p to be a particular integral, this result must be an identity (true for all x) and this is only possible if the coefficients of e^x and e^{-2x} on each side of the expression are the same.

1 Coefficients of e^x: $8A = 4$, so $A = 1/2$.
2 Coefficients of e^{-2x}: $5B = 1$, so $B = 1/5$.

Thus the required particular integral is

$$y_p = \frac{1}{2} e^x + \frac{1}{5} e^{-2x}.$$

The complementary function is the solution of the homogeneous equation

$$\frac{d^2y}{dx^2} + 2\frac{dy}{dx} + 5y = 0,$$

and this has the characteristic equation

$$\lambda^2 + 2\lambda + 5 = 0,$$

with the roots

$$\lambda = -1 \pm 2i.$$

Thus the complementary function is

$$y_c = e^{-x}(A \cos 2x + B \sin 2x),$$

and the general solution $y = y_c + y_p$ is

$$y = e^{-x}(A \cos 2x + B \sin 2x) + \frac{1}{2} e^x + \frac{1}{5} e^{-2x}.$$

SINES AND COSINES

If $f(x)$ has the general form

$$f(x) = P \cos nx + Q \sin nx,$$

we seek a particular integral of the form

$$y_p = A \cos nx + B \sin nx.$$

This follows because only by substituting a particular integral of this form into the left-hand side of the equation can the terms in the non-homogeneous term be generated. Let us apply this approach to the equation

$$\frac{d^2y}{dx^2} - 2\frac{dy}{dx} - 5y = 2\cos 3x - \sin 3x,$$

in order to find the particular integral. We set

$$y_p = A \cos 3x + B \sin 3x,$$

so

$$\frac{dy}{dx} = -3A \sin 3x + 3B \cos 3x,$$

$$\frac{d^2y}{dx^2} = -9A \cos 3x - 9B \sin 3x.$$

Substituting these expressions into the equation gives

$$-9(A \cos 3x + B \sin 3x) - 2(-3A \sin 3x + 3B + 3B \cos 3x)$$

$$-5(A \cos 3x + B \sin 3x) = 2\cos 3x - \sin 3x.$$

For y_p to be a particular integral this result must be an identity (true for all x) and this is only possible if the respective coefficients of the sines and cosines on either side of the expression are the same.

1 Coefficients of $\cos 3x$: $-14A - 6B = 2$.
2 Coefficients of $\sin 3x$: $6A - 14B = -1$.

Thus $A = -17/116$, $B = 1/116$, and the particular integral is thus

$$y_p = \frac{1}{116}(-17 \cos 3x + \sin 3x).$$

A routine calculation shows the complementary function is

$$y_c = A \exp[(1 + \sqrt{6})x] + B \exp[(1 - \sqrt{6})x],$$

so the general solution $y = y_c + y$ is

$$y = A \exp[(1 + \sqrt{6})x] + B \exp[(1 - \sqrt{6})x] + \frac{1}{116}(-17 \cos 3x + \sin 3x).$$

EXCEPTIONS

The previous methods fail if part or all of the non-homogeneous term is contained in the complementary function. The modification to the approach needed in such cases is illustrated in the following example.

Let us find the general solution of

$$\frac{d^2y}{dx^2} + 4y = 3 \sin 2x.$$

The complementary function is easily seen to be

$$y_c = A \cos 2x + B \sin 2x,$$

so the non-homogeneous term $3 \sin 2x$ is contained within the complementary function, so we cannot seek a particular integral of the form

$$y_p = C \cos 2x + D \sin 2x.$$

Instead, we seek it in the modified form

$$y_p = x(C \cos 2x + D \sin 2x).$$

Then

$$\frac{dy_p}{dx} = C \cos 2x + D \sin 2x + x(-2C \sin 2x + 2D \cos 2x)$$

and

$$\frac{d^2 y_p}{dx^2} = -4C \sin 2x + 4D \cos 2x + x(-4C \cos 2x - 4D \sin 2x).$$

Substituting into the differential equation gives

$$-4C \sin 2x + 4D \cos 2x + x(-4C \cos 2x - 4D \sin 2x)$$
$$+ 4x(C \cos 2x + D \sin 2x) = 3 \sin 2x.$$

For y_p to be a particular integral this must be an identity, and this is only possible if the respective coefficients of $\cos 2x$ and $\sin 2x$ on either side of this expression are equal.

1 Coefficients of $\cos 2x$: $4D = 0$, so $D = 0$.
2 Coefficients of $\sin 2x$: $-4C = 3$, so $C = -3/4$.

Thus the particular integral is

$$y_p = -\frac{3}{4} x \cos 2x,$$

and the general solution $y = y_c + y_p$ is

$$y = A \cos 2x + B \sin 2x - \frac{3}{4} x \cos 2x.$$

To summarize our approach, we remark that in this case, as the non-homogeneous term was contained in a complementary function of the form

$$y_c = A \cos nx + B \sin nx,$$

we looked for a particular integral of the form

$$y_p = x(C \cos nx + D \sin nx).$$

A different type of problem arises with an equation of the form

$$\frac{d^2 y}{dx^2} - \frac{dy}{dx} = x,$$

for here there is no undifferentiated term y in the equation, so we cannot seek a particular integral of the form

$$y_p = Ax + B$$

as in the subsection on polynomials above. Instead, noticing that the lowest order derivative of y is dy/dx and the highest is d^2y/dx^2, we seek a particular integral of the form

$$y_p = Ax^2 + Bx.$$

Substituting into the equation we find that

$$2A - (2Ax + B) = x,$$

which is only possible if $A = -1/2$ and $B = -1$, for only then does this expression become an identity. Thus

$$y_p = -\frac{1}{2}x^2 - x,$$

and the complementary function is seen to be

$$y_p = C + De^x,$$

so the general solution $y = y_c + y_p$ is

$$y = C + De^x - \frac{1}{2}x^2 - x.$$

INITIAL AND BOUNDARY VALUE PROBLEMS

If initial or boundary value problems are to be solved involving non-homogeneous constant coefficient linear differential equations the general solution must be found first, after which the arbitrary constants must be chosen to match the initial or boundary conditions.

SUMMARY OF RULES

The methods just outlined apply to non-homogeneous linear constant coefficient differential equations of any order. The general approach to the determination of particular integrals using undetermined coefficients can be summarized as follows.

Rules for determining a particular integral
It is required to find the form of a particular integral y_p of the nth order linear non-homogeneous equation

$$\frac{d^ny}{dx^n} + a_1\frac{d^{n-1}y}{dxn^{-1}} + \ldots + a_ny = f(x)$$

with real constant coefficients $a_1, a_2, \ldots, a_n$.
1 $f(x) =$ constant. Include in y_p the constant term K.
2 $f(x)$ is a polynomial in x of degree r.

(i) If the differential equation contains an undifferentiated term y, include in y_p terms of the form

$$A_0 x^r + A_1 x^{r-1} + \ldots + A_r.$$

(ii) If the differential equation does not contain an undifferentiated y, and $y^{(s)}$ is its lowest order derivative, include in y_p terms of the form

$$A_0 x^{r+s} + A_1 x^{r+s-1} + \ldots A_r x^s.$$

3 $f(x) = e^{ax}$.

(i) If e^{ax} is not contained in the complementary function, include in y_p the term $B e^{ax}$.

(ii) If the complementary function contains the terms $e^{ax}, xe^{ax}, \ldots, x^m e^{ax}$, include in y_p the term $B x^{m+1} e^{ax}$.

4 $f(x) = \cos qx$ and/or $\sin qx$.

(i) If $\cos qs$ and/or $\sin qx$ are not contained in the complementary function, include in y_p terms of the form

$$C \cos qx + D \sin qx.$$

(ii) If the complementary function contains the terms $x^s \cos qx$ and/or $x^s \sin qx$ with $s = 0, 1, 2, \ldots, m$, include in y_p terms of the form

$$x^{m+1}(C \cos qx + D \sin qx).$$

5 The form of the particular integral y_p is the sum of all the terms generated as a result of identifying each term in $f(x)$ with one of the special forms of $f(x)$ listed above in 1 to 4.

Example 78.1

Find the general solution of

$$\frac{d^3 y}{dx^2} - 3\frac{d^2 y}{dx^2} + 3\frac{dy}{dx} - y = x^2 + 2 \sin x + \cos x,$$

and hence solve the initial value problem for which

$$y(0) = y'(0) = 0 \quad \text{and} \quad y''(0) = 1.$$

Solution
The homogeneous equation is

$$\frac{d^3 y}{dx^2} - 3\frac{d^2 y}{dx^2} + 3\frac{dy}{dx} - y = 0,$$

and this has the characteristic equation

$$\lambda^3 - 3\lambda^2 + 3\lambda - 1 = 0 \quad \text{or} \quad (\lambda - 1)^3 = 0.$$

Thus the root $\lambda = 1$ has multiplicity 3 and so the complementary function is

$$y_c = (\tilde{A} + \tilde{B}x + \tilde{C}x^2) e^x.$$

The non-homogeneous right-hand side does not occur in the complementary function so we seek a particular integral of the form

$$y_p = Ax^2 + Bx + C + D \cos x + E \sin x.$$

In this expression the polynomial $Ax^2 + Bx + C$ has been included because of the term x^2 on the right-hand side, and the terms $D \cos x + E \sin x$ have been included because of the terms $2 \sin x + \cos x$ on the right-hand side. Thus differentiating y_p gives

$$\frac{dy_p}{dx} = 2Ax + B - D \sin x + E \cos x,$$

$$\frac{d^2 y}{dx} = 2A - D \cos x - E \sin x,$$

$$\frac{d^3 y_p}{dx^3} = D \sin x - E \cos x.$$

Substituting into the differential equation we find that

$$D \sin x - E \cos x - 3(2A - D \cos x - E \sin x) + 3(2Ax + B - D \sin x + E \cos x)$$

$$- (Ax^2 + Bx + C + D \cos x + E \sin x) = x^2 + 2 \sin x + \cos x.$$

Equating the coefficients of corresponding terms to make this an identity gives:
1 Coefficients of x^2: $-A = 1$, so $A = -1$.
2 Coefficients of x: $6A - B = 0$, so $B = -6$.
3 Coefficient of x^0; the constant terms: $-6A + 3B - C = 0$, so $C = -12$.
4 Coefficients of $\cos x$: $2E + 2D = 1$.
5 Coefficients of $\sin x$: $2E - 2D = 2$, so $D = -1/4, E = 3/4$.
The particular integral is thus

$$y_p = -x^2 - 6x - 12 - \frac{1}{4} \cos x + \frac{3}{4} \sin x,$$

and the general solution $y = y_c + y_p$ is

$$y = (\tilde{A} + \tilde{B}x + \tilde{C}x^2)e^x - x^2 - 6x - 12 - \frac{1}{4} \cos x + \frac{3}{4} \sin x.$$

To solve the initial value problem we must choose A, B and C such that $y(0) = y'(0) = 0$ and $y''(0) = 1$. Setting $y = 0$ when $x = 0$ in the general solution gives

$$0 = A - \frac{49}{4}, \quad \text{or} \quad A = \frac{49}{4}.$$

Similarly, differentiating y and setting $y' = 0$ when $x = 0$ gives

$$A + B = \frac{21}{4}, \quad \text{so} \quad B = -7.$$

Finally, differentiating y' and setting $y'' = 1$ when $x = 0$ gives

$$A + 2B + 2C - \frac{7}{4} = 1, \quad \text{so} \quad C = -9/4$$

and hence the solution to the initial value problem is

$$y = \frac{1}{4}(9x^2 - 28x + 49)e^x - x^2 - 6x - 12 - \frac{1}{4}\cos x + \frac{3}{4}\sin x. \qquad \blacktriangle$$

PROBLEMS 78

Find the general solution in problems 1 to 14.

1. $y'' - 4y' + 4y = x^2$.
2. $y'' - y' + y = x^3 + 6$.
3. $y'' + y' - 2y = 8\sin 2x$.
4. $y'' - 2y' + y = \sin x + \sinh x$.
5. $y'' + y' - 2y = 8\sin 2x$.
6. $y'' + y' - 6y = xe^{2x}$.
7. $y'' - y = e^x$.
8. $y'' - 2y' - 8y = e^x - 8\cos 2x$.
9. $y'' + 2y' + y = e^x + e^{-x}$.
10. $y'' - 3y' = x + \cos x$.
11. $y'' + 4y = 2\sin 2x - 3\cos 2x + 1$.
12. $y'' - y = xe^x$.
13. $y'' - 2y' = 3x + 2xe^x$.
14. $y'' - 2y' - 3y = x + xe^{3x}$.
15. Solve the initial value problem

$$y'' + 4y = \sin x,$$

given that $y(0) = 1$ and $y'(0) = 1$.
16. Solve the initial value problem

$$y'' - 2y' = e^{2x} + x^2 - 1,$$

given that $y(0) = 1/8$ and $y'(0) = 1$.

The differential equation

$$m\frac{d^2x}{dt^2} + D\frac{dx}{dt} + kx = f(t),$$

in which m, D and k are positive constants and $f(t)$ is a periodic function, describes the oscillatory behaviour of the variable $x(t)$, in which t is usually the time. It can, for example, describe the oscillation of a mass connected to a spring moving subject to a resistance proportional to the velocity, or the variation of electric charge in a circuit containing a capacitance, an inductance and a resistance. The function $f(t)$ is called the **forcing function**, and when $f(t) \equiv 0$ the physical system described by the homogeneous equation

$$m\frac{d^2x}{dt^2} + D\frac{dx}{dt} + kx = 0$$

is said to perform **free oscillations**. When $f(t)$ is a periodic function (not necessarily sinusoidal), the oscillations performed by the physical system described by the non-homogeneous equation are said to be **forced oscillations**.

In applications it is usual to set

$$\frac{D}{m} = 2\zeta\Omega_0 \quad \text{and} \quad \frac{k}{m} = \Omega_0^2$$

and to call ζ the **damping** and Ω_0 the **natural frequency** of the oscillations.

FREE OSCILLATIONS

The free oscillations of a physical system governed by a second order constant coefficient equation are described by

$$\frac{d^2x}{dt^2} + 2\zeta\Omega_0\frac{dx}{dt} + \Omega_0^2 x = 0.$$

The case of zero damping ($\zeta = 0$)
If there is no friction or electrical resistance removing energy from a physical system described by the above equation there is said to be no damping and $\zeta = 0$, so the equation reduces to

$$\frac{d^2x}{dt^2} + \Omega_0^2 x = 0$$

The characteristic equation for this differential equation is

$$\lambda^2 + \Omega_0^2 = 0, \quad \text{so} \quad \lambda = \pm i\Omega_0,$$

and the general solution (complementary function) is

$$x = A \sin \Omega_0 t + B \cos \Omega_0 t.$$

Let us rewrite this result as

$$x = (A^2 + B^2)^{1/2} \left[\frac{A}{(A^2 + B^2)^{1/2}} \sin \Omega_0 t + \frac{B}{(A^2 + B^2)^{1/2}} \cos \Omega_0 t \right],$$

and then set

$$a = (A^2 + B^2)^{1/2}, \quad \cos \varepsilon = \frac{A}{(A^2 + B^2)^{1/2}} \quad \text{and} \quad \sin \varepsilon = \frac{B}{(A^2 + B^2)^{1/2}},$$

so it becomes

$$x = a(\sin \Omega_0 t \cos \varepsilon + \cos \Omega_0 t \sin \varepsilon).$$

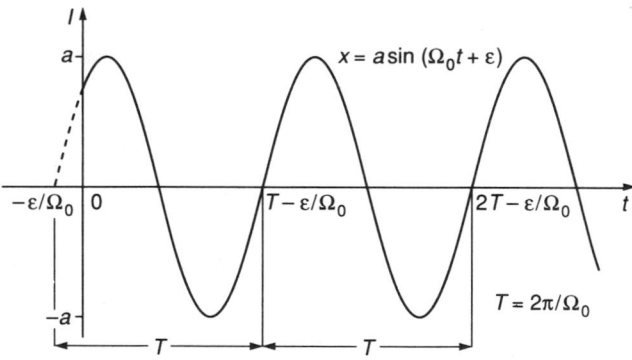

Fig. 154

Using the trigonometric identity

$$\sin(P + Q) = \sin P \cos Q + \cos P \sin Q$$

and setting $P = \Omega_0 t$, $Q = \varepsilon$ we see that

$$x = a \sin(\Omega_0 t + \varepsilon).$$

This form of the solution shows that x oscillates sinusoidally, with a the **amplitude** of the oscillation (the maximum magnitude of x), Ω_0 the **angular frequency**, $T = 2\pi/\Omega_0$ the **period** of the oscillation, $F = 1/T = \Omega_0/2\pi$ the **frequency** of the oscillation (the number of cycles in a unit time) and ε the **phase** of the oscillations. The relationship between a, T, Ω_0 and ε is shown in Fig. 154.

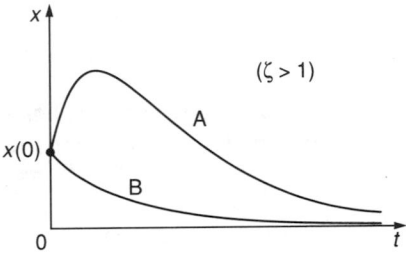

Fig. 155

The overdamped case ($\zeta > 1$)
When $\zeta > 1$, the physical system described by the homogeneous equation

$$\frac{d^2x}{dt^2} + 2\zeta\Omega_0 \frac{dx}{dt} + \Omega_0^2 = 0$$

is said to be **overdamped**. The characteristic equation for this differential equation is

$$\lambda^2 + 2\zeta\Omega_0\lambda + \Omega_0^2 = 0,$$

and because $\zeta > 1$ the roots are real and negative, with

$$\lambda = \Omega_0[-\zeta \pm (\zeta^2 - 1)^{1/2}].$$

Setting

$$\lambda_1 = \Omega_0[-\zeta - (\zeta^2 - 1)^{1/2}] \quad \text{and} \quad \lambda_2 = \Omega_0[-\zeta + (\zeta^2 - 1)^{1/2}]$$

the general solution of the differential equation becomes

$$x = Ae^{\lambda_1 t} + Be^{\lambda_2 t}.$$

This solution is not oscillatory, and the behaviour of a typical overdamped system is illustrated in Fig. 155. Depending on the initial conditions, there may be an initial overshoot as in line A of Fig. 155, or a pure decay as in B, though all solutions of this type will eventually decay to zero without oscillation.

The critically damped case ($\zeta = 1$)
When $\zeta = 1$, the physical system is said to be **critically damped**. The characteristic equation for such a system is

$$\lambda^2 + 2\Omega_0\lambda + \Omega_0^2 = 0, \quad \text{or} \quad (\lambda + \Omega_0)^2 = 0,$$

so there is only a single negative root $\lambda = -\Omega_0$ with multiplicity 2. The general solution in this case is thus

$$x = (A + Bt)\exp(-\Omega_0 t),$$

and again it is not oscillatory. The behaviour of a critically damped system is similar to that of an overdamped one.

The underdamped case $(\zeta < 1)$.

When $0 < \zeta < 1$ the physical system described by the homogeneous differential equation is said to be **underdamped**. The characteristic equation for such a system is

$$\lambda^2 + 2\zeta\Omega_0\lambda + \Omega_0^2 = 0,$$

so as $0 < \zeta < 1$ the roots are complex conjugates with negative real parts and they are given by

$$\lambda = \Omega_0[-\zeta \pm i\Omega_0(1 - \zeta^2)^{1/2}].$$

If we write $\Omega = \Omega_0(1 - \zeta^2)^{1/2}$, the general solution can be written as

$$x = \exp(-\zeta\Omega_0 t)(A \sin \Omega t + B \cos \Omega t).$$

Arguing as in the underdamped case, this can be re-expressed as

$$x = a\exp(-\zeta\Omega_0 t) \sin(\Omega t + \varepsilon)$$

where, as before,

$$a = (A^2 + B^2)^{1/2}, \quad \cos\varepsilon = \frac{A}{(A^2 + B^2)^{1/2}} \quad \text{and} \quad \sin\varepsilon = \frac{B}{(A^2 + B^2)^{1/2}},$$

but now the angular frequency is

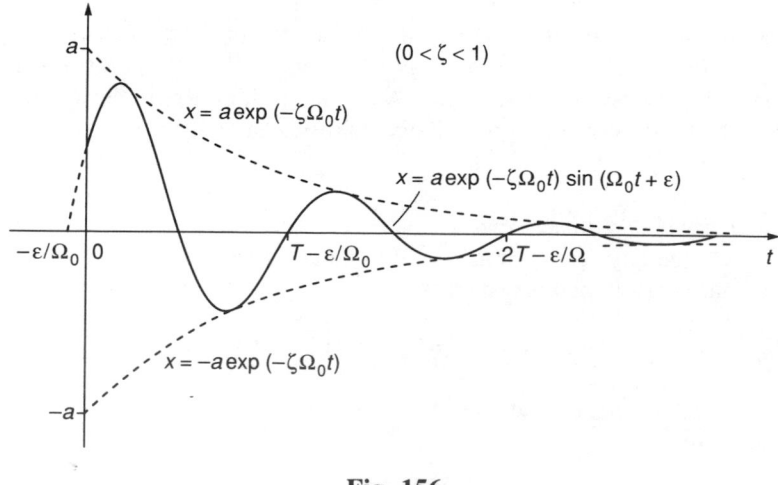

Fig. 156

$$\Omega = \Omega_0 (1 - \zeta^2)^{1/2}$$

Thus the solution for an underdamped system is sinusoidal in nature, it decays exponentially with time, its angular frequency is modified to Ω and its period to $T = 2\pi/\Omega$. The behaviour of a typical underdamped system is shown in Fig. 156.

FORCED OSCILLATIONS

We now consider the case of forced oscillations when the forcing function $f(t) = k \sin \omega t$. Thus the amplitude of the sinusoidal forcing function is k, and its frequency $F = \omega/2\pi$.

Forced oscillations in the absence of damping ($\zeta = 0$)
When there is no damping, the governing differential equation becomes

$$\frac{d^2 x}{dt^2} + \Omega_0^2 x = k \sin \omega t.$$

The complementary function of this differential equation is easily seen to be

$$x_c = A \cos \Omega_0 t + B \sin \Omega_0 t$$

or, equivalently,

$$x_c = a \sin(\Omega_0 t + \varepsilon)$$

where we may regard a and ε as the arbitrary constants instead of A and B.
Provided $\omega \neq \Omega_0$ the particular integral will be of the form

$$x_p = C \sin \omega t + D \cos \omega t.$$

Substituting this into the differential equation leads to the result

$$-C\omega^2 \sin \omega t - D\omega^2 \cos \omega t + \Omega_0^2 (C \sin \omega t + D \cos \omega t) = k \sin \omega t.$$

Equating corresponding coefficients of the sine and cosine functions on each side of this expression to make it an identity gives:
1 Coefficients of $\sin \omega t$: $C(\Omega_0^2 - \omega^2) = k$, so $C = k/(\Omega_0^2 - \omega^2)$.
2 Coefficients of $\cos \omega t$: $D(\Omega_0^2 - \omega^2) = 0$, so $D = 0$.
Thus the general solution $x = x_c + x_p$ is

$$x = a \sin(\Omega_0 t + \varepsilon) + \frac{k}{(\Omega_0^2 - \omega^2)} \sin \omega t, \quad \text{for} \quad \omega \neq \Omega_0.$$

If $\omega = \Omega_0$, the non-homogeneous term is contained in the complementary function, so the form of the particular integral involving undetermined coefficients must be modified to

$$x_p = t(C \sin \Omega_0 t + D\cos \Omega_0 t).$$

Determining the coefficients C and D in the usual manner gives

$$C = 0 \quad \text{and} \quad D = -k/(2\Omega_0),$$

so the particular integral then becomes

$$x_p = -\frac{k}{2\Omega_0} t \cos \Omega_0 t,$$

and the general solution $x = x_c + x_p$ is

$$x = a \sin(\Omega_0 t + \varepsilon) - \frac{k}{2\Omega_0} t \cos \Omega_0 t.$$

This is an oscillatory solution, but the amplitude of the oscillation due to the particular integral **increases linearly** with the time t. This phenomenon is called **resonance**, and it occurs when there is no damping and the forcing frequency equals the natural frequency of the undamped oscillations.

Forced oscillations with damping $(\zeta > 0)$
When damping is present the governing differential equation becomes

$$\frac{d^2 x}{dt^2} + 2\zeta\Omega_0 \frac{dx}{dt} + \Omega_0^2 x = k \sin \omega t.$$

The complementary function has been determined when considering the case of free oscillations, and in each case it was seen to decay to zero with increasing time. Thus, after a suitably long period of time, the forced oscillations will be determined by the particular integral. This solution is called the **steady-state solution**, in the sense that it is the limiting form of the oscillatory behaviour of the system.

The particular integral will have the form

$$x_p = C \sin \omega t + D \cos \omega t,$$

and proceeding in the usual manner it is easily shown that

$$C = \frac{k(\Omega_0^2 - \omega^2)}{[(\Omega_0^2 - \omega^2)^2 + (2\zeta\,\Omega_0\omega)^2]} \quad \text{and} \quad D = \frac{-k\,2\zeta\Omega_0\omega}{[(\Omega_0^2 - \omega)^2 + (2\zeta\,\Omega_0\omega)^2]},$$

so

$$x_p = \frac{k}{[(\Omega_0^2 - \omega^2)^2 + (2\zeta\,\Omega_0\omega)^2]} [(\Omega_0^2 - \omega^2) \sin \omega t - 2\zeta\Omega_0\omega \cos \omega t].$$

Thus, if we set

$$\cos \alpha = \frac{(\Omega_0^2 - \omega^2)}{[(\Omega_0^2 - \omega^2)^2 + (2\zeta\,\Omega_0\omega)^{1/2}]} \quad \text{and} \quad \sin \alpha = \frac{2\zeta\,\Omega_0\omega}{[(\Omega_0^2 - \omega^2)^2 + (2\zeta\,\Omega_0\omega^2)^2]^{1/2}}$$

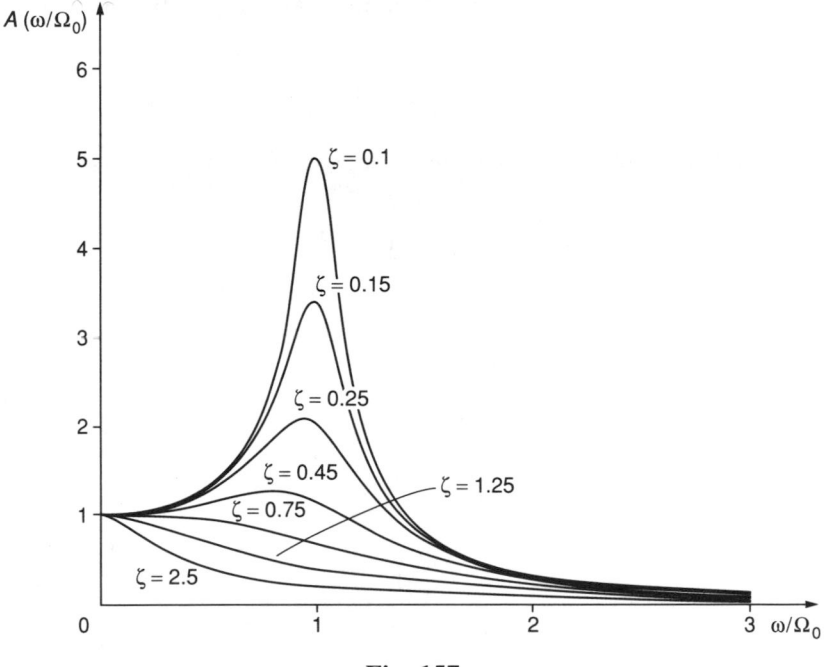

Fig. 157

we may write

$$x_p = \frac{k}{[(\Omega_0^2 - \omega^2)^2 + (2\zeta\Omega_0\omega^2)^2]^{1/2}} \sin(\omega t - \alpha).$$

This shows that the steady state solution is a sinusoid with the same angular frequency as the forcing function, but with a different amplitude and a phase lag α.

If this result is rewritten as

$$\frac{\Omega_0^2 x_p}{k} = \frac{\Omega_0^2}{[(\Omega_0^2 - \omega^2)^2 + (2\zeta\,\Omega_0\omega)^2]^{1/2}} \sin(\omega t - \alpha),$$

we see that the multiplier of $\sin(\omega t - \alpha)$ is the **amplification factor** for the forced oscillation. Dividing numerator and denominator of the amplification factor by Ω_0^2 shows it to be a function of the ratio ω/Ω_0. Denoting the amplification factor by $A(\omega/\Omega_0)$, we have

$$A(\omega/\Omega_0) = \frac{1}{\{[1 - (\omega/\Omega_0)^2]^2 + [2\zeta\,\omega/\Omega_0]^2\}^{1/2}}$$

Figure 157 shows the behaviour of $A(\omega/\Omega_0)$ for different values of the damping ζ. It is easily shown that the denominator of $A(\omega/\Omega_0)$ attains a minimum when $\omega^2 = \Omega_0^2(1 - 2\zeta^2)$, so the amplification factor $A(\omega/\Omega_0)$ will have a maximum at this frequency provided $\zeta < 1/\sqrt{2}$. The frequency

$\omega_R = \Omega_0 (1 - 2\zeta^2)^{1/2}$ is called the **resonant frequency in the presence of damping**. The maximum amplification factor attained when $\omega = \omega_R$ is

$$A_{\max} = \frac{1}{2\zeta (1 - \zeta^2)^{1/2}}, \quad \text{for} \quad \zeta < 1/\sqrt{2},$$

and the corresponding maximum amplitude $a_{\max}$ of the oscillation is

$$a_{\max} = \frac{k}{2\zeta \Omega_0^2 (1 - \zeta^2)^{1/2}}.$$

Simultaneous first order linear constant coefficient differential equations 80

In this section we offer a brief discussion of the solution of initial value problems for two simultaneous first order linear constant coefficient differential equations involving the dependent variables $x(t)$ and $y(t)$ and the independent variable t, which is often the time.

Such a system may be written

$$a_{11}\frac{\mathrm{d}x}{\mathrm{d}t} + a_{12}\frac{\mathrm{d}y}{\mathrm{d}t} + b_{11}x + b_{12}y = f(t),$$

$$a_{21}\frac{\mathrm{d}x}{\mathrm{d}t} + a_{22}\frac{\mathrm{d}y}{\mathrm{d}t} + b_{21}x + b_{22}y = g(t),$$

and it will be said to be **homogeneous** if $f(t) \equiv 0$ and $g(t) \equiv 0$.

If $f(t)$ and $g(t)$ are not both identically zero the system will be said to be **non-homogeneous**. We will illustrate a simple method for the solution of such systems by means of two examples.

A HOMOGENEOUS SYSTEM

Consider the solution of the homogeneous system

$$\frac{\mathrm{d}x}{\mathrm{d}t} + 2y + 3x = 0,$$

$$\frac{\mathrm{d}y}{\mathrm{d}t} + 3x - 2y = 0,$$

subject to the initial conditions $x(0) = 4$ and $y(0) = 0$.

Solving the first equation for y gives

$$y = -\frac{1}{2}\left(\frac{\mathrm{d}x}{\mathrm{d}t} + 3x\right),$$

and substitutiing this result into the second equation we find that

$$-\frac{1}{2}\left(\frac{d^2x}{dt^2}+3\frac{dx}{dt}\right)+3x+\left(\frac{dx}{dt}+3x\right)=0.$$

and so

$$\frac{d^2x}{dt^2}+\frac{dx}{dt}-12x=0.$$

This second order differential equation for x has the characteristic equation

$$\lambda^2+\lambda-12=0 \quad \text{or} \quad (\lambda+4)(\lambda-3)=0,$$

so $\lambda=-4$ or $\lambda=3$. The general solution (complementary function) for x is thus

$$x=Ae^{-4t}+Be^{3t}.$$

Substituting this expression for x into the first differential equation and solving it for y gives

$$y=-\frac{1}{2}(-4Ae^{-4t}+Be^{3t}+3Ae^{-4t}+3Be^{3t})\frac{1}{2}Ae^{-4t}-3Be^{3t}.$$

and so

$$y=\frac{1}{2}Ae^{-4t}-3Be^{3t}$$

It follows from this that the general solution, which is also the complementary function since the system is homogeneous, is

$$x=Ae^{-4t}+Be^{3t}$$

$$y=\frac{1}{2}Ae^{-4t}-3Be^{3t}.$$

To solve the initial value problem it is necessary to choose the arbitrary constants A and B such that $x(0)=4$ and $y(0)=0$. Setting $x=4$ when $t=0$ in the first equation, and $y=0$ when $t=0$ in the second equation, give

$$4=A+B$$

$$0=\frac{1}{2}A-3B.$$

These equations have the solution

$$A=\frac{24}{7} \quad \text{and} \quad B=\frac{4}{7},$$

so the solution of the initial value problem is

$$x=\frac{1}{7}(24e^{-4t}+4e^{3t}),$$

$$y=\frac{12}{7}(e^{-4t}-e^{3t}).$$

A NON-HOMOGENEOUS SYSTEM

Consider the solution of the non-homogeneous system

$$2\frac{dx}{dt}+\frac{dy}{dt}-2x-2y=5e^t \tag{A}$$

$$\frac{dx}{dt} + \frac{dy}{dt} + 4x + 2y = 5e^{-t}, \tag{B}$$

given that $x(0) = 2$ and $y(0) = 0$.

Substracting these equations gives

$$\frac{dx}{dt} - 6x - 4y = 5(e^t - e^{-t}), \tag{C}$$

and after differentiating this result with respect to t we find that

$$\frac{d^2x}{dt^2} - 6\frac{dx}{dt} - 4\frac{dy}{dt} = 5(e^t + e^{-t}). \tag{D}$$

Solving equation (B) for dy/dt gives

$$\frac{dy}{dt} = 5e^{-t} - \frac{dx}{dt} - 4x - 2y. \tag{E}$$

Substituting equation (E) into (D) gives

$$\frac{d^2x}{dt^2} - 6\frac{dx}{dt} - 4\left(5e^{-t} - \frac{dx}{dt} - 4x - 2y\right) = 5(e^t + e^{-t}),$$

or

$$\frac{d^2x}{dt^2} - 2\frac{dx}{dt} + 16x + 8y = 5e^t + 25e^{-t}. \tag{F}$$

Eliminating y between (C) and (F) shows that x satisfies the non-homogeneous equation

$$\frac{d^2x}{dt^2} + 4x = 15(e^t + e^{-t}). \tag{G}$$

This non-homogeneous equation is easily seen to have the complementary function

$$x_c = A\cos 2t + B\sin 2t. \tag{H}$$

Its particular integral will be of the form

$$x_p = Ce^t + De^{-t} \tag{I}$$

Substituting this into (G) gives

$$Ce^t + De^{-t} + 4(Ce^t + De^{-t}) = 15e^t + 15e^{-t}.$$

Equating the respective coefficients of e^t and e^{-t} on either side of this result to make it an identity gives:

1 Coefficients of e^t: $5C = 15$, so $C = 3$,
2 Coefficients of e^{-t}: $5D = 15$, so $D = 3$.

Thus the particular integral (I) becomes

$$x_p = 3e^t + 3e^{-t}, \tag{J}$$

so the general solution $x = x_c + x_p$ is

$$x = A\cos 2t + B\sin 2t + 3e^t + 3e^{-t}. \tag{K}$$

Substituting the expression for x in (K) into equation (C) and solving for y gives

$$y = \frac{1}{2}(B - 3A)\cos 2t - \frac{1}{2}(A + 3B)\sin 2t - 5e^t - 4e^{-t}. \tag{L}$$

The general solution of the system is given in equations (K) and (L). To solve the initial value problem, we must choose the arbitrary constants A and B such that $x(0) = 2$ and $y(0) = 0$. Setting $x = 2$ and $t = 0$ in equation (K), and $y = 0$ and $t = 0$ in equation (L) gives

$$2 = A + 6$$

and

$$0 = \frac{1}{2}(B - 3A) - 9.$$

These equations have the solution

$$A = -4 \quad \text{and} \quad B = 6,$$

so the solution of the initial value problem is

$$x = -4\cos 2t + 6\sin 2t + 3e^t + 3e^{-t},$$

and

$$y = 9\cos 2t - 7\sin 2t - 5e^t - 4e^{-t}.$$

PROBLEMS 80

In each of problems 1 to 6 find the general solution of the given system of equations.

1. $\dfrac{dx}{dt} = y$, $\dfrac{dy}{dt} = -x$.

2. $\dfrac{dx}{dt} = y - x$, $\dfrac{dy}{dt} = -x - 3y$.

3. $\dfrac{dx}{dt} - x - 2y = 0$, $\dfrac{dy}{dt} - y - 2x = 0$.

4. $\dfrac{dx}{dt} - x + y = 0$, $\dfrac{dy}{dt} - 3y - x = 0$.

5. $\dfrac{dx}{dt} + y = 0$, $\dfrac{dx}{dt} - \dfrac{dy}{dt} = 3x + y$.

6. $4\dfrac{dx}{dt} - \dfrac{dy}{dt} + 3x = \sin t$, $\dfrac{dx}{dt} + y = \cos t$.

In each of problems 7 to 10 find the general solution of the given system of equations and the solution to the initial value problem with the stated initial conditions.

7. $\dfrac{dx}{dt} + y - t = 0,$ $\dfrac{dy}{dt} - x + 2t = 0$; initial conditions $x(0) = 2, y(0) = -1$.

8. $\dfrac{dx}{dt} + x - y = e^t,$ $\dfrac{dy}{dt} - x + y = e^t$; initial conditions $x(0) = 1, y(0) = 3$.

9. $\dfrac{dx}{dt} + 2x + y = \sin t,$ $\dfrac{dy}{dt} - 4x - 2y = \cos t$; initial conditions $x(0) = 5, y(0) = 1$.

10. $5\dfrac{dx}{dt} - 2\dfrac{dy}{dt} + 4x - y = e^{-t},$ $\dfrac{dy}{dt} + 8x - 3y = 5\,e^{-t}$; initial conditions $x(0) = 2,$

$y(0) = 0$.

The Laplace transform and transform pairs

The Laplace transform is what is called an **integral transform**, and it transforms a function $f(t)$, in which t is often the time, into a related function $F(s)$, in which s is the **transform variable**. When applied to ordinary linear differential equations, the Laplace transform provides an efficient method for the solution of initial value problems. The Laplace transform approach is unlike the method just described in which both a complementary function and a particular integral need to be determined in order to form a general solution that must then be matched to the initial conditions. When using the Laplace transform to solve linear differential equations the initial conditions are incorporated at the time the transformation is carried out. As a result, the answer obtained is the solution to the given initial value problem, and so is free from arbitrary constants.

Before defining the Laplace transform we first need to introduce a new term. A function $f(t)$ is said to be **piecewise continuous** on the interval $a \leqslant t \leqslant b$ if the interval can be subdivided into smaller intervals on each of which $f(t)$ is continuous, but across each point separating adjacent sub-intervals $f(t)$ experiences a **finite jump**. A typical piecewise continuous function $f(t)$ is shown in Fig. 158, in which $f(t)$ is continuous for $a \leqslant t \leqslant b$ except at t_1 and t_2 where finite jumps occur.

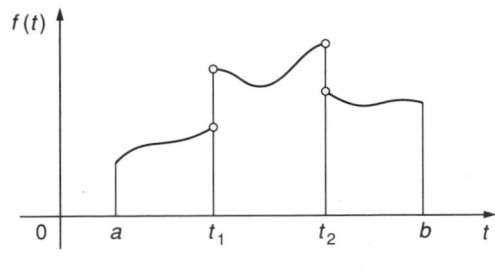

Fig. 158

The Laplace transform of $f(t)$
Let $f(t)$ be a piecewise continuous function of t which is defined for $t \geqslant 0$. Then, provided the improper integral exists, the **Laplace transform** $F(s)$ of $f(t)$ is defined as

$$F(s) = \int_0^\infty e^{-st} f(t) \, dt.$$

It is often convenient to use the notation $\mathscr{L}\{f(t)\}$ to signify the Laplace transform of $f(t)$, so that $F(s) = \mathscr{L}\{f(t)\}$. In what follows, we will use the convention that the function of t which is to be transformed will be denoted by a lower case letter, while the corresponding upper case letter will be used to denote the transformed function. Thus, for example, $F(s) = \mathscr{L}\{f(t)\}$, $Y(s) = \mathscr{L}\{y(t)\}$ and $X(s) = \mathscr{L}\{x(t)\}$.

SOME EXAMPLES OF LAPLACE TRANSFORMS

The Laplace transform operation involves an improper integral because the interval of integration is semi-infinite in length. Thus when evaluating the integral this fact must always be taken into account, and functions for which the integral does not converge will not have a Laplace transform.

1 If $f(t) = k$, with $k = $ constant,

$$\mathscr{L}\{k\} = \int_0^\infty k e^{-st} dt = \lim_{T \to \infty} \int_0^T k e^{-st} dt$$

$$= \lim_{T \to +\infty} \left(-\frac{k e^{-st}}{s} \right)\Big|_0^T = \lim_{T \to +\infty} \left(-\frac{k e^{-sT}}{s} \right) + \frac{k}{s}.$$

Provided $s > 0$ the limit on the right-hand side will be zero, and thus it follows that

$$\mathscr{L}\{k\} = \frac{k}{s}, \quad \text{for} \quad s > 0.$$

If $s < 0$ the integral will diverge and so the Laplace transform will not be defined for $s < 0$.

2 If $f(t) = t$, then

$$\mathscr{L}\{t\} = \int_0^\infty t e^{-st} dt = \lim_{T \to +\infty} \int_0^T t e^{-st} dt.$$

Integrating by parts gives

$$\mathscr{L}\{t\} = \lim_{T \to +\infty} \left(-\frac{t e^{-st}}{s} \right)\Big|_0^T + \lim_{T \to +\infty} \frac{1}{s} \int_0^T e^{-st} dt$$

$$= \lim_{T \to +\infty} \left(-\frac{T e^{-sT}}{s} \right) + \lim_{T \to +\infty} \left[\frac{1}{s} \left(-\frac{e^{-sT}}{s} \right) \right]\Big|_0^T$$

$$= \lim_{T \to +\infty} \left(-\frac{Te^{-sT}}{s} \right) - \lim_{T \to +\infty} \left(-\frac{e^{-sT}}{s} \right) + \frac{1}{s^2}.$$

It is a simple consequence of L'Hôpital's rule that

$$\lim_{T \to +\infty} (T^m e^{-sT}) = 0$$

for all $m \geq 0$, provided $s > 0$, so the first limit on the right-hand side is zero, while the second is also zero if $s > 0$, and thus we have shown that

$$\mathscr{L}\{t\} = \frac{1}{s^2}, \quad \text{for} \quad s > 0.$$

3 If $f(t) = e^{at}$, then

$$\mathscr{L}\{e^{at}\} = \int_0^\infty e^{at}e^{-st}dt = \lim_{T \to +\infty} \int_0^T e^{(a-s)t}dt$$

$$= \lim_{T \to +\infty} \left(\frac{e^{(a-s)t}}{(a-s)} \right)\Big|_0^T = \lim_{t \to +\infty} \left[\frac{e^{(a-s)T}}{(a-s)} \right] + \frac{1}{s-a}.$$

If $s < a$ the limit on the right-hand side is infinite, so the improper integral defining the Laplace transform diverges and the function has no Laplace transform. However, if $s > a$ the limit is zero and the improper integral defining the Laplace transform converges to $1/(s-a)$. Thus we have shown that

$$\mathscr{L}\{e^{at}\} = \frac{1}{s-a}, \quad \text{for} \quad s > a.$$

These typical examples show how a Laplace transform is determined from the definition, and how a condition on the transform variable s arises naturally from the requirement that the improper integral should be convergent. Clearly, a function $f(t)$ can only have a Laplace transform if $e^{-st}f(t)$ vanishes sufficiently rapidly as $t \to \infty$ for the defining integral to exist. It is this condition that determines whether or not function $f(t)$ has a Laplace transform. For example, the function e^{t^2} has no Laplace transform, because $e^{t^2}e^{-st} \to \infty$ for all s as $t \to +\infty$, so the defining improper integral is divergent for all s.

The function $f(t)$ and its Laplace transform $F(s) = \mathscr{L}\{f(t)\}$ are called a **Laplace transform pair** or, more simply, a **transform pair**. Thus k and k/s is an example of a transform pair, as are t and $1/s^2$, and e^{at} and $1/(s-a)$.

Any given function $f(t)$ for which the Laplace transform integral exists will have a unique Laplace transform $F(s)$. Conversely, with unimportant exceptions, a Laplace transform $F(s)$ corresponds to a unique function $f(t)$. These observations mean that if a table of pairs of functions $f(t)$ and $F(s)$ is constructed, by entering the table with a particular function $f(t)$, its Laplace transform $F(s)$ may be found. Conversely, by entering the table with a particular function $F(s)$, the function $f(t)$ with $F(s)$ as its Laplace transform may be found.

The operation of finding a function $f(t)$ of t which has a given function $F(s)$ as its Laplace transform is called performing the **inverse Laplace transform**, and it is convenient to denote it by the symbol $\mathscr{L}^{-1}$. Thus, if $F(s) = \mathscr{L}\{f(t)\}$, then $f(t) = \mathscr{L}^{-1}\{F(s)\}$. In particular, we have seen that

$$\mathscr{L}\{e^{at}\} = 1/(s-a), \quad \text{so} \quad \mathscr{L}^{-1}\{1/(s-a)\} = e^{at},$$

and

$$\mathscr{L}\{t\} = 1/s^2, \quad \text{so} \quad \mathscr{L}^{-1}\{1/s^2\} = t.$$

The linearity of the definite integral means that provided the integrals exist

$$\int_0^\infty \{af(t) + b\,g(t)\}\,dt = a\int_0^\infty f(t)\,e^{-st}dt + b\int_0^\infty g(t)\,e^{-st}dt,$$

where a, b are constants, and so

$$\mathscr{L}\{a\,f(t) + b\,g(t)\} = a\,\mathscr{L}\{f(t)\} + b\,\mathscr{L}\{g(t)\}.$$

Similarly,

$$\mathscr{L}^{-1}\{a\,F(s) + b\,G(s)\} = a\,\mathscr{L}^{-1}\{F(s)\} + b\,\mathscr{L}^{-1}\{G(s)\} = a\,f(t) + b\,g(t),$$

where $F(s) = \mathscr{L}\{f(t)\}$ and $G(s) = \mathscr{L}\{g(t)\}$.

These last results express the **linearity** of the Laplace transform and its inverse, and they are useful when finding both Laplace and inverse Laplace transforms.

Example 81.1

Find

(i) $\mathscr{L}\{3 + 4e^{2t}\}$; and

(ii) $\mathscr{L}^{-1}\left\{\dfrac{5}{s^2} + \dfrac{3}{s-1}\right\}$.

Solution

(i) $\mathscr{L}\{3 + 4e^{2t}\} = \mathscr{L}\{3\} + 4\,\mathscr{L}\{e^{2t}\}$,

but from example 1, $\mathscr{L}\{3\} = 3/s$, while from example $\mathscr{L}\{e^{2t}\} = 1/(s-2)$, so

$$\mathscr{L}\{3 + 4e^{2t}\} = \frac{3}{s} + \frac{4}{s-2}.$$

(ii) $\mathscr{L}^{-1}\left\{\dfrac{5}{s^2} + \dfrac{3}{s-1}\right\} = 5\,\mathscr{L}^{-1}(1/s^2) + 3\,\mathscr{L}^{-1}\{1/(s-1)\} = 5t + 3e^t$, where we

have made use of examples 2 and 3.   ▲

Partial fractions can be helpful when determining inverse Laplace transforms as shown by the next example.

Table 13 Laplace transform pairs

$f(t) = \mathcal{L}^{-1}\{F(s)\}$		$F(s) = \mathcal{L}\{f(t)\}$	
1.	k	$\dfrac{k}{s}$,	$s > 0$
2.	t	$\dfrac{1}{s^2}$,	$s > 0$
3.	t^n, n a positive integer	$\dfrac{n!}{s^{n+1}}$,	$s > 0$
4.	e^{at}	$\dfrac{1}{s-a}$,	$s > a$
5.	$t^n e^{at}$, n a positive intger	$\dfrac{n!}{(s-a)^{n+1}}$,	$s > a$
6.	$\sin at$	$\dfrac{a}{s^2+a^2}$,	$s > 0$
7.	$\cos at$	$\dfrac{s}{s^2+a^2}$,	$s > 0$
8.	$t \sin at$	$\dfrac{2as}{(s^2+a^2)^2}$,	$s > 0$
9.	$t \cos at$	$\dfrac{s^2-a^2}{(s^2+a^2)^2}$,	$s > 0$
10.	$e^{at} \sin bt$	$\dfrac{b}{(s-a)^2+b^2}$,	$s > a$
11.	$e^{at} \cos bt$	$\dfrac{s-a}{(s-a)^2+b^2}$,	$s > a$
12.	$\sinh at$	$\dfrac{a}{s^2-a^2}$,	$s > \|a\|$
13.	$\cosh at$	$\dfrac{s}{s^2-a^2}$,	$s > \|a\|$
14.	The Heaviside unit step function $f(t) = u_a(t) = \begin{cases} 0 & \text{for } t < a \\ 1 & \text{for } t > a \end{cases}$	$\dfrac{e^{-as}}{s}$,	$s > 0, a \geqslant 0$

Example 81.2

Find

$$\mathcal{L}^{-1}\left\{\frac{4s^2 - 3s - 9}{s^3 + 3s^2}\right\}.$$

Solution
The inverse transform is not immediately obvious, but by expressing the rational function of s whose inverse transform is to be found in terms of partial fractions we see that

$$\frac{4s^2 - 3s - 9}{s^3 + 3s^2} = \frac{4s^2 - 3s - 9}{s^2(s + 3)} = \frac{4}{s + 3} - \frac{3}{s^2}.$$

Thus,

$$\mathscr{L}^{-1}\left\{\frac{4s^2 - 3s - 9}{s^3 + 3s^2}\right\} = \mathscr{L}^{-1}\left\{\frac{4}{s + 3}\right\} + \mathscr{L}^{-1}\left\{\frac{-3}{s^2}\right\}$$

$$= 4e^{-3t} - 3t. \qquad \blacktriangle$$

Table 13 lists some commonly occurring functions $f(t)$ and their Laplace transforms $F(t)$. When used together with the linearity property and, where necessary, with a partial fraction decomposition, it will enable many Laplace and inverse Laplace transforms to be determined. The results of the table can be extended by reference to the second shift theorem of Section 83.

PROBLEMS 81

1. Find $\mathscr{L}\{3t^3\}$.
2. Find $\mathscr{L}\{\sin 4t\}$.
3. Find $\mathscr{L}\{e^{5t}\}$.
4. Find $\mathscr{L}\{te^t\}$.
5. Find $\mathscr{L}\{t\cos 3t\}$.
6. Find $\mathscr{L}\{e^{-2t}\sin 5t\}$.
7. Find $\mathscr{L}\{e^t\cos 2t\}$.
8. Find $\mathscr{L}\{\sinh 2t\}$.
9. Find $\mathscr{L}\{t^2 + 3\cos 2t\}$.
10. Find $\mathscr{L}\{te^{2t} + t^3\}$.
11. Find $\mathscr{L}\{t\cos t + 2\sin 2t\}$.
12. Find $\mathscr{L}\{e^{2t}\cos 3t + e^{2t}\sin 3t\}$.
13. Find $\mathscr{L}^{-1}\{3/s^5\}$.
14. Find $\mathscr{L}^{-1}\{5s/(s^2 + 4)^2\}$.
15. Find $\mathscr{L}^{-1}\{1/(s - 2)^2 + 3^2\}$.
16. Find $\mathscr{L}^{-1}\{3s/(s^2 - 9)\}$.

17. Find $\mathscr{L}^{-1}\left\{\dfrac{3}{s^3} + \dfrac{2}{s + 3}\right\}$.

18. Find $\mathscr{L}^{-1}\left\{\dfrac{4s}{s^2 + 4} + \dfrac{2}{s^2 + 9}\right\}$.

19. Find $\mathscr{L}^{-1}\left\{\dfrac{1}{s - 4} - \dfrac{3}{(s + 1)^3}\right\}$.

20. Find $\mathscr{L}^{-1}\left\{\dfrac{3s}{s^2 + 4} + \dfrac{1}{s^2 + 9}\right\}$.

Make use of partial fractions when evaluating the following inverse Laplace transforms.

21. Find $\mathscr{L}^{-1}\{(5s+10)/(s^2+3s-4)\}$.

22. Find $\mathscr{L}^{-1}\left\{\dfrac{s^2-6s-9}{(s-3)(s^2+9)}\right\}$.

23. Find $\mathscr{L}^{-1}\left\{\dfrac{2s+4}{s^2+2s+5}\right\}$.

24. Find $\mathscr{L}^{-1}\left\{\dfrac{4s^2+3s+29}{(s^2+9)(s+2)}\right\}$.

The Laplace transform of derivatives

82

When applying the Laplace transform to an ordinary linear differential equation it is necessary to transform derivatives. We now prove the basic result which is needed.

Let us determine $\mathscr{L}\{dy/dt\}$, where $y(t)$ is a function with the Laplace transform $Y(s)$, so that $\mathscr{L}\{y(t)\} = Y(s)$. By definition,

$$\mathscr{L}\{dy/dt\} = \int_0^\infty \left(\frac{dy}{dt}\right) e^{-st} dt = \lim_{T \to +\infty} \int_0^T \left(\frac{dy}{dt}\right) e^{-st} dt.$$

Applying integration by parts to this last result gives

$$\mathscr{L}\{dy/dt\} = \lim_{T \to +\infty} [y(t) e^{-st}]\Big|_0^T + \lim_{T \to +\infty} s \int_0^T y(t) e^{-st} dt$$

$$= \lim_{T \to +\infty} y(T) e^{-sT} - y(0) + s \mathscr{L}\{y(t)\}.$$

As $y(t)$ is assumed to have a Laplace transform the limit on the right-hand side must vanish, and so

$$\mathscr{L}\{dy/dt\} = s \mathscr{L}\{y(t)\} - y(0),$$

$$= s Y(s) - y(0).$$

This important result shows how, when transforming $y(t)$, the initial value $y(0)$ enters into the result.

A similar argument can be used to establish the following results, which we list for future reference.

Transformation of derivatives
When the Laplace transform $Y(s) = \mathscr{L}\{y(t)\}$ exists, then
1 $\mathscr{L}\{dy/dt\} = s Y(s) - y(0)$;
2 $\mathscr{L}\{d^2y/dt^2\} = s^2 Y(s) - y'(0) - s y(0)$;
3 $\mathscr{L}\{d^3y/dt^3\} = s^3 Y(s) - y''(0) - sy'(0) - s^2 y(0)$;
and, in general,
4 $\mathscr{L}\{d^ny/dt^n\} = s^n Y(s) - y^{(n-1)}(0) - s y^{(n-2)}(0) - s^2 y^{(n-3)}(0) - \ldots - s^{n-1} y(0)$,

where $y'(0) = (dy/dt)_{t=0}$, $y''(0) = (d^2y/dt^2)_{t=0}$, $y'''(0) = (d^3y/dt^3)|_{t=0}$, ..., and $y^{(r)}(0) = (d^r y/dt^r)_{t=0}$.

Example 82.1

Given that $\mathscr{L}\{y(t)\} = Y(s)$, find
(i) $\mathscr{L}\{y'\}$, given that $y(0) = 4$;
(ii) $\mathscr{L}\{y''\}$, given that $y(0) = -3$ and $y'(0) = 5$;
(iii) $\mathscr{L}\{y'''\}$, given that $y(0) = 1$, $y'(0) = -2$ and $y''(0) = 3$.

Solution
(i)   Using entry 1 of Table 13 gives $\mathscr{L}\{y'\} = \mathscr{L}\{dy/dt\} = sY(s) - y(0)$,
      but $y(0) = 4$, so

$$\mathscr{L}\{y'\} = sY(s) - 4.$$

(ii) Using entry 2 of Table 13 gives

$$\mathscr{L}\{y''\} = \mathscr{L}\{d^2y/dt^2\} = s^2Y(s) - y'(0) - sy(0),$$

      but $y'(0) = 5$ and $y(0) = -3$, so

$$\mathscr{L}\{y''\} = s^2Y(s) - 5 + 3s.$$

(iii) Using entry 3 of Table 13 gives

$$\mathscr{L}\{y'''\} = \{d^3y/dt^3\} = s^3Y(s) - y''(0) - s\,y'(0) - s^2y(0),$$

      but $y(0) = 1$, $y'(0) = -2$ and $y''(0) = 3$, so

$$\{y'''\} = s^2Y(s) - 3 + 2s - s^2. \qquad\blacktriangle$$

PROBLEM 82

In each of the following problems, find the Laplace transform of the required derivative of $y(t)$ in terms of $Y(s) = \mathscr{L}\{y(t)\}$ and the given initial conditions.

1. Find $\mathscr{L}\{y'\}$, given that $y(0) = -6$.
2. Find $\mathscr{L}\{y''\}$, given that $y(0) = 1$ and $y'(0) = 2$.
3. Find $\mathscr{L}\{y''\}$, given that $y(0) = 3$ and $y'(0) = 0$.
4. Find $\mathscr{L}\{y'''\}$, given that $y(0) = 2$, $y(0) = -1$ and $y''(0) = 4$.
5. Find $\mathscr{L}\{y'' + 3y' + y\}$, given that $y(0) = 3$ and $y'(0) = -1$.
6. Find $\mathscr{L}\{y'' - 2y' + 3y\}$, given that $y(0) = 0$ and $y'(0) = 0$.
7. Find $\mathscr{L}\{2y'' - 3y\}$, given that $y(0) = 1$ and $y'(0) = 2$.
8. Find $\mathscr{L}\{y'' + 4y' + 4y\}$, given that $y(0) = 2$ and $y'(0) = -2$.

There are two basic theorems, called **shift theorems**, which simplify the task of working with Laplace transforms. The first involves shifting the transform variable from s to $s - a$, and the second involves shifting the time variable t from t to $t - a$, where $a > 0$.

The first shift theorem
Let $\mathscr{L}\{f(t)\} = F(s)$ for $s > b$, then $\mathscr{L}\{e^{at}f(t)\} = F(s - a)$ for $s - a > b$.

Proof
By definition

$$F(s) = \int_0^\infty e^{-st} f(t)\,dt,$$

so

$$\mathscr{L}\{e^{at}f(t)\} = \int_0^\infty e^{-(s-a)t} f(t)\,dt = F(s - a).$$

Provided $F(s)$ exists for $s > b$, it follows that $F(s - a)$ exists for $s - a > b$. The result is proved.

The term 'shift' is used because multiplication of $f(t)$ by e^{at} shifts the transform variable s to $s - a$.

Example 83.1

Find
(i) $\mathscr{L}\{e^{3t}(\sinh t + 3\sin 2t)\}$;
(ii) $\mathscr{L}\{e^{2t}t\cos t\}$.

Solution
(i) By linearity we have

$$\mathscr{L}\{e^{3t}(\sinh t + 3\sin 2t)\} = \mathscr{L}\{e^{3t}\sinh t\} + 3\,\mathscr{L}\{e^{3t}\sin 2t\}.$$

Now from entry 12 in Table 13 with $a = 1$ we have

$$\mathscr{L}\{\sinh t\} = 1/(s^2 - 1).$$

Applying the first shift theorem with $a = 3$, we replace s by $s - 3$ in the above result to obtain

$$\mathscr{L}\{e^{3t} \sinh t\} = 1/[(s - 3)^2 - 1] = 1/(s^2 - 6s + 8).$$

Similarly, from entry 6 in Table 13 with $a = 2$ we have

$$\mathscr{L}\{\sin 2t\} = 2/(s^2 + 4).$$

Applying the first shift theorem with $a = 3$, we replace s by $s - 3$ in the above result to obtain

$$\mathscr{L}\{\sin 2t\} = 2/[(s - 3)^2 + 4] = 2/(s^2 - 6s + 13).$$

Thus, combining results, we find that

$$\mathscr{L}\{e^{3t}(\sinh t + 3 \sin 2t)\} = \frac{1}{s^2 - 6s + 8} + \frac{6}{s^2 - 6s + 13}.$$

(ii) From entry 9 in Table 13 with $a = 1$ we have

$$\mathscr{L}\{t \cos t\} = \frac{s^2 - 1}{(s^2 + 1)^2}.$$

Applying the first shift theorem with $a = 2$, we replace s by $s - 2$ in the above result to obtain

$$\mathscr{L}\{e^{2t} t \cos t\} = \frac{(s - 2)^2 - 1}{[(s - 2)^2 + 1]^2} = \frac{s^2 - 4s + 3}{(s^2 - 45 + 5)^2}. \qquad \blacktriangle$$

The first shift theorem can also be used to find inverse transforms, as shown in the next example.

Example 83.2

Find

(i) $\mathscr{L}^{-1}\left\{\dfrac{5}{s^2 - 2s + 1}\right\};$ and

(ii) $\mathscr{L}^{-1}\left\{\dfrac{6}{s^2 - 4s + 13}\right\}.$

Solution
(i) We have

$$\frac{5}{s^2 - 2s + 1} = 5 \cdot \left[\frac{1}{(s - 1)^2}\right],$$

but inspection of Table 13 shows that $\mathscr{L}\{t\} = 1/s^2$, so by the first shift theorem with $a = 1$, $\mathscr{L}\{e^t t\} = 1/(s - 1)^2$. Thus we see that $\mathscr{L}^{-1}\{1/(s - 1)^2\} = te^t$, and so

$$\mathscr{L}^{-1}\left\{\frac{5}{t^2 - 2t + 1}\right\} = 5te^t.$$

This result could, of course, have been deduced directly from entry 5 in Table 13 by setting $n = 1$ and $a = 1$.

(ii) By completing the square we have

$$\frac{6}{s^2 - 4s + 13} = \frac{6}{(s-2)^2 + 3^2}.$$

Inspection of Table 13 shows that

$$\mathscr{L}\{\sin 3t\} = \frac{3}{s^2 + 3^2}.$$

Applying the first shift theorem with $a = 2$ we see that

$$\mathscr{L}\{e^{2t}\sin 3t\} = \frac{3}{(s - 2^2)^2 + 3^2},$$

so

$$\mathscr{L}^{-1}\left\{\frac{3}{s^2 - 4s + 13}\right\} = e^{2t}\sin 3t,$$

and thus

$$\mathscr{L}^{-1}\left\{\frac{6}{s^2 - 4s + 13}\right\} = 2e^{2t}\sin 3t. \qquad \blacktriangle$$

The **second shift theorem** makes use of the **Heaviside unit step function** $u_a(t)$, which is defined as

$$u_a(t) = \begin{cases} 0 & \text{for} \quad t < a \\ 1 & \text{for} \quad t > a. \end{cases}$$

The name 'step function' arises from the fact that its graph shown in Fig. 159 jumps discontinuously at $t = a$, from the value zero for $t < a$ to the value unity when $t > a$ in a step-like manner, and thereafter remains constant. In physical problems a suitably scaled step function can be used to represent switching on or off a constant voltage at $t = a$, and it finds many other applications of a similar nature. An alternative notation for the step function which is often used is $H(t - a)$, with the understanding that $H(t - a) = u_a(t)$.

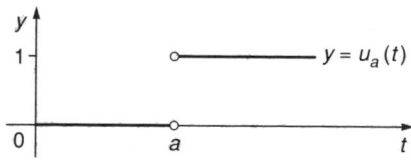

Fig. 159

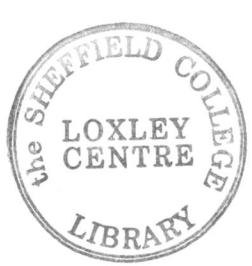

When used in conjunction with other functions, the Heaviside unit step function enables them to be 'switched on' and 'switched off'. These ideas are illustrated in the diagrams which follow. Figure 160(a) shows the function $f(t) = \cos t$, and Fig. 160(b) the function $f(t) = u_\pi(t) \cos t$, which is zero for $t < \pi$ and equals the cosine function for $t > \pi$. Thus $f(t) = u_\pi(t) \cos t$ is the zero function for $t < \pi$, after which the cosine function is 'switched on' and π becomes the function $\cos t$.

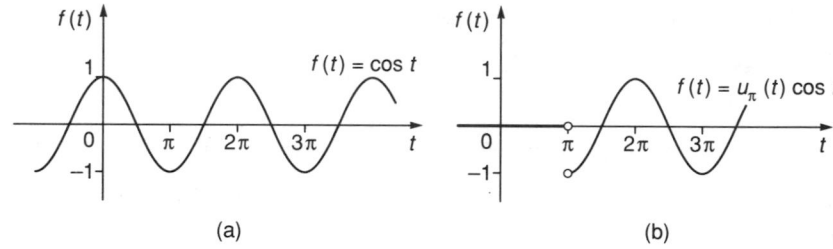

(a)   (b)

Fig. 160

Figure 161(a) shows the function $f(t) = \cos t$, Fig. 161(b) the function $f(t) = \cos(t - \pi)$ and Fig. 161(c) the function $f(t) = u_\pi(t) \cos(t - \pi)$. It is easily seen that Fig. 161(c) is the zero function for $t < \pi$ and the cosine function shifted by π for $t > \pi$.

When combined, Heaviside functions can be used to generate pulse-like functions. Thus in Fig. 162 the function

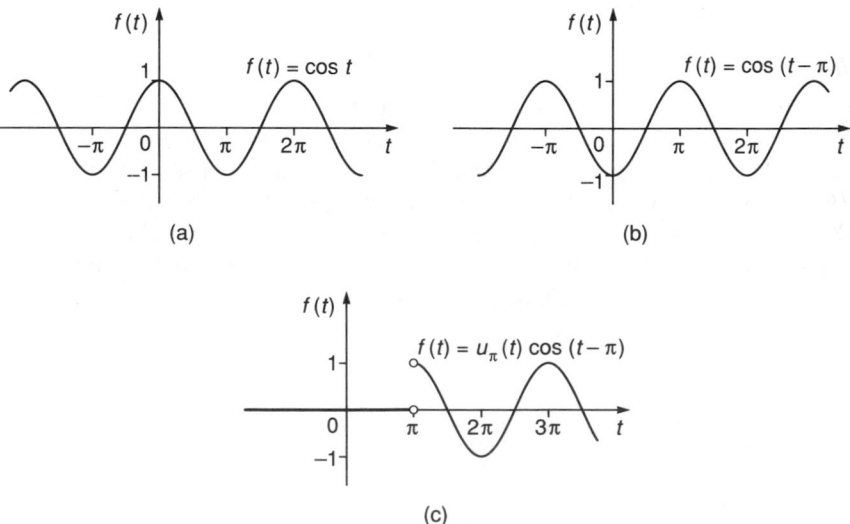

(a)   (b)

(c)

Fig. 161

$$f(t) = u_a(t) - u_b(t)$$

is seen to define a rectangular pulse of unit height, and width $b - a$, which may also be defined as

$$f(t) = \begin{cases} 0 & \text{for} & t < a \\ 1 & \text{for} & a < t < b \\ 0 & \text{for} & t > b. \end{cases}$$

Similarly, the function

$$f(t) = [u_a(t) - u_b(t)] g(t)$$

is such that

$$f(t) = \begin{cases} 0 & \text{for} & t < 0 \\ g(t) & \text{for} & a < t < b \\ 0 & \text{for} & t > b. \end{cases}$$

and the way in which the factor $[u_a(t) - u_b(t)]$ **samples** the function $g(t)$ in the interval $a < t < b$ can be seen by inspection of Fig. 163(a) and (b).

The Laplace transform of the Heaviside unit step function is contained as entry 14 in the table in Section 81. The result follows directly from the definition, because

$$\mathscr{L}\{u_a(t)\} = \int_0^\infty e^{-st} u_a(t)\, dt = \int_0^\infty e^{-st}\, dt = \frac{e^{-as}}{s}.$$

The Laplace transform of the rectangular pulse of unit height in the interval $a < t < b$ shown in Fig. 162 is

$$\mathscr{L}\{u_a(t) - u_b(t)\} = \mathscr{L}\{u_a(t)\} - \mathscr{L}\{u_b(t)\} = \frac{1}{s}(e^{-as} - e^{-bs}).$$

The second shift theorem
If $\mathscr{L}\{f(t)\} = F(s)$, then $\mathscr{L}\{u_a(t)f(t-a)\} = e^{-as}F(s)$ and, conversely,
$\mathscr{L}^{-1}\{e^{-as}F(s)\} = u_a(t)f(t-a)$.

Proof
By definition,

$$\mathscr{L}\{u_a(t)f(t-a)\} = \int_a^\infty e^{-st}f(t-a)\, dt.$$

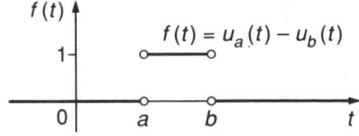

Fig. 162

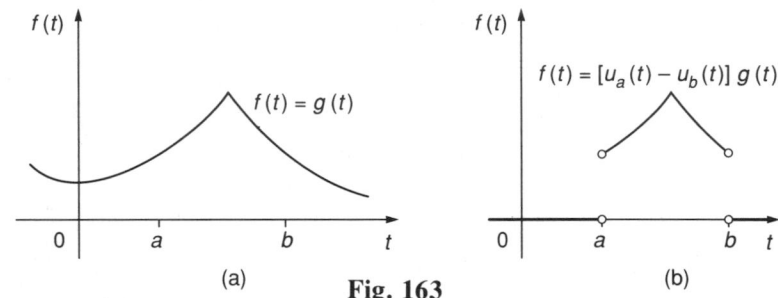

Fig. 163

If the variable in this integral is changed to $\tau = t - a$ it becomes

$$\mathscr{L}\{u_a(t)f(t-a)\} = \int_0^\infty e^{-s(a+\tau)}f(\tau)\,d\tau,$$

$$= e^{as}\int_0^\infty e^{st}f(\tau)\,d\tau$$

$$= e^{-as}F(s),$$

and the result is proved.

Example 83.3

Find
(i) the Laplace transform of $u_{\pi/3}(t)\,f(t-\pi/3)$, when $f(t)=t\cos t$;
(ii) the function $f(t)$ whose Laplace transform is

$$\frac{8se^{-2s}}{s^2+9},$$

(iii) the function $f(t)$ whose Laplace transform is

$$\frac{3e^{-3s}}{s^2} - \frac{5se^{-4s}}{(s^2+4)^2}.$$

Solution
(i) From entry 9 in Table 13 we have

$$\mathscr{L}\{t\cos t\} = \frac{s^2-1}{(s^2+1)^2}.$$

Thus applying the second shift theorem with $a=\pi/3$ we have

$$\mathscr{L}\left\{u_{\pi/3}(t)\left[\left(t-\frac{\pi}{3}\right)\cos\left(t-\frac{\pi}{3}\right)\right]\right\} = \frac{e^{-\pi s/3}(s^2-1)}{(s^2+1)^2}.$$

(ii) We must find the inverse Laplace transform of

$$\frac{8se^{-2s}}{s^2+9},$$

and because of the second shift theorem, the presence of the factor e^{-2s} in the numerator shows that a shift $a = 2$ is involved. We see from entry 7 in Table 13 that

$$\mathscr{L}\{\cos 3t\} = \frac{s}{s^2+9},$$

so by appeal to the second shift theorem with $a = 2$ we see that

$$\mathscr{L}^{-1}\left\{\frac{8se^{-2s}}{s^2+9}\right\} = 8u_2(t)\cos[3(t-2)].$$

(iii) In this example two separate applications of the second shift theorem are necessary. The factor e^{-3s} in the term $3e^{-3s}/s^2$ shows a shift $a = 3$ is involved.

As $\mathscr{L}\{t\} = 1/s^2$ it follows that

$$\mathscr{L}\{3t\} = 3/s^2, \quad \text{and thus} \quad \mathscr{L}^{-1}\{3/s^2\} = 3t,$$

so applying the second shift theorem with $a = 3$ gives

$$\mathscr{L}^{-1}\{3e^{-3s}/s^2\} = 3u_3(t)[t-3].$$

Similarly, the factor e^{-4s} in the term

$$\frac{-5se^{-4s}}{(s^2+4)^2}$$

indicates that a shift $a = 4$ is involved. We see from entry 8 in Table 13 that

$$\mathscr{L}\{t\sin 2t\} = \frac{4s}{(s^2+4)^2},$$

so

$$\mathscr{L}^{-1}\left\{\frac{-5s}{(s^2+4)^2}\right\} = -\frac{5}{4}t\sin 2t.$$

Applying the second shift theorem with $a = 4$ then gives

$$\mathscr{L}^{-1}\left\{\frac{-5se^{-4s}}{(s^2+4)^2}\right\} = -\frac{5}{4}u_4(t)\{(t-4)\sin[2(t-4)]\}.$$

Thus, combining results, we have

$$\mathscr{L}^{-1}\left\{\frac{3e^{-3s}}{s^2} - \frac{5se^{-4s}}{(s^2+4)^2}\right\} = 3u_3(t)[t-3] - \frac{5}{4}u_4(t)(t-4)\sin[2(t-4)]\}. \quad \blacktriangle$$

PROBLEMS 83

1. Show from the definition that

$$\mathscr{L}\{t^2\} = 2/s^3.$$

2. Show from the definition that
$$\mathscr{L}\{\sin at\} = a/(s^2 + a^2).$$

3. Show from the definition that
$$\mathscr{L}\{\cos at\} = s/(s^2 + a^2).$$

4. Show from the definition that
$$\mathscr{L}\{te^{at}\} = 1/(s - a)^2.$$

5. Find $\mathscr{L}\{e^{3t}\cos 3t\}$.
6. Find $\mathscr{L}\{e^{-2t} t^2\}$.
7. Find $\mathscr{L}\{e^{-t}\sinh 2t\}$.
8. Find $\mathscr{L}\{e^t t \sin t\}$.
9. Find $\mathscr{L}\{e^{2t} t \cos 2t\}$.
10. Find $\mathscr{L}\{e^{-3t} t \sin 2t\}$.

11. Find $\mathscr{L}^{-1}\left\{\dfrac{1}{s^2 - 4s + 20}\right\}$.

12. Find $\mathscr{L}^{-1}\left\{\dfrac{5}{s^2 + 4s + 20}\right\}$.

13. Find $\mathscr{L}^{-1}\left\{\dfrac{2(s - 1)}{(s^2 + 2s + 10)^2}\right\}$.

14. Find $\mathscr{L}^{-1}\left\{\dfrac{s^2 + 2s - 3}{2(s^2 + 2s + 5)^2}\right\}$.

15. Sketch the function
$$f(t) = u_1(t) - u_2(t) + u_3(t).$$

16. Sketch the function
$$f(t) = u_1(t) - 2u_2(t) + 3u_3(t).$$

17. Sketch the function
$$f(t) = u_{3\pi/2}(t) \cos t.$$

18. Sketch the function
$$f(t) = [u_{\pi/2}(t) - u_{3\pi/2}(t)] \sin t.$$

19. Sketch the function
$$f(t) = u_\pi(t) \sin(t - \pi).$$

20. Sketch the function
$$f(t) = u_1(t)(t - 1)^2.$$

21. Sketch the function
$$f(t) = u_2(t)e^{t-2}.$$

22. Sketch the function

$$f(t) = u_\pi(t) \cos [2(t - \pi)].$$

23. Find $\mathscr{L}\{u_{\pi/2}(t) \sin [3(t - \pi/2)]\}$.
24. Find $\mathscr{L}\{u_1(t) [(t - 1)^2 + 3(t - 1) + 4]\}$.
25. Find $\mathscr{L}\{u_2(t) e^{3(t-2)} \sin (t - 2)\}$.
26. Find $\mathscr{L}\{u_1(t) \cosh [3(t - 1)]\}$.

27. Find $\mathscr{L}^{-1}\left\{\dfrac{se^{-2s}}{s^2 + 4}\right\}$.

28. Find $\mathscr{L}^{-1}\left\{\dfrac{e^{-s}}{(s - 2)^2 + 2^2}\right\}$.

29. Find $\mathscr{L}^{-1}\left\{\dfrac{(s^2 - 9)e^{-4s}}{(s^2 + 9)^2}\right\}$.

30. Find $\mathscr{L}^{-1}\left\{\dfrac{(s - 1) e^{-2s}}{(s - 1)^2 + 3^2}\right\}$.

31. By expressing the rational function of s as the sum of two such functions find

$$\mathscr{L}^{-1}\left\{\frac{(s^2 + 6s - 9)e^{-s}}{(s^2 + 9)^2}\right\}.$$

32. By expressing the rational function of s as the sum of two such functions find

$$\mathscr{L}^{-1}\left\{\frac{3s - 8}{s^2 + 4}\right\}.$$

33. Use partial fractions to find

$$\mathscr{L}^{-1}\left\{\frac{(2s^2 + 3s + 2)e^{-3s}}{(s^2 + 1)(s - 1)}\right\}.$$

34. Use partial fractions to find

$$\mathscr{L}^{-1}\left\{\frac{(6s^2 + 20s + 24s)e^{-2s}}{(s^2 + 4)^3}\right\}.$$

We will now use the results of Sections 81 to 83 to illustrate the solution of initial value problems for linear ordinary differential equations by considering a number of examples.

Example 84.1

Solve the linear first order non-homogeneous differential equation

$$\frac{dy}{dt} + 3y = \sin t,$$

given that $y(0) = 2$.

Solution
Taking the Laplace transform of the differential equation, writing $Y(s) = \mathscr{L}\{y(t)\}$, using the fact that $\mathscr{L}\{y'\} = s\,Y(s) - y(0)$ and $\mathscr{L}\{\sin t\} = 1/(s^2 + 1)$ we have

$$s\,Y(s) - y(0) + 3Y(s) = \frac{1}{(s^2 + 1)},$$

but $y(0) = 2$ so

$$s\,Y(s) - 2 + 3Y(s) = \frac{1}{(s^2 + 1)}.$$

Solving for $Y(s)$ this becomes

$$Y(s) = \frac{2}{s + 3} + \frac{1}{(s + 3)(s^2 + 1)},$$

so as $y(t) = \mathscr{L}^{-1}\{Y(s)\}$ we see that

$$y(t) = \mathscr{L}^{-1}\left\{\frac{2}{s + 3} + \frac{1}{(s + 3)(s^2 + 1)}\right\}$$

$$= \mathscr{L}^{-1}\left\{\frac{2}{s + 3}\right\} + \mathscr{L}^{-1}\left\{\frac{1}{(s + 3)(s^2 + 1)}\right\}.$$

From entry 4 in Table 13 we have

$$\mathscr{L}^{-1}\left\{\frac{2}{s+3}\right\} = 2e^{-3t},$$

but to evaluate the other inverse Laplace transform we need to make use of partial fractions. Setting

$$\frac{1}{(s+3)(s^2+1)} = \frac{A}{s+3} + \frac{Bs+C}{(s^2+1)},$$

and multiplying by $(s+3)(s^2+1)$ gives

$$1 = A(s^2+1) + (Bs+C)(s+3).$$

Equating the coefficients of corresponding powers of s on each side of this result to make it an identity gives:

1 Coefficients of s^2: $A + B = 0$.
2 Coefficients of s: $3B + C = 0$.
3 Coefficients of s^0: $A + 3C = 1$

These equations have the solution

$$A = 1/10, \quad B = -1/10 \quad \text{and} \quad C = 3/10,$$

so

$$\frac{1}{(s+3)(s^2+1)} = \frac{1}{10}\left(\frac{1}{s+3}\right) - \frac{1}{10}\left(\frac{s}{s^2+1}\right) + \frac{3}{10}\left(\frac{1}{s^2+1}\right),$$

and thus

$$\mathscr{L}^{-1}\left\{\frac{1}{(s+3)(s^2+1)}\right\} = \frac{1}{10}\mathscr{L}^{-1}\left\{\frac{1}{s+3}\right\} - \frac{1}{10}\mathscr{L}^{-1}\left\{\frac{s}{s^2+1}\right\} + \frac{3}{10}\mathscr{L}^{-1}\left\{\frac{1}{s^2+1}\right\}.$$

Using entries 4, 7 and 6 in Table 13 then shows that

$$\mathscr{L}^{-1}\left\{\frac{1}{(s+3)(s^2+1)}\right\} = \frac{1}{10}[e^{-3t} - \cos t + 3\sin t].$$

Finally, combining results, we find that

$$y(t) = \mathscr{L}^{-1}\left\{\frac{2}{s+3}\right\} + \mathscr{L}^{-1}\left\{\frac{1}{(s+3)(s^2+1)}\right\}$$

$$= 2e^{-3t} + \frac{1}{10}[e^{-3t} - \cos t + 3\sin t],$$

and thus

$$y(t) = \frac{1}{10}[21\, e^{-3t} - \cos t + 3\sin t]. \qquad \blacktriangle$$

Example 84.2

Solve the linear second order homogeneous differential equation

$$\frac{d^2y}{dt^2} + 5\frac{dy}{dt} + 6y = 0,$$

given that $y(0) = 1$ and $y'(0) = -1$.

Solution
Taking the Laplace transform of the differential equation and using the results that $\mathscr{L}\{y'\} = sY(s) - y(0)$ and $\mathscr{L}\{y''\} = s^2Y(s) - y'(0) - sy(0)$, where $Y(s) = \mathscr{L}\{y(t)\}$, gives

$$s^2Y(s) - y'(0) - sy(0) + 5sY(s) - 5y(0) + 6Y(s) = 0.$$

Solving for $Y(s)$ and using the fact that $y(0) = 1$ and $y'(0) = -1$ this becomes

$$Y(s) = \frac{s+4}{s^2 + 5s + 6},$$

and so

$$y(t) = \mathscr{L}^{-1}\left\{\frac{s+4}{s^2 + 5s + 6}\right\}.$$

To find the inverse Laplace transform we express the rational function of s in terms of partial fractions by writing

$$\frac{s+4}{s^2 + 5s + 6} = \frac{A}{s+2} + \frac{B}{s+3},$$

from which it follows in the usual manner that $A = 2$ and $B = -1$, so

$$\frac{s+4}{s^2 + 5s + 6} = \frac{2}{s+2} - \frac{1}{s+3}.$$

Thus

$$y(t) = \mathscr{L}^{-1}\left\{\frac{2}{s+2}\right\} - \mathscr{L}^{-1}\left\{\frac{1}{s+3}\right\},$$

and after using entry 4 in Table 13 this becomes

$$y(t) = 2e^{-2t} - e^{-3t}. \qquad \blacktriangle$$

Example 84.3

Solve the linear second order non-homogeneous differential equation

$$\frac{d^2y}{dt^2} + 3\frac{dy}{dt} + 2y = 1,$$

given that $y(0) = 0$ and $y'(0) = 1$.

Solution
Taking the Laplace transform of the differential equation, and using the fact
that $\mathscr{L}\{1\} = 1/s$ gives

$$s^2 Y(s) - y'(0) - sy(0) + 3sY(s) - 3y(0) + 2Y(0) = 1/s,$$

where $Y(s) = \mathscr{L}\{y(t)\}$. Solving for $Y(s)$ after using the initial conditions
$y(0) = 0$ and $y'(0) = 1$ gives

$$Y(s) = \frac{1}{(s^2 + 3s + 2)} + \frac{1}{s(s^2 + 3s + 2)}.$$

Expanding these results by means of partial fractions in the usual manner
shows that

$$Y(s) = \underbrace{\frac{1}{s+1} - \frac{1}{s+2}}_{\text{first term}} + \underbrace{\frac{1}{2}\left(\frac{1}{s}\right) - \left(\frac{1}{s+1}\right) + \frac{1}{2}\left(\frac{1}{s+2}\right)}_{\text{second term}}$$

$$= \frac{1}{2}\left(\frac{1}{s}\right) + \frac{1}{2}\left(\frac{1}{s+2}\right).$$

Using results 1 and 4 in Table 13 gives the required solution:

$$y(t) = \frac{1}{2} + \frac{1}{2}e^{-2t}. \qquad\qquad \blacktriangle$$

Example 84.4
.

Solve the linear second order non-homogeneous differential equation

$$\frac{d^2 y}{dt^2} + 2\frac{dy}{dt} + y = e^{-t},$$

given that $y(0) = 0$ and $y'(0) = 1$.

Solution
Taking the Laplace transform of the differential equation as in Example 84.3,
using the initial conditions $y(0) = 0$ and $y'(0) = 1$ and the fact that $\mathscr{L}\{e^{-t}\} =
1/(s + 1)$, gives

$$s^2 Y(s) - 1 + 2sY(s) + Y(s) = \frac{1}{s+1},$$

and so

$$Y(s) = \frac{1}{(s + 1)^2} + \frac{1}{(s + 1)^3}.$$

Taking the inverse Laplace transform to find $y(t)$ we have

$$y(t) = \mathscr{L}^{-1}\left\{\frac{1}{(s + 1)^2}\right\} + \mathscr{L}^{-1}\left\{\frac{1}{(s + 1)^3}\right\}.$$

Entry 5 in Table 13 shows that

$$\mathcal{L}\{te^{-t}\} = \frac{1}{(s+1)^2} \quad \text{and} \quad \mathcal{L}\{t^2e^{-t}\} = \frac{2}{(s+1)^3},$$

and hence

$$\mathcal{L}^{-1}\left\{\frac{1}{(s+1)^2}\right\} = te^{-t} \quad \text{and} \quad \mathcal{L}^{-1}\left\{\frac{1}{(s+1)^3}\right\} = \tfrac{1}{2}t^2e^{-t}.$$

The required solution is thus

$$y(t) = t\left(1 + \frac{1}{2}t\right)e^{-t}.$$

Notice that the solution using the Laplace transform was obtained easily, yet had the differential equation been solved by the method of undermined coefficients it would have given difficulty. This is so because the characteristic equation is

$$\lambda^2 + 2\lambda + 1 = 0 \quad \text{or} \quad (\lambda + 1)^2 = 0,$$

so the complementary function must be

$$y_c(t) = Ae^{-t} + Bte^{-t}.$$

When seeking a particular integral a difficulty would have arisen because the non-homogeneous term e^{-t} is contained in $y_c(t)$, as is te^{-t}. Thus, for a particular integral, it would have been necessary to seek one of the form

$$y_p(t) = Ct^2e^{-t}.$$

All these considerations have been avoided by using the Laplace transform, which proceeded in a straightforward manner, as with the other examples considered. ▲

Example 84.5

Solve the linear second order non-homogeneous differential equation

$$\frac{d^2y}{dt^2} + y = \sin t,$$

given that $y(0) = 1$ and $y'(0) = 0$.

Solution
Taking the Laplace transform of the differential equation we have

$$s^2Y(s) - y'(0) - sy(0) + Y(s) = 1/(s^2 + 1),$$

where $Y(s) = \mathcal{L}\{y(t)\}$ and we have used the result that $\mathcal{L}\{\sin t\} = 1/(s^2 + 1)$. Inserting the initial conditions $y(0) = 1$, $y'(0) = 0$ and solving for $Y(s)$ gives

$$Y(s) = \frac{s}{s^2 + 1} + \frac{1}{(s^2 + 1)^2}.$$

As $y(t) = \mathcal{L}^{-1}\{Y(s)\}$ we have

$$y(t) = \mathcal{L}^{-1}\left\{\frac{s}{s^2+1}\right\} + \mathcal{L}^{-1}\left\{\frac{1}{(s^2+1)^2}\right\}$$

$$= \cos t + \mathcal{L}^{-1}\left\{\frac{1}{(s^2+1)^2}\right\},$$

where the first inverse Laplace transform was found from Table 13. The remaining inverse Laplace transform is not contained in the table, but inspection of entry 9 suggests that we rewrite $1/(s^2+1)^2$ as

$$\frac{1}{(s^2+1)^2} = \frac{1}{2}\left\{\frac{(s^2+1)-(s^2-1)}{(s^2+1)^2}\right\}$$

$$= \frac{1}{2}\left(\frac{1}{s^2+1}\right) - \frac{1}{2}\left(\frac{s^2-1}{(s^2+1)^2}\right).$$

Thus

$$\mathcal{L}^{-1}\left\{\frac{1}{(s^2+1)^2}\right\} = \frac{1}{2}\mathcal{L}^{-1}\left\{\frac{1}{(s^2+1)}\right\} - \frac{1}{2}\mathcal{L}^{-1}\left\{\frac{s^2-1}{(s^2+1)^2}\right\},$$

so from entries 6 and 9 in Table 13 we have

$$\mathcal{L}^{-1}\left\{\frac{1}{(s^2+1)^2}\right\} = \frac{1}{2}\sin t - \frac{1}{2}t\cos t.$$

The required solution

$$y(t) = \cos t + \mathcal{L}^{-1}\left\{\frac{1}{(s^2+1)^2}\right\}$$

becomes

$$y(t) = \cos t + \frac{1}{2}\sin t - \frac{1}{2}t\cos t.$$

This differential equation provides an example of resonance without damping, of the type considered in Section 79. In this case the unbounded growth of the solution as t increases occurs because of the term $-\frac{1}{2}t\cos t$. ▲

The last second order differential equation we consider has a more complicated non-homogeneous term comprising the sum of a cosine function and a step function.

Example 84.6

Solve the linear second order non-homogeneous differential equation

$$\frac{d^2y}{dt^2} + 2\frac{dy}{dt} + 5y = 3\cos t + 2u_3(t),$$

given that $y(0) = 0$ and $y'(0) = 0$.

Solution

Taking the Laplace transform of the differential equation in the usual manner, incorporating the initial conditions, and using the fact that $\mathscr{L}\{3\cos t\} = 3s/(s^2 + 1)$ and $\mathscr{L}\{2u_3(t)\} = 2e^{-3s}/s$, gives

$$s^2 Y(s) + 2sY(s) + 5Y(s) = \frac{3s}{s^2 + 1} + \frac{2e^{-3}}{s}.$$

Thus

$$Y(s) = \frac{3s}{(s^2 + 2s + 5)(s^2 + 1)} + \frac{2e^{-3s}}{s(s^2 + 2s + 5)},$$

and so

$$y(t) = \mathscr{L}^{-1}\left\{\frac{3s}{(s^2 + 2s + 5)(s^2 + 1)}\right\} + \mathscr{L}^{-1}\left\{\frac{2e^{-3s}}{s(s^2 + 2s + 5)}\right\}.$$

We must now determine these two inverse Laplace transforms with the help of partial fraction decompositions and, in the case of the second inverse transform, the second shift theorem. A routine calculation shows that

$$\frac{3s}{(s^2 + 2s + 5)(s^2 + 1)} = \frac{3}{5}\left(\frac{s}{s^2 + 1}\right) + \frac{3}{10}\left\{\frac{1}{s^2 + 1}\right\} - \frac{3}{10}\left(\frac{2s + 5}{s^2 + 2s + 5}\right),$$

so taking the inverse Laplace transform gives

$$\mathscr{L}^{-1}\left\{\frac{3s}{(s^2 + 2s + 5)(s^2 + 1)}\right\} = \frac{3}{5}\,\mathscr{L}^{-1}\left\{\frac{s}{s^2 + 1}\right\} + \frac{3}{10}\,\mathscr{L}^{-1}\left\{\frac{1}{s^2 + 1}\right\}$$

$$- \frac{3}{10}\,\mathscr{L}^{-1}\left\{\frac{2s + 5}{s^2 + 2s + 5}\right\}.$$

The first two inverse Laplace transforms on the right-hand side follow from Table 13 and we have

$$\mathscr{L}^{-1}\left\{\frac{3s}{(s^2 + 2s + 5)(s^2 + 1)}\right\} = \frac{3}{5}\cos t + \frac{3}{10}\sin t - \frac{3}{10}\,\mathscr{L}^{-1}\left\{\frac{2s + 5}{s^2 + 2s + 5}\right\}.$$

To determine the last inverse transform we complete the square in the denominator by writing $s^2 + 2s + 5 = (s + 1)^2 + 2^2$, and then, because of the form of the denominator, we rewrite the rational function of s in the form of entries 10 and 11 in Table 13. As a result we have

$$\frac{2s + 5}{s^2 + 2s + 5} = \frac{2(s + 1) + 3}{(s + 1)^2 + 2^2} = 2\left(\frac{s + 1}{(s + 1)^2 + 2^2}\right) + \frac{3}{2}\left(\frac{2}{(s + 1)^2 + 2^2}\right),$$

and so

$$- \frac{3}{10}\,\mathscr{L}^{-1}\left\{\frac{2s + 5}{s^2 + 2s + 5}\right\} = -\frac{3}{5}\,\mathscr{L}^{-1}\left\{\frac{s + 1}{(s + 1)^2 + 2^2}\right\} - \frac{9}{20}\,\mathscr{L}^{-1}\left\{\frac{2}{(s + 1)^2 + 2^2}\right\}.$$

Direct appeal to entries 10 and 11 in Table 13 then shows that

$$-\frac{3}{10}\mathcal{L}^{-1}\left\{\frac{2s+5}{s^2+2s+5}\right\}=-\frac{3}{5}e^{-t}\cos 2t-\frac{9}{20}e^{-t}\sin 2t,$$

so combining terms gives

$$\mathcal{L}^{-1}\left\{\frac{3s}{(s^2+2s+5)(s^2+1)}\right\}=\frac{3}{5}\cos t+\frac{3}{10}\sin t-\frac{3}{5}e^{-t}\cos 2t-\frac{9}{20}e^{-t}\sin 2t.$$

Another straightforward calculation shows that

$$\frac{2}{s(s^2+2s+5)}=\frac{2}{5}\left(\frac{1}{s}\right)-\frac{2}{5}\left(\frac{s+2}{s^2+2s+5}\right)$$

$$=\frac{2}{5}\left(\frac{1}{s}\right)-\frac{2}{5}\left(\frac{(s+1)+1}{(s+1)^2+2^2}\right)$$

$$=\frac{2}{5}\left(\frac{1}{s}\right)-\frac{2}{5}\left(\frac{s+1}{(s+1)^2+2^2}\right)-\frac{1}{5}\left(\frac{2}{(s+1)^2+2^2}\right).$$

Thus multiplying by e^{-3s} and taking the inverse Laplace transform we have

$$\mathcal{L}^{-1}\left\{\frac{2e^{-3s}}{s(s^2+2s+5)}\right\}=\frac{2}{5}\mathcal{L}^{-1}\left\{\frac{e^{-3s}}{s}\right\}-\frac{2}{5}\mathcal{L}^{-1}\left\{\frac{(s+1)e^{-3s}}{(s+1)^2+2^2}\right\}$$

$$-\frac{1}{5}\mathcal{L}^{-1}\left\{\frac{2e^{-3s}}{(s+1)^2+2^2}\right\}.$$

An appeal to entries 1, 10 and 11 in Table 13 together with the second shift theorem then shows that

$$\mathcal{L}^{-1}\left\{\frac{2e^{-3s}}{s(s^2+2s+5)}\right\}=\frac{2}{5}u_3(t)-\frac{2}{5}u_3(t)e^{-(t-3)}\cos[2(t-3)]$$

$$-\frac{1}{5}u_3(t)e^{-(t-3)}\sin[2(t-3)].$$

The required solution

$$y(t)=\mathcal{L}^{-1}\left\{\frac{3s}{(s^2+2s+5)(s^2+1)}\right\}+\mathcal{L}^{-1}\left\{\frac{2e^{-3s}}{s(s^2+2s+5)}\right\}$$

is thus seen to be

$$y(t)=\frac{3}{5}\cos t+\frac{3}{10}\sin t-\frac{3}{5}e^{-t}\cos 2t-\frac{9}{20}e^{-t}\sin 2t$$

$$+\frac{1}{5}u_3(t)\{2-2e^{-(t-3)}\cos[2(t-3)]-e^{-(t-3)}\sin[2(t-3)]\}.$$

Inspection of the form of the solution shows, as would be expected, that the step function in the non-homogeneous term only influences the solution when

$t > 3$. The determination of this solution without the aid of the Laplace transform would have involved a far more complicated form of argument.

▲

The last example involves the solution of two simultaneous first order linear non-homogeneous differential equations of the type considered in Section 80. The Laplace transform provides an alternative approach to the solution of initial value problems for such equations.

Example 84.7

Solve the simultaneous differential equations

$$\frac{dx}{dt} = 2y + \sin t \quad \text{and} \quad \frac{dy}{dt} = x + y,$$

given that $x(0) = 0$ and $y(0) = 0$.

Solution
To solve these simultaneous differential equations for $x(t)$ and $y(t)$ it is necessary to introduce the two Laplace transforms

$$X(s) = \mathscr{L}\{x(t)\} \quad \text{and} \quad Y(s) = \mathscr{L}\{y(t)\}.$$

Taking the Laplace transform of each differential equation gives

$$sX(s) - x(0) = 2Y(s) + \frac{1}{s^2 + 1} \quad \text{and} \quad sY(s) = X(s) + Y(s),$$

but $x(0) = 0$ and $y(0) = 0$, so

$$sX(s) = Y(s) + \frac{1}{s^2 + 1} \quad \text{and} \quad sY(s) - y(0) = X(s) + Y(s),$$

Solving the second equation for $X(s)$ gives

$$X(s) = (s - 1)Y(s),$$

so using this result to eliminate $X(s)$ from the first equation we have

$$s(s - 1)Y(s) = 2Y(s) + \frac{1}{s^2 + 1}.$$

Solving this equation for $Y(s)$ gives

$$Y(s) = \frac{1}{(s^2 - s - 2)(s^2 + 1)},$$

and so

$$y(t) = \mathscr{L}^{-1}\left\{\frac{1}{(s^2 - s - 2)(s^2 + 1)}\right\}.$$

A partial fractions expansion shows that

$$\frac{1}{(s^2 - s - 2)(s^2 + 1)} = \frac{1}{10}\left(\frac{s}{s^2 + 1}\right) - \frac{3}{10}\left(\frac{1}{s^2 + 1}\right) - \frac{1}{6}\left(\frac{1}{s + 1}\right) + \frac{1}{15}\left(\frac{1}{s - 2}\right),$$

so from entries 4, 6 and 7 in Table 13 we have

$$y(t) = \mathcal{L}^{-1}\left\{\frac{1}{(s^2 - s - 2)(s^2 + 1)}\right\}$$

$$= \frac{1}{10}\cos t - \frac{3}{10}\sin t - \frac{1}{6}e^{-t} + \frac{1}{15}e^{2t}.$$

To find $x(t)$, we may either solve the two transformed equations for $X(s)$ and determine it from $x(t) = \mathcal{L}^{-1}\{X(s)\}$, or substitute $y(t)$ into the second differential equation and determine it from

$$x = \frac{dy}{dt} - y.$$

In this case the second approach is simpler so we will use it. As a result we find that

$$x(t) = \left[-\frac{1}{10}\sin t - \frac{3}{10}\cos t + \frac{1}{6}e^{-t} + \frac{2}{15}e^{2t}\right]$$
$$- \left[\frac{1}{10}\cos t - \frac{3}{10}\sin t - \frac{1}{6}e^{-t} + \frac{1}{15}e^{2t}\right].$$

where the first in brackets is dy/dt. Thus,

$$x(t) = \frac{1}{5}\sin t - \frac{2}{5}\cos t + \frac{1}{3}e^{-t} + \frac{1}{15}e^{2t}.$$

Thus the required solution is

$$x(t) = \frac{1}{5}\sin t - \frac{2}{5}\cos t + \frac{1}{3}e^{-t} + \frac{1}{15}e^{2t},$$

$$y(t) = \frac{1}{10}\cos t - \frac{3}{10}\sin t - \frac{1}{6}e^{-t} + \frac{1}{15}e^{2t}.$$

PROBLEMS 84

Solve the following initial value problems.

1. $y'' - 3y' + 2y = 0$, with $y(0) = 0$, $y'(0) = 1$.
2. $y'' - 4y = 0$, with $y(0) = 1$, $y'(0) = -1$.
3. $y'' - y' - 2y = 0$, with $y(0) = 2$, $y'(0) = -1$.
4. $y'' + 2y' + 4y = 0$, with $y(0) = 1$, $y'(0) = 0$.
5. $y'' - 4y' + 5y = 0$, with $y(0) = 1$, $y'(0) = 0$.
6. $y'' + 2y' + 10y = 0$, with $y(0) = -1$, $y'(0) = 1$.
7. $y'' - 2y' + y = 0$, with $y(0) = 3$, $y'(0) = 0$.

8. $y''' - 3y'' + 3y' - y = 0$, with $y(0) = 1, y'(0) = 0, y''(0) = 1$.
9. $y''' - y'' + y' - y = 0$, with $y(0) = 4, y'(0) = 0, y''(0) = 0$.
10. $y'' + y = 3 \sin x$, with $y(0) = 0, y'(0) = 1$.
11. $y'' - y = e^t - t$, with $y(0) = 1, y'(0) = 0$.
12. $y'' - 3y' + 2y = 3 \cos t$, with $y(0) = 1, y'(0) = 0$.
13. $y'' - 2y' + y = t\,e^t$, with $y(0) = 0, y'(0) = 1$.
14. $y'' - 4y = 1 + u_1(t)$, with $y(0) = 0, y'(0) = 1$.
15. $y'' + 4y = \cos t + u_{\pi/2}(t)$, with $y(0) = 0, y'(0) = 0$.
16. $y'' + y' - 2y = t + u_2(t)$, with $y(0) = 1, y'(0) = 0$.
17. $y'' + 3y' + 2y = 1 - u_1(t)$, with $y(0) = 1, y'(0) = 0$.

18. $\dfrac{dx}{dt} = 2x + y$, $\dfrac{dy}{dt} = 3x + 4y$, with $x(0) = 1, y(0) = 0$.

19. $\dfrac{dx}{dt} = x + y$, $\dfrac{dy}{dt} = -2x + 3y$, with $x(0) = 1, y(0) = 2$.

20. $\dfrac{dx}{dt} = 2x + y$, $\dfrac{dy}{dt} = -x + 4y$, with $x(0) = 0, y(0) = -1$.

21. $\dfrac{dx}{dt} = -3x + 2y$, $\dfrac{dy}{dt} = -2x + y$, with $x(0) = 2, y(0) = 1$.

22. $\dfrac{dx}{dt} = x + 2y$, $\dfrac{dy}{dt} = x - 5 \sin t$, with $x(0) = 1, y(0) = 1$.

23. $\dfrac{dx}{dt} = y - 2t$, $\dfrac{dy}{dt} = -x + t$, with $x(0) = 2, y(0) = 1$.

Enlarging the list of Laplace transform pairs

Applications of the Laplace transform to the solution of initial value problems can often be simplified if Table 13, the list of Laplace transform pairs, in Section 81 is enlarged. This can be accomplished in many ways as, for example, by using the shift theorems, but one of the simplest additional methods involves the differentiation of a transform.

Differentiation of a transform
Let $\mathscr{L}\{f(t)\} = F(s)$, for $s > s_0$. Then,

$$\mathscr{L}\{(-t)^n f(t)\} = \frac{d^n F(s)}{ds^n}, \quad \text{for} \quad s > s_0.$$

Proof
We have

$$F(s) = \int_0^\infty e^{-st} f(t)\, dt \quad \text{for} \quad s > s_0,$$

so differentiating with respect to s and assuming that this operation can be taken under the integral sign (this can be justified) gives

$$\frac{dF(s)}{ds} = \int_0^\infty \frac{\partial}{\partial s} [e^{-st} f(t)]\, dt \quad \text{for} \quad s > s_0.$$

The partial derivative with respect to s is required under the integral sign because $e^{-st} f(t)$ is a function of the two variables s and t. Performing the indicated differentiation gives

$$\frac{dF(s)}{ds} = \int_0^\infty e^{-st} (-t) f(t)\, dt$$

$$= \mathscr{L}\{(-t) f(t)\} \quad \text{for} \quad s > s_0,$$

and the result is proved for $n = 1$.

A repetition of the argument establishes the general result

$$F^{(n)}(s) = \mathscr{L}\{(-t)^n f(t)\} \quad \text{for} \quad s > s_0,$$

where $F^{(n)}(s) = d^n F/ds^n$.

Example 85.1

Given that $\mathscr{L}\{\cos at\} = \dfrac{s}{s^2 + a^2}$, show that

$$\mathscr{L}\{t \cos at\} = (s^2 - a^2)/(s^2 + a^2)^2.$$

Solution
Applying the theorem with $n = 1$ gives

$$\mathscr{L}\{-t \cos at\} = \frac{d}{ds}\left[\frac{s}{s^2 + a^2}\right] = \frac{a^2 - s^2}{(s^2 + a^2)^2},$$

and so

$$\mathscr{L}\{t \cos at\} = \frac{s^2 - a^2}{(s^2 + a^2)^2}.$$

Thus we have derived entry 9 in Table 13 from entry 7.   ▲

Example 85.2

Given that $\mathscr{L}\{e^{at}\} = 1/(s - a)$, show that

$$\mathscr{L}\{t^2 e^{at}\} = 2/(s - a)^3.$$

Solution
Applying the theorem with $n = 2$ gives

$$\mathscr{L}\{(-t)^2 e^{at}\} = \frac{d^2}{ds^2}\left(\frac{1}{s - a}\right) = \frac{2}{(s - a)^2},$$

and so

$$\mathscr{L}\{t^2 e^{at}\} = \frac{2}{(s - a)^2}.$$

Here, we have derived a special case of entry 5 in Table 13 from entry 4.   ▲

Example 85.3

Show from entries 6 and 9 in Table 13 that

$$\mathscr{L}\{\sin at - at \cos at\} = \frac{2a^3}{(s^2 + a^2)^2}.$$

Use this result to find

$$\mathscr{L}\{t \sin at - at^2 \cos at\}.$$

Solution

Starting from the results

$$\mathscr{L}\{\sin at\} = \frac{a}{s^2 + a^2}$$

and

$$\mathscr{L}\{t\cos at\} = \frac{s^2 - a^2}{(s^2 + a^2)^2}$$

we have

$$\mathscr{L}\{\sin at - at\cos at\} = \frac{a}{s^2 + a^2} - \frac{a(s^2 - a^2)}{(s^2 + a^2)^2} = \frac{2a^3}{(s^2 + a^2)^2}.$$

Applying the theorem with $n = 1$ to this result gives

$$\mathscr{L}\{(-t)[\sin at - at\cos at]\} = \frac{d}{ds}\frac{2a^3}{(s^2 + a^2)^2} = \frac{-8a^3 s}{(s^2 + a^2)^3},$$

and so

$$\mathscr{L}\{t\sin at - at^2\cos at\} = \frac{8a^3 s}{(s^2 + a^2)^3}.$$

This result is not contained in the table of Laplace transform pairs, and would have necessitated a considerable amount of calculation had it been derived by direct integration using the definition of a Laplace transform. ▲

PROBLEMS 85

1. Given that $\mathscr{L}\{1\} = 1/s$, show by induction that
$$\mathscr{L}\{t^n\} = n!/s^{n+1}, \quad \text{for } n = 1, 2, \dots.$$

2. Given that $\mathscr{L}\{e^{at}\} = 1/(s - a)$, show by induction that
$$\mathscr{L}\{t^n e^{at}\} = n!/(s - a)^{n+1}, \quad \text{for } n = 1, 2, \dots.$$

3. Given that $\mathscr{L}\{\sinh at\} = a/(s^2 - a^2)$, find $\mathscr{L}\{t\sinh at\}$.
4. Given that $\mathscr{L}\{\cosh at\} = s/(s^2 - a^2)$, find $\mathscr{L}\{t\cosh at\}$.
5. Use Table 13 to show that

$$\mathscr{L}\{1 - \cos at\} = \frac{a^2}{s(s^2 + a^2)}.$$

Use this result to find

$$\mathscr{L}\{t - t\cos at\}.$$

6. Use Table 13 to show that

$$\mathscr{L}\{at - \sin at\} = \frac{a^3}{s^2(s^2 + a^2)}.$$

Use this result to find

$$\mathcal{L}\{at^2 - t\sin at\}.$$

7. Use Table 13 to show that

$$\mathcal{L}\{\sin at + at\cos at\} = \frac{2as^2}{(s^2 + a^2)^2}.$$

Use this result to find

$$\mathcal{L}\{t\sin at + at^2\cos at\}.$$

8. Use Table 13 to show that

$$\mathcal{L}\{\sinh at - \sin at\} = \frac{2a^3}{s^4 - s^4}.$$

Use this result to find

$$\mathcal{L}\{t\sinh at - t\sin at\}.$$

Answers

PROBLEMS 1

1.   −1   3

2.   2   4

3.   −1   2

4.   −2   1   3

5.   −2   3   ; $x < -2$ and $x > 3$.

6.   2   3   ; $-2 \leqslant x \leqslant 3$.

7.   1   2   ; $x < 1, \; x > 2$.

8.   1   2   ; $1 < x < 2$.

9.   1   3   ; $1 < x \leqslant 3$.

10.   0   2   ; $0 < x < 2$.

11.   −16   −2   2   6   ; $-16 \leqslant x \leqslant -2$ and $2 \leqslant x \leqslant 6$.

12.   −4   −3   1   2   ; $-4 \leqslant x \leqslant -3$ and $1 \leqslant x \leqslant 2$.

13. $(a+b)/2 - a = (b-a)/2 > 0$ since $b > a$, so $a < (a+b)/2$.

Also $b - (a+b)/2 = (b-a)/2 > 0$, so $b > (a+b)/2$.

14. $\dfrac{b+k}{a+k} - \dfrac{b}{a} = \dfrac{(a-b)k}{a(a+k)} > 0$, because $a > b$, and thus $\dfrac{b}{a} < \dfrac{b+k}{a+k}$. The other
result allows in a similar fashion by considering the other difference.

15. Proceed as shown in the answer to problem 14.

16. (a) $|a+b| = |3-4| = 1 \leqslant |a| + |b| = |3| + |-4| = 7$;

$||a| - |b|| = |3-4| = 1 \leqslant |3 - (-4)| = 7$.

(b) $|a+b| = |4+1| = 5 \leqslant |4| + |1| = |5|$;

$||a| - |b|| = |4-1| = 3 \leqslant |4-1| = 3$.

(c) $|a+b| = |-3-5| = 8 \leqslant |-3| + |-5| = 8$;

$||a| - |b|| = |3-5| \leqslant 2 = |-3 - (-5)| = 2$.

(d) $|a+b| = |-1+1| = 0 < |-1| + |1| = 2$;

$||a| - |b|| = |1-1| = 0 \leqslant |-1-1| = 2$.

17. From Example 1.4 it follows that

$$|a+b| \leqslant |a| + |b|$$

and

$$|a+b| = |a - (-b)| \geqslant ||a| - |b||.$$

Thus

$$\frac{1}{|a| + |b|} \leqslant \left|\frac{1}{a+b}\right| \leqslant \frac{1}{||a| - |b||},$$

and the result follows from this because

$$\left|\frac{1}{a+b}\right| = \frac{1}{|a+b|}.$$

18. $\left|x^3 - 4x - 6\right| \leqslant |x|^3 + 4|x| + 6$ and max. $|x| = 3$, so $\left|x^3 - 4x - 6\right| \leqslant$
$3^3 + 4 \cdot 3 + 6 = 45$. So the result is true for $M \geqslant 45$.

19. $\left|x^4 - 2x^3 + 1\right| \leqslant |x|^4 + 2|x|^3 + 1$ and max. $|x| = 2$, so $\left|x^4 - 2x + 1\right| \leqslant$
$2^4 + 2 \cdot 3^3 + 1 = 33$. So the result is true for $M \geqslant 33$.

20. $\dfrac{a + |a|}{a\,|b|} = \dfrac{1}{|a|} + \dfrac{1}{a} = \begin{cases} 2/a & \text{if } a > 0 \\ 0 & \text{if } a < 0. \end{cases}$

21. The result follows directly from the inequalities $ma_1 + ma_2 + \ldots + ma_n$ $\leqslant k_1a_1 + k_2a_2 + \ldots + k_na_n \leqslant Ma_1 + Ma_2 + \ldots + Ma_n$ combined with fact that $b_1 + b_2 + \ldots + b_n > 0$.

22. The signs of $a^p - b^p$ and $a^q - b^q$ are the same, so $(a^p - b^p)(a^q - b^q) \geqslant 0$, and thus $a^{p+q} - a^pb^q - a^qb^p + b^{p+q} \geqslant 0$, from which the result then follows.

23. $(a + b)^2 - (a - b)^2 = 4ab > 0$, so $(a + b)^2 \geqslant 4ab$, and hence $\dfrac{a+b}{2} \geqslant \sqrt{ab}$.

24. If $\sqrt{2} = m/n$, where m, n have no common factor, squaring shows that $2 = m^2/n^2$, and so $m^2 = 2n^2$. As m, n are integers this asserts that m^2 is even (it is divisible by 2) and thus m must be even, so we may set $m = 2p$. The result $\sqrt{2} = m/n$ now becomes $\sqrt{2} = 2p/n$ or, after squaring, $n^2 = 2p^2$. This shows that this is even, and hence n is even, so we may set $n = 2q$. As $m = 2p$ and $n = 2q$, the assumption that $\sqrt{2}$ is rational shows that, contrary to hypothesis, m and n have a common factor (it is 2). This contradiction implies that $\sqrt{2}$ cannot be represented as a rational number, and so it is irrational.

PROBLEMS 2

1. Range $1 \leqslant y \leqslant 10$.

2. Range $1 \leqslant y \leqslant 10$.

3. Range $-1 \leqslant y \leqslant 1$.

4. Range $-1 \leqslant y \leqslant 1/\sqrt{2}$ (with positive square root).

5. Range $-1 \leqslant x \leqslant \infty$.

6. Range $-1/\sqrt{2} \leqslant y \leqslant 1$ (with positive square root).

7. Range $0 \leqslant y \leqslant 8$.

8. Range $1/2 \leqslant y \leqslant 3/2$.

9. One–one (monotonic increasing).

10. Many–one.

11. Many–one (it is a function because $|\sqrt{x}|$ is non-negative).

12. One–one (monotonic decreasing).

13. One–many mapping.

14. One–many mapping.

15. One–one (monotonic increasing).

16. One–one (monotonic increasing).

17. Many–one.

18. One–one (monotonic decreasing).

19. Domain $-\infty < x < \infty$ and range $-\infty < y < \infty$.

20. Domain $-\infty < x < \infty$ and range $0 \leqslant y \leqslant 3$.

21. Domain $-\infty < x < \infty$ and range $-1 \leqslant y \leqslant 1$.

22. Domain $x \leqslant \infty$ and range $-1 < y \leqslant 1$.

PROBLEMS 3

1. $(-3, 3)$, $R = 4$; $(x + 3)^2 + (y - 3)^2 = 16$.

2. $(2, 4)$, $R = 2$; $(x - 2)^2 + (y - 4)^2 = 4$.

3. $(2, 4)$, $R = 3$; $(x - 2)^2 + (y - 4)^2 = 9$.

4. $(-2, -3)$, $R = 3$; $(x + 2)^2 + (y + 3)^2 = 9$.

5. $(4, -1)$, $R = 1$; $(x - 4)^2 + (x + 1)^2 = 1$.

6. $(-2, 3)$, $R = 5$; $(x + 2)^2 + (y - 3)^2 = 25$.

7. $(2, -1)$, semi-major axis $= 3$, semi-minor axis $= 2$;
$$[(x - 2)^2/4] + [(y + 1)^2/9] = 1; \text{ vertical.}$$

8. $(-1, 2)$, semi-major axis $= 4$, semi-minor axis $= 2$;
$$[(x + 1)^2/16] + [(y - 2)^2/4] = 1; \text{ horizontal.}$$

9. $(0, -3)$, semi-major axis $= 3$, semi-minor axis $= 1$;
$$x^2/9 + (y + 3)^2 = 1; \text{ horizontal.}$$

10. $(1, -2)$, semi-major axis $= 2$, semi-minor axis $= 1$;
$$[(x - 1)^2/4] + (y + 2)^2 = 1; \text{ horizontal.}$$

11. $(1, -2)$, semi-major axis $= 4$, semi-minor axis $= 3$;
$$[(x - 1)^2/9] + [(y + 2)^2/16] = 1; \text{ vertical.}$$

12. $(-4, -2)$, semi-major axis $= 2$, semi-minor axis $= 1$;
$$(x + 4)^2 + [(y + 2)^2/4] = 1; \text{ vertical.}$$

13. $(1, -2)$; $[(x - 1)^2/4] - [(y + 2)^2/9] = 1$; horizontal; $y = -2 \pm (3/2)(x - 1)$.

14. $(-2, -1)$; $(x + 2)^2 - [(y + 1)^2/9] = 1$; horizontal ; $y = -1 \pm 3(x + 2)$.

15. $(3, -1)$; $[(y - 3)^2/4] - [(x + 1)^2/9] = 1$; vertical; $y = -1 \pm (2/3)(x + 1)$.

16. $(1, -3)$; $[(y-1)^2/16] - [(x+3)^2/4] = 1$; vertical; $y = -3 \pm 2(x+3)$.

17. $(2, -4)$; $[(x-2)^2/9] - [(y+4)^2/4] = 1$; horizontal; $y = 2 \pm (2/3)(x-2)$.

18. $(-1, -1)$; $[(y+1)^2/4] - (x+1)^2 = 1$; vertical; $y = -1 \pm 2(x+1)$.

19. Vertical; vertex $(2, -2)$; focus $(2, -4)$; $(x-2)^2 = -8(y+2)$; concave-down.

20. Horizontal; vertex $(1, 3)$; focus $(4, 3)$; $(y-3)^2 = 12(x-1)$; concave to the right.

21. Horizontal; vertex $(-2, -4)$; focus $(-3, -4)$; $(y+4)^2 = -4(x+2)$; concave to the left.

22. Vertical; vertex $(3, 5)$; focus $(3, 8)$; $(x-3)^2 = 12(y-5)$; concave-up.

23. Vertical; vertex $(-3, 1)$; focus $(-3, -1)$; $(x+3)^2 = -8(y-1)$; concave to the left.

24. Horizontal; vertex $(0, 3)$; focus $(3, 3)$; $(y-3)^2 = 12x$; concave to the right.

25. $x = -1/2$ and $y = -2$.

26. $y = -(3/2)x$.

27. $x = -1$ and $y = x - 1$.

28. $x = 3/2$ and $y = -5/2$.

29. $x = \pm 2$, $x = \pm \sqrt{2}$ and $y = 0$.

30. $x = \pm 1$ and $y = 1 + x$.

31. $y = 2(x-1)$ and $y = -2(x+1)$.

PROBLEMS 4

1. (a) $x = 3/\sqrt{2}$, $y = 3/\sqrt{2}$;

    (b) $x = 0$, $y = -4$;

    (c) $x = -3.0311$, $y = 1.75$;

    (d) $x = 5.5433$, $y = -2.2961$.

2. (a) $r = 5$, $\theta = -0.25$ rad;

    (b) $r = 3.5$, $\theta = 1.0472$ rad;

    (c) $r = 2$, $\theta = 2.7489$ rad;

    (d) $r = 3$, $\theta = 3.5343$ rad.

3. $x = a$; a straight line.

4. $x^2 + y^2 = 2ay$; a circle.

5. $y = k/x$; a rectangular hyperbola.

6. $y = 2a - x$; a straight line.

7. $(x^2 + y^2 - ax)^2 = a^2(x^2 + y^2)$; a cardioid.

8. $\dfrac{x^2}{25} + \dfrac{y^2}{9} = 1$; an ellipse.

9. $\dfrac{x^2}{16} - \dfrac{y^2}{9} = 1$; a hyperbola.

10. $y^2 = 6x$; a parabola.

11. A heart-shaped curve lying on its side, which is symmetrical about the polar axis, has a cusp at the origin and lies mainly to the left of the origin.

12. A spiral starting from the origin and winding around the origin infinitely many times as θ increases (or decreases) from the value $\theta = 0$. The spiral winds anticlockwise around the origin when $\theta \geq 0$ and clockwise when $\theta \leq 0$.

13. A spiral about the origin which grows slower than the corresponding spiral of Archimedes.

14. A curve with four symmetrically positioned loops centred on the origin with their only points in common being at the origin (like two figures eight at right angles to one another).

PROBLEMS 6

2. $\begin{pmatrix} 7 \\ 2 \end{pmatrix} = \dfrac{7!}{5!\,2!} = 21,$ $\begin{pmatrix} 8 \\ 3 \end{pmatrix} = \dfrac{8!}{5!\,3!} = 56,$

$\begin{pmatrix} 5 \\ 4 \end{pmatrix} = \dfrac{5!}{1!\,4!} = 5,$ $\begin{pmatrix} 9 \\ 3 \end{pmatrix} = \dfrac{9!}{6!\,3!} = 84.$

3. $-\begin{pmatrix} 9 \\ 7 \end{pmatrix} = -36$; the negative sign ocurs because when b is replaced by $-b$ the term $a^2(-b)^7 = -a^2 b^7$; and $\begin{pmatrix} 9 \\ 6 \end{pmatrix} = 84.$

4. $\begin{pmatrix} 8 \\ 6 \end{pmatrix} = 28$ and $\begin{pmatrix} 8 \\ 4 \end{pmatrix} = 70.$

PROBLEMS 7

1. $f + g = 2(1 + x) + \sin x$; domain $(-\infty, \infty)$,
    $f - g = 2(1 - x) + \sin x$; domain $(-\infty, \infty)$,

$fg = 2x(2 + \sin x)$; domain $(-\infty, \infty)$,

$f/g = (2 + \sin x)/2x$; domain $(-\infty, \infty)$, $x \neq 0$.

2. $f + g = 3 + 2x^2$; domain $(-\infty, \infty)$,

$f - g = -1$; domain $(-\infty, \infty)$,

$fg = (1 + x^2)(2 + x^2) = x^4 + 3x^2 + 2$; domain $(-\infty, \infty)$,

$f/g = (1 + x^2)/(2 + x^2)$; domain $(-\infty, \infty)$.

3. $f + g = \sin x(1 + \sin x)$; domain $(-\infty, \infty)$,

$f - g = \sin x(\sin x - 1)$; domain $(-\infty, \infty)$,

$fg = \sin^3 x$; domain $(-\infty, \infty)$,

$f/g = \sin x$; domain $(-\infty, \infty)$.

4. $f + g = \sin x(1 + \sin x)$; domain $(-\infty, \infty)$,

$f - g = \sin x(1 - \sin x)$; domain $(-\infty, \infty)$,

$fg = \sin^3 x$; domain $(-\infty, \infty)$,

$f/g = 1/\sin x$; domain $(-\infty, \infty)$, $x \neq \pm n\pi$ for $n = 0, 1, 2, \ldots$.

5. $f + g = \sin x^2 + 1/(1 + x^2)$; domain $(-\infty, \infty)$,

$f - g = \sin^2 x - 1/(1 + x^2)$; domain $(-\infty, \infty)$,

$fg = \sin^2 x/(1 + x^2)$; domain $(-\infty, \infty)$,

$f/g = (1 + x^2) \sin^2 x$; domain $(-\infty, \infty)$.

6. $f + g = \cos x^2 + 1/(1 - x^2)$; domain $(-\infty, \infty)$ with $x \neq \pm 1$,

$f - g = \cos x^2 - 1/(1 - x^2)$; domain $(-\infty, \infty)$ with $x \neq \pm 1$,

$fg = \cos x^2/(1 - x^2)$; domain $(-\infty, \infty)$ with $x \neq \pm 1$,

$f/g = (1 - x^2) \cos x^2$; domain $(-\infty, \infty)$ with $x \neq \pm 1$.

7. $f + g = x^2 + \sqrt{(4 - x)}$; domain $x \leq 4$,

$f - g = x^2 - \sqrt{(4 - x)}$; domain $x \leq 4$,

$fg = x^2 \sqrt{(4 - x)}$; domain $x \leq 4$,

$f/g = x^2/\sqrt{(4 - x)}$; domain $x < 4$.

8. $f + g = \sqrt{|1 - x|} + x$; domain $(-\infty, \infty)$,

$f - g = \sqrt{|1 - x|} - x$; domain $(-\infty, \infty)$,

$fg = x \sqrt{|1 - x|}$; domain $(-\infty, \infty)$,

$f/g = (\sqrt{|1 - x|})/x$; domain $(-\infty, \infty)$, $x \neq 0$.

9. $f(g(x)) = 2x^3$, $g(f(x)) = 2(x - 1)^3 + 1 = 2x^3 - 6x^2 + 6x + 1$; domains $(-\infty, \infty)$;.

$f(g(x)) \neq g(f(x))$.

10. $f(g(x)) = |2x + 1|$, $g(f(x)) = \sqrt{|2x^2 + 1|}$; domains $(-\infty, \infty)$; $f(g(x)) \neq g(f(x))$.

11. $f(g(x)) = g(f(x)) = x$; domain $(-\infty, \infty)$.

12. $f(g(x))$ is not defined; $g(f(x)) = 7 - x$; domain $(-\infty, 9)$.

13. $f(g(x)) = g(f(x)) = x$; domain $(-\infty, \infty)$, $x \neq -2$, $x \neq 4$.

14. $f(g(x)) = x^2 + 3$; domain $(-\infty, \infty)$; $g(f(x)) = x^2 + 6|x| + 9$;
     domain $(-\infty, \infty)$.

15. $f(g(x)) = x/(2 - x)$; domain $(-\infty, \infty)$, $x \neq 0$, $x \neq 1, 2,$
     $g(f(x)) = 2(x - 1)$; domain $(-\infty, \infty)$, $x \neq 0$, $x \neq 1$.

PROBLEMS 8

1.   Odd.

2.   Neither.

3.   Even.

4.   Neither.

5.   Even.

6.   Neither.

7.   Odd.

8.   Even.

9.   Odd.

10. Neither.

11. $f(-x) = f(x)$, $f(-x) = g(x)$, so $f(-x)\,g(-x) = f(x)\,g(x)$.

12. $f(-x) = -f(x)$, $g(-x) = -g(x)$, so $f(-x)\,g(-x) = f(x)\,g(x)$.

13. $f(-x) = f(x)$, $g(-x) = -g(x)$, so $f(-x)\,g(-x) = -f(x)\,g(x)$.

14. $y = (4 - x)/2$.

15. $y = (x - 11)/5$.

16. $y = x - 2$; the original line, and hence the reflected line, are parallel to
     $y = x$.

17. $y = (x + 1)/3$.

18. $y = (6 - x)/4$.

19. 2π.

20. $\pi..$

21. 4π ; this is the smallest period common to both functions.

22. 4π ; this is the smallest period common to both functions.

23. 6π ; this is the smallest period common to both functions.

24. 8π ; this is the smallest period common to both functions.

25. 3π ; this is the smallest period common to both functions.

PROBLEMS 9

1. $f^{-1}(x) = (x - 16)/3.$

2. $f^{-1}(x) = y = 2 - x.$

3. $f^{-1}(x) = 9 - x^2,\ x \geqslant 0.$

4. $f^{-1}(x) = 4 + x^2,\ x \geqslant 4.$

5. $f^{-1}(x) = 1/x,\ \text{ for } -\infty < x < \infty,\ x \neq 0.$

6. $f^{-1}(x) = 1 - 1/x,\ \text{ for } x \neq 0.$

7. $f^{-1}(x) = x/(2 - x),\ \text{ for } x \neq 2.$

8. $f^{-1}(x) = (3x - 2)/(1 + x),\ \text{ for } x \neq 1.$

9. $\arcsin(-1/\sqrt{2}) = -\pi/4.$

10. $\arctan(-\sqrt{3}) = \pi/3.$

11. $\arccos 0.3 = 1.266\,10$ radians.

12. $\arctan 2 = 1.107\,15$ radians.

13. $x = -2.$

14. $x = \dfrac{3}{4} + \dfrac{1}{4\sqrt{2}}.$

15. $x = \dfrac{1}{2} - \dfrac{1}{2\sqrt{2}}.$

16. $x = -0.078\,39.$

PROBLEMS 10

1. (a) $-i$; (b) 1; (c) i; (d) -1; (e) -1; (f) 1; (g) $-i$.

2. (a) $3i$; (b) $5i$; (c) $7i$; (d) $i\pi$.

3. (a) $4 - i$; (b) $2 + 3i$; (c) $1 + 2i$; (d) $4 - 2i$.

4.   (a) $5 - 5i$;   (b) $-4 + 12i$;   ·(c) $5 + 5i$.

5.   (a) $4 - 14i$;   (b) $39 - 33i$;   (c) $28 - 45i$.

6.   (a) $(1 + 7i)/5$;   (b) $(1 - 7i)/10$;   (c) $-\dfrac{1}{2} - \dfrac{1}{4}i$.

7.   (a) $(6 - 2i)/5$;   (b) $(13 - i)/34$;   (c) i.

8.   (a) $20 + 20i$;   (b) $15 - 15i$;   (c) $-32 - 24i$.

9.   (a) $-28 - 96i$;   (b) $\dfrac{3}{16} + \dfrac{1}{4}i$;   (c) $\dfrac{1}{64}i$.

10.   (a) $11 - 27i$;   (b) $41 - 23i$.

11.   Equating real parts gives $a - 2b = 1$. Equating imaginary parts gives $b - 2a = 2$, so $a = -5/3$, $b = -4/3$.

12.   Equating real parts gives $a + 2b = 2$. Equating imaginary parts gives $6b - a = 1$, so $a = 5/4$, $b = 3/8$.

13.   Equating real parts gives $(3a + 4b)/13 = 1$. Equating imaginary parts gives $(6b - 2a)/13 = 2$, so $a = -1$, $b = 4$.

14.   Equating real parts gives $(a - 2b)/5 = 1$. Equating imaginary parts gives $(b + 2a)/5 = 2$, so $a = 5$, $b = 0$.

15. $x = 1$ by inspection, so $(x - 1)$ is a factor.

$$(x^3 - 1)/(x - 1) = x^2 + x + 1,$$

remaining roots are roots of $x^2 + x + 1 = 0$, namely

$$x = (-1 - i\sqrt{3})/2$$

and

$$x = (-1 + i\sqrt{3})/2.$$

16. $x = 2$ by inspection, so $(x - 2)$ is a factor.

$$(x^3 - 2x^2 + 5x - 10)/(x - 2) = x^2 + 5,$$

remaining roots are roots of $x^2 + 5 = 0$, namely

$$x = -i\sqrt{5}$$

and

$$x = +i\sqrt{5}.$$

17. $x = -1$ by inspection, so $(x + 1)$ is a factor.

$$(2x^3 + 3x^2 + 6x + 5)/(x + 1) = 2x^2 + x + 5,$$

remaining roots are roots of $2x^2 + x + 5 = 0$, namely

$$x = (-1 - i\sqrt{39})/4$$

and

$$x = (-1 + i\sqrt{39})/4.$$

18. $x = 1$ by inspection, so $(x - 1)$ is a factor.

$$(x^3 - x^2 + 8x - 8)/(x - 1) = x^2 + 8,$$

remaining roots are roots of $x^2 + 8 = 0$, namely

$$x = -i\sqrt{8}$$

and

$$x = i\sqrt{8}.$$

PROBLEMS 11

1. $z_1 + z_2 = 5 + 3i$, $z_1 - z_2 = 1 - i$.

2. $z_1 + z_2 = 3 - 5i$, $z_1 - z_2 = 5 - i$.

3. $z_1 + z_2 = 4$, $z_1 - z_2 = -2i$.

4. $z_1 + z_2 = 1 - 5i$, $z_1 - z_2 = -3 + i$.

5. $z_1 + z_2 = 3 + 5i$, $z_1 - z_2 = 3 - 3i$.

6. $z_1 + z_2 = -3 + 3i$, $z_1 - z_2 = -3 - 3i$.

7.   (a) $|z| = \sqrt{20}$;   (b) $|z| = \sqrt{5}$;   (c) $|z| = \sqrt{2}$.

8.   (a) $|\bar{z}| = \sqrt{10}$;   (b) $|\bar{z}| = \sqrt{5}$;   (c) $|\bar{z}| = \sqrt{5}$.

9.   (a) $\left|z_1\right| = 5$, $\left|z_2\right| = \sqrt{2}$, $\left|z_1 + z_2\right| = 5$, $\left|z_1 - z_2\right| = \sqrt{29}$, so

$$\left|z_1 + z_2\right| = 5 < \left|z_1\right| + \left|z_2\right| = \sqrt{5} + \sqrt{2}$$

and

$$\left|\left|z_1\right| - \left|z_2\right|\right| = |5 - \sqrt{2}| = 5 - \sqrt{2} < \left|z_1 - z_2\right| = \sqrt{29}.$$

(b) $\left|z_1\right| = \sqrt{20}$, $\left|z_2\right| = \sqrt{5}$, $\left|z_1 + z_2\right| = \sqrt{45}$, $\left|z_1 - z_2\right| = \sqrt{5}$, so

$$\left|z_1 + z_2\right| = \sqrt{45} = \left|z_1\right| + \left|z_2\right| = \sqrt{20} + \sqrt{5}$$

and

$$\left|\left|z_1\right| - \left|z_2\right|\right| = \sqrt{20} - \sqrt{5} = \left|z_1 - z_2\right| = \sqrt{5}.$$

(c) $\left|z_1\right| = \sqrt{52}$, $\left|z_2\right| = \sqrt{13}$, $\left|z_1 + z_2\right| = \sqrt{13}$, $\left|z_1 - z_2\right| = \sqrt{117}$, so

$$\left|z_1 + z_2\right| = \sqrt{13} < \left|z_1\right| + \left|z_2\right| = \sqrt{52} + \sqrt{13}$$

and

$$\left| \left| z_1 \right| - \left| z_2 \right| \right| = \sqrt{52} - \sqrt{13} < \left| z_1 - z_2 \right| = \sqrt{117}.$$

PROBLEMS 12

1. $x = 3 \cos (3\pi/4)$, $y = 3 \sin (3\pi/4)$, so $x = -(3/\sqrt{2})$, $y = 3/\sqrt{2}$.

2. $x = \sqrt{5} \cos (-3\pi/4)$, $y = \sqrt{5} \sin (-3\pi/4)$, so $x = \sqrt{(5/2)}$, $y = -\sqrt{(5/2)}$.

3. $x = 4 \cos (2\pi/3)$, $y = 4 \sin (2\pi/3)$, so $x = -2$, $y = 2\sqrt{3}$.

4. $x = 2 \cos (-\pi/4)$, $y = 2 \sin (-\pi/4)$, so $x = \sqrt{2}$, $y = -\sqrt{2}$.

5. $x = 7 \cos (5\pi/6)$, $y = 7 \sin (5\pi/6)$, so $x = -(7\sqrt{3}/2)$, $y = 7/2$.

6. $x = 6 \cos (\pi/6)$, $y = 6 \sin (\pi/6)$, so $x = 3\sqrt{3}$, $y = 3$.

7. $r = |z| = \sqrt{8}$, $\theta = \arg z = \pi/4$..

8. $r = |z| = 11$, $\theta = \arg z = \pi/2$..

9. $r = |z| = [(-3\sqrt{3})^2 + (-3)^2]^{1/2} = 6$,

$$\theta = \arg z$$

$$= \arctan \left(\frac{-3}{-3\sqrt{3}} \right) - \pi$$

$$= \arctan \left(\frac{1}{\sqrt{3}} \right) - \pi = -5\pi/6.$$

10. $r = |z| = [(-3)^2 + 3^2]^{1/2} = 3\sqrt{2}$,

$$\theta = \arg z$$

$$= \pi - \arctan \left| \frac{3}{-3} \right|$$

$$= \pi - \arctan 1 = 3\pi/4.$$

11. $r = |z| = [3^2 + (-2)^2]^{1/2} = \sqrt{13}$,

$$\theta = \arg z$$

$$= -\arctan \left| \frac{-2}{3} \right|$$

$$= -0.5880 \, \text{rad}.$$

12. $r = |z| = 4$, $\theta = \arg z = \pi$.

13. (a) $z_1 z_2 = 6\left[\cos\left(\dfrac{\pi}{4} + \dfrac{\pi}{3}\right) + i \sin\left(\dfrac{\pi}{4} + \dfrac{\pi}{3}\right)\right],$

$\qquad = 6\left[\cos\dfrac{7\pi}{12} + i \sin\dfrac{7\pi}{12}\right].$

(b) $z_1/z_2 = \dfrac{3}{2}\left[\cos\left(-\dfrac{\pi}{12}\right) + i \sin\left(-\dfrac{\pi}{12}\right)\right],$

$\qquad = \dfrac{3}{2}\left[\cos\dfrac{\pi}{12} - i \sin\dfrac{\pi}{12}\right].$

14. (a) $z_1 = 4\left(\cos\dfrac{\pi}{6} - i \sin\dfrac{\pi}{6}\right) = 4\left[\cos\left(-\dfrac{\pi}{6}\right) + i \sin\left(-\dfrac{\pi}{6}\right)\right],$

so $z_1 z_2 = 12\left[\cos\left(-\dfrac{\pi}{6} + \dfrac{\pi}{3}\right) + i \sin\left(-\dfrac{\pi}{6} + \dfrac{\pi}{3}\right)\right]$

$\qquad = 12\left(\cos\dfrac{\pi}{6} + i \sin\dfrac{\pi}{6}\right) = 6\sqrt{3} + 6i.$

(b) $z_1/z_2 = \dfrac{4}{3}\left[\cos\left(-\dfrac{\pi}{6} - \dfrac{\pi}{3}\right) + i \sin\left(-\dfrac{\pi}{6} - \dfrac{\pi}{3}\right)\right],$

$\qquad = \left[\cos\left(-\dfrac{\pi}{2}\right) + i \sin\left(-\dfrac{\pi}{2}\right)\right] = \dfrac{-4i}{3}.$

15. (a) $z_2 = 5\left(\cos\dfrac{\pi}{4} - i \sin\dfrac{\pi}{4}\right) = 5\left[\cos\left(-\dfrac{\pi}{4}\right) + i \sin\left(-\dfrac{\pi}{4}\right)\right],$

so $z_1 z_2 = 20\left[\cos\left(\dfrac{\pi}{3} - \dfrac{\pi}{4}\right) + i \sin\left(\dfrac{\pi}{3} - \dfrac{\pi}{4}\right)\right]$

$\qquad = 20\left[\cos\dfrac{\pi}{12} + i \sin\dfrac{\pi}{13}\right].$

(b) $z_1/z_2 = \dfrac{4}{5}\left[\cos\left(\dfrac{\pi}{3} + \dfrac{\pi}{4}\right) + i \sin\left(\dfrac{\pi}{3} + \dfrac{\pi}{4}\right)\right]$

$\qquad = \dfrac{4}{5}\left[\cos\dfrac{7\pi}{12} + i \sin\dfrac{7\pi}{12}\right].$

16. $(1 + i)^{30} = \left[\sqrt{2}\left(\cos\dfrac{\pi}{4} + i \sin\dfrac{\pi}{4}\right)\right]^{30}$

$\qquad = 2^{15}\left[\cos\dfrac{30\pi}{4} + i \sin\dfrac{30\pi}{4}\right]$

$\qquad = 2^{15}\left(\cos\dfrac{3\pi}{2} + i \sin\dfrac{3\pi}{2}\right) = -2^{15} i.$

17. $\left(\dfrac{1+i}{\sqrt{3}-i}\right)^5 = \dfrac{(1+i)^5}{(\sqrt{3}-i)^5}$.   Now $1+i=\sqrt{2}\left(\cos\dfrac{\pi}{4}+i\sin\dfrac{\pi}{4}\right)$ and

$$\sqrt{3}-i=2\left(\dfrac{\sqrt{3}}{2}-\dfrac{i}{2}\right)=2\left[\cos\left(-\dfrac{\pi}{6}\right)+i\sin\left(-\dfrac{\pi}{6}\right)\right],$$

so

$$\left(\dfrac{1+i}{\sqrt{3}-i}\right)^5 = \dfrac{\left[\sqrt{2}\left(\cos\dfrac{\pi}{4}+i\sin\dfrac{\pi}{4}\right)\right]^5}{\left\{2\left[\cos\left(-\dfrac{\pi}{6}\right)+i\sin\left(-\dfrac{\pi}{6}\right)\right]\right\}^5}$$

$$=\dfrac{1}{2^{5/2}}\dfrac{\left[\cos\dfrac{5\pi}{4}+i\sin\dfrac{5\pi}{4}\right]}{\left[\cos\left(-\dfrac{5\pi}{6}\right)+i\sin\left(-\dfrac{5\pi}{6}\right)\right]}$$

$$=\dfrac{1}{2^{5/2}}\left\{\cos\left[\dfrac{5\pi}{4}-\left(-\dfrac{5\pi}{6}\right)\right]+i\sin\left[\dfrac{5\pi}{4}-\left(-\dfrac{5\pi}{6}\right)\right]\right\}$$

$$=\dfrac{1}{2^{5/2}}\left[\cos\dfrac{50\pi}{24}+i\sin\dfrac{50\pi}{24}\right]=\dfrac{1}{2^{5/2}}\left[\cos\dfrac{\pi}{12}+i\sin\dfrac{\pi}{12}\right]$$

18. Proceed as in the answer to problem 17, using the facts that

$$1+i\sqrt{3}=2\left(\cos\dfrac{\pi}{3}+i\sin\dfrac{\pi}{3}\right)$$

and

$$1-i=\sqrt{2}\left[\cos\left(-\dfrac{\pi}{4}\right)+i\sin\left(-\dfrac{\pi}{4}\right)\right],$$

to show that

$$\left(\dfrac{1+i\sqrt{3}}{1-i}\right)^{20}=512(1-i\sqrt{3}).$$

19. $\dfrac{1+i\tan\theta}{1-i\tan\theta}=\dfrac{\cos\theta+i\sin\theta}{\cos\theta-i\sin\theta}$, so

$$\left(\dfrac{1+i\tan\theta}{1-i\tan\theta}\right)^n=\dfrac{(\cos\theta+i\sin\theta)^n}{[\cos(-\theta)+i\sin(-\theta)]^n}$$

$$=\dfrac{\cos n\theta+i\sin n\theta}{\cos(-n\theta)+i\sin(-n\theta)}$$

$$= \frac{\cos n\theta + i \sin n\theta}{\cos n\theta - i \sin n\theta}$$

The result then follows after division by $\cos n\theta$.

20. $z = \dfrac{\cos \theta + i \sin \theta}{\cos \theta - i \sin \theta} = \dfrac{(\cos \theta + i \sin \theta)(\cos \theta + i \sin \theta)}{(\cos \theta - i \sin \theta)(\cos \theta + i \sin \theta)}$

$$= (\cos \theta + i \sin \theta)^2 = \cos 2\theta + i \sin 2\theta.$$

Thus $|z| = 1$, so $\left| z^n \right| = 1$ and

$$z^n = (\cos 2\theta + i \sin 2\theta)^n = \cos 2n\theta + i \sin 2n\theta$$

so that $\arg z^n = 2n\theta$.

PROBLEMS 13

1. $1,\ i,\ -1,\ -i.$

2. $w_k = 2^{1/6}\left[\cos \dfrac{(12k+11)\,\pi}{6} + i \sin \dfrac{(12k+11)\,\pi}{6} \right],$

    with $k = 0, 1, \ldots, 5.$

3. $w_k = 5^{1/6}\left[\cos\left(0.1545 + \dfrac{2k\pi}{3}\right) + i \sin\left(0.1545 + \dfrac{2k\pi}{3}\right) \right],$

    with $k = 0, 1, \ldots, 5.$

4. $w_k = 29^{1/8}\left[\cos\left(0.2976 + \dfrac{k\pi}{2}\right) + i \sin\left(0.2976 + \dfrac{k\pi}{2}\right) \right],$

    with $k = 0, 1, 2, 3.$

5. $w_k = 10^{1/6}\left[\cos\left(\dfrac{2k\pi}{3} - 0.1073\right) + i \sin\left(\dfrac{2k\pi}{3} - 0.1073\right) \right],$

    with $k = 0, 1, 2.$

6. $w_k = 2^{1/2}\left[\cos \dfrac{(2k+1)\,\pi}{4} + i \sin \dfrac{(2k+1)\,\pi}{4} \right],$

    with $k = 0, 1, 2, 3$. Thus $w_0 = 1 + i,\ w_1 = -1 + i,\ w_2 = -1 - i$ and $w_3 = 1 - i.$

7. $w_k = \cos \dfrac{(1 + 4k)\,\pi}{12} + i \sin \dfrac{(1 + 4k)\,\pi}{12},$

    with $k = 0, 1, 2, \ldots, 5.$

8. $w_k = \cos \dfrac{2k\pi}{n} + i \sin \dfrac{2k\pi}{n},$

    with $n = 0, 1, \ldots, n - 1$. These are called the nth roots of unity.

PROBLEMS 14

1. 11/7.

2. 0.

3. $\lim\limits_{x \to 2} \left[\dfrac{(x-2)(x+3)}{(x-2)(2x+1)} \right] = \lim\limits_{x \to 2} \left(\dfrac{x+3}{2x+1} \right) = 1.$

4. 4/3

5. − 3.

6. $3x^2.$

7. 6.

8. 2.

9. 0.

10. 2 √2/3.

11. 3/2 .

12. 1/16.

13. 5/7.

14. $\lim\limits_{x \to 4} \left[\dfrac{x^4 - 64x}{(x-1)\ \tan 3(x-4)} \right] = \lim\limits_{x \to 4} \left[\left(\dfrac{x}{x-1} \right) \dfrac{(x^3 - 64)}{\tan 3(x-4)} \right]$

$= \lim\limits_{x \to 4} \left(\dfrac{x}{x-1} \right) \cdot \lim\limits_{x \to 4} \left\{ (x^2 + 4x + 16) \left[\dfrac{x-4}{\tan 3(x-4)} \right] \right\}$

$= \dfrac{4}{3} \cdot \dfrac{48}{3} = \dfrac{64}{3}.$

15. Write $\dfrac{\sin mx}{\sin nx} = \left(\dfrac{\sin mx}{x} \right)\left(\dfrac{x}{\sin nx} \right)$, and then $\lim\limits_{x \to 0} \left[\dfrac{\sin mx}{\sin nx} \right] = \dfrac{m}{n}.$

16. 1.

17. − 7.

18. Use the fact that $\sin \pi\,(x-1) = \sin \pi x\ \cos \pi - \cos \pi x\ \sin \pi = -\sin \pi x$ to write

$$\dfrac{x-1}{\sin \pi x} = \dfrac{-(x-1)}{\sin \pi\,(x-1)}.$$

Then setting $u = x - 1$,

$$\lim\limits_{x \to 1} \left[\dfrac{x-1}{\sin \pi x} \right] = \lim\limits_{x \to 1} \left[\dfrac{-(x-1)}{\sin \pi\,(x-1)} \right] = \lim\limits_{u \to 0} \left[\dfrac{-u}{\sin \pi u} \right] = \dfrac{-1}{\pi}.$$

19. Write

$$\frac{x - \sin 2x}{x - \sin 5x} = \frac{(x/\sin 5x) - (\sin 2x/\sin 5x)}{(x/\sin 5x) - 1}$$

so

$$\lim_{x \to 0} \left[\frac{x - \sin 2x}{x - \sin 5x} \right] = \lim_{x \to 0} \left[\frac{(x/\sin 5x) - (\sin 2x/\sin 5x)}{(x/\sin 5x) - 1} \right]$$

$$= \frac{(1/5) - (2/5)}{(1/5) - 1} = \frac{1}{4}$$

20. Write

$$\frac{\sin x}{\sin 6x - \sin 7x} = \frac{(\sin x/\sin 7x)}{(\sin 6x/\sin 7x) - 1},$$

then

$$\lim_{x \to 0} \left[\frac{\sin x}{\sin 6x - \sin 7x} \right] = \lim_{x \to 0} \left[\frac{(\sin x/\sin 7x)}{(\sin 6x/\sin 7x) - 1} \right]$$

$$= \frac{(1/7)}{(6/7) - 1} = -1.$$

21. Use the trigonometric identity $\cos(A - B) - \cos(A + B) = 2 \sin A \sin B$ and set $A - B = 3x$, $A + B = 7x$. Then $A = 5x$, $B = 2x$ and so $\cos 3x - \cos 7x = 2 \sin 5x \sin 2x$.

Then

$$\lim_{x \to 0} \left[\frac{\cos 3x - \cos 7x}{x^2} \right] = 2 \left[\lim_{x \to 0} \left(\frac{\sin 5x}{x} \right) \right] \cdot \left[\lim_{x \to 0} \left(\frac{\sin 2x}{x} \right) \right]$$

$$= 2 \times 5 \times 2 = 20.$$

PROBLEMS 15

1. (a) 1/6; (b) 1/6; removable discontinuity; continuous for all x if we define $f(3) = 1/6$.

2. (a) 0; (b) not defined.

3. (a) 0; (b) 0.

4. (a) 0; (b) 1; jump discontinuity.

5. (a) -3; (b) 3; jump discontinuity.

6. (a) 0; (b) 3; jump discontinuity.

7. (a) 0; (b) ∞; infinite jump.

8. (a) $2\sqrt{2}/3$; (b) $2\sqrt{2}/3$; removable discontinuity; continuous at $x = 4$ if we define $f(4) = 2\sqrt{2}/3$.

9.   (a) $-5/3$;   (b) $5/3$; jump discontinuity.

10.   (a) 0;   (b) 2; jump discontinuity.

11.   Continuous for $-3 \leqslant x \leqslant 4$.

12.   Continuous for $-1 \leqslant x \leqslant 2$.

13.   Discontinuous at $x = 2$.

14.   Discontinuities at $x = 2, 3, 4, \ldots$. No discontinuity at $x = 1$ because $f(x) = 1$ for $0 \leqslant x \leqslant 1$ and $f(x) = x$ for $1 \leqslant x < 2$, so $f(1) = 1$.

15.   Continuous for $-\pi/4 \leqslant x \leqslant \pi/4$.

16.   Discontinuous at $x = \pm 2$.

17.   Discontinuous at $x = -5$.

18.   Continuous for all x.

19.   Discontinuous at $x = n\pi/2$, for $n = 0, \pm 1, \pm 2, \ldots$.

20.   Continuous for all x.

PROBLEMS 16

1. $df/dx = -3 \sin x + 7 \cos x$; $f^{(1)}(\pi/4) = 2\sqrt{2}$.

2. $df/dx = 4x^3 - 6x + 1$; $f^{(1)}(1) = -1$.

3. $df/dx = \dfrac{2}{3} x^{-1/3} + 2$; $f^{(1)}(2) = \left(\dfrac{2}{3}\right)\dfrac{1}{2^{1/3}} + 2$.

4. $\dfrac{df}{dx} = \dfrac{1 - x^2}{(1 + x^2)^2}$; $f^{(1)}(-1) = 0$.

5. $\dfrac{df}{dx} = \sqrt{(1 + x)} + \dfrac{x}{2\sqrt{(1 + x)}}$; $f^{(1)}(0) = 1$.

6. $\dfrac{df}{dx} = \sqrt{(1 + x^2)} + \dfrac{x^2}{2\sqrt{(1 + x^2)}}$; $f^{(1)}(0) = 1$.

7. $\dfrac{df}{dx} = \dfrac{-2x^2 - 6x + 25}{(x^2 - 5x + 5)^2}$; $f^{(1)}(1) = 17$.

8. $\dfrac{df}{dx} = \dfrac{1 - 4x}{x^2(2x - 1)^2}$; $f^{(1)}(-1) = \dfrac{5}{9}$.

9. $\dfrac{df}{dx} = 3x^2 \sin 2x + 2x^3 \cos 2x$; $f^{(1)}(\pi) = 2\pi^3$.

10. $\dfrac{df}{dx} = \dfrac{-2}{(\sin x - \cos x)^2}$; $f^{(1)}(0) = -2$.

11. $\dfrac{df}{dx} = \dfrac{1}{\sqrt{x}(1 - \sqrt{x})^2}$; $f^{(1)}(2) = \dfrac{1}{\sqrt{2}(1 - \sqrt{2})^2}$.

12. $\dfrac{df}{dx} = \dfrac{6 - x^{2/3}}{6\sqrt{x}\,(2 + x^{2/3})^2}$; $f^{(1)}(1) = \dfrac{5}{54}$.

13. $y^{(1)}(x) = 3x^2 + 8x$, so the gradient when $x = 3$ is $y^{(1)}(3) = 3 \times 3^2 + 8 \times 3$, or $y^{(1)}(3) = 51$. $y(3) = 3^3 + 4 \times 3^2 - 3 = 60$ so the tangent line $y = mx + c$ through the point $(3, 60)$ has gradient 51. Hence $60 = 51 \times 3 + c$, giving $c = -93$ and thus the tangent line is $y = 51x - 93$.

14. $y^{(1)}(x) = 1/(2x^{1/2}) + 1/(3x^{2/3}) + 1/(4x^{3/4})$, so the gradient when $x = 1$ is $y^{(1)}(1) = \tfrac{1}{2} + \tfrac{1}{3} + \tfrac{1}{4} = 13/12$. $y(1) = 3$ so the tangent line $y = mx + c$ through the point $(1, 3)$ has gradient 13/12. Hence

$$3 = \frac{13}{12} \times 1 + c, \quad \text{giving } c = \frac{23}{12}$$

and thus the tangent line is $y = (13/12)x + 23/12$.

15. $y^{(1)}(x) = 5(\cos x - x \sin x)$, so the gradient when $x = \pi/2$ is $y^{(1)}(\pi/2) = -5\pi/2$. $y(\pi/2) = 0$ so the tangent line $y = mx + c$ through the point $(\pi/2, 0)$ has gradient $-5\pi/2$. Hence

$$0 = -\frac{5\pi}{2} \cdot \frac{\pi}{2} + c, \quad \text{giving } c = \frac{5\pi^2}{4}$$

and thus the tangent line is $y = -(5\pi/2)x + (5\pi^2/4)$.

16. $dy/dx = 6x^2 + 2x$, so when $y^{(1)}(x) = 4$ it follows that x must satisfy the equation $4 = 6x^2 + 2x$ or, equivalently, $3x^2 + x - 2 = 0$. The roots of this equation are $x = -1$ and $x = 2/3$. We have $y(-1) = 0$ and $y(2/3) = 55/27$, so the required points are $(-1, 0)$ and $(2/3, 55/27)$.

17. $y(\tfrac{1}{2}) = 1$, so P is the point $(\tfrac{1}{2}, 1)$. Now $dy/dx = 2\pi \cos 2\pi x - 3\pi \sin 3\pi x$, so $y^{(1)}(\tfrac{1}{2}) = \pi$ and thus the tangent to the curve at P has gradient π. Thus the gradient of the line normal (perpendicular) to the tangent at P (and thus normal to the curve itself at P) must be $-1/\pi$ (see Section 3). Consequently the required line $y = mx + c$ through the point $(\tfrac{1}{2}, 1)$ has gradient $m = -1/\pi$, and thus $1 = -1/\pi \cdot \tfrac{1}{2} + c$, so that $c = 1 + (1/2\pi)$. The required line is thus

$$y = -\frac{1}{\pi} x + 1 + \frac{1}{2}\pi .$$

18. $y(1) = -2$, so P is the point $(1, -2)$. Now $dy/dx = 6x - 2$, so $y^{(1)}(1) = 4$ and thus the tangent to the curve at P has gradient 4. Thus the gradient of the line normal to the tangent at P must be $-1/4$. Consequently the required line $y = mx + c$ through the point $(1, -2)$ has gradient $m = -1/4$, and thus

$$-2 = -1/4 \cdot 1 + c, \quad \text{so that } c = -(7/4).$$

The required line is thus $y = -\dfrac{1}{4}x - 7/4$.

19. Set $u = 5x$ and differentiate $\tan u$ to obtain

$$\frac{d}{dx}[\tan 5x] = \sec^2 u \frac{du}{dx} = 5 \sec^2 5x,$$

or write $\tan 5x = \sin 5x/\cos 5x$ and differentiate the quotient.

20. Set $u = x^2$ and differentiate $\cot u$ to obtain

$$\frac{d}{dx}[\cot x^2] = - \operatorname{cosec}^2 u \frac{du}{dx} = - 2x \operatorname{cosec}^2 x^2.$$

21. Set $u = (1 + x^2)^{1/2}$ and differentiate $\sec u$ to obtain

$$\frac{d}{dx}[\sec(1 + x)^{1/2}] = \sec u \tan u \frac{du}{dx}$$

$$= \frac{x}{(1 + x)^{1/2}} \sec(1 + x^2)^{1/2} \tan(1 + x^2)^{1/2}.$$

22. $\dfrac{df}{dx} = \dfrac{3 \cos 3x}{\cos 2x} + \dfrac{2 \sin 2x \sin 3x}{\cos^2 2x}.$

23. $\dfrac{df}{dx} = 6 \tan 3x + 6 \tan^3 3x = 6 \tan 3x \ \sec^2 3x.$

24. $\dfrac{df}{dx} = -\dfrac{2x \cos 2x}{(1 + x^2)^2} - \dfrac{2 \sin 2x}{1 + x^2}.$

25. Set $u = \cos 3x$ and differentiate $\sin u$ to obtain

$$\frac{df}{dx} = -3 \sin 3x \cos(\cos 3x).$$

26. $\dfrac{df}{dx} = -\dfrac{3x(1 + \cos 5x)}{(x^2 - 1)^{5/2}} - \dfrac{5 \sin 5x}{(x^2 - 1)^{3/2}}.$

27. Set $u = 5x + 1$ and differentiate $3 \cos 2x \ \sin^3 u$ to obtain

$$\frac{df}{dx} = 45 \cos 2x \sin^2(5x + 1) \cos(5x + 1) - 6 \sin x \sin^3(5x + 1).$$

28. Set $u = 2x + 1$ and $v = \sin u$ and differentiate $f(x) = (2 - v^2)^{1/2}$, using the repeated chain rule $\dfrac{df}{dx} = \dfrac{df}{dv}\dfrac{dv}{du}\dfrac{du}{dx}$, to obtain

$$\frac{df}{dx} = \frac{-2 \sin(2x + 1) \cos(2x + 1)}{[3 - \sin^2(2x + 1)]^{1/2}}.$$

29. Set $u = x^2 + 2$ and $v = \cos u$ and differentiate $f(x) = (4 + v^2)^{3/2}$, using the repeated chain rule as in the above answer, to obtain

$$\frac{df}{dx} = -3x \sin(x^2 + 2)[4 + \cos(x^2 + 2)]^{1/2}.$$

30. Set $u = 2x$ and $v = 1 + \sin u$ and differentiate $f(x) = (3 + v^2)^{1/2}$, to obtain

$$\frac{df}{dx} = \frac{2(1 + \sin 2x) \cos 2x}{(\sin^2 2x + 2 \sin 2x + 4)^{1/2}}.$$

31. $\dfrac{df}{dx} = \dfrac{-2x}{(x^2 - 9)^2}, \quad \dfrac{d^2f}{dx^2} = \dfrac{6(x^2 + 3)}{(x^2 - 9)^3}, \quad \dfrac{d^3f}{dx^3} = \dfrac{-24x(x^2 + 9)}{(x^2 - 9)^4}.$

32. $\dfrac{df}{dx} = 4 \cos 4x, \quad \dfrac{d^2f}{dx^2} = -16 \sin 4x, \quad \dfrac{d^3f}{dx^3} = -64 \cos 4x.$

33. $\dfrac{df}{dx} = \sin x + x \cos x, \quad \dfrac{d^2f}{dx^2} = 2 \cos x - x \sin x, \quad \dfrac{d^3f}{dx^3} = -3 \sin x - x \cos x.$

34. $\dfrac{df}{dx} = \dfrac{1}{(x + 4)^{1/2}}, \quad \dfrac{d^2f}{dx^2} = \dfrac{-1}{4(x + 4)^{3/2}}, \quad \dfrac{d^3f}{dx^3} = \dfrac{3}{8(x + 4)^{5/2}}.$

35. $\dfrac{df}{dx} = \cos 3x - 3x \sin 3x, \quad \dfrac{d^2f}{dx^2} = -6 \sin 3x - 9x \cos 3x,$

$$\frac{d^3f}{dx^3} = -27 \cos 3x + 27x \sin 3x.$$

36. $\dfrac{df}{dx} = 12x^2(1 + x^3)^3, \quad \dfrac{d^2f}{dx^2} = 12x(2 + 11x^3)(1 + x^3)^2,$

$$\frac{d^3f}{dx^3} = 24(55x^6 + 29x^3 + 1)(1 + x^3).$$

37. $\dfrac{df}{dx} = \cos x \cos 2x - 2 \sin x \sin 2x,$

$$\frac{d^2f}{dx^2} = -5 \sin x \cos 2x - 4 \cos x \sin 2x,$$

$$\frac{d^3f}{dx^3} = 14 \sin x \sin 2x - 13 \cos x \cos 2x.$$

38. $\dfrac{df}{dx} = \dfrac{\cos x}{1 + x} - \dfrac{\sin x}{(1 + x)^2},$

$$\frac{d^2f}{dx^2} = \frac{-2 \cos x}{(1 + x)^2} - \frac{(x^2 + 2x - 1) \sin x}{(1 + x)^3},$$

$$\frac{d^3f}{dx^3} = \frac{3(x^2 + 2x - 1) \sin x}{(1 + x)^4} - \frac{(x^2 + 2x - 5) \cos x}{(1 + x)^3}.$$

PROBLEMS 17

1. $\dfrac{d}{dx}[\sin kx] = k \cos kx = k \sin\left(kx + \dfrac{\pi}{2}\right),$

$\dfrac{d^2}{dx^2}[\sin kx] = \dfrac{d}{dx}[k \cos kx] = -k^2 \sin kx = k^2 \sin(kx + \pi),$

$\dfrac{d^3}{dx^3}[\sin kx] = \dfrac{d}{dx}[-k^2 \sin kx] = -k^3 \cos kx = k^3 \sin\left(kx + \dfrac{3\pi}{2}\right),$

$\dfrac{d^4}{dx^4}[\sin kx] = \dfrac{d}{dx}[-k^3 \cos kx] = k^4 \sin kx = k^4 \sin(kx + 2\pi),$

and so as this pattern repeats itself with further differentiation

$$\dfrac{d^n}{dx^n}[\sin kx] = k^n \sin\left(kx + \dfrac{n\pi}{2}\right),$$

for $n = 1, 2, 3, \ldots$.

2. Proceed as in the above answer.

3. Set $f(x) = x^2$, $g(x) = \sin kx$ to obtain

$$\dfrac{d^n}{dx^n}[x^2 \sin kx] = x^2 k^n \sin\left(kx + \dfrac{n\pi}{2}\right) + 2nk^{n-1}x \sin\left[kx + \left(\dfrac{n-1}{2}\right)\pi\right]$$
$$+ n(n-1)k^{n-2} \sin\left[kx + \left(\dfrac{n-2}{2}\right)\pi\right],$$

for $n = 1, 2, \ldots$.

4. Set $f(x) = x^2$, $g(x) = \cos kx$ to obtain

$$\dfrac{d^n}{dx^n}[x^2 \cos kx] = x^2 k^n \cos\left(kx + \dfrac{n\pi}{2}\right) + 2nk^{n-1}x \cos\left[kx + \left(\dfrac{n-1}{2}\right)\pi\right]$$
$$+ n(n-1)k^{n-2} \cos\left[kx + \left(\dfrac{n-2}{2}\right)\pi\right],$$

for $n = 1, 2, \ldots$.

5. $1 = (1 + kx)g(x)$, so set $f(x) = 1 + kx$.

Then

$$\dfrac{d^n}{dx^n}[1] = 0 = (1 + kx)\dfrac{d^n g}{dx^n} + nk\dfrac{d^{n-1}g}{dx^{n-1}},$$

and so

$$\dfrac{d^n}{dx^n}\left[\dfrac{1}{1 + kx}\right] = -\dfrac{kn}{(1 + kx)}\dfrac{d^{n-1}}{dx^{n-1}}\left[\dfrac{1}{1 + kx}\right].$$

As $dg/dx = -k/(1 + kx)^2$, setting $n = 2$ gives

$$\frac{d^3g}{dx^2} = -\left(\frac{2k}{1 + kx}\right)\left[\frac{-k}{(1 + kx)^2}\right] = \frac{2k^2}{(1 + kx)^3} = \frac{(-1)^2k^2 2!}{(1 + kx)^3}.$$

Similarly, setting $n = 3$ gives

$$\frac{d^3g}{dx^3} = \frac{-3k}{(1 + kx)} \frac{k^2 2!}{(1 + kx)^3} = \frac{(-1)^3k^3 3!}{(1 + kx)^4},$$

from which it can be seen by inspection that, in general,

$$\frac{d^ng}{dx^n} = \frac{(-1)^nk^n n!}{(1 + kx)^{n+1}}, \quad \text{for } n = 1, 2, \ldots .$$

This last result can be proved rigorously by using mathematical induction.

6.   Write

$$1 = (1 - 2x^2)g(x),$$

and setting $f(x) = 1 - 2x^2$ proceed as in Example 17.2 using the fact that $df/dx = -4x$, $d^2f/dx^2 = -4$ and $d^nf/dx^n = 0$ for $n > 2$ to obtain

$$(1 - 2x^2)\frac{d^ng}{dx^n} - 4nx\frac{d^{n-1}g}{dx^{n-1}} - 2n(n-1)\frac{d^{n-2}g}{dx^{n-2}} = 0,$$

for $n \geqslant 2$.

Direct differentiation shows that

$$\frac{dg}{dx} = \frac{4x}{(1 - 2x^2)^2},$$

so using this result with $n = 2$ gives

$$\frac{d^2g}{dx^2} = \frac{-4(6x^2 + 1)}{(1 - 2x^2)^3},$$

so setting $n = 3$ and using dg/dx and d^2g/dx^2 gives

$$\frac{d^3}{dx^3}\left[\frac{1}{1 - 2x^2}\right] = \frac{96x(2x^2 + 1)}{(1 - 2x^2)^4}.$$

PROBLEMS 18

1. $dy = \dfrac{3}{2}x^{1/2}\,dx.$

2. $dy = 4\cos(4x - 1)\,dx.$

3. $dy = 5x(1 + x^2)^{3/2}dx.$

4. $dy = [\cos(5x - 3) - 5x \sin(5x - 1)]\,dx.$

5. $dy = \left[2x(1 - x^2)^{1/2} - \dfrac{x^3}{(1 - x^2)^{1/2}}\right]dx.$

6. $dy = [\cos(3x^2 - 6) - 6x^2 \sin(3x^2 - 6)]\,dx.$

7. $dy = \left[\dfrac{3x^2 \sin 4x - 4x^3 \cos 4x}{\sin^2 4x}\right]dx.$

8. $dy = -\left[\dfrac{8 \sin 2x}{(2 \cos 2x + 1)^2}\right]dx.$

9. $dy = [\cos x \tan 4x + 4 \sin x \sec^2 4x]\,dx.$

10. $dy = [10x + \sin x + x \cos x]\,dx.$

11. $dy = [(x \cos x + \sin x)\cos 2x - 2x \sin x \sin 2x]\,dx.$

12. $dy = -\left[\dfrac{16}{(x - 9)^2}\right]dx.$

13. $dy = \left[\dfrac{1}{2x^{1/2}} - \dfrac{1}{4x^{5/4}}\right]dx.$

14. $dy = [\sec x + x \sec x \tan x]\,dx.$

15. $dT = (\pi/\sqrt{g})(1/l^{1/2})dl$, so the fractional change in T is $dT/T = (1/2l)dl$.
     Thus the percentage change in T is $100\,dT/T = (50/l)dl$.

     (a) $dl = 0.03l$, so $100\,dT/T = (50/l) \times 0.03l = 1.5\%$ (increase).
     (b) $dl = -0.05l$, so $100\,dT/T = (50/l) \times (-0.05l) = -2.5\%$ (decrease).

16. $dM = 3\rho\, l^2 dl$, so the fractional change in mass is $dM/M = (3/l)dl$. Thus the percentage change in M is $100\,dM/M = (300/l)dl$.

     (a) $dl = -0.02l$, so $100\,dM/M = (300/l)(-0.02l) = -6\%$ (decrease).
     (b) $dl = 0.03l$, so $100dM/M = (300/l) \times (0.03l) = 9\%$ (increase).

17. $dF = (3/2\, k_1 v^{1/2} + 2k_2 v)\,dv$, so the fractional change in F is

$$\frac{dF}{F} = \left(\frac{\frac{3}{2}k_1 v^{1/2} + 2k_2 v}{k_1 v^{3/2} + k_2 v^2}\right)dv = \frac{1}{2}\left(\frac{3k_1 + 4k_2 v^{1/2}}{k_1 v + k_2 v^{3/2}}\right)dv.$$

PROBLEMS 19

1. $\dfrac{df}{dx} = \dfrac{4}{16x^2 + 1}$.

2. $\dfrac{df}{dx} = \arcsin 3x + \dfrac{3x}{(1 - 9x^2)^{1/2}}$.

3. $\dfrac{df}{dx} = (1 - x^2)^{1/2} - 2x \ \arcsin x.$

4. $\dfrac{df}{dx} = 6x \ \text{arcsec} \ 3x + \dfrac{3x^2}{|x| \ (9x^2 - 1)^{1/2}}.$

5. $\dfrac{df}{dx} = \dfrac{1}{\sqrt{[(4 - x) \ (x - 2)]}}.$

6. $\dfrac{df}{dx} = \dfrac{1}{2 \sqrt{x}(x + 1)}.$

7. $\dfrac{df}{dx} = \dfrac{-x}{|x| \ (81 - x^2)^{1/2}}.$

8. $\dfrac{df}{dx} = \dfrac{x}{|x| \ \sqrt{[(x^2 + 1) \ (x^2 + 2)]}}.$

9. $\dfrac{df}{dx} = \arctan (1 + x^2) + \dfrac{2x^2}{x^4 + 2x^2 + 2}.$

10. $\dfrac{df}{dx} = \dfrac{-2x}{|x| \ \sqrt{[(x^2 + 1) \ (x^2 + 2)]}}.$

11. $\dfrac{df}{dx} = \arctan \left[\dfrac{\sqrt{x}}{2} \right] + \dfrac{1 + x}{\sqrt{x}(4 + x)}.$

12. $\dfrac{df}{dx} = 3x^2 \ \arcsin \sqrt{x} + \dfrac{x^{5/2}}{2 \sqrt{(1 - x)}}.$

PROBLEMS 20

1. $\dfrac{dy}{dx} = \dfrac{1 - 2x - 3y}{3x + 2y}; \quad \left(\dfrac{dy}{dx} \right)_{(1, 1)} = -\dfrac{4}{5}.$

2. $\dfrac{dy}{dx} = -\left(\dfrac{2x + 2xy^2}{2x^2y + 3y^2} \right); \quad \left(\dfrac{dy}{dx} \right)_{(1, 2)} = -\dfrac{5}{8}.$

3. $\dfrac{dy}{dx} = -\left(\dfrac{2x + y}{2y + x} \right); \quad \left(\dfrac{dy}{dx} \right)_{(4, 3)} = -\dfrac{11}{10}.$

4. $\dfrac{dy}{dx} = \dfrac{2x - 2xy^3}{3x^2y^2 + 3}; \quad \left(\dfrac{dy}{dx} \right)_{(3, 1)} = 0.$

5. $\left(\dfrac{dy}{dx} \right)_{(1, 0)} = -2; \quad \left(\dfrac{d^2y}{dx^2} \right)_{(1, 0)} = -\dfrac{2}{3}.$

6. $\cos(x+y)\left[1+\dfrac{dy}{dx}\right]+3y+3x\dfrac{dy}{dx}=0,$ so $\left(\dfrac{dy}{dx}\right)_{\left(\frac{\pi}{2},\frac{\pi}{2}\right)}=-1;$

$-\sin(x+y)\left[1+\dfrac{dy}{dx}\right]^2+\cos(x+y)\dfrac{d^2y}{dx^2}+6\dfrac{dy}{dx}+3x\dfrac{d^2y}{dx^2}=0,$

so

$$\left(\dfrac{d^2y}{dx^2}\right)_{\left(\frac{\pi}{2},\frac{\pi}{2}\right)}=\dfrac{12}{3\pi-2}.$$

PROBLEMS 21

1. $\dfrac{dy}{dx}=-1.$

2. $\dfrac{dy}{dx}=-\dfrac{b}{a}\cot t.$

3. $\dfrac{dy}{dx}=1-\dfrac{3}{t}+\dfrac{9}{t^2}.$

4. $\dfrac{dy}{dx}=\cot\left(\tfrac{1}{2}t\right).$

5. $\dfrac{dy}{dx}=t.$

6. $\dfrac{dy}{dx}=\dfrac{t+1}{t(t^2+1)}.$

7. $\dfrac{dy}{dx}=-\dfrac{b}{a}.$

8. $\dfrac{dy}{dx}=-\dfrac{b}{a}\tan t.$

9. $\dfrac{dy}{dx}=\dfrac{t(2-t^3)}{1-2t^3}.$

10. $\dfrac{dy}{dx}=\tan t.$

11. $\left(\dfrac{dy}{dx}\right)_{t=\pi/4}=1,\ \left(\dfrac{d^2y}{dx^2}\right)_{t=\pi/4}=2^{3/2}.$

12. $\left(\dfrac{dy}{dx}\right)_{t=-2}=-5/9,\ \left(\dfrac{d^2y}{dx^2}\right)_{t=-2}=-\dfrac{4}{243}.$

13. $\left(\dfrac{dy}{dx}\right)_{t=\pi/3} = \sqrt{3}, \left(\dfrac{d^2y}{dx^2}\right)_{t=\pi/3} = -\dfrac{4}{a}$.

14. $\left(\dfrac{dy}{dx}\right)_{t=-2} = -\dfrac{4}{5}, \left(\dfrac{d^2y}{dx^2}\right)_{t=-2} = -\dfrac{27}{250}$.

15. $\dfrac{d^3y}{dx^3} = \dfrac{-3\cos t}{a^2 \sin^5 t}$.

16. $\dfrac{d^3y}{dx^3} = \dfrac{\cos^2 t - 4\sin^2 t}{9a^2 \cos^7 t \sin^3 t}$.

PROBLEMS 22

1. $e^{-1/4}$.

2. $e^{2/5}$.

3. $\lim\limits_{n \to \infty}\left(3^n + \dfrac{4}{3^{n+1}}\right)^{3^n} = \lim\limits_{n \to \infty}\left(3^n + \dfrac{4}{3}\dfrac{1}{3^n}\right)^{3^n} = e^{4/3}$.

4. $\lim\limits_{n \to \infty}\left(5^n - \dfrac{1}{5^{n+1}}\right)^{5^n} = \lim\limits_{n \to \infty}\left(5^n - \dfrac{1}{5}\dfrac{1}{5^n}\right)^{5^n} = e^{-1/5}$.

5. e^{2x}.

6. $\lim\limits_{n \to \infty}\left(2^n - \dfrac{\cos x}{2^{n+2}}\right)^{2^n} = \lim\limits_{n \to \infty}\left(2^n - \dfrac{\cos x}{x}\dfrac{1}{2^n}\right)^{2^n} = \exp(-\cos x/4)$.

7. $\dfrac{dy}{dx} = -\sin e^{\cos x}, \dfrac{d^2y}{dx^2} = (\sin^2 x - \cos x)e^{\cos x}$.

8. $\dfrac{dy}{dx} = 3x^2 e^{x^3}, \dfrac{d^2y}{dx^2} = 3x(2 + 3x^3)e^{x^3}$.

9. $\dfrac{dy}{dx} = \dfrac{-1}{x^2}e^{1/x}, \dfrac{d^2y}{dx^2} = \left(\dfrac{2x+1}{x^4}\right)e^{1/x}$.

10. $y = e^x \cdot e^{x^2} = e^{x+x^2}, \dfrac{dy}{dx} = (1 + 2x)e^{x+x^2}$,

$$\dfrac{d^2y}{dx^2} = [2 + (1 + 2x)^2]\,e^{x+x^2} = (3 + 4x + 4x^2)\,e^{x+x^2}.$$

11. $\dfrac{dy}{dx} = \dfrac{k}{2}(e^{kx} - e^{-kx}), \dfrac{d^2y}{dx^2} = \dfrac{k^2}{2}(e^{kx} + e^{-kx})$.

12. $\dfrac{dy}{dx} = \dfrac{k}{2}(e^{kx} + e^{-kx}), \quad \dfrac{d^2y}{dx^2} = \dfrac{k^2}{2}(e^{kx} - e^{-kx}).$

13. $\dfrac{dy}{dx} = \dfrac{1}{2\sqrt{x}}e^{\sqrt{x}}, \quad \dfrac{d^2y}{dx^2} = \dfrac{(\sqrt{x}-1)}{4x^{3/2}}e^{\sqrt{x}}.$

14. $\dfrac{dy}{dx} = -2x\,\exp(1-x^2), \quad \dfrac{d^2y}{dx^2} = (4x^2-2)\,\exp(1-x^2).$

15. Find dy/dx from

$$2xe^y + x^2e^y\,\dfrac{dy}{dx} + 3 - 2y\,\dfrac{dy}{dx} = 0.$$

16. Find dy/dx from

$$e^{y^2} + 2xye^{y^2}\dfrac{dy}{dx} + 5y + 5x\dfrac{dy}{dx} + 2x + \dfrac{dy}{dx} = 0.$$

PROBLEMS 23

1. $\log_7 4 = \ln 4/\ln 7 = 1.386\,29/1.945\,91 = 0.712\,41.$

2. $(1+4x)^2.$

3. $x^{3/2}$

4. $27x^6.$

5. $x + \sin x.$

6. $\dfrac{1}{2}x^2.$

7. $\sin x - \cos x + x.$

8. $\sin^2 x + \cos^2 x = 1$ for all $x.$

9. $x = \pm\,(e^{3/2} + 1)^{1/2}.$

10. $-5/2.$

11. $1/(x+1).$

12. $1/x.$

13. $\left(2\ln(3x) + \dfrac{1}{x}\right)e^{2x}.$

14. $(e^x - 2\sin x \cos x)/(2 + \cos^2 x + e^x).$

15. $(8x + \cos x)/(4x^2 + \sin x).$

16. $-\tan x.$

17. $2(\cot 2x + \tan 2x).$

18. $\tan x.$

19. $2 \cos 2x \ln (\cos 2x) - \dfrac{2 \sin^2 2x}{\cos 2x}$.

20. $\dfrac{2x \, e^{x^2}[1 + (x^2 + 1) \ln (x^2 + 1)]}{x^2 + 1}$.

21. $\dfrac{-(x + 1)(3x^2 + 10x - 6)}{(x^2 + 3)^{7/2}}$.

22. $\dfrac{3(x - 3)^2 (3x + 1)}{(x^2 + 1)^{5/2}}$.

23. $\dfrac{e^x}{e^x + 3} - \dfrac{e^x(e^x + 2)}{(e^x + 3)^2}$.

24. $\dfrac{-x(2x^2 + 3)}{(x^2 + 3)^{5/2}(x^2 + 2)^{1/2}}$.

25. $\left(\ln^2 x + \ln x + \dfrac{1}{x} \right) \exp (x^x \ln x + x \ln x)$.

26. $(x \cos x + 1) \, e^{\sin x}$.

27. $\dfrac{2[2 \sin x \cos x + x]}{(x^2 - 2 \cos^2 x)}$.

28. $\dfrac{e^x + e^{-x}}{e^x - e^{-x}}$.

29. $\dfrac{3x^2 - 4 \sin x \cos x}{x^3 - 2 \sin^2 x + 1}$.

30. $\dfrac{1}{x \ln x - 1}$.

31. $\dfrac{x + (x \ln x - 1)e^{-x}}{x(x - e^{-x} \ln x)}$.

32. $\dfrac{1 - x}{x(\ln x - x)}$.

33. $\dfrac{1}{x(1 - x^2)}$.

34. $\dfrac{\tan x}{1 + \cos x}$.

35. $\dfrac{-x}{\sqrt{(x^2 + 3x)}}$.

36. $\dfrac{2e^{2x}}{\sqrt{(e^{4x} + 1)}}$.

37. $\dfrac{2}{e^{4x} + 1}$.

38. $- \tan x \sin^2 x$.

39. $\dfrac{dy}{dx} = \dfrac{dy/dx}{dt/dt} = \dfrac{2 \cos t \sin t/2}{\sin t \cos t/2}$. Using the identities $\sin t = 2 \sin t/2 \cos t/2$ and

$\cos^2 t/2 = \dfrac{1}{2}(1 + \cos t)$ this simplifies to

$$\dfrac{dy}{dx} = \dfrac{2 \cos t}{1 + \cos t}.$$

40. $\dfrac{dy}{dx} = - e^{-t}$.

PROBLEMS 24

1.   Substitute $\tanh x = (e^x - e^{-x})/(e^x + e^{-x})$ and $\operatorname{sech} x = 2/(e^x + e^{-x})$ into the left-hand side and simplify to reduce it to unity. If the identity $\cosh^2 x - \sinh^2 x = 1$ is accepted as true, the result also follows by dividing this identity by $\cosh^2 x$ and rearranging terms.

2.   Substitute $\coth x = (e^x + e^{-x})/(e^x - e^{-x})$ and $\operatorname{cosech} x = 2/(e^x - e^{-x})$ into the left-hand side and simplify to reduce it to unity. If the identity $\cosh^2 x - \sinh^2 x = 1$ is accepted as true, the result also follows by dividing this identity by $\sinh^2 x$ and rearranging terms.

3.   Substitute for the functions on the right-hand side and simplify to show it reduces to $(e^{(x-y)} + e^{-(x-y)})/2 = \cosh(x - y)$.

4.   Substitute for the functions on the right-hand side and simplify to show it reduces to $(e^{2x} + e^{-2x})/2 = \cosh 2x$.

The second result follows by substituting $\cosh^2 x = 1 + \sinh^2 x$.

The third result follows by substituting $\sinh^2 x = \cosh^2 x - 1$.

5.   Establish by evaluating $\dfrac{d}{dx}\left[\dfrac{\sinh x}{\cosh x}\right]$.

6.   Establish by evaluating $\dfrac{d}{dx}\left[\dfrac{\cosh x}{\sinh x}\right]$.

7.   Establish by evaluating $\dfrac{d}{dx}\left[\dfrac{1}{\cosh x}\right]$.

8.   Establish by evaluating $\dfrac{d}{dx}\left[\dfrac{1}{\sinh x}\right]$.

9. $2 \cosh (2x + 1)$.

10. $(6x + 1) \sinh (3x^2 + x - 1)$.

11. $\tanh \sqrt{x} + (\sqrt{x}/2) \operatorname{sech}^2 \sqrt{x}$.

12. $-(e^x + 1) \operatorname{sech} (e^x + x + 1) \tanh (e^x + x + 1)$.

13. $\dfrac{-2x}{(2x^2 + 3)^{1/2}} \operatorname{cosech}^2 (2x^2 + 3)^{1/2}$.

14. $-(e^x + 2x + 3) \operatorname{cosech} (e^x + x^2 + 3) \coth (e^x + x^2 + 3)$.

15. $-\dfrac{1}{x^2} \sinh \sqrt{(x^2 + 1)} + \dfrac{1}{\sqrt{(x^2 + 1)}} \cosh \sqrt{(x^2 + 1)}$.

16. $\left(1 + \dfrac{1}{x}\right) \operatorname{sech} (3x + 1) - 3(x + \ln x) \operatorname{sech} (3x + 1) \tanh (3x + 1)$.

17. $\dfrac{\mathrm{d}x}{\mathrm{d}t} = \operatorname{sech}^2 t$, $\dfrac{\mathrm{d}y}{\mathrm{d}t} = \sinh t$ so

$$\frac{\mathrm{d}y}{\mathrm{d}x} = \frac{\sinh t}{\operatorname{sech}^2 t} = \sinh t \cosh^2 t.$$

However, $\sinh 2t = 2 \sinh t \cosh t$, so

$$\frac{\mathrm{d}y}{\mathrm{d}x} = \frac{1}{2} \sinh 2t \cosh t.$$

As $\tanh^2 t + \operatorname{sech}^2 t = 1$ the explicit equation of the curve is

$$x^2 + \frac{1}{y^2} = 1.$$

18. $\dfrac{\mathrm{d}x}{\mathrm{d}t} = t \sinh t$, $\dfrac{\mathrm{d}y}{\mathrm{d}t} = t \cosh t$, so

$$\frac{\mathrm{d}y}{\mathrm{d}x} = \frac{\mathrm{d}y}{\mathrm{d}t} \bigg/ \frac{\mathrm{d}x}{\mathrm{d}t} = \coth t.$$

$$\frac{\mathrm{d}^2 y}{\mathrm{d}x^2} = \frac{\mathrm{d}}{\mathrm{d}x}\left(\frac{\mathrm{d}y}{\mathrm{d}x}\right) = \frac{\mathrm{d}t}{\mathrm{d}x} \frac{\mathrm{d}}{\mathrm{d}t}\left(\frac{\mathrm{d}y}{\mathrm{d}x}\right)$$

$$= \frac{1}{t \sinh t} \frac{\mathrm{d}}{\mathrm{d}t} (\coth t) = \frac{-1}{t \sinh^3 t}.$$

19. $\dfrac{\mathrm{d}x}{\mathrm{d}t} = a \sinh t$, $\dfrac{\mathrm{d}y}{\mathrm{d}t} = a \cosh t$, so

$$\frac{\mathrm{d}y}{\mathrm{d}x} = \frac{\mathrm{d}y}{\mathrm{d}t} \bigg/ \frac{\mathrm{d}x}{\mathrm{d}t} = \coth t.$$

Now

$$\frac{d^2y}{dx^2} = \frac{d}{dx}\left(\frac{dy}{dx}\right) = \frac{dt}{dx}\frac{d}{dt}\left(\frac{dy}{dx}\right)$$

$$= \frac{1}{a \sinh t}\frac{d}{dt}(\coth t) = \frac{-1}{a \sinh^3 t} .$$

so

$$\frac{d^3y}{dx^3} = \frac{d}{dx}\left(\frac{d^2y}{dx^2}\right) = \frac{dt}{dx}\frac{d}{dt}\left(\frac{-1}{a \sinh t}\right) = \left(\frac{1}{a \sinh t}\right)\frac{d}{dt}\left(\frac{-1}{a \sinh^3 t}\right)$$

$$= \frac{3 \cosh t}{a^2 \sinh^5 t}.$$

PROBLEMS 25

1. Start from the result $x = \cosh y = (e^y + e^{-y})/2$ and solve for e^y, hence find $y = \text{arcosh}\, x$.

2. Start from the result $x = \tanh y = (e^y - e^{-y})/(e^y + e^{-y})$ and solve for e^y, hence find $y = \text{artanh}\, x$.

8. $\dfrac{3}{(9x^2 + 30x + 26)^{1/2}} .$

9. $\sec x.$

10. $\dfrac{2x}{(4 - x^2)^{1/2}(x^2 - 2)^{1/2}} .$

11. $\text{artanh}\,[\tanh (\sin^2 x)] = \sin^2 x$, so

$$\frac{d}{dx}[\text{artanh}\,\{\tanh (\sin^2 x)\}] = \frac{d}{dx}[\sin^2 x] = 2 \sin x \cos x.$$

12. $\dfrac{2 \cos x}{(1 + 4 \sin^2 x)^{1/2}} .$

13. $\text{arcosh}\,[\cosh (x^2 + 1)] = x^2 + 1$, so

$$\frac{d}{dx}[\text{arcosh}\,\{\cosh (x^2 + 1)\}] = \frac{d}{dx}[x^2 + 1] = 2x.$$

14. $1/x.$

15. Differentiating the equation implicitly with respect to x gives

$$4xy + 2x^2 \frac{dy}{dx} + \text{artanh}\left(\frac{3 - y^2}{y^2 + 3}\right) + x\frac{d}{dx}\left[\text{artanh}\left(\frac{3 - y^2}{y^2 + 3}\right)\right] = 0,$$

and so

$$4xy + 2x^2 \frac{dy}{dx} + \operatorname{artanh}\left(\frac{3 - y^2}{y^2 + 3}\right) + x \frac{dy}{dx} \frac{d}{dy}\left[\operatorname{artanh}\left(\frac{3 - y^2}{y^2 + 3}\right)\right] = 0,$$

and thus

$$4xy + 2x^2 \frac{dy}{dx} + \operatorname{artanh}\left(\frac{3 - y^2}{y^2 + 3}\right) + x \frac{dy}{dx}\left(-\frac{1}{y}\right) = 0.$$

The required derivative follows by solving this equation for dy/dx.

PROBLEMS 26

1. Max. at $x = 0$, min. at $x = 2$.

2. Max. at $x = \pm\sqrt{3}$, min. at $x = 0$.

3. Max. at $x = 0$, min. at $x = 2$; asymptotes $x = 1$ and $y = x - 1$.

4. Max. at $x = -1$, min. at $x = 1$; asymptote $x = 0$.

5. Max. at $x = 0$; asymptotes $x = \pm 2$, $y = 0$.

6. Max. at $x = 4$, asymptotes $x = 2$, $y = 0$.

7. Min. at $x = -2$.

8. Max. at $x = -1$.

9. Max. at $x = 1$, asymptote $y = 0$.

10. Min. at $x = a/e$.

11. Max. at $x = (\pi/4) + 2k\pi$, min. at $x = (5\pi/4) + 2k\pi$ with $k = 0, \pm 1, \pm 2, \ldots$.

12. Min. at $x = 6$, stationary point at $x = 0$ across which the function is monotonic increasing; asymptotes $x = 2$ and $y = \frac{1}{4}x + 1$.

13. Max. at $x = -1$, min. at $x = 0$.

14. Max. at $x = 0$, min. at $x = \pm 1$.

15. Max. at $x = 0$.

16. Max. at $x = -2\sqrt{3}$, min. at $x = 2\sqrt{3}$.

17. 1.

18. 6.

19. 2/3.

20. $-1/\sqrt{2}$.

21. 1/2.

22. 2/3.

23. 1.

24. 1.

25. $-6\sqrt{2}$.

26. 1/2.

27. 0.

28. 0.

29. − 1/2

30. 4.

31. 0.

32. 0.

33. 3.

34. 0.

35. 2.

36. 0.

37. 1/2.

38. To combine the terms multiply numerator and denominator by $\sqrt{(x^2 + x + 1)} + \sqrt{(x^2 - x)}$ before proceeding to the limit to obtain the value 1.

39. 1/4.

40. 1/2.

PROBLEMS 27

1.

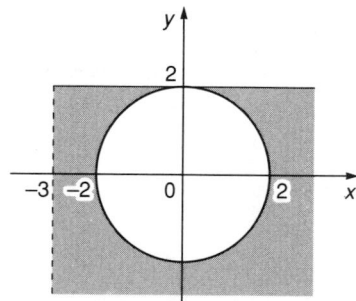

2.

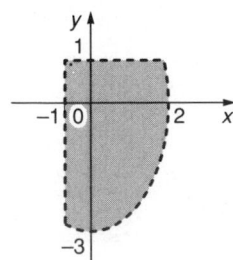

3.

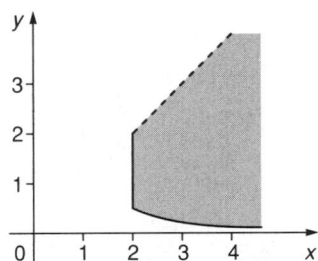

4.

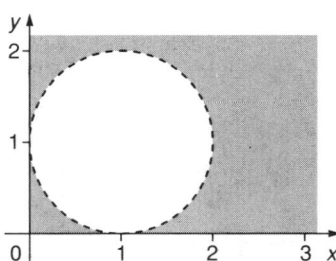

5.   The logarithmic function is only defined for positive arguments, so
      $f(x, y)$ is defined in the interior of the ellipse $x^2 + 2y^2 = 1$.

6. $f(x, y)$ is defined throughout the entire (x, y)-plane.

7.   The function artanh w is only defined for $|w| \leqslant 1$, so we require
      $(x^2 + 6)/(x^2 + y^2 + 4) \leqslant 1$ or, equivalently, $y^2 \leqslant 2$. Thus $f(x, y)$ is defined
      for $-\infty < x < \infty$ and $-\sqrt{2} \leqslant y \leqslant \sqrt{2}$.

8.   The logarithmic function is only defined for positive arguments, so
      $f(x, y)$ is defined provided sinh $(xy) > 0$, which is equivalent to $xy > 0$.
      Thus $f(x, y)$ is defined inside the first quadrant corresponding to $x > 0$,
      $y > 0$ and inside the third quadrant corresponding to $x < 0$, $y < 0$.

9.   The square root function is only real if its argument is non-negative, so
      $f(x, y)$ will be defined outside the circle $x^2 + y^2 = 1$.

10.   The square root function is only defined for non-negative arguments, so
      $[(x - 1)^2 + (y - 1)^2 - 4]^{1/2}$ is defined outside the circle $(x - 1)^2 + (y - 1)^2 = 4$
      (centre at (1, 1) and radius 2). The logarithmic function is only defined
      for positive arguemnts, so $\ln(1 - x^2 - y^2)$ is defined inside the circle
      $x^2 + y^2 = 1$ (centre at (0, 0) and radius 1). Thus $f(x, y)$ will be defined in
      the region common to these two circles shown as the shaded crecent-
      shaped area in the diagram

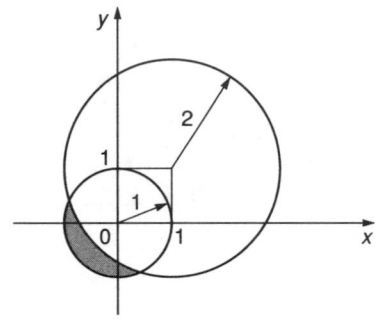

11. The equation of the contour lines when projected on to the (x, y)-plane is

$$\frac{x^2}{4} - \frac{y^2}{16} = \text{constant},$$

which describes a family of hyperbolas. Cutting the saddle-shaped surface shown in Fig. 78 by the plane $z = \text{const.}$ $(z > 0)$ is seen to generate these curves.

12. The equation of the contour lines when projected on to the (x, y)-plane is

$$x^2 + 2xy + y^2 = \text{const.} = k \text{ (say)},$$

which is equivalent to

$$x + y = \sqrt{k} \quad (k > 0).$$

Thus when projected on to the (x, y)-plane, the contour lines are the straight lines

$$y = -x + \sqrt{k}.$$

This is in agreement with the u-shaped surface shown in Fig. 79, which can be visualized as a sheet of paper bent in a U-shape with the bottom of the bend lying along the line $y = -x$ (i.e. corresponding to $k = 0$). This surface is an example of what is called a **ruled surface**, because it is generated by a family of straight lines.

PROBLEMS 28

1. 9.
2. 0.
3. 1/3.
4. 3/22.
5. 0.
6. 0.

7.   Limit does not exist.

8.   Limit does not exist because when x, y are small, $\sin xy \approx xy$, so setting $y = kx$ shows that

$$\lim_{(x, y) \to (0, 0)} \left[\frac{\sin xy}{x^2 + y^2} \right] = \lim_{x \to 0} \left[\frac{kx^2}{x^2 + k^2 x^2} \right] = \frac{k}{1 + k^2},$$

which depends on the gradient k of the direction of approach of (x, y) to $(0, 0)$.

9.   The numerator is always positive but the denominator vanishes on the circle $x^2 + y^2 = 1$. Thus $f(x, y)$ is continuous everywhere except for points on this circle on which it is discontinuous.

10. The exponential function depends continuously on its argument, so as $2xy + 1$ is a continuous function for all (x, y), so also is $f(x, y)$. Thus $f(x, y)$ is never discontinuous.

11. The denominator vanishes on the parabola $y = x^2$, while the numerator is always non-negative. Thus $f(x, y)$ is continuous everywhere except on the parabola on which it is discontinuous.

12. The logarithmic function is only defined for positive arguments and is infinte when the argument is zero, so $f(x, y)$ is continuous in the half-plane $x > 0$, but discontinuous on the y-axis.

PROBLEMS 29

1. $\dfrac{\partial f}{\partial x} = 3x^2 + 6xy^2, \quad \dfrac{\partial f}{\partial y} = 6x^2 y - 3y^2.$

2. $\dfrac{\partial f}{\partial x} = \dfrac{2x}{x^2 + y^2}, \quad \dfrac{\partial f}{\partial y} = \dfrac{2y}{x^2 + y^2}.$

3. $\dfrac{\partial f}{\partial x} = \dfrac{-y^2}{(x - y)^2}, \quad \dfrac{\partial f}{\partial y} = \dfrac{x^2}{(x - y)^2}.$

4. $\dfrac{\partial f}{\partial x} = \dfrac{y}{x^2 + y^2}, \quad \dfrac{\partial f}{\partial y} = \dfrac{-x}{x^2 + y^2}.$

5. $\dfrac{\partial f}{\partial x} = -3 \sin (3x - 4y), \quad \dfrac{\partial f}{\partial y} = 4 \sin (3x - 4y).$

6. $\dfrac{\partial f}{\partial x} = \dfrac{5t}{(x + 2t)^2}, \quad \dfrac{\partial f}{\partial t} = \dfrac{-5x}{(x + 2t)^2}.$

7. $\dfrac{\partial f}{\partial r} = \dfrac{\theta}{2 \sqrt{(r - r^2 \theta^2)}}, \quad \dfrac{\partial f}{\partial \theta} = \sqrt{\left(\dfrac{r}{1 - r\theta^2} \right)}.$

8. $\dfrac{\partial f}{\partial x} = \cot (x - 2y), \quad \dfrac{\partial f}{\partial y} = -2 \cot (x - 2y).$

9. $\dfrac{\partial f}{\partial x} = \dfrac{3y}{(3y-2x)^2}$, $\dfrac{\partial f}{\partial y} = \dfrac{-3x}{(3y-2x)^2}$.

10. The result follows from the fact that

$$\frac{\partial w}{\partial x} = \frac{1}{2\sqrt{x}(\sqrt{x}+\sqrt{y})} \quad \text{and} \quad \frac{\partial w}{\partial y} = \frac{1}{2\sqrt{y}(\sqrt{x}+\sqrt{y})} .$$

11. The result follows from the fact that

$$\frac{\partial u}{\partial x} = e^{x/y^2}/y^2 \quad \text{and} \quad \frac{\partial u}{\partial y} = -2x\, e^{x/y^2}/y^3.$$

12. The result follows from the fact that

$$\frac{\partial u}{\partial x} = \frac{\sin(y/x)}{2\sqrt{x}} - \frac{y\cos(y/x)}{x^{3/2}} \quad \text{and} \quad \frac{\partial u}{\partial y} = \frac{\cos(y/x)}{\sqrt{x}} .$$

13. $\dfrac{\partial^2 w}{\partial x^2} = 2y^3$, $\quad \dfrac{\partial^2 w}{\partial x\,\partial y} = 6xy^2 + 2$, $\quad \dfrac{\partial^2 w}{\partial y^2} = 6x^2 y + 2.$

14. $\dfrac{\partial^2 u}{\partial x\,\partial y} = \dfrac{xy}{(2xy+y^2)^{3/2}}$.

15. $\dfrac{\partial^2 u}{\partial x\,\partial y} = 0.$

16. Show that

$$\frac{\partial f}{\partial x} = \frac{\sqrt{(y/x)}}{2\sqrt{x}\,\sqrt{(x-y)}} , \quad \text{so} \quad \frac{\partial}{\partial y}\left(\frac{\partial f}{\partial x}\right) = \frac{1}{4\sqrt{y}(x-y)^{3/2}} .$$

and

$$\frac{\partial f}{\partial y} = \frac{-1}{2\sqrt{y}\,\sqrt{(x-y)}} , \quad \text{so} \quad \frac{\partial}{\partial x}\left(\frac{\partial f}{\partial y}\right) = \frac{1}{4\sqrt{y}(x-y)^{3/2}} .$$

17. The result follows by showing that

$$\frac{\partial^2 u}{\partial t^2} = -Ac^2\lambda^2 \sin(c\lambda t + \omega)\sin \lambda x$$

and

$$\frac{\partial^2 u}{\partial x^2} = -A\lambda^2 \sin(c\lambda t + \omega)\sin \lambda x.$$

18. The result follows by showing that

$$\frac{\partial u}{\partial x} = \frac{x}{(x^2 + y^2 + z^2)^{1/2}} ,$$

$$\frac{\partial u}{\partial y} = \frac{y}{(x^2 + y^2 + z^2)^{1/2}} ,$$

$$\frac{\partial u}{\partial z} = \frac{z}{(x^2 + y^2 + z^2)^{1/2}},$$

substituting into the left-hand side of the equation and using the definition of u.

19. $\dfrac{\partial^3 f}{\partial x \, \partial y^2} = - xy \cos (xy) - 2x \sin (xy).$

20. The result follows by showing that

$$\frac{\partial^2 u}{\partial t^2} = 9a^2 \exp [3(x + at)] + a^2 \exp (x - at)$$

and

$$\frac{\partial^2 u}{\partial x^2} = 9 \exp [3(x + at)] + \exp (x - at).$$

PROBLEMS 30

1. If $z = f(x, y)$, then $dz = (2x + 3y^2)dx + (6xy - 3y^2)dy.$

2. If $z = f(x, y)$, then $dz = (y \cos (xy) + 2x)dx + (x \cos (xy) - 3)dy.$

3. If $z = f(x, y)$, then $dz = (\cosh x \cos xy - y \sinh x \sin (xy) + 2x)dx$
   $+ (2y - x \sinh x \sin (xy))dy.$

4. If $z = f(x, y)$, then $dz = \left(\dfrac{2x}{x^2 + y^2} + y \right) dx - \left(\dfrac{2y}{x^2 + y^2} + x \right) dy.$

5. If $z = f(r, \theta, \varphi)$, then

   $$dz = (2r \sin \theta + \cos \varphi) \, dr + (r^2 \cos \theta + \cos \theta \, \sin \varphi) \, d\theta$$
   $$- (r \sin \theta - \sin \theta \, \cos \varphi) \, d\varphi .$$

6. If $z = f(u, v, w)$, then

   $$dz = (2u \sin v + v^2 \cos u + vw^2)du + (u^2 \cos v + 2v \sin u + uw^2)dv$$
   $$+ 2uv \, w \, dw.$$

7. $\dfrac{\partial f}{\partial u} = \dfrac{2uv^{1/2}}{w^{1/2}}, \quad \dfrac{\partial f}{\partial v} = \dfrac{u^2}{2v^{1/2}w^{1/2}}, \quad \dfrac{\partial f}{\partial w} = -\dfrac{u^2v^{1/2}}{2w^{3/2}}, \quad$ so

   $$100 \, \frac{df}{f} = 100 \left(\frac{2}{u} \, du + \frac{1}{2v} \, dv - \frac{1}{2w} \, dw \right).$$

8. $\dfrac{\partial f}{\partial x} = \dfrac{1}{2x^{1/2}y^{1/2}}, \quad \dfrac{\partial f}{\partial y} = -\dfrac{x^{1/2}}{2y^{3/2}}, \quad$ so

$$100 \frac{df}{f} = 100 \left(\frac{1}{2x} dx - \frac{1}{2y} dy \right)$$

$$= 50 \left(\frac{1}{x} dx - \frac{1}{y} dy \right).$$

9. $\dfrac{dy}{du} = - \left[\dfrac{9x^2y - 2y^2 + 2x}{3x^3 - 4xy + 2y} \right].$

10. $\dfrac{dy}{dx} = - \left[\dfrac{\sinh(x + 2y + 1) - 2x}{2 \sinh(x + 2y + 1) - 4y} \right].$

11. Setting $f(x, y, z) = x + 2yz^2 + \cos(x + 2y - z)$,

$$\frac{\partial z}{\partial x} = - \left(\frac{\partial f}{\partial x} \right) \Big/ \left(\frac{\partial f}{\partial z} \right) \quad \text{and} \quad \frac{\partial z}{\partial y} = - \left(\frac{\partial f}{\partial y} \right) \Big/ \left(\frac{\partial f}{\partial z} \right)$$

follow from the fact that

$$\frac{\partial f}{\partial x} = 1 - \sin(x + 2y - z), \quad \frac{\partial f}{\partial y} = 2z^2 - 2 \sin(x + 2y - z)$$

and

$$\frac{\partial f}{\partial z} = 4yz + \sin(x + 2y - z).$$

12. Setting $f(x, y, z) = z \ln(x^2 + 2y^2 + 1) - 2xyz^2 + 3x$,

$$\frac{\partial z}{\partial x} = - \left(\frac{\partial f}{\partial x} \right) \Big/ \left(\frac{\partial f}{\partial z} \right) \quad \text{and} \quad \frac{\partial z}{\partial y} = - \left(\frac{\partial f}{\partial y} \right) \Big/ \left(\frac{\partial f}{\partial z} \right)$$

follow from the fact that

$$\frac{\partial f}{\partial x} = \frac{2xz}{x^2 + 2y^2 + 1} - 2yz^2 + 3, \quad \frac{\partial f}{\partial y} = \frac{4yz}{x^2 + 2y^2 + 1} - 2xz^2$$

and

$$\frac{\partial f}{\partial z} = \ln(x^2 + 2y^2 + 1) - 4xyz.$$

PROBLEMS 31

1. $\dfrac{dw}{dt} = \left(4t + \dfrac{3}{t^2} \right) \exp\left(2t^2 - \dfrac{3}{t} \right).$

2. $\dfrac{dw}{dt} = \dfrac{6t}{(1 - t^2)^2} \cosh\left[\dfrac{4 - t^2}{1 - t^2} \right].$

3. $\dfrac{dw}{dt} = 3t^2 + 4 \sin t \cos t - 8 \tan t \sec^2 t.$

4. $\dfrac{dw}{dt} = \dfrac{1 - t^3}{(t^3 + 2)^2}.$

5. Set $f(x, y) = \sin x + \sinh (x^2 + y)$, so

$$\frac{\partial f}{\partial x} = \cos x + 2x \cosh (x^2 + y), \quad \frac{\partial f}{\partial y} = \cosh (x^2 + y)$$

and $g(x, y) = \cosh (x - y) - x^3$, so

$$\frac{\partial g}{\partial x} = \sinh (x - y) - 3x^2, \quad \frac{\partial g}{\partial x} = - \sinh (x - y).$$

Find dw/dx by substituting into

$$\frac{dw}{dx} = \frac{\partial f}{\partial x} - \left(\frac{\partial f}{\partial y}\right)\left(\frac{\partial g}{\partial x}\right) \Big/ \left(\frac{\partial g}{\partial y}\right).$$

6. Set $f(x, y) = \ln (xy + 4)$, so

$$\frac{\partial f}{\partial x} = \frac{y}{xy + 4}, \quad \frac{\partial f}{\partial y} = \frac{x}{xy + 4} \quad \text{and} \quad g(x, y) = xy + \ln (x^2 + y), \text{ so}$$

$$\frac{\partial g}{\partial x} = y + \frac{2x}{x^2 + y}, \quad \frac{\partial g}{\partial y} = x + \frac{1}{x^2 + y}.$$

Find dw/dx as in the answer to problem 5.

PROBLEMS 32

1. $\dfrac{\partial F}{\partial u} = 2u \dfrac{\partial f}{\partial x} + 2v \dfrac{\partial f}{\partial y}, \quad \dfrac{\partial F}{\partial v} = 2v \dfrac{\partial f}{\partial x} + 2u \dfrac{\partial f}{\partial y},$

from which the first result follows after making use of the fact that $x = u^2 + v^2$ and $y = 2uv$. The last part follows by using the same form of reasoning as in Example 32.2 after making use of the fact that

$$\frac{\partial}{\partial u} \equiv 2u \frac{\partial}{\partial x} + 2v \frac{\partial}{\partial y}.$$

2. $\dfrac{\partial F}{\partial s} = (3s^2 + 2) \dfrac{\partial f}{\partial x} + t \dfrac{\partial f}{\partial y} \quad \text{and} \quad \dfrac{\partial F}{\partial t} = s \dfrac{\partial f}{\partial y}. \text{ Thus } \dfrac{\partial}{\partial t} \equiv s \dfrac{\partial}{\partial y}, \text{ and so}$

$$\frac{\partial^2 F}{\partial t \partial s} = \frac{\partial}{\partial t}\left[\frac{\partial F}{\partial s}\right] = \frac{\partial}{\partial t}\left[(3s^2 + 2) \frac{\partial f}{\partial x} + t \frac{\partial f}{\partial y}\right]$$

$$= (3s^2 + 2) \frac{\partial}{\partial t}\left(\frac{\partial f}{\partial x}\right) + \frac{\partial f}{\partial y} + t \frac{\partial}{\partial t}\left(\frac{\partial f}{\partial y}\right)$$

$$= (3s^2 + 2) s \frac{\partial}{\partial y}\left(\frac{\partial f}{\partial x}\right) + \frac{\partial f}{\partial y} + ts \frac{\partial}{\partial y}\left(\frac{\partial f}{\partial y}\right)$$

$$= \frac{\partial f}{\partial y} + (3s^3 + 2x) \frac{\partial^2 f}{\partial x \partial y} + ts \frac{\partial^2 f}{\partial y^2}.$$

3. $$\frac{\partial F}{\partial u} = 2u \frac{\partial f}{\partial x} + v \frac{\partial f}{\partial y}, \quad \frac{\partial F}{\partial v} = -2v \frac{\partial f}{\partial x} + u \frac{\partial f}{\partial y}$$

$$\frac{\partial}{\partial u} \equiv 2u \frac{\partial}{\partial x} + v \frac{\partial}{\partial y}, \text{ so}$$

$$\frac{\partial^2 F}{\partial u^2} = \frac{\partial}{\partial u} \left(\frac{\partial F}{\partial u} \right) = \frac{\partial}{\partial u} \left[2u \frac{\partial f}{\partial x} + v \frac{\partial f}{\partial y} \right]$$

$$= 2 \frac{\partial f}{\partial x} + 2u \frac{\partial}{\partial u} \left(\frac{\partial f}{\partial x} \right) + v \frac{\partial}{\partial u} \left(\frac{\partial f}{\partial y} \right)$$

$$= 2 \frac{\partial f}{\partial x} + 2u \left[2u \frac{\partial}{\partial x} + v \frac{\partial}{\partial y} \right] \left(\frac{\partial f}{\partial x} \right) + v \left[2u \frac{\partial}{\partial x} + v \frac{\partial}{\partial y} \right] \left(\frac{\partial f}{\partial y} \right)$$

$$= 2 \frac{\partial f}{\partial x} + 4u^2 \frac{\partial^2 f}{\partial x^2} + 4uv \frac{\partial^2 f}{\partial x \partial y} + v^2 \frac{\partial^2 f}{\partial y^2}.$$

4. $$\frac{\partial^2 F}{\partial r^2} = \frac{\partial}{\partial r} \left(\cos \theta \frac{\partial f}{\partial x} + \sin \theta \frac{\partial f}{\partial y} \right) = \cos \theta \frac{\partial}{\partial r} \left(\frac{\partial f}{\partial x} \right) + \sin \theta \frac{\partial}{\partial r} \left(\frac{\partial f}{\partial y} \right),$$

and the first result then follows from the fact that

$$\frac{\partial}{\partial r} = \cos \theta \frac{\partial}{\partial x} + \sin \theta \frac{\partial}{\partial y}.$$

$$\frac{\partial^2 F}{\partial \theta^2} = \frac{\partial}{\partial \theta} \left[-r \sin \theta \frac{\partial f}{\partial x} + r \cos \theta \frac{\partial f}{\partial y} \right]$$

$$= -r \cos \theta \frac{\partial f}{\partial x} - r \sin \theta \frac{\partial}{\partial \theta} \left(\frac{\partial f}{\partial x} \right) - r \sin \theta \frac{\partial f}{\partial y} + r \cos \theta \frac{\partial}{\partial \theta} \left(\frac{\partial f}{\partial y} \right).$$

The expression for $\partial^2 F / \partial \theta^2$ then follows after using the fact that

$$\frac{\partial}{\partial \theta} = -r \sin \theta \frac{\partial}{\partial x} + r \cos \theta \frac{\partial}{\partial y}.$$

together with the fact that

$$-r \left(\cos \theta \frac{\partial f}{\partial x} + \sin \theta \frac{\partial f}{\partial y} \right) = -r \frac{\partial F}{\partial r}.$$

The last result follows by adding the expresssions for

$$\frac{\partial^2 F}{\partial r^2} \quad \text{and} \quad \frac{1}{r} \frac{\partial F}{\partial r} + \frac{1}{r^2} \frac{\partial^2 F}{\partial \theta^2}.$$

5. $$\frac{\partial F}{\partial u} = 2u \frac{\partial f}{\partial x} + 2v \frac{\partial f}{\partial y}, \quad \frac{\partial F}{\partial v} = -2v \frac{\partial f}{\partial x} + 2u \frac{\partial f}{\partial y}.$$

The first result now follows by squaring and adding these results. It follows from the above results that

$$u\frac{\partial F}{\partial u} - v\frac{\partial F}{\partial v} = 2(u^2 + v^2)\frac{\partial f}{\partial x}.$$

However, if

$$u\frac{\partial F}{\partial u} - v\frac{\partial F}{\partial v} = 0,$$

it must follow that $2(u^2 + v^2)\partial f/\partial x = 0$. The factor $2(u^2 + v^2) > 0$, so $\partial f/\partial x = 0$, which implies the f is a function of y only.

6. $\dfrac{\partial v}{\partial x} = \dfrac{\partial V}{\partial s}\dfrac{\partial s}{\partial x} + \dfrac{\partial V}{\partial t}\dfrac{\partial t}{\partial x} = \dfrac{2x}{x^2 + y^2}\dfrac{\partial V}{\partial s} + 2xe^{x^2 - y^2}\dfrac{\partial V}{\partial t}$

$$= 2x\left(e^{-s}\frac{\partial V}{\partial s} + t\frac{\partial V}{\partial t}\right),$$

from which the result for $(1/2x)(\partial V/\partial x)$ follows.

Similarly,

$$\frac{\partial v}{\partial y} = \frac{\partial V}{\partial s}\frac{\partial s}{\partial y} + \frac{\partial V}{\partial t}\frac{\partial t}{\partial y} = \frac{2y}{x^2 + y^2}\frac{\partial V}{\partial s} - 2ye^{x^2 - y^2}\frac{\partial V}{\partial t}$$

$$= 2y\left(e^{-s}\frac{\partial V}{\partial s} - t\frac{\partial V}{\partial t}\right),$$

from which the result for $(1/2y)(\partial v/\partial y)$ follows.

If $y(\partial v/\partial x) + x(\partial v/\partial y) = 0$, it follows from the above results that

$$e^{-s}\frac{\partial V}{\partial s} = 0,$$

and hence that $\partial V/\partial s = 0$. Thus V depends only on t, and hence on $x^2 - y^2$.

7. $\dfrac{\partial F}{\partial x} = \dfrac{\partial f}{\partial u}\dfrac{\partial u}{\partial x} + \dfrac{\partial f}{\partial v}\dfrac{\partial v}{\partial x}$ and $\dfrac{\partial F}{\partial y} = \dfrac{\partial f}{\partial u}\dfrac{\partial u}{\partial y} + \dfrac{\partial f}{\partial v}\dfrac{\partial v}{\partial y},$

so

$$\frac{\partial F}{\partial x} = \frac{y^2 - x^2}{(x^2 + y^2)^2}\frac{\partial f}{\partial u} + \frac{2xy}{(x^2 + y^2)^2}\frac{\partial f}{\partial v}$$

$$= (v^2 - u^2)\frac{\partial f}{\partial u} - 2uv\frac{\partial f}{\partial v}$$

$$\frac{\partial F}{\partial y} = \frac{-2xy}{(x^2 + y^2)^2}\frac{\partial f}{\partial u} + \frac{y^2 - x^2}{(x^2 + y^2)^2}\frac{\partial f}{\partial v}$$

$$= 2uv\frac{\partial f}{\partial u} + (v^2 - u^2)\frac{\partial f}{\partial v}.$$

If $f(u, v)$ is independent of v we must have $\partial f/\partial v = 0$. Setting $\partial f/\partial v = 0$ and eliminating $\partial f/\partial u$ gives

$$2xy \frac{\partial F}{\partial x} + (y^2 - x^2) \frac{\partial F}{\partial y} = 0.$$

PROBLEMS 33

1. $\dfrac{1}{3} x^3 + \dfrac{3}{2} x^2 - x^2 - x + C.$

2. Using the fact that $(x - 3)/x^3 = (1/x^2) - (3/x^3)$ to arrive at the solution

    $$\frac{3}{2} x^2 - \frac{1}{x} + C.$$

3. $\dfrac{2}{3} x^{3/2} + \dfrac{12}{5} x^{5/4} + C.$

4. $\dfrac{1}{7} x^{7x} + x + C.$

5. $\dfrac{\sin 4x}{4} + \dfrac{4}{3} x^{3/2} + C.$

6. Use the fact that $(x^3 + 5x + 3)/x^2 = x + (5/x) + (3/x^2)$ to arrive at the solution

    $$5 \ln |x| + \frac{x^2}{2} - \frac{3}{x} + C.$$

7. $\dfrac{4}{3} \arctan \dfrac{x}{3} + C.$

8. $-\dfrac{1}{4} \cos 2x + C = -\dfrac{1}{4} (\cos^2 x - \sin^2 x) + C$

    $$= -\frac{1}{4} (1 - 2 \sin^2 x) + C$$

    $$= \frac{1}{2} \sin^2 x + C - \frac{1}{4}$$

    $$= \frac{1}{2} \sin^2 x + C'.$$

9. Proceed as in Example 33.7 to arrive at the solution

    $$\frac{(1 + x^2)^4}{8} + C.$$

10. $5 \arcsin \dfrac{x}{2} + C.$

11. $\dfrac{3}{(9-4x^2)^{1/2}} = \dfrac{3}{2}\,\dfrac{1}{[\,(9/4)-x^2\,]^{1/2}}$,

so

$$\int \dfrac{3}{(9-4x^2)^{1/2}} = \dfrac{3}{2}\arcsin\left(\dfrac{2x}{3}\right) + C.$$

12. $\dfrac{1}{2\sqrt{10}}\ln\left|\dfrac{x-\sqrt{10}}{x+\sqrt{10}}\right| + C.$

13. Express the integrand as the sum of two terms and then integrate to obtain

$$\dfrac{3x^{7/6}(8-7x^{1/6})}{28} + C.$$

14. Multiply the two factors in the integrand and then integrate the result to obtain

$$\dfrac{2x^{5/2}}{5} + x + C.$$

15. $\cosh 2x = \cosh^2 x + \sinh^2 x = 1 + 2\sinh^2 x$,

so

$$\sinh^2 x = \dfrac{1}{2}(\cosh 2x - 1).$$

Thus

$$\int \sinh^2 x = \int \dfrac{1}{2}(\cosh 2x - 1)\mathrm{d}x$$

$$= \dfrac{1}{2}\int \cosh 2x\,\mathrm{d}x - \dfrac{1}{2}\int 1\cdot \mathrm{d}x$$

$$= \dfrac{1}{4}\sinh 2x - \dfrac{1}{2}x + C.$$

As $\sinh 2x = 2\sinh x\cosh x$, this may also be written

$$\int \sinh^2 x\,\mathrm{d}x = \dfrac{1}{2}\sinh x\cosh x - \dfrac{1}{2}x + C.$$

16. $\cos 4x = \cos^2 2x + \sin^2 2x = 2\cos^2 2x - 1$, so

$$\cos^2 2x = \dfrac{1}{2}(1 + \cos 4x).$$

Thus

$$\int \cos^2 2x \, dx = \int \frac{1}{2} (1 + \cos 4x) dx$$

$$= \frac{1}{2} \int 1 \cdot dx + \frac{1}{2} \int \cos 4x \, dx$$

$$= \frac{1}{2} x + \frac{1}{8} \sin 4x + C.$$

As $\sin 4x = 2 \sin 2x \cos 2x$ this may also be written

$$\int \cos^2 2x \, dx = \frac{1}{2} x + \frac{1}{4} \sin 2x \cos 2x + C.$$

17. Base your approach on the solution to problem 16, and hence show that

$$\int \sin^2 2x \, dx = \frac{1}{2} x - \frac{1}{8} \sin 4x + C = \frac{1}{2} x - \frac{1}{4} \sin 2x \cos 2x + C.$$

18. $\sinh x = \frac{1}{2} (e^x - e^{-x})$, so $e^{-x} \sinh x = \frac{1}{2} (1 - e^{-2x})$ and thus

$$\int e^{-x} \sinh x \, dx = \int \frac{1}{2} (1 - e^{-2x}) dx$$

$$= \frac{1}{2} \int 1 \cdot dx - \frac{1}{2} \int e^{-2x} dx$$

$$= \frac{1}{2} x + \frac{1}{4} e^{-2x} + C.$$

19. Use the result that $\cosh (7x + 3) = \cosh 7x \cosh 3 + \sinh 7x \sinh 3$ to show that

$$\int \cosh (7x + 3) dx = \frac{1}{7} (\sinh 7x \cosh 3 + \cosh 7x \sinh 3) + C$$

$$= \frac{1}{7} \sinh (7x + 3) + C.$$

20. Use the result that $\sin (2x - 1) = \sin 2x \cos 1 - \cos 2x \sin 1$ to show that

$$\int \sin (2x - 1) dx = \frac{-1}{2} (\cos 2x \cos 1 + \sin 2x \sin 1) + C$$

$$= \frac{-1}{2} \cos (2x - 1) + C.$$

PROBLEMS 34

1. $2 \ln |x + 3| + C.$

2. $-3 \ln |x - 2| + C.$

3. $\frac{1}{6} \sinh (6x + 3) + C.$

4. $\frac{3}{5} (x + 5)^{5/3} + C.$

5. $\frac{1}{2} \cos (3 - 2x) + C.$

6. $-\frac{1}{4} \cosh (1 - 4x) + C.$

7. $\frac{1}{30} (5x + 4)^6 + C;$ set $u = 5x + 4.$

8. $\frac{1}{24} (1 + x^3)^8 + C;$ set $u = 1 + x^3.$

9. $-\frac{1}{24} (1 - 2x^2)^6 + C;$ set $u = 1 - 2x^2.$

10. $\frac{1}{3} \sqrt{(2x^3 - 5)} + C;$ set $u = 2x^3 - 5.$

11. $\frac{1}{3} \ln |3 \sin x + 5| + C;$ set $u = 3 \sin x + 5.$

12. $-2 \ln |2 \cos x + 7| + C;$ set $u = 2 \cos x + 7.$

13. $-\frac{1}{2} \exp (4 - x^2) + C;$ set $u = 4 - x^2.$

14. $\frac{5}{4} \ln |2x^2 + 3| + C;$ set $u = 2x^2 + 3.$

15. $\frac{2}{5} \sqrt{(5x - 3)} + C;$ set $u = 5x - 3.$

16. $\frac{1}{2} \ln [x^2 + \sqrt{(1 + x^4)}] + C;$ set $u = x^2$ to reduce the integral to

$$\frac{1}{2} \int \frac{du}{\sqrt{(1 + u^2)}} = \frac{1}{2} \operatorname{arcsinh} u + C = \frac{1}{2} \ln [x^2 + \sqrt{(1 + x^4)}] + C.$$

17. $\frac{1}{3} \ln \left| x^3 + \sqrt{(x^6 - 1)} \right| + C;$ set $u = x^3$ to reduce the integral to

$$\frac{1}{3} \int \frac{du}{\sqrt{(u^2 - 1)}} = \frac{1}{3} \ln \left| x^3 + \sqrt{(x^6 - 1)} \right| + C.$$

18. $\frac{1}{2} (\ln x)^2 + C;$ set $u = \ln x.$

19. $\frac{1}{2} \ln x \ln 3 + \frac{1}{4} (\ln x)^2;$ write integral as

$$\int \frac{\ln 3x}{2x} \, dx = \frac{1}{2} \int \left(\frac{\ln 3 + \ln x}{x} \right) dx$$

$$= \frac{\ln 3}{2} \int \frac{dx}{x} + \frac{1}{2} \int \frac{\ln x}{x} \, dx$$

and then use the result of problem 18.

20. $-\cos(\ln x) + C$; set $u = \ln x$.

21. $\sqrt{(x^2 + 1)} + \ln\left|x + \sqrt{(x^2 + 1)}\right| + C$; write integral as

$$\int \frac{x}{\sqrt{(x^2 + 1)}}\,dx + \int \frac{dx}{\sqrt{(1 + x^2)}} = \int \frac{x}{\sqrt{(x^2 + 1)}}\,dx + \operatorname{arsinh} x + C.$$

Then set $u = x^2 + 1$ in the first intgral and use logarithmic form of arsinh.

22. $\arcsin x - \sqrt{(1 - x^2)} + C$; proceed in similar fashion to answer in problem 21.

23. $-\dfrac{1}{\ln|x|} + C$; set $u = \ln x$.

24. $-\dfrac{2}{\sqrt{e^x}} + C$; set $u = e^x$.

25. $-\dfrac{2}{3e^{3x/2}} + C$; set $u = e^{3x}$.

26. $-\exp\left(\dfrac{1}{2} - x\right) + C$; set $u = 2x - 1$.

27. $\dfrac{2}{\sqrt{7}}\arctan\left[\dfrac{4x - 1}{\sqrt{7}}\right] + C$; complete square in denominator and then make a change of variable.

28. $\dfrac{1}{2\sqrt{7}}\ln\left|\dfrac{x - \sqrt{7} + 2}{x + \sqrt{7} + 2}\right| + C$; complete square in denominator and then make a change of variable.

29. $\ln\left|2\sqrt{(x^2 + x + 1)} + 2x + 1\right| + C$; complete square under the square root and then make a change of variable.

30. $\ln\left|2\sqrt{(x^2 + 2x - 4)} + x + 1\right| + C$; complete square under the square root and then make a change of variable.

31. $\arcsin\left[\dfrac{1}{\sqrt{5}}(x - 1)\right] + C$; complete square under the square root and then make a change of variable.

32. $\arcsin\left[\dfrac{1}{\sqrt{5}}(x + 1)\right] + C$; complete square under the square root and then make a change of variable.

33. $(1/\sqrt{2})\arcsin(4x - 1) + C$; complete square under the square root and then make a change of variable.

34. $\frac{1}{2}\ln\left|4\sqrt{[x(4x + 1)]} + 8x + 1\right| + C$; complete square under the square root and then make a change of variable.

35. $4 \arcsin\left[\dfrac{1}{\sqrt{5}}(x-2)\right] - 2\sqrt{(1+4x-x^2)} + C$; complete square under the square root and then make a change of variable.

36. $\dfrac{1}{2}\ln\left[\dfrac{\sqrt{(x^2+1)}-1}{\sqrt{(x^2+1)}+1}\right] + C$; obtained by setting $u^2 = x^2 + 1$.

37. $\arctan\left(\sqrt{(x^2-1)}\right) + C$; obtained by setting $u^2 = x^2 - 1$.

38. $\dfrac{1}{2}\arcsin x - \dfrac{1}{2}x\sqrt{(1-x^2)} + C$; obtained by setting $x = \sin u$ to give

$$\int \frac{x^2}{\sqrt{(1-x^2)}}\, dx = \int \sin^2 u\, du$$

$$= \frac{1}{2}\int (1 - \cos 2u)\,du$$

$$= \frac{1}{2}u - \frac{1}{4}\sin 2u + C$$

$$= \frac{1}{2}u - \frac{1}{2}\sin u \cos u + C$$

$$= \frac{1}{2}\arcsin x - \frac{1}{2}x\sqrt{(1-x^2)} + C.$$

39. $-\dfrac{2}{3}\sec h^3\sqrt{x} + C$; obtained by setting $u = \cosh\sqrt{x}$ to give

$$\int \frac{\sinh\sqrt{x}\,\operatorname{sech}^4\sqrt{x}}{\sqrt{x}}\, dx = \int \frac{2}{u^4}\, du = -\frac{2}{3u^3} + C$$

$$= -\frac{2}{3}\operatorname{sech}^3\sqrt{x} + C.$$

40. $\dfrac{1}{2}\arcsin\sqrt{(x-1)} - \dfrac{1}{8}\sin\left[4\arcsin\sqrt{(x-1)}\right] + C$; obtained by setting $x = 1 + \sin^2 u$ to give

$$\int \sqrt{[(x-1)(2-x)]}\, dx = 2\int \sin^2 u \cos^2 u\, du$$

$$= \frac{1}{2}\int \sin^2 2u\, du$$

$$= \frac{1}{2}\int (1 - \cos 4u)\,du$$

$$= \frac{1}{2} u - \frac{1}{8} \sin 4u + C$$

$$= \frac{1}{2} \arcsin \sqrt{(x - 1)} - \frac{1}{8} \sin \left[4 \arcsin \sqrt{(x - 1)} \right] + C.$$

41. $\dfrac{1}{\sqrt{3}} \arctan (\sqrt{3} \tan x) + C$; obtained by rewriting integral as

$$\int \frac{\sec^2 x}{1 + 3 \tan^2 x} \, dx = \int \frac{dx}{(\cos^2 x + 3 \sin^2 x)}$$

and then using the substitution $t = \tan x$.

42. $\dfrac{1}{2} \tan \dfrac{1}{2} x + \dfrac{1}{6} \tan^3 \dfrac{1}{2} x + C$; set $t = \tan \dfrac{x}{2}$.

43. $\dfrac{1}{2} x - \dfrac{1}{2} \ln |\sin x + \cos x| + C$; set $t = \tan \dfrac{x}{2}$.

44. $\dfrac{1}{3} \arctan (3 \tan x) + C$; set $t = \tan x$.

45. $\dfrac{1}{4} \ln \left| \dfrac{\tan x + 2}{\tan x - 2} \right| + C$; set $t = \tan x$.

46. $\dfrac{1}{8} x - \dfrac{1}{24} \arctan (3 \tan x) + C$; set $t = \tan x$.

47. $\dfrac{1}{2\sqrt{5}} \arctan \left[\dfrac{2}{\sqrt{5}} \tan x \right] + C$; set $t = \tan x$.

48. $\dfrac{x}{2} + \dfrac{1}{2} \ln |\sin x - \cos x| + C$; rewrite integral as

$$\int \frac{\sin x}{\sin x - \cos x} \, dx$$

and set $t = \tan \dfrac{x}{2}$.

PROBLEMS 35

1. $\dfrac{1}{28} \sin^7 4x + C.$

2. $-\dfrac{1}{8} \cos^4 2x + C.$

3. $\dfrac{1}{24} \cosh^8 3x + C.$

4. $\dfrac{1}{25} \sinh^5 5x + C.$

5. $\dfrac{1}{4} \tanh^4 x + C.$

6. $\dfrac{1}{16} (x^2 + 6x + 1)^8 + C.$

7. $\dfrac{1}{15} (3x^3 - 6x + 1)^5 + C.$

8. $\dfrac{1}{2} \ln \left| x^2 + 4x + 1 \right| + C.$

9. $\ln \left| 2x^2 - x + 1 \right| + C.$

10. $\dfrac{1}{4} \ln |\sin 4x| + C.$

11. $\dfrac{1}{3} \ln \cosh 3x + C.$

12. $\dfrac{1}{6} \ln |\sinh 6x| + C.$

13. $\dfrac{1}{4} e^{x^4} + C.$

14. $\dfrac{1}{2} e^{\sin 2x} + C.$

15. $\dfrac{1}{2} \exp (x^2 + 2x - 3) + C.$

16. $\dfrac{1}{2} e^{\tan 2x} + C.$

17. $\dfrac{1}{2} (1 + \cos 2x) = \cos^2 x$, so

$$\int \sin x \cos x \exp \left[\frac{1}{2} (1 + \cos 2x) \right] dx = \int \sin x \cos x \, e^{\cos^2 x} \, dx = -\frac{1}{2} e^{\cos^2 x} + C.$$

18. $1 + \tan^2 = \sec^2 x = d[\tan x]/dx$, so

$$\int \frac{1 + \tan^2 x}{\tan x} \, dx = \int \frac{\sec^2 x}{\tan x} \, dx = \ln |\tan x| + C.$$

PROBLEMS 36

1. $x \sin x + \cos x + C$; set $u = x$.

2. $(x - 1) e^x + C$; set $u = x$.

3. $-(x + 1) e^{-x} + C$; set $u = x$.

4. $\dfrac{1}{2} e^x(\sin x - \cos x) + C$ set $u = e^x$.

5. $\dfrac{1}{5} e^{2x}(\sin x + 2 \cos x) + C$ set $u = e^{2x}$.

6. $\dfrac{1}{2} x^2 \ln |x| - \dfrac{1}{4} x^2 + C$; set $u = \ln |x|$.

7. $-\dfrac{\ln |x|}{x} - \dfrac{1}{x} + C$; set $u = \ln |x|$.

8. $(x^2/4) - (x/2) \sin x \cos x - (1/8) \cos 2x + C$; write
     $x \sin^2 x = x \sin x \, d/dx \, [- \cos x]$ and show that

$$\int x \sin^2 x \, dx = - x \sin x \cos x + \int \sin x \cos x \, dx + \int x \cos^2 x \, dx$$

$$= - x \sin x \cos x - \frac{1}{4} \cos 2x + \int x(1 - \sin^2 x) dx$$

$$= - x \sin x \cos x - \frac{1}{4} \cos 2x + \frac{x^2}{2} - \int x \sin^2 x + C,$$

so

$$\int x \sin^2 x \, dx = \frac{x^2}{4} - \frac{x}{2} \sin x \cos x - \frac{1}{8} \cos 2x + C.$$

9. $\dfrac{1}{2} (x^2 \arctan x + \arctan x - x) + C$; set $u = \arctan x$.

10. $e^x(x^2 - 2x + 2) + C$; set $u = e^x$.

11. $x \ln (x^2 + 1) - 2x + 2 \arctan x + C$; set $u = \ln (x^2 + 1)$.

12. $(x/2)[\cos (\ln |x|) + \sin (\ln |x|)] + C$; write
     $\cos (\ln |x|) = \cos (\ln |x|) d/dx[x]$.

13. $\dfrac{x^2}{2} \arcsin x - \dfrac{1}{4} \arcsin x + \dfrac{x}{4} \sqrt{(1 - x^2)} + C$; set $u = \arcsin x$.

14. $\dfrac{1}{9} \left[2x \sin 3x - \dfrac{1}{3} (9x^2 - 2) \cos 3x \right] + C$; set $u = \sin 3x$.

15. $\frac{x}{2}$ [sin (ln $|x|$) $-$ cos (ln $|x|$)] $+ C$; write sin (ln $|x|$) $=$ sin (ln $|x|$) $\frac{d}{dx}$ [x].

16. $\frac{-1}{2^x}\left[\frac{x}{\ln x}+\frac{1}{(\ln x)^2}\right]+C$; write $2^{-x}=e^{-x\ln 2}$ and set $u=x$.

17. Proceed as in Example 36.7.

18. Set $u=(1+\sin^2 x)^n$.

19. Set $u=\sec^{n-2} x$, $v=\tan x$ and use the identity $\sec^2 x=1+\tan^2 x$.

20. Set $u=x\cos^{n-1} x$, $v=\sin x$ and use the identity $\sin^2 x=1-\cos^2 x$.

PROBLEMS 37

1. $\ln|2x+1|-3\ln|x-1|+C$;

   partial fractions $\dfrac{2}{2x+1}-\dfrac{3}{x-1}$.

2. $4\ln|x+1|+3\ln|x-1|+C$;

   partial fractions $\dfrac{4}{x+1}+\dfrac{3}{x-1}$.

3. $\dfrac{1}{3}\ln|x+2|-\dfrac{1}{2}\ln|x+1|+\dfrac{1}{6}\ln|x-1|+C$;

   partial fractions $\dfrac{1}{3(x+2)}-\dfrac{1}{2(x+1)}+\dfrac{1}{6(x-1)}$.

4. $\ln|x-1|-2\ln|x+1|-\dfrac{2}{x+1}+C$;

   partial fractions $\dfrac{1}{x-1}-\dfrac{2}{x+1}+\dfrac{2}{(x+1)^2}$.

5. $\dfrac{-(4x+5)}{8(2x+1)^2}+C$;

   partial fractions $\dfrac{1}{2(2x+1)^2}+\dfrac{3}{2(2x+1)^3}$.

6. $\ln|x+1|+\dfrac{2x+3}{2(x+1)^2}+C$;

   partial fractions $\dfrac{1}{x+1}-\dfrac{1}{(x+1)^2}-\dfrac{1}{(x+1)^3}$.

7. $5\ln|x-2|-\ln|x+1|+\dfrac{1}{2}x^2+3x+C$;

   partial fractions $\dfrac{5}{x-2}-\dfrac{1}{x+1}+x+3$.

8. $\dfrac{7}{\sqrt{3}}$ arctan $[(2x + 1)/\sqrt{3}] + \dfrac{1}{2}$ ln $\left| x^2 + x + 1 \right| + x^2 - 3x + C$;

partial fractions $\dfrac{x}{x^2 + x + 1} + \dfrac{4}{x^2 + x + 1} + 2x - 3$.

9. $\dfrac{1}{8}$ arctan $(x/2) + \dfrac{1}{2}$ ln $\left| x^2 + 4 \right| - \dfrac{(3x - 8)}{4(x^2 + 4)} + C$;

partial fractions $\dfrac{-4x}{(x^2 + 4)^2} - \dfrac{6}{(x^2 + 4)^2} + \dfrac{x}{x^2 + 4} + \dfrac{1}{x^2 + 4}$.

10. -2 arctan $(2x + 1) - \dfrac{3}{4}$ ln $\left| 2x^2 + 2x + 1 \right| + 2$ ln $\left| x + 1 \right| + \dfrac{x}{2} + C$;

partial fractions $\dfrac{-3x}{2x^2 + 2x + 1} - \dfrac{7}{2(2x^2 + 2x + 1)} + \dfrac{2}{x + 1} + \dfrac{1}{2}$.

11. 4 ln $\left| x - 1 \right| - 4$ ln $\left| x - 2 \right| - \dfrac{(7x - 6)}{(x - 1)(x - 2)} + C$;

partial fractions $\dfrac{-1}{(x - 1)^2} + \dfrac{4}{x - 1} + \dfrac{8}{(x - 2)^2} - \dfrac{4}{x - 2}$.

12. -4 ln $\left| x + 1 \right| - \dfrac{1}{x + 1} + \dfrac{x^3}{3} - x^2 + 3x + C$;

partial fractions $\dfrac{1}{(x + 1)^2} - \dfrac{4}{x + 1} + x^2 - 2x + 3$.

13. $\dfrac{15}{4}$ ln $\left| x + 2 \right| - \dfrac{7}{3}$ ln $\left| x + 1 \right| - \dfrac{5}{12}$ ln $\left| x - 2 \right| + C$;

partial fractions $\dfrac{15}{4(x + 2)} - \dfrac{7}{3(x + 1)} - \dfrac{5}{12(x - 2)}$.

14. $\dfrac{2}{\sqrt{3}}$ arctan $[(2x + 1)/\sqrt{3}] + x + C$;

partial fractions $1 + \dfrac{1}{x^2 + x + 1}$.

15. $\dfrac{7\sqrt{11}}{33}$ arctan $[(2x + 1)/\sqrt{11}] - \dfrac{1}{6}$ ln $\left| x^2 + x + 3 \right| + \dfrac{1}{3}$ ln $\left| x + 1 \right| + C$;

partial fractions $\dfrac{-x}{3(x^2 + x + 3)} + \dfrac{1}{x^2 + x + 3} + \dfrac{1}{3(x + 1)}$.

16. $\dfrac{-(9x + 1)}{6(x + 1)^3} + C$;

partial fractions $\dfrac{3}{(x + 1)^3} - \dfrac{4}{(x + 1)^4}$.

PROBLEMS 39

1.   15/4.

2. $2 + \cosh 3 - \cosh 1$.

3. $3 + \pi^2/4$.

4. $3 \cdot 2^{2/3} + 16 \sqrt{2}/5$.

5. $1/\sqrt{5} \arctan (\sqrt{65}/13) + \sqrt{13}/18$.

6. $-\dfrac{1}{2} \ln 2 + \ln (1 + \sqrt{3}) + \sqrt{3}/2$.

7. $\ln 3 - \dfrac{1}{2} \ln 5$.

8. $\ln 2$.

9. $\ln (4 + \sqrt{17})$; write $5 + 4x + x^2 = 1 + (x + 2)^2$ and set $u = x + 2$.

10. $\dfrac{1}{2} \pi - 2 \arctan (1/2)$; write $1 + 4x - x^2 = 5 - (x - 2)^2$ and set $u = x - 2$.

11. $4\sqrt{6}$; set $u = x - 2$.

12. $2\sqrt{3}$; set $u = x - 1$.

13. $\arctan \pi/4$.

14. $\ln 3 - \dfrac{1}{2} \ln 5$; write $\dfrac{1}{x^2 - 1} = \dfrac{1}{2}\left[\dfrac{1}{x - 1} - \dfrac{1}{x + 1} \right]$.

15. $\arctan 3 - \arctan 2$; write $\dfrac{1}{x^2 + 4x + 5} = \dfrac{1}{(x + 2)^2 + 1}$ and set $u = x + 2$.

16. $\ln 4/3$; write $\dfrac{1}{x^2 - 3x + 2} = \dfrac{1}{x - 2} - \dfrac{1}{x - 1}$.

17. $\pi/12$; set $u = y^3$.

18. $\pi/4$.

19. $\pi/8 + 1/4$; use $\cos^2 \theta = \dfrac{1}{2} (1 + \cos 2\theta)$.

20. $\pi/8 - 1/4$; use $\sin^2 \theta = \dfrac{1}{2} (1 - \cos 2\theta)$.

21. 0.

22. $\arctan e - \pi/4$; set $u = e^x$.

23. $\pi/6 - \sqrt{3}/32$; use $\sin^2 4x = \dfrac{1}{2} (1 - \cos 8x)$.

24. $\ln (1 + \sqrt{2})$; use $\displaystyle\int \dfrac{dx}{\sqrt{(1 + x^2)}} = \ln \left| \sqrt{(x^2 + 1)} + x \right|$.

25. $\ln 2 - \ln\left(1 + \dfrac{1}{e}\right) = \ln 2 + 1 - \ln (1 + e)$; set $u = e^{-x}$

26. $2 \ln 2 - 1$; integrate by parts with $u = \ln (1 + x)$, $v = x$.

27. $\dfrac{1}{2} [\sqrt{2} + \ln (1 + \sqrt{2})]$; set $x = \sinh u$ to obtain

$$\int_0^1 \sqrt{(1 + x^2)}\,dx = \int_0^{\text{arcsin } 1} \cosh^2 u\, du, \text{ and then use}$$

$$\cosh^2 u = \dfrac{1}{2} [1 + \cosh 2u],$$

$$\sinh 2u = 2 \sinh u \cosh u, \text{arsinh } 1 = \ln (1 + \sqrt{2}),$$

$$\sinh (\text{arsinh } 1) = 1 \text{ and } \cosh (\text{arsinh } 1) = \sqrt{2}.$$

28. $\pi/4 - 1/2$; set $x = \sin^2 u$.

29. $2 - \ln 2$; set $u^2 = 2x + 1$.

30. $\pi/2 - 1$; integrate by parts with $u = \text{arc sin } x$, $v = x$.

31. $\pi/2 - \dfrac{1}{2} \ln 2$; integrate by parts with $u = \arctan x$, $v = x$.

32. $\pi/8$; integrate by parts with $u = \arcsin x$, $v = \dfrac{1}{2} x^2$.

33. $\pi/4 - \dfrac{1}{2}$; integrate by parts with $u = \arctan x$, $v = \dfrac{1}{2} x^2$.

34. π; set $u = 2 \sin u$ to obtain $16 \displaystyle\int_0^{\pi/2} \sin^2 u \cos^2 u\, du$, and then use

$$\sin^2 u = \dfrac{1}{2} (1 - \cos 2u), \cos^2 u = \dfrac{1}{2} (1 + \cos 2u) \text{ and}$$

$$\cos^2 2u = \dfrac{1}{2} (1 + \cos 4u).$$

35. 1; integrate by parts.

36. $\sqrt{2}\pi/8 + 1/\sqrt{2} - 1$; integrate by parts.

37. $\dfrac{1}{4} (e^2 + 1)$; integrate by parts.

38. $2 - 10/e^2$; integrate by parts.

39. $9 \ln 3 - (8/3) \ln 2 - 19/9$; integrate by parts twice.

40. $-2 \ln 3 + 3 \ln 2 + 1/6$; use partial fractions.

41. $7/48 - \dfrac{1}{4} \ln (3/2)$; use partial fractions.

42. $\pi/4 - \arctan (1/2) - \ln 5 + 3 \ln 2$; use partial fractions.

43. $3\pi/4 - (3/2) \arctan (1/2) - \dfrac{3}{4} \ln 5 + \dfrac{1}{2} \ln 3$; use partial fractions.

44. $\dfrac{1}{2} \arctan (1/2) + \dfrac{1}{4} \ln 3$; use partial fractions.

45. $J_2 = \pi/4$, $J_4 = 3\pi/16$, $J_6 = 5\pi/32$.

46. $J_2 = \pi/4$, $J_4 = 3\pi/16$, $J_6 = 5\pi/32$.

47. $J_3 = \dfrac{\pi}{3} - \dfrac{7}{9}$, $J_4 = \dfrac{3\pi^2}{64} - \dfrac{1}{4}$.

48. $J_4 = 4/3$, $J_6 = 28/15$.

PROBLEMS 40

1.   Convergent to 1.

2.   Convergent to 2.

3.   Convergent to $2\sqrt{2}$; set $u = 2 - x$.

4.   Divergent; set $u = x - 2$ and consider

$$\int_{-2}^{2} \frac{du}{u^2} = \lim_{\varepsilon \to 0} \int_{-2}^{-\varepsilon} \frac{du}{u} + \lim_{\delta \to 0} \int_{\delta}^{2} \frac{du}{u} = -1 + \lim_{\varepsilon \to 0} \frac{1}{\varepsilon} + \lim_{\delta \to 0} \frac{1}{\delta}.$$

This is indeterminate since ε and δ tend to zero independently of each other.

5.   Convergent to $\pi/4 - \dfrac{1}{2} \arctan (1/2)$.

6.   Divergent; integrate by parts.

7.   Convergent to $\pi/2$; a standard integral.

8.   Convergent to $1/2$; integrate by parts.

9.   Convergent to $\dfrac{1}{3} \ln (5/2)$; use partial fractions.

10. Convergent to $\pi/2$; write $\left(\dfrac{1 + 2x}{1 - 2x} \right)^{1/2} = \dfrac{(1 + 2x)^{1/2} \times (1 + 2x)^{1/2}}{(1 - 2x)^{1/2} \times (1 + 2x)^{1/2}}$

$$= \frac{1 + 2x}{\sqrt{(1 - 4x^2)}}.$$

11.   Divergent for $0 < \lambda \leqslant 1$ and convergent to $1/(\lambda - 1)$ for $\lambda > 1$; consider
      seperately the cases $0 < \lambda < 1$, $\lambda = 1$ and $\lambda > 1$.

12.   Convergent to 0; write

$$\int_{-\infty}^{\infty} xe^{-x^2}dx = \lim_{R_1 \to +\infty} \int_{-R_1}^{0} xe^{-x^2} + \lim_{R_2 \to +\infty} \int_{0}^{R_2} xe^{-x^2}dx$$

and set $u = x^2$.

13.   Divergent; consider

$$\int_{0}^{2} \frac{dx}{1-x^2} = \lim_{\varepsilon \to 0} \int_{0}^{1-\varepsilon} \frac{dx}{1-x^2} + \lim_{\delta \to 0} \int_{1+\delta}^{2} \frac{dx}{1-x^2}$$

and then write

$$\frac{1}{1-x^2} = \frac{1}{2}\left[\frac{1}{x+1} - \frac{1}{x-1}\right],$$

and thus obtain

$$\int_{0}^{2} \frac{dx}{1-x^2} = \frac{1}{2}\ln 3 + \lim_{\substack{\varepsilon \to 0 \\ \delta \to 0}} \frac{1}{2}\ln\left(\frac{\delta}{\varepsilon}\right).$$

The last limit is not defined since ε and δ tend to zero independently
of each other, so the quotient δ/ε is indeterminate.

14.   Divergent; set $x = e^y$.

PROBLEMS 41

1. $\int_{1}^{3} \frac{dx}{x} = \ln 3 - \ln 1 = \ln 3$; $I_{\text{trap}} = 1.103\,21$ (eight strips); $I_{\text{simp}} = 1.098\,73$

     (eight strips) .

2. $I_{\text{trap}} = 5.709\,43$ (six strips); $I_{\text{simp}} = 5.720\,84$ (six strips)

$$I = (2\arctan x + x\ln(1+x^2) - 2x)\Big|_{1}^{4} = 5.720\,54.$$

3. $I_{\text{simp}} = 1.547\,53$ (four strips); $I_{\text{simp}} = 1.549\,80$ (eight strips); remember x is
     in radians.

4. $I_{\text{trap}} = 8.400\,38$ (eight strips); $I_{\text{simp}} = 8.389\,79$ (eight strips)

$$I = (xe^x - e^x)\Big|_{0}^{2} = 8.389\,04.$$

5. $I_{simp} = 0.697\,31$ (four strips); $I_{simp} = 0.364\,01$ (eight strips); $\sin 3x$ oscillates in the interval and Simpson's rule with four strips cannot represent the integrand with sufficient accuracy. The result with eight strips is reasonably good but in practice the calculation would be repeated with 16 strips to determine the increase in accuracy. Remember x is in radians.

6. $I_{simp} = 3.801\,47$ (eight strips);

$$\int_{-1}^{2} \left(\frac{3+x}{3-x}\right)^{1/2} dx = \left\{ 6 \arctan\left[\left(\frac{3+x}{3-x}\right)^{1/2} \right] + (x-3)\left(\frac{3+x}{3-x}\right)^{1/2} \right\} \Bigg|_{-1}^{2} = 3.801\,05.$$

7. $I_{simp} = 1.910\,59$ (six strips); remember x is in radians.

8. $I_{simp} = -1.891\,15.$

PROBLEMS 42

1. $A = \displaystyle\int_{0}^{\pi} \left(3\sin 2x - \frac{1}{2}\cos x \right) dx = 3\pi.$

2. $A = 2\sqrt{2}$; $\cos x \geqslant \sin x$ in $0 \leqslant x \leqslant \pi/4$ and $\sin x \geqslant \cos x$ in $\pi/4 \leqslant x \leqslant \pi$,
so

$$A = \int_{0}^{\pi/4} (\cos x - \sin x) \, dx + \int_{\pi/4}^{\pi} (\sin x - \cos x) \, dx = 2\sqrt{2}.$$

3. $s = \sinh 3 - \sinh 1$; $s = \displaystyle\int_{1}^{3} \sqrt{(1 + \sinh^2 x)} \, dx = \int_{1}^{3} \cosh x \, dx = \sinh 3 - \sinh 1.$

4. $s = \dfrac{2}{27}(10\sqrt{10} - 1)$; $s = \displaystyle\int_{0}^{1} \sqrt{(1 + 9x)} \, dx = \dfrac{2}{27}(1 + 9x)^{3/2} \Big|_{0}^{1} = \dfrac{2}{27}(10\sqrt{10} - 1).$

5. $s = -\ln|\cos \pi/4| = 0.3466$; $dy/dx = \sec x$ so

$$s = \int_{0}^{\pi/4} \sqrt{(1 + \sec^2 x)} \, dx = \int_{0}^{\pi/4} \tan x \, dx$$

$$= (-\ln|\cos x|) \Big|_{0}^{\pi/4} = -\ln|\cos \pi/4|.$$

6. $s = 9866/405$; $s = \displaystyle\int_{1}^{3} \left(\frac{1 + x^8}{2\,x^4}\right)^{1/2} dx = \left(\frac{3x^8 - 5}{30x^4}\right) \Big|_{1}^{3} = \frac{9866}{405}.$

7.   Arc length between points corresponidng to $\theta = 0$ and $\theta = \pi/2$ is $3a/2$. Because of symmetry, and the fact the astroid has four arcs, the total length is $6a$; $X' = -3a \sin \theta \, \cos^2 \theta$, $Y' = 3a \cos \theta \, \sin^2 \theta$ so

$$\int_0^{\pi/2} \sqrt{\left[1 + \left(\frac{-\cos \theta \, \sin^2 \theta}{\sin \theta \, \cos^2 \theta} \right)^2 \right]} (-3a \sin \theta \, \cos^2 \theta) \, d\theta$$

$$= -3a \int_0^{\pi/2} \sqrt{(1 + \tan^2 \theta)} \, (\sin \theta \, \cos^2 \theta) \, d\theta.$$

As $\sec^2 \theta = 1 + \tan^2 \theta$ this becomes

$$s = -3a \int_0^{\pi/2} \sqrt{(\sec^2 \theta)} \, (\sin \theta \, \cos \theta) \, d\theta.$$

Now if s is to increase with θ we select the negative square root to obtain

$$s = 3a \int_0^{\pi/2} \sin \theta \, \cos \theta \, d\theta = \frac{3a}{2} \int_0^{\pi/2} \sin 2\theta \, d\theta = 3a/2.$$

8. $S = \dfrac{1}{2} \pi \, (2 + \sinh 4 - \sinh 2)$;

$$S = 2\pi \int_1^2 \cosh x \, \sqrt{(1 + \sinh^2 x)} \, dx$$

$$= 2\pi \int_1^2 \cosh^2 x \, dx$$

$$= 2\pi \int_1^2 \frac{1}{2} (1 + \cosh 2x) \, dx$$

$$= \frac{1}{2} \pi \, (2 + \sinh 4 - \sinh 2).$$

9. $S = \dfrac{5\pi}{27} [29 \sqrt{145} - 2 \sqrt{10}]$;

$$S = 2\pi \int_1^2 x^3 \sqrt{(1 + 9x^4)} \, dx$$

$$= \frac{\pi}{27} (1 + 9x^4)^{3/2} \Big|_1^2 = \frac{5\pi}{27} (29\sqrt{145} - 2\sqrt{10});$$

(set $u = 1 + 9x^4$).

10. $S = 4\pi \sqrt{2};\ S = 2\pi \int_1^3 (3-x) \sqrt{2}\ dx = 4\pi \sqrt{2}.$

11. $V = \dfrac{1}{4} \pi (4 + \sinh 4);\ V = \pi \int_0^2 \cosh^2 x\ dx;$ set $\cosh^2 x = \dfrac{1}{2}(1 + \cosh 2x).$

12. $V = \dfrac{1}{8} \pi (2 + \pi);\ V = \pi \int_{\pi/4}^{\pi/2} \sin^2 x\ dx;$ set $\sin^2 x = \dfrac{1}{2}(1 - \cos 2x).$

13. $V = \dfrac{1}{4} \pi (\pi^2 - 8);\ V = \pi \int_0^1 (\arcsin x)^2\ dx$

$$= \pi\ [x(\arcsin x)^2 + 2 \sqrt{(1 - x^2)}\ \arcsin x - 2x]\ \Big|_0^1$$

$$= \dfrac{1}{4} \pi (\pi^2 - 8);$$

integrate by parts twice starting with $u = (\arcsin x)^2$ and $v = x.$

14. $V = 2\pi \{[(\ln (2 + \sqrt{5})]^2 - \sqrt{5} \ln (2 + \sqrt{5}) + 2\};$

$$V = \pi \int_0^2 [\text{arsinh}\ x]^2\ dx$$

$$= \pi \{x[\ln (\sqrt{(x^2 + 1)} + x)]^2 - 2 \sqrt{(x^2 + 1)} \ln (\sqrt{(x^2 + 1)} + x) + 2x\}\ \Big|_0^2;$$

integrate by parts twice, starting with $u = (\text{arsinh}\ x)^2$ and $v = x.$

PROBLEMS 43

1. $\bar{x} = 13a/10,\ \bar{y} = 9a/10.$

2. $\bar{x} = 7a/3,\ \bar{y} = 0.$

3. $\bar{x} = a/3,\ \bar{y} = a/3;$ the hypotenuse of the triangle has the equation $y = a - x,$ so $f(x) = a - x,\ g(x) = 0$ for $0 \leqslant x \leqslant a$ and $\rho(x) = \rho_0.$

4. $\bar{x} = 2a/\sqrt{3},\ \bar{y} = a/3;$ the hypotenuse of the triangle has the equation $y = x/\sqrt{3},$ so $f(x) = x/\sqrt{3},\ g(x) = 0$ for $0 \leqslant x \leqslant a\sqrt{3}$ and $\rho(x) = \rho_0.$

5. $\bar{x} = 4R/3\pi,\ \bar{y} = 0;\ M_y = \int_0^R 2\rho_0 x \sqrt{(R^2 - x^2)}\ dx$ so setting $u^2 = R^2 - x^2$ (or $x = R \sin \theta$) it follows that $M_y = 2\rho_0 R^3/3.\ M = \tfrac{1}{2} \rho_0 \pi R^2,$ so $\bar{x} = M_y/M = 4R/3\pi.$

6. $\bar{x} = [b(a + 2c)]/[3(a + c)],\ \bar{y} = 0;$ the equation of the top of the trapezium is $y = a - [(a - c)/b]\ x$ and the equation of the bottom of the trapezium is

$y = -a + [(a-c)/b]x$ so $f(x) = a - [(a-c)/b]x$ and $g(x) = -a + [(a-c)/b]x$ for $0 \leqslant x \leqslant b$ and $\rho(x) = \rho_0$.

7. $\bar{x} = 0$, $\bar{y} = 8a^2/5$; here $f(x) = 4a^2 - x^2$, $g(x) = 0$ for $-2a \leqslant x \leqslant 2a$ and $\rho(x) = \rho_0$.

8. $\bar{x} = 3a/8$, $\bar{y} = 8a^2/5$; here $f(x) = 4a^2 - x^2$, $g(x) = 0$ for $0 \leqslant x \leqslant 2a$ and $\rho(x) = \rho_0$.

9. $\bar{x} = \dfrac{b}{2}\left[\dfrac{a(2+bk) + c(4+3bk)}{a(3+bk) + c(3+2bk)}\right]$, $\bar{y} = 0$; $f(x)$ and $g(x)$ are as in problem 6

but now $\rho(x) = \rho_0(1+kx)$;

$$M_y = \int_0^b 2x\rho_0(1+kx)\left[a - \left(\frac{a-c}{b}\right)x\right]dx$$

$$= \frac{\rho_0}{6}b^2[a(2+bk) + c(4+3bk)]$$

and

$$M = \int_0^b \rho_0 2(1+kx)\left[a - \left(\frac{a-c}{b}\right)x\right]dx$$

$$= \frac{\rho_0}{3}b[a(3+bk) + c(3+2bk)].$$

10. $\bar{x} = 4ka^2/5$, $\bar{y} = 8a^2/5$; $f(x)$ and $g(x)$ are as in problem 7 but now $\rho(x) = \rho_0(1+kx)$;

$$M_x = \frac{1}{2}\int_{-2}^{2a} \rho_0(1+kx)(4a^2 - x^2)^2\,dx = 256\,\rho_0 a^5/15,$$

$$M_y = \frac{1}{2}\int_{-2}^{2a} x\,\rho_0(1+kx)(4a^2 - x^2)\,dx = 128\,\rho_0 ka^5/15,$$

and

$$M = \int_{-2}^{2a} \rho_0(1+kx)(4a^2 - x^2)\,dx = 32\,\rho_0 a^3/3.$$

PROBLEMS 44

1. Centre of pressure lies on the vertical centre line of the plate at a depth $d = h + \frac{1}{3}b^2/h$ below the surface.

2. Let the vertical distance from the edge in the surface to the vertex below
    it be h. Then the centre of pressure lies at a depth $h/2$ below the surface
    on the median drawn from the submerged vertex.

3. The centre of pressure lies on the vertical centre line of the semicircle at
    a depth at a distance $3\pi R/16$ below the surface; the centroid lies on this
    same line at a distance $4R/3\pi$ below the surface.

4. Centre of pressure lies on vertical line of plate at $y = d$, with

$$d = -\left[\frac{32\,Rh + 3\pi(R^2 + 4h^2)}{4(4R - 3h)}\right];$$

    proceed as in Example 44.2 but integrate over the semicircle from
    $y = -R$ to $y = 0$, though now the integral of the odd function $y\sqrt{(R^2 - y^2)}$
    will not vanish because the limits are from $y = -R$ to $y = 0$,

$$F = 2\rho \int_{-R}^{0} (h - y)\,\sqrt{(R^2 - y^2)}\,dy$$

$$= 2\rho h \int_{-R}^{0} \sqrt{(R^2 - y^2)}\,dy - 2\rho \int_{-R}^{0} y\,\sqrt{(R^2 - y^2)}\,dy$$

$$= \frac{1}{2}\,\rho R^2 h - \frac{2\rho a^3}{3} = \frac{1}{6}\,\rho(3R^2 h - 4a^3),$$

$$M_L = 2\rho \int_{-R}^{0} (h - y)^2\,\sqrt{(R^2 - y^2)}\,dy$$

$$= 2\rho h \int_{-R}^{0} \sqrt{(R^2 - y^2)}\,dy - 4\rho h \int_{-R}^{0} y\,\sqrt{(R^2 - y^2)}\,dy + 2\rho \int_{-R}^{0} y^2\,\sqrt{(R^2 - y^2)}\,dy$$

$$= \frac{1}{2}\,\pi\rho R^2 h^2 + \frac{4}{3}\,\rho R^3 h + \frac{\pi\rho a^4}{8},$$

    and $d = M_L / F$

PROBLEMS 45

1. $I_y = Ma^2/3$ and $k_y = a/\sqrt{3}$; the mass per unit length $\rho(x) = M/(2a)$.

2. $I_y = 7Ma^2/12$ and $k_y = a\,\sqrt{(7/12)}$.

3. $I_L = \int_{-a/2}^{a/2} mx^2\left(1 + \frac{2x}{a}\right)dx = \frac{ma^3}{12}$,

$$\text{mass of rod } M = \int_{-a/2}^{a/2} mx^2 \left(1 + \frac{2x}{a}\right) dx = am, \text{ so}$$

$$k_L = a/\sqrt{12}.$$

4. $$I_L = 2\pi m \int_0^a r^3 \left(1 + \frac{r}{a}\right) dr = \frac{9\pi m a^2}{10},$$

    $$\text{mass of disc } M = 2\pi m \int_0^a r \left[1 + (r/a)\right] dr = (5\pi ma^2)/3, \text{ so}$$

    $$k_L = (I_L/M)^{1/2} = \frac{3}{5} \sqrt{\frac{3}{2}} \, a = \frac{3\sqrt{6}a}{10}.$$

5. $I = Ma^2/3$; argue as in Example 45.1 but with $\rho(x) = M/a^2$ the mass per unit area and consider a strip parallel to the edge about which the moment of inertia is required.

6. $I_L = M(R_1^2 + R_2^2)/2$; mass per unit area is $M/[\pi(R_2^2 - R_1^2)]$, so

    $$\Delta M = \frac{2Mr}{(R_2^2 - R_1^2)} \Delta r$$

    and hence

    $$\Delta I_L = \frac{2Mr^3}{(R_2^2 - R_1^2)} \Delta r.$$

    In the limit as $\Delta r \to 0$, by integrating over the annulus we have

    $$I_L = \frac{2M}{(R_2^2 - R_1^2)} \int_{R_1}^{R_2} r^3 \, dr = M(R_1^2 + R_2^2)/2.$$

PROBLEMS 46

1. Convergent to 1.

2. Convergent to 0.

3. Divergent; the terms oscillate boundedly between ± 1.

4. Divergent; $\lim_{n \to \infty} u_n = 1$ for n even and $\lim_{n \to \infty} u_n = -1/3$ for n odd.

5. Convergent to 0.

6. Convergent to zero for $|x| < 1$ and divergent for $|x| \geq 1$; the term $\sin(2n+1)\pi/2$ alternates in sign between ± 1.

7.   Divergent; as $n \to \infty$ so $u_n \approx \sin nx$ which has no limit.

8.   Convergent to 0.

9.   Dinvergent for $x \neq 0$, because $\cos n^2 x$ oscillates boundedly between ± 1 but convergent to 1 if $x = 0$.

10. Convergent to 0 for any finite x.

PROBLEMS 47

1.   Divergent by nth term test.

2.   Divergent by nth term test; because $\lim_{n \to \infty} [1 + (1/n)]^n = e$.

3.   Convergent; a geometric series with $r = 3/4$.

4.   Divergent; because $\Sigma (1/3)^n$ is a convergent geometric series but $\Sigma (6/5)^n$ is a divergent geometric series.

5.   Divergent by comparison with $\Sigma (1/n)$.

6.   Convergent; it is the sum of two convergent geometric series.

7.   Divergent by nth term test.

8.   Divergent by nth term test.

9.   Convergent by comparison with $\Sigma (1/2)^n$.

10. Divergent because $S_n = \ln 2 + \sum_{r=2}^{n} \ln \left(\dfrac{r+1}{r-1} \right) = \ln [n(n+1)]$ and $\lim_{n \to \infty} S_n = \infty$.

11. Convergent because by partial fractions and telescoping

$$S_n = \frac{1}{2} \left(1 + \frac{1}{2} - \frac{1}{n+1} - \frac{1}{n+2} \right) \text{ and } \lim_{n \to \infty} S_n = \frac{3}{4}.$$

12. Convergent because by partial fractions and telescoping

$$S_n = \frac{1}{2} \left(1 - \frac{1}{2n+1} \right) \text{ and } \lim_{n \to \infty} S_n = \frac{1}{2}.$$

13. Convergent by ratio test.

14. Ratio test fails, but divergent by nth term test.

15. Convergent by ratio test.

16. Convergent by alternating series test.

17. Convergent by alternating series test.

18. Absolutely convergent by ratio test.

19. Absolutely convergent by ratio test.

20. Ratio test fails; convergent by alternating series test but not absolutely convergent because the series of absolute values is divergent by comparison with $\Sigma\,(1/n)$.

21. $a_n = 1/\sqrt{(n+3)}$; ratio test fails but divergent by comparison with $\Sigma\,(1/n)$.

22. Convergent by nth root test.

23. Convergent by nth root test.

24. Convergent by integral test; $\displaystyle\int_1^\infty \frac{x\,\mathrm{d}x}{(x+1)^3} = 3/8.$

25. Divergent by integral test; $\displaystyle\int_1^\infty \frac{x\,\mathrm{d}x}{1+x^2} = \infty$; also seen to be divergent by comparison with $\Sigma\,(1/n)$.

26. Convergent by integral test;

$$\int_1^\infty \frac{\mathrm{d}x}{(2x+1)^2 - 1} = \left[\frac{1}{4}\ln\left(\frac{x}{x+1}\right)\right]_1^\infty = \frac{1}{4}\ln 2.$$

27. $\dfrac{n}{n^4+1} < \dfrac{1}{n^3}$ and $\Sigma\, 1/n^3$ is convergent as it is a p-series with $p = 3$. So series is convergent by comparison with $\Sigma\,(1/n^3)$.

28. Absolutely convergent by ratio test.

29. Absolutely convergent by nth root test; because

$$\left|a_n\right|^{1/n} = \frac{1}{\ln(2n+1)} \text{ and } \lim_{n\to\infty}\left|a_n\right|^{1/n} = 0.$$

30. Convergent by nth root test; because

$$\left|a_n\right|^{1/n} = \frac{\ln n}{n} \text{ and } \lim_{n\to\infty}\left|a_n\right|^{1/n} = 0;$$

to see this apply L'Hôpital's rule (Section 26) to

$$\lim_{n\to\infty}\left(\frac{\ln x}{x}\right) \text{ to show } \lim_{n\to\infty}\left(\frac{\ln x}{x}\right) = 0,$$

and then let $x \to \infty$ through integral values.

PROBLEMS 48

1. $r = 1$, $-1 < x < 1$.

2. $r = 3$, $-3 < x < 3$.

3. $r = 2$, $-2 < x < 2$.

4. $r = 2$, $-1 < x < 3$.

5. $r = 4$, $-5 < x < 3$.

6. $r = 1$, $1 < x < 3$.

7. $r = 0$; converges only when $x = 0$.

8. $r = e$; $-e < x < e$; use $\lim_{n \to \infty} [1 + (1/n)]^n = e$.

9. $r = \infty$, $-\infty < x < \infty$.

10. $r = 2$, $-2 < x < 2$.

11. $r = \infty$, $-\infty < x < \infty$.

12. $r = 1/10$, $-1/10 < x < 1/10$.

13. $r = 1$, $3 < x < 5$.

14. $r = 2$, $-2 < x < 2$.

15. $r = \sqrt{5}/2$, $-\sqrt{5}/2 < x < \sqrt{5}/2$.

16. $r = \sqrt{3}/2$, $-\sqrt{3}/2 < x < \sqrt{3}/2$.

17. $r = 1/e$, $-2 - (1/e) < x < -2 + (1/e)$; use the formula for r based on the nth root test and $\lim_{n \to \infty} [1 + (1/n)]^n = e$.

18. $r = 9/4$, $-5/4 < x < 13/4$; use the formula for r based on the nth root test.

19. $r = \sqrt{5}$, $-\sqrt{5} < x < \sqrt{5}$; write as

$$x \left[\frac{1}{5\sqrt{2}} - \frac{x^2}{5^2\sqrt{2}} + \frac{x^4}{5^3\sqrt{2}} - \cdots \right] = x \sum_{n=1}^{\infty} \frac{(-1)^{n+1} z^{n-1}}{5^n \sqrt{(n+1)}}$$

with $z = x^2$.

20. $r = 1$, $0 < x < 2$; write as

$$(x - 1) \sum_{n=1}^{\infty} \frac{z^{n-1}}{2n - 1}$$

with $z = (x - 1)^2$.

21. $r = 5$; $-2 < x < 8$.

22. $r = 0$; converges only when $x = -5$; use formula for r based on nth root test.

23. $r = 2$, $-2 < x < r$; set $z = x^2$.

24. $r = \sqrt{3}$, $-\sqrt{3} < x < \sqrt{3}$; write as

$$x \sum_{n=1}^{\infty} \frac{z^{n-1}}{3^n}$$

with $z = x^2$.

25. $r = 1,\ -1 < x < 1$; set $z = x^2$.

26. $r = 1,\ -1 < x < 1$; work from first principles and consider

$$\lim_{n \to \infty} \left| \frac{x^{n!}}{x^{(n+1)!}} \right| < 1.$$

PROBLEMS 49

1. $x + x^2 + \dfrac{x^3}{2} + \dfrac{x^4}{6}.$

2. $1 - 2x^2 + \dfrac{2x^4}{3} - \dfrac{4x^6}{45}.$

3. $1 + \alpha x + \dfrac{\alpha(\alpha - 1)}{2!} x^2 + \dfrac{\alpha(\alpha - 1)(\alpha - 2)}{3!} x^3.$

   (Do you recognize the binomial theorem?)

4. $1 + \dfrac{9}{2} x^2 + \dfrac{27}{8} x^4 + \dfrac{81}{80} x^6.$

5. $\dfrac{1}{2} x + \dfrac{1}{48} x^3 + \dfrac{1}{3840} x^5 + \dfrac{1}{645\,120} x^7.$

6. $\dfrac{2}{3} x - \dfrac{2}{9} x^2 + \dfrac{8}{81} x^3 - \dfrac{4}{81} x^4.$

7. $\sqrt{x} - \dfrac{x}{2} + \dfrac{x^{3/2}}{3} - \dfrac{x^2}{4}.$

8. $1 - \dfrac{x^2}{2} + \dfrac{3x^4}{8} - \dfrac{5x^6}{16}.$

9. $x + x^2 + \dfrac{x^3}{3} - \dfrac{x^5}{30}.$

10. $x + 2x^2 + \dfrac{13}{6} x^3 + \dfrac{5}{3} x^4.$

11. $-x + \dfrac{x^2}{2} - \dfrac{x^3}{3} - \dfrac{3}{40} x^5.$

12. $x + \dfrac{x^2}{2} + \dfrac{3}{8} x^3 + \dfrac{5}{16} x^4.$

13. $1 + x \ln a + \dfrac{x^2}{2} (\ln a)^2 + \dfrac{x^3}{6} (\ln a)^3$.

14. $x^2 - \dfrac{1}{3} x^4 + \dfrac{2}{45} x^6 - \dfrac{1}{315} x^8$.

15. $x - \dfrac{1}{3} x^3 + \dfrac{2}{15} x^5 - \dfrac{17}{315} x^7$.

16. $1 + \dfrac{1}{2} x^2 + \dfrac{5}{24} x^4 + \dfrac{61}{720} x^6$.

17. $\dfrac{1}{2} + \dfrac{\sqrt{3}}{2} x - \dfrac{1}{4} x^2 - \dfrac{\sqrt{3}}{13} x^3$.

18. $x - \dfrac{1}{6} x^3 + \dfrac{3}{40} x^5 - \dfrac{5}{112} x^7$.

19. $\dfrac{1}{4} x - \dfrac{1}{16} x^3 + \dfrac{1}{64} x^5 - \dfrac{1}{256} x^7$.

20. $1 + 4x + 7x^2 + 10x^3$

21. $(x - 1) - \dfrac{(x - 1)^2}{2} + \dfrac{(x - 1)^3}{3} - \dfrac{(x - 1)^4}{4}$.

22. $1 - (x - 1) + (x - 1)^2 - (x - 1)^3$.

23. $1 + 2(x + 1) + 3(x + 1)^2 + 4(x + 1)^3$.

24. $e^{-2} \left[1 + (x + 2) + \dfrac{(x + 2)^2}{2} + \dfrac{(x + 2)^3}{6} \right]$.

25. $2 + \dfrac{1}{4} (x - 4) - \dfrac{1}{64} (x - 4)^2 + \dfrac{1}{512} (x - 4)^3$.

26. $-\left(x - \dfrac{\pi}{2} \right) + \dfrac{1}{6} \left(x - \dfrac{\pi}{2} \right)^3 - \dfrac{1}{120} \left(x - \dfrac{\pi}{2} \right)^5 + \dfrac{1}{5040} \left(x - \dfrac{\pi}{2} \right)^7$.

27. $\displaystyle\int_0^x \dfrac{\sin t}{t}\, dt = x - \dfrac{x^3}{18} + \dfrac{x^5}{600} - \dfrac{x^7}{35\,280} + \ldots$

28. $\displaystyle\int_0^x \left(\dfrac{1 - \cos t}{t^2} \right) dt = \dfrac{1}{2} x - \dfrac{1}{72} x^3 + \dfrac{1}{360} x^5 - \dfrac{1}{282\,240} x^7 + \ldots$

29. $\displaystyle\int_0^x \dfrac{\ln (1 + 2t)}{t}\, dt = 2x - x^2 + \dfrac{8}{9} x^3 - x^4 + \dfrac{32}{25} x^5 - \ldots$

30. $\displaystyle\int_0^x (1 + t^2)^{1/3}\, dt = x + \dfrac{1}{9} x^3 - \dfrac{1}{45} x^5 + \dfrac{5}{567} x^7 - \ldots$

31. $\int_0^x \left(\frac{1 - e^{-t^2}}{t^2} \right) dt = x - \frac{1}{6} x^3 + \frac{1}{30} x^5 - \frac{1}{168} x^7 + \dots$

32. $\int_0^x \left(\frac{\cosh 2t - 1}{t^2} \right) dt = 2x + \frac{2}{9} x^3 + \frac{4}{225} x^5 + \frac{2}{2205} x^7 + \dots$

33. $\ln \left(\frac{1 + x}{1 - x} \right) = \ln (1 + x) - \ln (1 - x)$, so subtracting the series gives

$$\ln \left(\frac{1 + x}{1 - x} \right) = 2 \left(x + \frac{x^3}{3} + \frac{x^5}{5} + \frac{x^7}{7} + \dots \right)$$

34. $x^2 - \frac{1}{90} x^6$.

35. $1 + x + \frac{1}{2} x^2$.

36. $e \left(1 - \frac{1}{2} x^2 + \frac{1}{6} x^4 \right)$.

37. $x^2 - \frac{1}{3} x^4 + \frac{2}{45} x^6$.

38. $e \left(1 - x^2 + \frac{5}{6} x^4 \right)$.

39. 1.4958.

40. 1.3242.

41. 0.8019.

42. 1.1052.

43. − 0.4642.

44. 1.1058.

45. − 4.6369.

46. (a) 0.125; (b) 0.125; (c) 0.25.

PROBLEMS 50

1. $f(x, y) = 1 + x + \frac{1}{2} (x^2 - y^2) + \frac{1}{6} (x^3 - 3xy^2) + \dots$.

2. $f(x, y) = 1 + x + xy + \frac{1}{2} x^2 y + \dots$; to determine the partial derivatives take logarithms and differentiate $\ln f = (1 + y) \ln (1 + x)$.

3. $f(x, y) = 1 + (x - 2) + (y + 2) + \dfrac{[(x - 2) + (y + 2)]^2}{2} + \dfrac{[(x - 2) + (y + 2)]^3}{6} + \dots$

4. $f(x, y) = 1 - \dfrac{1}{2!}\left[x + \left(y - \dfrac{\pi}{2}\right)\right]^2 + \dfrac{1}{4!}\left[x + \left(y - \dfrac{\pi}{2}\right)\right]^4 + \dots$.

5. $(1, -2)$ is a local minimum.

6. $(1, 2)$ is a saddle point.

7. $(0, 1)$ is a local maximum.

8. $(-1/2, 0)$ is a local minimum.

9. $(0, 0)$ is a saddle point and $(1, -1)$ is a local minimum.

10. $(0,1)$ and $(0, -1)$ are saddle points.

11. $(1, 2)$ and $(1, -2)$ are saddle points, $(2, 1)$ is a local minimum and $(-2, -1)$ is a local maximum.

12. $(0, 0)$ is a local minimum, $(5, 6)$, $(5, -6)$, $(-5, 6)$ and $(-5, -6)$ are saddle points;

$$f_x = 0 \text{ implies } x(4x^2 - 3y^2 + 8) = 0$$

$$f_y = 0 \text{ implies } y(-3x^2 + 2y^2 + 3) = 0.$$

Stationary points occur when $x = 0$, $y = 0$, when $x = 0$ and $-3x^2 + 2y^2 + 3 = 0$, when $y = 0$ and $4x^2 - 3y^2 + 8 = 0$ and when $4x^2 - 3y^2 + 8 = 0$ and $-3x^2 + 2y^2 + 3 = 0$; thus at $(0, 0)$ and at the solutions of

$$4x^2 - 3y^2 + 8 = 0 \quad \text{and} \quad -3x^2 + 2y^2 + 3 = 0.$$

The solutions of $x = 0$ and $-3x^2 + 2y^2 + 3 = 0$ and of $y = 0$ and $4x^2 - 3y^2 + 8 = 0$ are complex and so must be discarded.

13. $(0, 0)$ the test fails, $(2/3, 0)$, $(0, 1/3)$ and $(2/9, 1/9)$ are saddle points.

$$f_x = 0 \text{ implies } 2y(3x + 3y - 1) = 0,$$

$$f_y = 0 \text{ implies } x(3x + 12y - 2) = 0.$$

Stationary points occur when $x = 0$ and $y = 0$, when $y = 0$ and $3x + 12y - 2 = 0$, when $x = 0$ and $3x + 3y - 1 = 0$ and when $3x + 3y - 1 = 0$ and $3x + 12y - 2 = 0$. In fact $(0, 0)$ is a saddle point, as can be seen by considering the behaviour of $f(x, y)$ along $x = y$ and $x = -y$.

14. $(0, 0)$ saddle point, test fails at $(1, 1)$, $(1, -1)$, $(-1, 1)$ and $(-1, -1)$; $f_x = y(1 - x^2) \exp\left[-\frac{1}{2}(x^2 + y^2)\right]$ and $f_y = x(1 - y^2) \exp\left[-\frac{1}{2}(x^2 + y^2)\right]$ so as $\exp\left[-\frac{1}{2}(x^2 + y^2)\right] \neq 0$ the stationary points are found by solving simultaneously

$$y(1 - x^2) = 0 \text{ and } x(1 - y^2) = 0.$$

PROBLEMS 51

1. $\dfrac{1}{2} + \dfrac{2}{\pi} \displaystyle\sum_{n=1}^{\infty} \dfrac{\sin (2n-1)x}{(2n-1)}.$

2. $\dfrac{1}{2} + \dfrac{2}{\pi} \displaystyle\sum_{n=1}^{\infty} (-1)^{n+1} \dfrac{\cos (2n-1)x}{(2n-1)}.$

3. $\dfrac{\pi}{4} + \sin x - \dfrac{2 \cos x}{\pi} - \dfrac{\sin 2x}{2} + \dfrac{\sin 3x}{3} - \dfrac{2 \cos 3x}{9\pi} - \dfrac{2 \sin 4x}{4} + \dfrac{\sin 5x}{5}$
   $- \dfrac{2 \cos 5x}{25\pi} - \dots .$

4. $\dfrac{\pi}{4} + \dfrac{4}{\pi} \displaystyle\sum_{n=1}^{\infty} \dfrac{\cos (2n-1)x}{(2n-1)^2}.$

5. $\dfrac{3\sqrt{3}}{2\pi} + \dfrac{3\sqrt{3}}{\pi} \displaystyle\sum_{n=1}^{\infty} (-1)^{n+1} \dfrac{\cos nx}{(9n^2-1)}.$

   The function is continuous at $x = 0$ with the value 1, so the series converges to 1, and thus

   $$1 = \dfrac{3\sqrt{3}}{2\pi} + \dfrac{3\sqrt{3}}{\pi} \sum_{n=1}^{\infty} \dfrac{(-1)^{n+1}}{(9n^2-1)},$$

   so

   $$\sum_{n=1}^{\infty} \dfrac{(-1)^{n+1}}{(9n^2-1)} = \dfrac{\pi}{3\sqrt{3}} - \dfrac{1}{2}.$$

6. $\dfrac{\pi^2}{3} + 4 \displaystyle\sum_{n=1}^{\infty} (-1)^n \dfrac{\cos nx}{n^2}$

   (a) The function is continuous at $x = 0$ with the value 0, so the series converges to 0, and thus

   $$\sum_{n=1}^{\infty} \dfrac{(-1)^{n+1}}{n^2} = \dfrac{\pi^2}{12}.$$

   (b) The function and its periodic extension are continuous at $x = \pi$ with the value π^2, so the series converges to π^2, and thus

   $$\dfrac{2}{3}\pi^2 = 4 \sum_{n=1}^{\infty} \dfrac{(-1)^n \cos nx}{n^2} = 4 \sum_{n=1}^{\infty} \dfrac{1}{n^2},$$

so

$$\sum_{n=1}^{\infty} \frac{1}{n^2} = \frac{\pi^2}{6}.$$

7. $\frac{1}{3\pi} + \frac{1}{2}\sin 3x + \frac{2}{\pi}\left[\frac{3}{5}\cos 2x - \frac{3}{7}\cos 4x - \frac{1}{9}\cos 6x - \frac{3}{55}\cos 8x \right.$

$\left. - \frac{3}{91}\cos 10x - \frac{1}{45}\cos 12x - \dots \right].$

8. $\frac{1}{\pi} + \frac{1}{2}\sin x - \frac{2}{\pi}\left[\frac{\cos 2x}{3} + \frac{\cos 4x}{15} + \frac{\cos 6x}{35} + \dots \right].$

9. $\frac{1}{2} + \frac{1}{2}\cos x + \frac{2}{\pi}\sum_{n=1}^{\infty}\frac{1}{(4n^2 - 1)}[2n\sin 2nx - (2n + 1)\sin (2n - 1)x].$

10. $\frac{2}{\pi} + \frac{4}{\pi}\sum_{n=1}^{\infty}(-1)^{n+1}\frac{\cos 2nx}{(4n^2 - 1)}.$

11. $\frac{2}{\pi} + \frac{2}{\pi}\sum_{n=1}^{\infty}\left(\frac{1 + (-1)^n}{1 - n^2}\right)\cos nx.$

12. $\frac{\pi}{4} - \frac{2}{\pi}\sum_{n=1}^{\infty}\frac{1}{(2n - 1)^2}\cos (4n - 2)x.$

PROBLEMS 52

1. 6.

2. 1.

3. $-5a.$

4. $-1 + 6i.$

5. $\lambda^2 - 5\lambda + 2.$

6. 1 (because $\sin^2 x + \cos^2 x = 1$).

7. 1 (because $\cosh^2 x - \sinh^2 x = 1$).

8. $-2.$

9. $M_{11} = \begin{vmatrix} 1 & 2 \\ 0 & 5 \end{vmatrix} = 5, \quad M_{12} = \begin{vmatrix} 2 & 2 \\ 1 & 5 \end{vmatrix} = 8, \quad M_{13} = \begin{vmatrix} 2 & 1 \\ 1 & 0 \end{vmatrix} = -1,$

$M_{21} = \begin{vmatrix} 3 & -1 \\ 0 & 5 \end{vmatrix} = 15, \quad M_{22} = \begin{vmatrix} 1 & -1 \\ 1 & 5 \end{vmatrix} = 6, \quad M_{23} = \begin{vmatrix} 1 & 3 \\ 1 & 0 \end{vmatrix} = -3,$

$$M_{31} = \begin{vmatrix} 3 & -1 \\ 1 & 2 \end{vmatrix} = 7, \quad M_{32} = \begin{vmatrix} 1 & -1 \\ 2 & 2 \end{vmatrix} = 4, \quad M_{33} = \begin{vmatrix} 1 & 3 \\ 2 & 1 \end{vmatrix} = -5.$$

10. $M_{11} = \begin{vmatrix} 2 & 1 \\ 1 & 3 \end{vmatrix} = 5, \quad M_{12} = \begin{vmatrix} 1 & 1 \\ -1 & 3 \end{vmatrix} = 4, \quad M_{13} = \begin{vmatrix} 1 & 2 \\ -1 & 1 \end{vmatrix} = 3,$

$$M_{21} = \begin{vmatrix} 1 & -2 \\ 1 & 3 \end{vmatrix} = 5, \quad M_{22} = \begin{vmatrix} -2 & -2 \\ -1 & 3 \end{vmatrix} = -8, \quad M_{23} = \begin{vmatrix} -2 & 1 \\ -1 & 1 \end{vmatrix} = -1,$$

$$M_{31} = \begin{vmatrix} 1 & -2 \\ 2 & 1 \end{vmatrix} = 5, \quad M_{32} = \begin{vmatrix} -2 & -2 \\ 1 & 1 \end{vmatrix} = 0, \quad M_{33} = \begin{vmatrix} -2 & 1 \\ 1 & 2 \end{vmatrix} = -5.$$

11. $C_{11} = 6, \quad C_{12} = -1, \quad C_{13} = -8,$
$C_{21} = -3, \quad C_{22} = 1, \quad C_{23} = 4,$
$C_{31} = -5, \quad C_{32} = 1, \quad C_{33} = 7.$

12. $C_{11} = -3, \quad C_{12} = 2, \quad C_{13} = -1,$
$C_{21} = 3, \quad C_{22} = 2, \quad C_{23} = -7,$
$C_{31} = 0, \quad C_{32} = -8, \quad C_{33} = 4.$

13. (a) $(-1) \begin{vmatrix} -2 & 3 \\ 2 & -3 \end{vmatrix} + 4 \begin{vmatrix} 4 & 3 \\ 2 & -3 \end{vmatrix} - \begin{vmatrix} 4 & -2 \\ 2 & 2 \end{vmatrix} = -60;$

(b) $3 \begin{vmatrix} 1 & 4 \\ 2 & 2 \end{vmatrix} + \begin{vmatrix} 4 & -2 \\ 2 & 2 \end{vmatrix} + (-3) \begin{vmatrix} 4 & -2 \\ 1 & 4 \end{vmatrix} = -60.$

14. (a) $3 \begin{vmatrix} 1 & 0 \\ -4 & 3 \end{vmatrix} + (2)(-1) \begin{vmatrix} 4 & -1 \\ -4 & 3 \end{vmatrix} + (-2) \begin{vmatrix} 4 & -1 \\ 1 & 0 \end{vmatrix} = -9;$

(b) $(4)(-1) \begin{vmatrix} 2 & 0 \\ -2 & 3 \end{vmatrix} + \begin{vmatrix} 3 & -1 \\ -2 & 3 \end{vmatrix} + (-4)(-1) \begin{vmatrix} 3 & -1 \\ 2 & 0 \end{vmatrix} = -9.$

15. $-\lambda^3 + 6\lambda^2 - 7\lambda - 3.$

16. $-\lambda^3 + 5\lambda^2 - 3\lambda + 6.$

17. (a) $\begin{vmatrix} 1 & 2 & 3 \\ 4 & 2 & 1 \\ 1 & 0 & 2 \end{vmatrix} = 2 \begin{vmatrix} 1 & 1 & 3 \\ 4 & 1 & 1 \\ 1 & 0 & 2 \end{vmatrix}$ (remove factor 2 from column (2))

$$= 2 \begin{vmatrix} 1 & 4 & 3 \\ 4 & 2 & 1 \\ 1 & 2 & 2 \end{vmatrix}$$ add column (3) to column (2)

$$= 2 \times (-8) = -16.$$

(b) $\begin{vmatrix} 1 & 4 & 3 \\ 0 & 2 & 1 \\ 4 & 2 & 1 \end{vmatrix} = (-1) \begin{vmatrix} 1 & 4 & 3 \\ 4 & 2 & 1 \\ 0 & 2 & 1 \end{vmatrix}$ interchange rows (2) and (3)

$$= (-1) \begin{vmatrix} 1 & 4 & 3 \\ 4 & 2 & 1 \\ -1 & -2 & -2 \end{vmatrix}$$ subtract row(2) from row (3)

$$= (-1)(-1) \begin{vmatrix} 1 & 4 & 3 \\ 4 & 2 & 1 \\ 1 & 2 & 2 \end{vmatrix} \qquad \text{remove factor } -1 \text{ from row (3)}$$

$$= -8.$$

18. $(a-b)(a-c)(a-d)(b-c)(b-d)(c-d)$

(proceed as in Example 52.12 and use the result that

$p^3 - q^3 = (p-q)(p^2 + pq + q^2)$).

19. This is an alternant with $a = 2$, $b = -3$ and $c = 4$, so from Example 52.12 we have

$$\Delta = (c-b)(c-a)(b-a) = [4-(-3)](4-2)(-3-2) = -70.$$

20. This is an alternant with $a = p+q$, $b = p+r$ and $c = p+s$, so from Example 52.12 we have

$$\Delta = (c-b)(c-a)(b-a) = (s-r)(s-q)(r-q).$$

21. $\Delta = -9$, $\Delta_1 = -9$, $\Delta_2 = -9$, $\Delta_3 = -18$, so $x_1 = 1$, $x_2 = 1$, $x_3 = 2$.

22. $\Delta = -6$, $\Delta_1 = 6$, $\Delta_2 = -27$, $\Delta_3 = -57$, so $x_1 = -1$, $x_2 = 9/2$, $x_3 = 19/2$.

23. $\Delta = 16$, $\Delta_1 = 20$, $\Delta_2 = -9$, $\Delta_3 = 5$, so $x_1 = 5/4$, $x_2 = -9/16$, $x_3 = 5/16$.

24. $\Delta = -3$, $\Delta_1 = -1$, $\Delta_2 = -6$, $\Delta_3 = 2$, so $x_1 = 1/3$, $x_2 = -2$, $x_3 = -2/3$.

PROBLEMS 53

1. $A+B = \begin{bmatrix} 1 & -1 \\ 5 & 5 \end{bmatrix}$, $A-B = \begin{bmatrix} 3 & 3 \\ 1 & 3 \end{bmatrix}$, $2A+3B = \begin{bmatrix} 1 & -4 \\ 12 & 11 \end{bmatrix}$.

2. $A+B = \begin{bmatrix} 6 & -1 & 5 \\ 0 & 0 & 1 \end{bmatrix}$, $A-B = \begin{bmatrix} -2 & 3 & 3 \\ -4 & 2 & -1 \end{bmatrix}$, $A-2B = \begin{bmatrix} -6 & 5 & 2 \\ -6 & 3 & -2 \end{bmatrix}$.

3. $A+C = \begin{bmatrix} 1 & 3 \\ 5 & -3 \end{bmatrix}$, $A-C = \begin{bmatrix} 3 & -1 \\ 1 & -1 \end{bmatrix}$, $B+D = \begin{bmatrix} -1 & 3 \\ 5 & 4 \\ 2 & -2 \end{bmatrix}$, $B-D = \begin{bmatrix} 3 & 1 \\ 1 & -2 \\ 0 & 2 \end{bmatrix}$;

$A \pm B$ and $C \pm D$ are not defined.

4. $a = -1$, $b = 4$, $c = 7$, $d = 3$, $e = -1$.

5. $a = 1$, $b = 2$, $c = 4$, $d = 14$, $e = -8$.

6. $\begin{bmatrix} \sin A \cos B + \cos A \sin B & \cos A \cos B + \sin A \sin B \\ \cosh A \cosh B + \sinh A \sinh B & \sinh A \cosh B - \cosh A \sinh B \end{bmatrix}$

$$= \begin{bmatrix} \sin (A+B) & \cos (A-B) \\ \cosh (A+B) & \sinh (A-B) \end{bmatrix}.$$

7. $A^T = \begin{bmatrix} 1 & 7 & 9 \\ 4 & 6 & 2 \\ 2 & 1 & 4 \end{bmatrix}$, $B^T = \begin{bmatrix} 1 & 5 & -9 \\ 5 & 0 & 6 \\ -9 & 6 & 3 \end{bmatrix}$ (**B** is symmetric).

8. $A^T = \begin{bmatrix} 1 & 0 \\ 3 & 2 \\ 7 & 5 \\ 2 & 3 \end{bmatrix}$, $B^T = \begin{bmatrix} 0 & -5 & -6 & -1 \\ 5 & 0 & 3 & 2 \\ 6 & -3 & 0 & -1 \\ 1 & -2 & 1 & 0 \end{bmatrix} = -B$ (**B** is skew-symmetric).

PROBLEMS 54

1. $AB = \begin{bmatrix} -6 & 9 \\ 8 & 32 \end{bmatrix}$, $BA = \begin{bmatrix} 32 & 18 \\ 4 & -6 \end{bmatrix}$.

2. $AB = \begin{bmatrix} 7 & 2 \\ 14 & -24 \\ 13 & 21 \end{bmatrix}$.

3. $AB = 4$, $BA = \begin{bmatrix} 2 & 8 & -6 & 4 \\ -1 & -4 & 4 & -2 \\ 2 & 8 & -6 & 4 \\ 6 & 24 & -18 & 12 \end{bmatrix}$.

4.   **AB** is not defined.

$BA = \begin{bmatrix} 10 & 10 & 1 & 22 \\ 2 & 0 & 0 & 26 \end{bmatrix}$.

5. $AB = 0$, $AC = 6$, $BD = \begin{bmatrix} 1 & 3 & -2 \\ 1 & 3 & -2 \\ 1 & 3 & -2 \\ 0 & 0 & 0 \end{bmatrix}$.

6. $AB = \begin{bmatrix} 11 & -11 \\ 21 & -26 \end{bmatrix}$, $BA = \begin{bmatrix} 4 & -13 \\ 5 & -19 \end{bmatrix}$.

7. $AB = \begin{bmatrix} 7 + 5i & 4 + 6i \\ 1 + 15i & -1 + 3i \end{bmatrix}$, $BA = \begin{bmatrix} 5 + 7i & -9 + i \\ 8 - 6i & 1 + i \end{bmatrix}$.

8. $AB = \begin{bmatrix} 7 - x^2 & x + 1 \\ 2 - 2x^2 & -x^2 - 4x + 1 \end{bmatrix}$, $BA = \begin{bmatrix} -x^2 - 4x + 1 & 1 - x \\ 2(x + 1)^2 & 7 - x^2 \end{bmatrix}$.

9.   **AB, BA,** and **CB** are not defined.

$AC = \begin{bmatrix} 31 & 12 \\ 10 & 4 \end{bmatrix}$, $CA = \begin{bmatrix} 7 & -1 & 8 \\ 16 & 2 & 20 \\ 20 & 5 & 26 \end{bmatrix}$, $BC = \begin{bmatrix} 15 & 7 \\ 0 & 5 \\ 9 & 7 \\ 33 & 10 \end{bmatrix}$.

10. **AB, AC, CA, BC** and **CB** are not defined.

$$BA = \begin{bmatrix} -21 & -1 & 26 & 19 \\ 8 & 9 & 22 & 2 \\ 11 & 0 & 13 & 5 \end{bmatrix}.$$

11. $A^3 = \begin{bmatrix} 30 & 9 & 43 \\ 25 & 80 & -9 \\ 9 & -25 & 30 \end{bmatrix}.$

12. $A^2 = \begin{bmatrix} 1 & 0 & 0 \\ 0 & 1 & 0 \\ 0 & 0 & 1 \end{bmatrix}, \quad A^3 = \begin{bmatrix} 0 & 0 & 1 \\ 0 & 1 & 0 \\ 1 & 0 & 0 \end{bmatrix}.$

As A^2 is the unit matrix, it follows that $A^n = A$ when n is odd and $A^n = I$ when n is even.

13. $A(B + C) = AB + AC = \begin{bmatrix} 18 & 0 \\ -9 & 0 \end{bmatrix}.$

14. $A(BC) = (AB)C = \begin{bmatrix} 22 & -22 \\ -11 & 11 \end{bmatrix}.$

15. $A^T B = \begin{bmatrix} -4 & 8 \\ 9 & 10 \end{bmatrix}, \quad B^T A = \begin{bmatrix} -4 & 9 \\ 8 & 10 \end{bmatrix}.$

16. $AB = \begin{bmatrix} -13 & 0 & 0 \\ 0 & -13 & 0 \\ 0 & 0 & -13 \end{bmatrix} = -13 \begin{bmatrix} 1 & 0 & 0 \\ 0 & 1 & 0 \\ 0 & 0 & 1 \end{bmatrix} = -13I.$

17. $A^2 = \begin{bmatrix} 1 - 2\cos^2 x & -2\sin x \cos x \\ 2\sin x \cos x & 2\cos^2 x - 1 \end{bmatrix} = \begin{bmatrix} -\cos 2x & -\sin 2x \\ \sin 2x & -\cos 2x \end{bmatrix}.$

18. $A^2 = \begin{bmatrix} 2\cos^2 x - 1 & 2\sin x \cos x \\ -2\sin x \cos x & 2\cos^2 x - 1 \end{bmatrix} = \begin{bmatrix} \cos 2x & \sin 2x \\ -\sin 2x & \cos 2x \end{bmatrix}.$

19. $AB = \begin{bmatrix} 4 & 5 & 6 \\ 7 & 8 & 9 \\ 1 & 2 & 3 \end{bmatrix}$; premultiplication of **B** by **A**, which is matrix obtained

from the unit matrix **I** by interchanging its rows, has interchanged the rows of **A** in the **same** order.

20. $3x + 4y + 7z = -19$

$-2x + z = 6$

$4x + 3y - 2z = 4.$

21. $A = \begin{bmatrix} 1 & 6 & -7 & 8 \\ 3 & -1 & 4 & 9 \\ 1 & 0 & 2 & 1 \\ 0 & 4 & -6 & 7 \end{bmatrix}, \quad X = \begin{bmatrix} x \\ y \\ z \\ u \end{bmatrix}, \quad B = \begin{bmatrix} -1 \\ 3 \\ -14 \\ 0 \end{bmatrix}.$

22. $QA = \begin{bmatrix} 1 & 0 \\ 0 & 1 \end{bmatrix}$. The system is $AX = B$, with

$$A = \begin{bmatrix} 4 & 1 \\ 3 & 2 \end{bmatrix}, \quad X = \begin{bmatrix} x \\ y \end{bmatrix} \text{ and } B = \begin{bmatrix} 1 \\ -1 \end{bmatrix}.$$

Thus $QAX = QB$, but $QA = I$ and $IX = X$, so $X = QB$.

Substituting for X, Q and B gives

$$\begin{bmatrix} x \\ y \end{bmatrix} = \begin{bmatrix} 2/5 & -1/5 \\ -3/5 & 4/5 \end{bmatrix} \begin{bmatrix} 1 \\ -1 \end{bmatrix}$$

$$= \begin{bmatrix} 3/5 \\ -7/5 \end{bmatrix},$$

and so $x = 3/5$, $y = -7/5$.

23. $x^2 + 6xy + 8xz - 2y^2 + 2yz + 2z^2$.

24. $2x^2 - 2xy + 6xz + y^2 - 4yz + 5z^2$.

PROBLEMS 55

1. $A^{-1} = \begin{bmatrix} 2/29 & 3/29 \\ 9/29 & -1/29 \end{bmatrix}$.

2. $A^{-1} = \begin{bmatrix} -1/21 & 5/21 \\ 5/21 & -4/21 \end{bmatrix}$.

3. $A^{-1} = \begin{bmatrix} 1/16 & 3/8 \\ -1/8 & 1/4 \end{bmatrix}$.

4. $A^{-1} = \begin{bmatrix} -2/19 & 7/19 \\ 1/19 & 6/19 \end{bmatrix}$.

5. $A^{-1} = \begin{bmatrix} -(1+8i)/13 & (-1+5i)/13 \\ (3-2i)/13 & (3-2i)/13 \end{bmatrix}$.

6. $A^{-1} = \begin{bmatrix} (1+i)/6 & -(1+3i)/6 \\ 1/3 & (-1+i)/6 \end{bmatrix}$.

7. $A^{-1} = \begin{bmatrix} 2/7 & 5/14 & -18/7 \\ -1/7 & 1/14 & 9/7 \\ 1/7 & -1/14 & -2/7 \end{bmatrix}$.

8. $A^{-1} = \begin{bmatrix} 0 & -1 & 1 \\ 0 & 1 & 0 \\ 1 & 0 & 0 \end{bmatrix}$.

9. $A^{-1} = \begin{bmatrix} -1/3 & 1/3 & 1/3 \\ 0 & 1/2 & 0 \\ 1/3 & -4/3 & 2/3 \end{bmatrix}$.

10. $A^{-1} = \begin{bmatrix} 1/32 & 11/32 & -5/32 \\ -1/4 & 1/4 & 1/4 \\ 3/16 & 1/16 & 1/16 \end{bmatrix}$.

11. $A^{-1} = \begin{bmatrix} -1/6 & 1/3 & 1/6 \\ 1/2 & 0 & -1/2 \\ -2/3 & -2/3 & 5/3 \end{bmatrix}$, so $(A^{-1})^T = \begin{bmatrix} -1/6 & 1/2 & -2/3 \\ 1/3 & 0 & -2/3 \\ 1/6 & -1/2 & 5/3 \end{bmatrix}$,

$A^T = \begin{bmatrix} 2 & 3 & 2 \\ 4 & 1 & 2 \\ 1 & 0 & 1 \end{bmatrix}$, so $(A^T)^{-1} = \begin{bmatrix} -1/6 & 1/2 & -2/3 \\ 1/3 & 0 & -2/3 \\ 1/6 & -1/2 & 5/3 \end{bmatrix}$.

12. $(AB)^{-1} = \begin{bmatrix} 5 & 9 & 12 \\ 3 & 2 & 4 \\ 7 & 6 & 29 \end{bmatrix}^{-1} = \begin{bmatrix} -2/9 & -1/3 & 4/9 \\ 1/27 & -13/9 & 16/27 \\ 4/27 & 11/9 & -17/27 \end{bmatrix}$,

$B^{-1}A^{-1} = \begin{bmatrix} 1/3 & 0 & -1/3 \\ -2/9 & 2/3 & -1/9 \\ 1/9 & -1/3 & 5/9 \end{bmatrix} \begin{bmatrix} 1/3 & 0 & 2/3 \\ 0 & -2 & 1 \\ 1/3 & 1 & -2/3 \end{bmatrix}$

$= \begin{bmatrix} -2/9 & -1/3 & 4/9 \\ 1/27 & -13/9 & 16/27 \\ 4/27 & 11/9 & -17/27 \end{bmatrix}$.

13. $(ABC)^{-1} = C^{-1}B^{-1}A^{-1} = \dfrac{1}{210}\begin{bmatrix} 23 & -36 \\ 2 & 6 \end{bmatrix}$.

14. $((AB)^T)^{-1} = \begin{bmatrix} 1 & -3 \\ 15 & -1 \end{bmatrix}^{-1} = \begin{bmatrix} -1/44 & 3/44 \\ -15/44 & 1/44 \end{bmatrix}$.

$(A^{-1})^T (B^{-1})^T = \begin{bmatrix} 2/11 & -3/11 \\ 1/11 & 4/11 \end{bmatrix}^T \begin{bmatrix} 1/4 & -3/4 \\ 1/4 & 1/4 \end{bmatrix}^T$

$= \begin{bmatrix} 2/11 & 1/11 \\ -3/11 & 4/11 \end{bmatrix} \begin{bmatrix} 1/4 & 1/4 \\ -3/4 & 1/4 \end{bmatrix} = \begin{bmatrix} -1/44 & 3/44 \\ -15/44 & 1/44 \end{bmatrix}$,

and so we have verified that

$$((AB)^T)^{-1} = (A^{-1})^T(B^{-1})^T.$$

15. $A^{-1} = \begin{bmatrix} -1/19 & 11/19 & -4/19 \\ 3/19 & 5/19 & -7/19 \\ 2/19 & -3/19 & 8/19 \end{bmatrix}$, so $\begin{bmatrix} x \\ y \\ z \end{bmatrix} = A^{-1}\begin{bmatrix} 1 \\ 3 \\ -5 \end{bmatrix} = \begin{bmatrix} 52/19 \\ 53/19 \\ -47/19 \end{bmatrix}$,

and thus $x = 52/19$, $y = 53/19$, $z = -47/19$.

16. $A^{-1} = \begin{bmatrix} -1/6 & 11/18 & -1/18 \\ 1/3 & -2/9 & 1/9 \\ -1/6 & -1/18 & 5/18 \end{bmatrix}$, so $\begin{bmatrix} x \\ y \\ z \end{bmatrix} = A^{-1} \begin{bmatrix} 2 \\ 1 \\ 4 \end{bmatrix} = \begin{bmatrix} 1/18 \\ 8/9 \\ 13/18 \end{bmatrix}$,

and thus $x = 1/18$, $y = 8/9$, $z = 13/18$.

PROBLEMS 56

1. $x = -5/16$, $y = -7/16$.

2. $x = 19/21$, $y = 5/21$.

3. $x = -11/31$, $y = 39/31$.

4. $x = 11/17$, $y = -8/17$.

5. $x = 2.8925$, $y = -0.2842$.

6. $x = -0.1220$, $y = 0.8537$.

7. $x = -2$, $y = -9/5$, $z = -13/5$.

8. $x = 16/9$, $y = 7/9$, $z = -5/3$.

9. $x = -71/49$, $y = 1/7$, $z = 74/49$.

10. $x = -32/3$, $y = 97/3$, $z = -10/3$.

11. $x = 0.4660$, $y = 11.6104$, $z = 8.8083$.

12. $x = -0.2231$, $y = 1.5252$, $z = -0.7089$.

13. $x = 0.3070$, $y = 0.2958$, $z = 0.0270$.

14. $x = 0.7026$, $y = 0.1922$, $z = 0.8373$.

15. No solution.

16. $x = -9/8$, $y = 5/8$, $z = 0$.

17. $x = (10k - 8)/7$, $y = -(8k - 5)/7$, $z = k$ (k a parameter).

18. No solution.

19. Only solution is $x = y = z = 0$.

20. $x = 7k/5$, $y = k/5$, $z = k$ (k a parameter).

21. $x = -k/7$, $y = -10k/7$, $z = k$ (k a parameter).

22. $x = -k$, $y = 0$, $z = k$ (k a parameter).

23. No solution if $p \neq 3$; unique solution, $x = 2$, $y = -3$ if $p = 1/3$.

24. No solution if $p \neq 19/7$; $x = 9k/10$, $y = -7k/10$, $z = k$ if $p = 19/7$ (k a parameter).

PROBLEMS 57

1. System is already in diagonally dominant form.

(a)

n	$x_1^{(n)}$	$x_2^{(n)}$
0	0	0
1	1.2390	-0.1642
2	1.1590	-0.1367
3	1.1724	-0.1413
4	1.1701	-0.1405
5	1.1705	-0.1407

(b)

n	$x_1^{(n)}$	$x_2^{(n)}$
0	1	1
1	1.7262	-0.3320
2	1.0772	-0.1086
3	1.1861	-0.1460
4	1.1678	-0.1397
5	1.1709	-0.1408

2. Interchange the equations to bring them into diagonally dominant form.

(a)

n	$x_1^{(n)}$	$x_2^{(n)}$
0	0	0
1	0.3683	-0.4699
2	0.5705	-0.4185
3	0.5484	-0.4241
4	0.5508	-0.4235
5	0.5505	-0.4236

(b)

n	$x_1^{(n)}$	$x_2^{(n)}$
0	1	1
1	-0.0621	-0.5794
2	0.6176	-0.4065
3	0.5432	-0.4254
4	0.5514	-0.4233
5	0.5505	-0.4236

3. Interchange the equations to bring them into diagonally dominant form.

(a)

n	$x_1^{(n)}$	$x_2^{(n)}$
0	0	0
1	0.8020	-0.7408
2	0.9736	-0.8125
3	0.9903	-0.8194
4	0.9919	-0.8201
5	0.9920	-0.8201

(b)

n	$x_1^{(n)}$	$x_2^{(n)}$
0	1	1
1	0.5702	-0.6440
2	0.9512	-0.8031
3	0.9881	-0.8185
4	0.9917	-0.8200
5	0.9920	-0.8201

4. System is already in diagonally dominant form.

(a)

n	$x_1^{(n)}$	$x_2^{(n)}$
0	0	0
1	-0.5753	-0.9776
2	-0.2494	-0.9110
3	-0.2716	-0.9156
4	-0.2701	-0.9152
5	-0.2702	-0.9153

(b)

n	$x_1^{(n)}$	$x_2^{(n)}$
0	1	1
1	-0.9086	-1.0458
2	-0.2267	-0.9064
3	-0.2731	-0.9159
4	-0.2700	-0.9152
5	-0.2702	-0.9153

5. Interchange the equations to bring them into diagonally dominant form.

	n	$x_1^{(n)}$	$x_2^{(n)}$
	0	0	0
	1	-0.9086	-1.0458
(a)	2	0.1323	-0.7024
	3	-0.0044	-0.7683
	4	0.0315	-0.7510
	5	0.0221	-0.7555

Working with the equations in their original non-diagonally dominant form.

	n	$x_1^{(n)}$	$x_2^{(n)}$
	0	0	0
	1	1.5887	-3.6232
(b)	2	-5.9243	10.1508
	3	22.6373	-42.2123
	4	-85.9424	156.8505
	5	326.8329	-599.9042

6. Write first equation last to express system in diagonally dominant form.

n	$x_1^{(n)}$	$x_2^{(n)}$	$x_3^{(n)}$
0	0	0	0
1	0.2456	1.5527	0.8288
2	-0.6591	1.5529	1.0164
3	-0.7104	1.5080	1.0038
4	-0.6873	1.5052	0.9976
5	-0.9844	1.5064	0.9976

7. Write last equation first to express system in diagonally dominant form.

n	$x_1^{(n)}$	$x_2^{(n)}$	$x_3^{(n)}$
0	0	0	0
1	0.5880	0.0088	-0.0706
2	0.6195	-0.0259	-0.0779
3	0.6158	-0.0260	-0.0786
4	0.6160	-0.0263	-0.0787
5	0.6160	-0.0263	-0.0787

8. Write first equation last to express system in diagonally dominant form.

n	$x_1^{(n)}$	$x_2^{(n)}$	$x_3^{(n)}$
0	0	0	0
1	1.3205	-0.2898	0.1741
2	1.1618	-0.1847	0.1708
3	1.1996	-0.2000	0.1682
4	1.1951	-0.1990	0.1688
5	1.1953	-0.1989	0.1687

9. Write first equation second to express system in diagonally dominant form.

n	$x_1^{(n)}$	$x_2^{(n)}$	$x_3^{(n)}$
0	0	0	0
1	0.2654	-0.4106	0.0494
2	0.3513	-0.3716	-0.0061
3	0.3544	-0.3855	-0.0037
4	0.3571	-0.3840	-0.0055
5	0.3572	-0.3845	-0.0054

10. Write second equation third to express system in diagonally dominant form.

n	$x_1^{(n)}$	$x_2^{(n)}$	$x_3^{(n)}$
0	0	0	0
1	0.2883	-0.4808	-0.3931
2	0.3378	-0.6143	-0.3642
3	0.3809	-0.5969	-0.3813
4	0.3725	-0.6044	-0.3766
5	0.3755	-0.6023	-0.3781

PROBLEMS 58

1. $\lambda^2 - 7\lambda + 6 = 0$; $\lambda_1 = 1$, $\lambda_2 = 6$;

$$X_1 = \begin{bmatrix} 1 \\ -1 \end{bmatrix}, \ X_2 = \begin{bmatrix} 4 \\ 1 \end{bmatrix}, \ \hat{X}_1 = \frac{(\pm 1)}{\sqrt{2}} \begin{bmatrix} 1 \\ -1 \end{bmatrix}, \ \hat{X}_2 = \frac{(\pm 1)}{\sqrt{17}} \begin{bmatrix} 4 \\ 1 \end{bmatrix}.$$

2. $\lambda^2 - 3\lambda - 4 = 0$; $\lambda_1 = -1$, $\lambda_2 = 4$;

$$X_1 = \begin{bmatrix} 1 \\ -1 \end{bmatrix},\ X_2 = \begin{bmatrix} 2 \\ 3 \end{bmatrix},\ \hat{X}_1 = \frac{(\pm 1)}{\sqrt{2}} \begin{bmatrix} 1 \\ -1 \end{bmatrix},\ \hat{X}_2 = \frac{(\pm 1)}{\sqrt{13}} \begin{bmatrix} 2 \\ 3 \end{bmatrix}.$$

3. $\lambda^2 - 4\lambda - 5 = 0$; $\lambda_1 = -1$, $\lambda_2 = 5$;

$$X_1 = \begin{bmatrix} 1 \\ -1 \end{bmatrix},\ X_2 = \begin{bmatrix} 1 \\ 2 \end{bmatrix},\ \hat{X}_1 = \frac{(\pm 1)}{\sqrt{2}} \begin{bmatrix} 1 \\ -1 \end{bmatrix},\ \hat{X}_2 = \frac{(\pm 1)}{\sqrt{5}} \begin{bmatrix} 1 \\ 2 \end{bmatrix}.$$

4. $\lambda^2 - 7\lambda + 10 = 0$; $\lambda_1 = 2$, $\lambda_2 = 5$;

$$X_1 = \begin{bmatrix} 1 \\ -2 \end{bmatrix},\ X_2 = \begin{bmatrix} 1 \\ 1 \end{bmatrix},\ \hat{X}_1 = \frac{(\pm 1)}{\sqrt{5}} \begin{bmatrix} 1 \\ -2 \end{bmatrix},\ \hat{X}_2 = \frac{(\pm 1)}{\sqrt{2}} \begin{bmatrix} 1 \\ 1 \end{bmatrix}.$$

5. $\lambda^3 - 10\lambda^2 + 27\lambda - 18 = 0$; as $\lambda = 3$ is a root of the charateristic equation, $(\lambda - 3)$ is a factor, so division by $(\lambda - 3)$ shows the other eigenvalues to be roots of $\lambda^2 - 7\lambda + 6 = 0$. Thus the other eigenvalues are $\lambda = 1$ and $\lambda = 6$, and hence the eigenvalues are $\lambda_1 = 1$, $\lambda_2 = 3$, $\lambda_3 = 6$;

$$X_1 = \begin{bmatrix} 1 \\ -1 \\ 0 \end{bmatrix},\ X_2 = \begin{bmatrix} 1 \\ -1 \\ -2 \end{bmatrix},\ X_3 = \begin{bmatrix} 1 \\ 2 \\ 1 \end{bmatrix};$$

$$\hat{X}_1 = \frac{(\pm 1)}{\sqrt{2}} \begin{bmatrix} 1 \\ -1 \\ 0 \end{bmatrix},\ \hat{X}_2 = \frac{(\pm 1)}{\sqrt{6}} \begin{bmatrix} 1 \\ -1 \\ -2 \end{bmatrix},\ \hat{X}_3 = \frac{(\pm 1)}{\sqrt{6}} \begin{bmatrix} 1 \\ 2 \\ 1 \end{bmatrix}.$$

6. $\lambda^3 - 10\lambda^2 + 23\lambda - 14 = 0$; as $\lambda = 1$ is a root, $(\lambda - 1)$ is a factor, so division by $(\lambda - 1)$ shows the other eigenvalues to be roots of $\lambda^2 - 9\lambda + 14 = 0$. Thus the other eigenvalues are $\lambda = 2$ and $\lambda = 7$, and hence the eigenvalues are $\lambda_1 = 1$, $\lambda_2 = 2$, $\lambda_3 = 7$;

$$X_1 = \begin{bmatrix} 1 \\ 2 \\ -2 \end{bmatrix},\ X_2 = \begin{bmatrix} -2 \\ 1 \\ 2 \end{bmatrix},\ X_3 = \begin{bmatrix} 1 \\ 2 \\ 4 \end{bmatrix};$$

$$\hat{X}_1 = \frac{(\pm 1)}{3} \begin{bmatrix} 1 \\ 2 \\ -2 \end{bmatrix},\ \hat{X}_2 = \frac{(\pm 1)}{3} \begin{bmatrix} -2 \\ 1 \\ 2 \end{bmatrix},\ \hat{X}_3 = \frac{(\pm 1)}{\sqrt{21}} \begin{bmatrix} 1 \\ 2 \\ 4 \end{bmatrix}.$$

7. $\lambda^3 - 6\lambda^2 + 11\lambda - 6 = 0$; as $\lambda = 1$ is a root of the charateristic equation, $(\lambda - 1)$ is a factor. Division by $(\lambda - 1)$ shows the other eigenvalues to be roots of $\lambda^2 - 5\lambda + 6 = 0$. Thus the other eigenvalues are $\lambda = 2$ and $\lambda = 3$, and hence the eigenvalues are $\lambda_1 = 1$, $\lambda_2 = 2$, $\lambda_3 = 3$;

$$X_1 = \begin{bmatrix} 2 \\ -1 \\ 1 \end{bmatrix},\ X_2 = \begin{bmatrix} 3 \\ -1 \\ 2 \end{bmatrix},\ X_3 = \begin{bmatrix} 2 \\ -1 \\ 2 \end{bmatrix};$$

$$\hat{X}_1 = \frac{(\pm 1)}{\sqrt{6}} \begin{bmatrix} 2 \\ -1 \\ 1 \end{bmatrix}, \ \hat{X}_2 = \frac{(\pm 1)}{\sqrt{14}} \begin{bmatrix} 3 \\ -1 \\ 2 \end{bmatrix}, \ \hat{X}_3 = \frac{(\pm 1)}{3} \begin{bmatrix} 2 \\ -1 \\ 2 \end{bmatrix}.$$

8. $\lambda^3 + 2\lambda^2 - \lambda - 2 = 0$; as $\lambda = -1$ is a root of the charateristic equation, $(\lambda + 1)$ is a factor. Division by $(\lambda + 1)$ shows the other eigenvalues to be roots of $\lambda^2 + \lambda - 2 = 0$. Thus the other eigenvalues are $\lambda = 1$ and $\lambda = -2$, and hence the eigenvalues are $\lambda_1 = -2$, $\lambda_2 = -1$ and $\lambda_3 = 1$;

$$X_1 = \begin{bmatrix} 1 \\ -2 \\ 4 \end{bmatrix}, \ X_2 = \begin{bmatrix} 1 \\ -1 \\ 1 \end{bmatrix}, \ X_3 = \begin{bmatrix} 1 \\ 1 \\ 1 \end{bmatrix};$$

$$\hat{X}_1 = \frac{(\pm 1)}{\sqrt{21}} \begin{bmatrix} 1 \\ -2 \\ 4 \end{bmatrix}, \ \hat{X}_2 = \frac{(\pm 1)}{\sqrt{3}} \begin{bmatrix} 1 \\ -1 \\ 1 \end{bmatrix}, \ \hat{X}_3 = \frac{(\pm 1)}{\sqrt{3}} \begin{bmatrix} 1 \\ 1 \\ 1 \end{bmatrix}.$$

9. $\lambda^3 - \lambda = 0$; $\lambda_1 = -1$, $\lambda_2 = 0$, $\lambda_3 = 1$;

$$X_1 = \begin{bmatrix} 1 \\ -2 \\ -3 \end{bmatrix}, \ X_2 = \begin{bmatrix} 2 \\ -1 \\ 4 \end{bmatrix}, \ X_3 = \begin{bmatrix} 1 \\ 0 \\ -1 \end{bmatrix};$$

$$\hat{X}_1 = \frac{(\pm 1)}{\sqrt{14}} \begin{bmatrix} 1 \\ -2 \\ -3 \end{bmatrix}, \ \hat{X}_2 = \frac{(\pm 1)}{\sqrt{21}} \begin{bmatrix} 2 \\ -1 \\ 4 \end{bmatrix}, \ \hat{X}_3 = \frac{(\pm 1)}{\sqrt{2}} \begin{bmatrix} 1 \\ 0 \\ -1 \end{bmatrix}.$$

10. $\lambda^3 - 17\lambda^2 - 156\lambda - 288 = 0$; as $\lambda = -3$ is a root of the charateristic equation, $(\lambda + 3)$ is a factor. Division by $(\lambda + 3)$ shows the other eigenvalues to be roots of $\lambda^2 - 20\lambda - 96 = 0$. Thus the other eigenvalues are $\lambda = -4$ and $\lambda = 24$, and hence the eigenvalues are $\lambda_1 = -4$, $\lambda_2 = -3$, $\lambda_3 = 24$;

$$X_1 = \begin{bmatrix} 1 \\ 0 \\ -1 \end{bmatrix}, \ X_2 = \begin{bmatrix} 1 \\ 1 \\ 1 \end{bmatrix}, \ X_3 = \begin{bmatrix} 1 \\ -2 \\ 1 \end{bmatrix};$$

$$\hat{X}_1 = \frac{(\pm 1)}{\sqrt{2}} \begin{bmatrix} 1 \\ 0 \\ -1 \end{bmatrix}, \ \hat{X}_2 = \frac{(\pm 1)}{\sqrt{3}} \begin{bmatrix} 1 \\ 1 \\ 1 \end{bmatrix}, \ \hat{X}_3 = \frac{(\pm 1)}{\sqrt{6}} \begin{bmatrix} 1 \\ -2 \\ 1 \end{bmatrix}.$$

11. $\lambda^3 + 5\lambda^2 + 6\lambda = 0$; $\lambda_1 = -3$, $\lambda_2 = -2$, $\lambda_3 = 0$;

$$X_1 = \begin{bmatrix} 1 \\ 0 \\ -1 \end{bmatrix}, \ X_2 = \begin{bmatrix} 2 \\ -1 \\ 0 \end{bmatrix}, \ X_3 = \begin{bmatrix} 0 \\ 1 \\ -1 \end{bmatrix};$$

$$\hat{X}_1 = \frac{(\pm 1)}{\sqrt{2}} \begin{bmatrix} 1 \\ 0 \\ -1 \end{bmatrix}, \ \hat{X}_2 = \frac{(\pm 1)}{\sqrt{5}} \begin{bmatrix} 2 \\ -1 \\ 0 \end{bmatrix}, \ \hat{X}_3 = \frac{(\pm 1)}{\sqrt{2}} \begin{bmatrix} 0 \\ 1 \\ -1 \end{bmatrix}.$$

12. $\lambda^3 - 6\lambda^2 + 3\lambda + 10$; as $\lambda = 5$ is a root, $(\lambda - 5)$ is a factor, so division by $(\lambda - 5)$ shows the other eigenvalues to be roots of $\lambda^2 - \lambda - 2 = 0$. Thus the other eigenvalues are $\lambda = -1$ and $\lambda = 2$, and hence the eigenvalues are $\lambda_1 = -1$, $\lambda_2 = 2$ and $\lambda_3 = 5$;

$$X_1 = \begin{bmatrix} 1 \\ 0 \\ 0 \end{bmatrix}, \; X_2 = \begin{bmatrix} 0 \\ 2 \\ 1 \end{bmatrix}, \; X_3 = \begin{bmatrix} -1 \\ 5 \\ 3 \end{bmatrix};$$

$$\hat{X}_1 = (\pm 1) \begin{bmatrix} 1 \\ 0 \\ 0 \end{bmatrix}, \; \hat{X}_2 = \frac{(\pm 1)}{\sqrt{5}} \begin{bmatrix} 0 \\ 2 \\ 1 \end{bmatrix}, \; \hat{X}_3 = \frac{(\pm 1)}{\sqrt{35}} \begin{bmatrix} -1 \\ 5 \\ 3 \end{bmatrix}.$$

PROBLEMS 59

1.

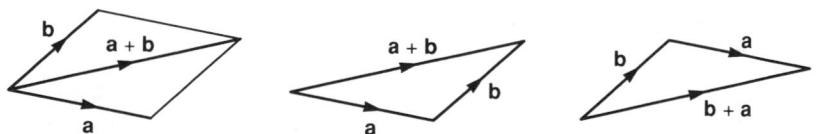

2. By Pythogoras' theorem the magnitude of its final displacement is $\sqrt{(3^2 + 3^2)} = \sqrt{18}$ miles. The direction of the displacement is south east.

3. $\mathbf{a} + \mathbf{x} = \mathbf{b}$, so $\mathbf{x} = \mathbf{b} - \mathbf{a}$.

4. $\mathbf{a} + (-\mathbf{x}) = \mathbf{b} + \mathbf{c}$, so $\mathbf{x} = \mathbf{a} - \mathbf{b} - \mathbf{c}$.

5.

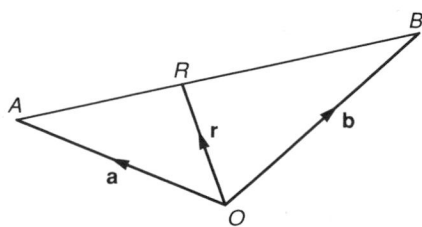

$\underline{OA} = \mathbf{a}$, $\underline{OB} = \mathbf{b}$, $\underline{OR} = \mathbf{r}$ and $\dfrac{AR}{RB} = \dfrac{m}{n}$, so $nAR = mRB$ and hence $n\underline{AR} = m\underline{RB}$. However $\underline{AR} = \mathbf{r} - \mathbf{a}$ and $\underline{RB} = \mathbf{b} - \mathbf{r}$, so $n\mathbf{r} + m\mathbf{r} = n\mathbf{a} + m\mathbf{b}$ and thus $\mathbf{r} = (n\mathbf{a} + m\mathbf{b})/(n + m)$.

6.

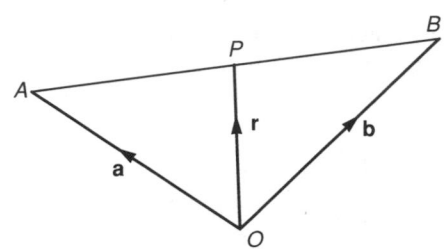

$\underline{AB} = \mathbf{b} - \mathbf{a}$, so $\underline{OP} = \mathbf{r} = \underline{OA} + \underline{AP} = \mathbf{a} + \dfrac{1}{2}\underline{AB} = \dfrac{1}{2}(\mathbf{a} + \mathbf{b})$. Thus

$\mathbf{x} = -2\mathbf{r} = -(\mathbf{a} + \mathbf{b})$.

7. $\underline{OM} = \mathbf{x} = \underline{OP} + \dfrac{1}{2}\underline{PB}$, but $\underline{OP} = \underline{OA} + \dfrac{1}{2}\underline{AC} = \mathbf{a} + \dfrac{1}{2}(\mathbf{c} - \mathbf{a}) = \dfrac{1}{2}(\mathbf{a} + \mathbf{c})$.

Now $\underline{PB} = \mathbf{b} - \underline{OP} = \mathbf{b} - \dfrac{1}{2}(\mathbf{a} + \mathbf{c})$, so $\dfrac{1}{2}\underline{PB} = \dfrac{1}{2}\mathbf{b} - \dfrac{1}{4}(\mathbf{a} + \mathbf{c})$, so

$\mathbf{x} = \dfrac{1}{2}(\mathbf{a} + \mathbf{c}) + \dfrac{1}{2}\mathbf{b} - \dfrac{1}{4}(\mathbf{a} + \mathbf{c}) = \dfrac{1}{2}\mathbf{b} + \dfrac{1}{4}(\mathbf{a} + \mathbf{c})$.

8. The forces are mutually perpendicular, so by Pythogoras' theorem, the magnitude of the sum of the forces of magnitudes 1 and 2 is $\sqrt{(1^2 + 2^2)} = \sqrt{5}$. This resultant force lies in the plane of the forces of magnitudes 1 and 2, and so is perpendicular to the force of magnitude 3. A further application of Pythogoras' theorem shows the magnitude of the resultant of all three forces is thus $\sqrt{[(\sqrt{5})^2 + 3^2]} = \sqrt{14}$. The direction of the resultant force R is as shown in the diagram.

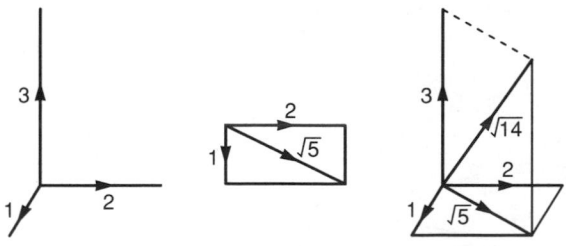

PROBLEMS 60

1. $|\mathbf{a}| = \sqrt{29}$, $|\mathbf{b}| = \sqrt{14}$, $\hat{\mathbf{a}} = \dfrac{1}{\sqrt{29}}(4\mathbf{i} - 2\mathbf{j} + 3\mathbf{k})$, $\hat{\mathbf{b}} = \dfrac{1}{\sqrt{14}}(-2\mathbf{i} + 3\mathbf{j} + \mathbf{k})$,

$3\mathbf{a} - 2\mathbf{b} = 16\mathbf{i} - 12\mathbf{j} + 7\mathbf{k}$.

2. $|\mathbf{a}| = \sqrt{41},\ |\mathbf{b}| = \sqrt{21},\ \hat{\mathbf{a}} = \dfrac{1}{\sqrt{41}}(6\mathbf{i} + 2\mathbf{j} + \mathbf{k}),\ \hat{\mathbf{b}} = \dfrac{1}{\sqrt{21}}(-\mathbf{i} - 4\mathbf{j} + 2\mathbf{k}),$

   $2\mathbf{a} + \mathbf{b} = 11\mathbf{i} + 4\mathbf{k}.$

3. $|\mathbf{a}| = \sqrt{29},$ so $l = 3/\sqrt{29},\ m = 4/\sqrt{29},\ n = -2/\sqrt{29}.$

4. $2\mathbf{a} - \mathbf{b} = 7\mathbf{j} - 4\mathbf{k},$ so $|2\mathbf{a} - \mathbf{b}| = \sqrt{65}$ and hence $l = 0,\ m = 7/\sqrt{65},\ n = -4/\sqrt{65}.$

5. $|\mathbf{a}| = \sqrt{74},\ |\mathbf{b}| = \sqrt{184},\ \mathbf{a} + \mathbf{b} = 9\mathbf{i} + 5\mathbf{j} + 8\mathbf{k},\ |\mathbf{a} + \mathbf{b}| = \sqrt{170}$ so $l = 9/\sqrt{170},$

   $m = 5/\sqrt{170},\ n = 8/\sqrt{170}.$

6. (a) $\underline{AB} = \mathbf{i} - 2\mathbf{j} - \mathbf{k},$ (b) $\underline{CO} = -\mathbf{i} + \mathbf{j} + 2\mathbf{k}.$

7. $\underline{AB} = \mathbf{i} - \mathbf{j} + 2k,\ \underline{CD} = 4\mathbf{i} + 4\mathbf{j} - 2\mathbf{k},\ \underline{AB} + \underline{CD} = 5\mathbf{i} + 3\mathbf{j}.$ Length of

   $\underline{AB} + \underline{CD}$ is $|\underline{AB} + \underline{CD}| = \sqrt{34}.$

8. Resultant is $\mathbf{R} = 9\mathbf{i} + 13\mathbf{j} - 8\mathbf{k},\ |\mathbf{R}| = \sqrt{314},$ so $l = 9/\sqrt{314},\ m = 13/\sqrt{314},$

   $n = -8/\sqrt{314}$ and hence $\alpha = \arccos l = 59.48°,\ \beta = \arccos m = 42.8°,$

   $\gamma = \arccos n = 116.83°.$

9. $\mathbf{R} = \left(\dfrac{2}{\sqrt{14}} - \dfrac{5}{\sqrt{6}}\right)\mathbf{i} + \left(\dfrac{1}{\sqrt{14}} - \dfrac{1}{\sqrt{6}}\right)\mathbf{j} + \left(-\dfrac{3}{\sqrt{14}} + \dfrac{8}{\sqrt{6}}\right)\mathbf{k}$ or

   $\mathbf{R} = -1.507\,\mathbf{i} - 0.141\,\mathbf{j} + 2.464\,\mathbf{k};\ |\mathbf{R}| = 2.8918$ so $l = -0.5211,$

   $m = -0.0488,\ n = 0.8521.$

10. $\underline{PQ} = 2\mathbf{i} - 9\mathbf{j} + 11\mathbf{k},\ l = 0.1393,\ m = -0.6269,\ n = 0.7663.$

11. (a) $2\mathbf{i} + 2\sqrt{3}\,\mathbf{j};$ (b) $(3/\sqrt{2})\mathbf{i} - (3/\sqrt{2})\mathbf{j};$ (c) $-(5\sqrt{3}/2)\mathbf{i} - (5/2)\mathbf{j}.$

12. (a) $5\sqrt{2}$ miles N E (45°); (b) 5 miles N 30° W (330°).

13. If $\mathbf{i},\ \mathbf{j}$ represent 1 mile to E and N, respectively,

   Displacement is $\left(3 - \dfrac{1}{\sqrt{2}} + \dfrac{5\sqrt{3}}{4}\right)\mathbf{i} - \left(\dfrac{5}{4} + \dfrac{1}{\sqrt{2}}\right)\mathbf{j}$

   or $4.458\,\mathbf{i} - 1.957\,\mathbf{j}.$ Magnitude 4.869 miles and direction 113.7°.

14. $\underline{AC} = \mathbf{a} + 3\mathbf{b},\ \underline{DB} = -\mathbf{a} + 3\mathbf{b},\ \underline{BC} = 2\mathbf{a} + 2\mathbf{b},\ \underline{CA} = -\mathbf{a} - 3\mathbf{b}.$

15. Position vectors at 1, 3, 5 and 7s are, respectively, $(\sqrt{3}/2)\mathbf{i} + (1/2)\mathbf{j},\ \mathbf{j},$

   $-(\sqrt{3}/2)\mathbf{i} + (1/2)\mathbf{j}$ and $-(\sqrt{3}/2)\mathbf{i} - (1/2)\mathbf{j}.$

   Particle velocity vectors at 3/2, 3 and 5s are, respectively,

   $\pi/(6\sqrt{2})(\mathbf{j} - \mathbf{i}),\ -(\pi/6)\mathbf{i}$ and $-(\pi/12)(\mathbf{i} + \sqrt{3}\mathbf{j}).$

16. Velocity is $4\mathbf{i} + \mathbf{j},$ speed is $\sqrt{17}$ km/h at an angle arctan 4.

17.   Resultant $\mathbf{R} = (1/\sqrt{2})(5\mathbf{i} + 4\mathbf{j} + 3\mathbf{k})$; $|\mathbf{R}| = 5$ kg; $l = 1/\sqrt{2}$, $m = 4/(5\sqrt{2})$, $n = 3/(5\sqrt{2})$, so $\alpha = \arccos l = 45°$, $\beta = \arccos m = 55.55°$, $n = \arccos n = 64.9°$.

18. $\mathbf{r} = 3\mathbf{i} - 3\mathbf{j} - \mathbf{k}$.

19. $-\mathbf{i} + \mathbf{j}$.

20.   Take the origin to be located at vertex C and let the position vectors of vertices A and B relative to C be $\mathbf{a}$ and $\mathbf{b}$, respectively.

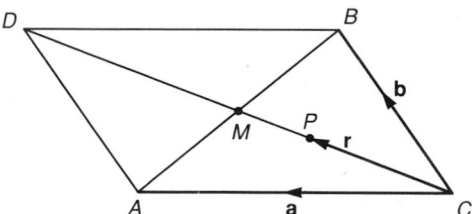

Then the position vector $\mathbf{r}$ of the centroid is $\mathbf{r} = \dfrac{m\mathbf{a} + m\mathbf{b} + m\mathbf{c}}{3m} = \dfrac{1}{3}(\mathbf{a} + \mathbf{b})$,

where m is the particle mass. However, $\mathbf{a} + \mathbf{b} = \underline{CD}$, so $\mathbf{r} = \dfrac{1}{3}\underline{CD} = \dfrac{2}{3}\underline{CM}$.

The argument is identical for any choice of vertex as origin.

PROBLEMS 61

1. $\dfrac{x - (1/4)}{(3/4)} = \dfrac{y + 3}{2} = \dfrac{z - 1}{4}$; $\mathbf{a} = (1/4)\mathbf{i} - 3\mathbf{j} + \mathbf{k}$, $\mathbf{b} = (3/4)\mathbf{i} + 2\mathbf{j} + 4\mathbf{k}$.

2. $\dfrac{x + (7/3)}{-3} = \dfrac{y - (3/2)}{2} = \dfrac{z - (5/3)}{-(1/3)}$; $\mathbf{a} = -(7/3)\mathbf{i} + (3/2)\mathbf{j} + (5/3)\mathbf{k}$,
      $\mathbf{b} = -3\mathbf{i} + 2\mathbf{j} - (1/3)\mathbf{k}$.

3. $\dfrac{x + (3/2)}{1} = \dfrac{z - (9/4)}{-(3/4)}$; $\mathbf{a} = (-3/2)\mathbf{i} + (9/4)\mathbf{k}$, $\mathbf{b} = \mathbf{i} - (3/4)\mathbf{k}$.

4. $\dfrac{x + 9}{4} = \dfrac{y + 6}{2} = \dfrac{z - 16}{5}$; $\mathbf{a} = -9\mathbf{i} - 6\mathbf{j} + 16\mathbf{k}$, $\mathbf{b} = 4\mathbf{i} + 2\mathbf{j} + 5\mathbf{k}$.

5.   The point $(1, 1, 1)$ is on L so we may set $\mathbf{a} = \mathbf{i} + \mathbf{j} + \mathbf{k}$. The vector from $(1, 1, 1)$ to $(-2, -1, 3)$ is $-3\mathbf{i} - 2\mathbf{j} + 2\mathbf{k}$, so this is a vector $\mathbf{b}$ directed along L. Hence the vector equation of L is

$$\mathbf{r} = (\mathbf{i} + \mathbf{j} + \mathbf{k}) + \lambda(-3\mathbf{i} - 2\mathbf{j} + 2\mathbf{k}).$$

The Cartesian equations are thus

$$\frac{x-1}{-3} = \frac{y-1}{-2} = \frac{z-1}{2} \quad (=\lambda).$$

Had we taken the point $(-2, -1, 3)$ as the point **a** on the line we would have obtained the equivalent set of equations

$$\frac{x+2}{-3} = \frac{y-1}{-2} = \frac{z-3}{2}.$$

6. $x = 2 + 3\lambda$, $y = -1 + 2\lambda$, $z = 1 - 3\lambda$; so $\lambda = -1$ corresponds to $(-1, -3, 4)$, $\lambda = 1$ corresponds to $(5, 1, -2)$, and $\lambda = 2$ corresponds to $(8, 3, -5)$.

7.   We set $\mathbf{a} = \mathbf{i} + 2\mathbf{j} + 3\mathbf{k}$. The vector joining $(2, 3, 1)$ to $(5, 4, 2)$ is $3\mathbf{i} + \mathbf{j} + \mathbf{k}$, so we may set $\mathbf{b} = 3\mathbf{i} + \mathbf{j} + \mathbf{k}$. Thus inspection shows that the Cartesian equations of L are

$$\frac{x-1}{3} = \frac{y-2}{1} = \frac{z-3}{1}.$$

8. $\dfrac{x-3}{3} = \dfrac{y+1}{2} = \dfrac{z-2}{-6}.$

PROBLEMS 62

1. $\mathbf{a} \cdot \mathbf{b} = 6$; $\cos\theta = 6/(\sqrt{11}\sqrt{6})$, so $\theta = 0.7399\,\text{rad}\ (42.39°)$.

2. $\mathbf{a} \cdot \mathbf{b} = -9$; $\cos\theta = -9/(3\sqrt{26})$, so $\theta = 2.1998\,\text{rad}\ (126.04°)$.

3. $\mathbf{a} \cdot \mathbf{b} = -28$; $\cos\theta = -28/(\sqrt{14}\sqrt{56}) = -1$, so $\theta = \pi\,\text{rad}\ (180°)$.

4. $\mathbf{a} \cdot \mathbf{b} = 8$; $\cos\theta = 8/(\sqrt{14}\sqrt{21})$, so $\theta = 1.0854\,\text{rad}\ (62.19°)$.

5.   Two vectors $\mathbf{u}$ and $\mathbf{v}$ will be orthogonal (perpendicular) if $\mathbf{u} \cdot \mathbf{v} = 0$;

$$\mathbf{a} \cdot \mathbf{b} = -6,\ \mathbf{a} \cdot \mathbf{c} = 0,\ \mathbf{a} \cdot \mathbf{d} = 0,$$

$$\mathbf{b} \cdot \mathbf{c} = 10,\ \mathbf{b} \cdot \mathbf{d} = 25,\ \mathbf{c} \cdot \mathbf{d} = 13,$$

so **a** and **c** are orthogonal and **a** and **d** are orthogonal.

6. $\mathbf{a} \cdot (\mathbf{b} + \mathbf{c}) = (5\mathbf{i} + 3\mathbf{j} - 4\mathbf{k}) \cdot (3\mathbf{i} + 3\mathbf{j} + 2\mathbf{k}) = 16$

$\mathbf{a} \cdot \mathbf{b} = (5\mathbf{i} + 3\mathbf{j} - 4\mathbf{k}) \cdot (2\mathbf{i} + \mathbf{j} - \mathbf{k}) = 17$ and

$\mathbf{a} \cdot \mathbf{c} = (5\mathbf{i} + 3\mathbf{j} - 4\mathbf{k}) \cdot (\mathbf{i} + 2\mathbf{j} + 3\mathbf{k}) = -1$, so

$$\mathbf{a} \cdot \mathbf{b} + \mathbf{a} \cdot \mathbf{c} = 17 - 1 = 16 = \mathbf{a} \cdot (\mathbf{b} + \mathbf{c}).$$

7. $\mathbf{a} \cdot \mathbf{b} = 10 + 5\alpha$, so $\mathbf{a} \cdot \mathbf{b} = 0$ when $\alpha = -2$.

8. $W = \dfrac{8}{\sqrt{3}} (\mathbf{i}+\mathbf{j}+\mathbf{k}) \cdot \dfrac{5}{\sqrt{14}} (2\mathbf{i}-\mathbf{j}+3\mathbf{k})$

$= \dfrac{40}{\sqrt{42}} (2 - 1 + 3) = \dfrac{160}{\sqrt{42}}$ work units.

9. (a) The projection of **a** in the direction of **b** is

$$\mathbf{a} \cdot \hat{\mathbf{b}} = (\mathbf{i}+\mathbf{j}+\mathbf{k}) \cdot \dfrac{1}{\sqrt{29}} (3\mathbf{i} - 2\mathbf{j} + 4\mathbf{k}) = \dfrac{5}{\sqrt{29}}.$$

(b) The projection of **b** in the direction of **a** is

$$\hat{\mathbf{a}} \cdot \mathbf{b} = \dfrac{1}{\sqrt{3}} (\mathbf{i}+\mathbf{j}+\mathbf{k}) \cdot (3\mathbf{i} - 2\mathbf{j} + 4\mathbf{k}) = \dfrac{5}{\sqrt{3}}.$$

10. (a) The length of the projection of **a** in the direction of **b** is

$$|\mathbf{a} \cdot \hat{\mathbf{b}}| = \left| (-4\mathbf{i} + 2\mathbf{j} + 2\mathbf{k}) \cdot \dfrac{1}{\sqrt{14}} (3\mathbf{i} - 2\mathbf{j} + \mathbf{k}) \right|$$

$$= \left| \dfrac{-14}{\sqrt{14}} \right| = \sqrt{14}.$$

(b) The length of the projection of **b** in the direction of **a** is

$$|\hat{\mathbf{a}} \cdot \mathbf{b}| = \left| \dfrac{1}{\sqrt{24}} (-4\mathbf{i} + 2\mathbf{j} + 2\mathbf{k}) \cdot (3\mathbf{i} - 2\mathbf{j} + \mathbf{k}) \right|$$

$$= \left| \dfrac{-14}{\sqrt{24}} \right| = \dfrac{14}{\sqrt{24}}.$$

11. We require $\mathbf{n} \cdot \mathbf{a} = 0$ and $\mathbf{n} \cdot \mathbf{b} = 0$, so

$$n_1 - n_2 + n_3 = 0 \text{ and } 3n_1 + 2n_2 - 2n_3 = 0.$$

Thus n_1, n_2 and n_3 must satisfy

$$n_1 - n_2 + n_3 = 0$$
$$3n_1 + 2n_2 - 2n_3 = 0.$$

Using Gaussian elimination to eliminate n_1 from the second equation gives

$$n_1 - n_2 + n_3 = 0$$
$$5n_2 - 5n_3 = 0.$$

Setting $n_3 = \mu$, back-substitution shows that $n_2 = \mu$ and $n_1 = 0$. Thus the required vector is

$$\mathbf{n} = \mu\mathbf{j} + \mu\mathbf{k},$$

with $\mu \neq 0$ arbitrary.

PROBLEMS 63

1. $3x + y + 2z = 6.$

2. $7x - y + 3z = 2.$

3. $3x + 6y - 4z = 0.$

4. The normals $\mathbf{N}_1$ and $\mathbf{N}_2$ to the planes are $\mathbf{N}_1 = 2\mathbf{i} - \mathbf{j} + \mathbf{k}$ and $\mathbf{N}_2 = \mathbf{i} + 4\mathbf{j} + 3\mathbf{k}$, thus the angle θ between the planes is such that

$$\cos\theta = \frac{\mathbf{N}_1 \cdot \mathbf{N}_2}{|\mathbf{N}_1|\,|\mathbf{N}_2|} = \frac{-1}{\sqrt{6}\sqrt{26}},$$

so $\theta = 94.59°.$

5. $\mathbf{N} = 4\mathbf{i} - 2\mathbf{j} + 5\mathbf{k}$; $d = 4/|\mathbf{N}| = 4/\sqrt{45}.$

6. $\hat{\mathbf{n}} = (3\mathbf{i} + 4\mathbf{j} - 2\mathbf{k})/[3^2 + 4^2 + (-2)^2]^{1/2} = (1/\sqrt{29})(3\mathbf{i} + 4\mathbf{j} - 2\mathbf{k})$; $d = 0.$

7. In the notation already introduced, $\mathbf{a} = \mathbf{i} + \mathbf{j} - \mathbf{k}$, $\mathbf{b} = 2\mathbf{i} + \mathbf{j} - 3\mathbf{k}$,

    $\mathbf{N} = \mathbf{i} + 2\mathbf{j} + \mathbf{k}$, and so

$$d = \frac{|\mathbf{a} \cdot \mathbf{N} - \mathbf{b} \cdot \mathbf{N}|}{|\mathbf{N}|} = \frac{|2 - 1|}{\sqrt{6}} = \frac{1}{\sqrt{6}}.$$

8. The normal to the plane is $2\mathbf{i} + 3\mathbf{j} - \mathbf{k}$ and the point $\mathbf{a} = 2\mathbf{i} + 3\mathbf{j} - \mathbf{k}$, so the equation of the plane is

    $$\mathbf{r} \cdot \mathbf{a} = \mathbf{a} \cdot \mathbf{a},$$

    or

    $$2x + 3y - z = 14.$$

9. Apply the formula for d without the absolute value signs, first to the point at the origin $(0, 0, 0)$ and then to the point $(2, 3, -5)$. The points will be on the same side of the plane if these results have the same sign and on opposite sides if the signs are different. The absolute values of each result will, of course, be d. For the point at the origin $(\mathbf{a} \cdot \mathbf{N} - \mathbf{b} \cdot \mathbf{N})/|\mathbf{N}| = 3$ and for the point $(2, 3, -5)$ $(\mathbf{a} \cdot \mathbf{N} - \mathbf{b} \cdot \mathbf{N})/|\mathbf{N}| = -3$, so the points are both distance 3 from the plane, but on opposite sides.

PROBLEMS 64

1. $\mathbf{a} \times \mathbf{b} = -\mathbf{j} + 7\mathbf{k}$, $\mathbf{a} \times \mathbf{c} = 2\mathbf{i} + \mathbf{j} + 3\mathbf{k}$, $\mathbf{b} \times \mathbf{c} = -4\mathbf{i} + 5\mathbf{j} + \mathbf{k}.$

2. $\mathbf{u} = -5\mathbf{j} + 5\mathbf{k}$, $\mathbf{v} = -8\mathbf{i} - \mathbf{j} + 5\mathbf{k}$, $\mathbf{u} \times \mathbf{v} = -20\mathbf{i} - 40\mathbf{j} - 40\mathbf{k}.$

3. $S = \sqrt{185}.$

4. $S = 4\sqrt{38}$.

5. $\mathbf{a} \times (\mathbf{b} + \mathbf{c}) = (3\mathbf{i} + 2\mathbf{j} - \mathbf{k}) \times (2\mathbf{i} - 5\mathbf{j}) = -5\mathbf{i} - 2\mathbf{j} - 19\mathbf{k}$,

   $\mathbf{a} \times \mathbf{b} = -4\mathbf{i} + 8\mathbf{j} + 4\mathbf{k}$, $\mathbf{a} \times \mathbf{c} = -\mathbf{i} - 10\mathbf{j} - 23\mathbf{k}$, so

   $$\mathbf{a} \times \mathbf{b} + \mathbf{a} \times \mathbf{c} = -5\mathbf{i} - 2\mathbf{j} - 19\mathbf{k}.$$

6. $\pm(-14\mathbf{i} + 7\mathbf{k})/(7\sqrt{5})$; the result is unique apart from its sign.

7. -21.

8. 18.

9. α must be such that $\mathbf{a} \cdot (\mathbf{b} \times \mathbf{c}) = 0$, so it must satisfy

   $$\begin{vmatrix} 2 & -2 & 3 \\ 1 & 1 & 4 \\ 1 & -1 & \alpha \end{vmatrix} = 0$$

   which is equivalent to $4\alpha - 6 = 0$, so $\alpha = 3/2$.

10. $(\mathbf{a} \times \mathbf{b}) \times \mathbf{c} = (\mathbf{a} \cdot \mathbf{c})\mathbf{b} - (\mathbf{b} \cdot \mathbf{c})\mathbf{a} = 12\mathbf{b} + 4\mathbf{a} = 16\mathbf{i} + 8\mathbf{j} - 56\mathbf{k}$,

    $\mathbf{a} \times (\mathbf{b} \times \mathbf{c}) = -(\mathbf{b} \times \mathbf{c}) \times \mathbf{a} = -[(\mathbf{b} \cdot \mathbf{a})\mathbf{c} - (\mathbf{c} \cdot \mathbf{a})\mathbf{b}]$

    $$= -[-23\mathbf{c} - 12\mathbf{b}] = 58\mathbf{i} + 69\mathbf{j} - 49\mathbf{k}.$$

11. $(\mathbf{a} \times \mathbf{b}) \times \mathbf{c} = (\mathbf{a} \cdot \mathbf{c})\mathbf{b} - (\mathbf{b} \cdot \mathbf{c})\mathbf{a} = \mathbf{b} - 0\mathbf{a} = \mathbf{i} - \mathbf{j} - \mathbf{k}$,

    $\mathbf{a} \times (\mathbf{b} \times \mathbf{c}) = -(\mathbf{b} \times \mathbf{c}) \times \mathbf{a}$

    $$= -[(\mathbf{b} \cdot \mathbf{a})\mathbf{c} - (\mathbf{c} \cdot \mathbf{a})\mathbf{b}]$$

    $$= 2\mathbf{c} + \mathbf{b}$$

    $$= 3\mathbf{i} - 3\mathbf{j}.$$

12. Vector $\mathbf{c}$ will be orthogonal to both $\mathbf{a}$ and $\mathbf{b}$ if $(\mathbf{a} \times \mathbf{b}) \times \mathbf{c} = \mathbf{0}$. Thus $(\mathbf{a} \cdot \mathbf{c})\mathbf{b} - (\mathbf{b} \cdot \mathbf{c})\mathbf{a} = 0$, and so $(\alpha - 2)\mathbf{b} - (4 - 2\alpha)\mathbf{c} = \mathbf{0}$. This last result is only possible if $\alpha = 2$.

13. The vector addition of $\mathbf{a}$, $\mathbf{b}$ and $\mathbf{c}$ brings us back to the initial point of $\mathbf{a}$, so the total displacement is zero.

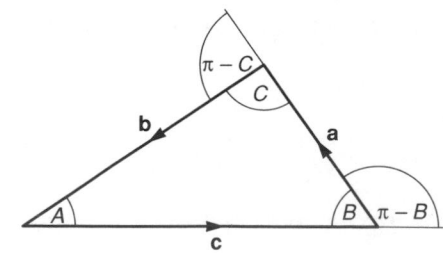

$$\mathbf{a} \times (\mathbf{a} + \mathbf{b} + \mathbf{c}) = \mathbf{a} \times \mathbf{0},$$

so forming the vector product with $\mathbf{a}$ gives

$$\mathbf{a} \times \mathbf{b} + \mathbf{a} \times \mathbf{c} = \mathbf{0}, \text{ because } \mathbf{a} \times \mathbf{a} = \mathbf{0}.$$

If $\hat{\mathbf{n}}$ is the unit vector normal to the plane of the triangle and such that $\mathbf{a}$, $\mathbf{b}$ and $\hat{\mathbf{n}}$ form a right-handed set, the above result becomes

$$|\mathbf{a}| \, |\mathbf{b}| \, \sin(\pi - C) \, \hat{\mathbf{n}} + |\mathbf{a}| \, |\mathbf{c}| \, \sin(\pi - B)(-\hat{\mathbf{n}}) = \mathbf{0},$$

or

$$ab \sin C - ac \sin B = 0,$$

so

$$\frac{\sin A}{a} = \frac{\sin B}{b}.$$

The remainder of the sine rule follows in similar fashion after forming the vector product with $\mathbf{b}$.

14.   Form the vector product of $\mathbf{a}$ with $\mathbf{a} + \mathbf{b} + \mathbf{c} = \mathbf{0}$ to obtain

$$\mathbf{a} \times \mathbf{b} + \mathbf{a} \times \mathbf{c} = \mathbf{0} \quad (\mathbf{a} \times \mathbf{a} = \mathbf{0}).$$

Now take the scalar product of this result with $\mathbf{c}$ to obtain

$$(\mathbf{a} \times \mathbf{b}) \cdot \mathbf{c} + (\mathbf{a} \times \mathbf{c}) \cdot \mathbf{c} = 0.$$

However, the second triple scalar product is zero because two of the vectors involved in it are identical, so

$$(\mathbf{a} \times \mathbf{b}) \cdot \mathbf{c} = 0.$$

PROBLEMS 65

1. $\hat{\mathbf{n}} = (\pm 1)(-3\mathbf{i} + 5\mathbf{j} + 11\mathbf{k})/\sqrt{155}$; $\sin\theta = \sqrt{155}/(\sqrt{6}\sqrt{26})$ so $\theta = 85.4°$; to find unit vectors in the plane of and perpendicular to the given vectors form the vector product of each vector with $\hat{\mathbf{n}}$ and then normalize the result to obtain $(\pm 1)(-16\mathbf{i} - 25\mathbf{j} + 7\mathbf{k})/\sqrt{930}$ and $(\pm 1)(49\mathbf{i} - 30\mathbf{j} + 27\mathbf{k})/\sqrt{4030}$.

2.   In standard form the line is

$$\frac{x + 2}{3} = \frac{y + 1}{2} = \frac{z - 3}{-2},$$

so the vector along the line is $\mathbf{b} = 3\mathbf{i} + 2\mathbf{j} - 2\mathbf{k}$. The plane through $(2, 1, 1)$ with $\mathbf{b}$ as its normal is

$$3x + 2y - 2z = 6.$$

3. The equation of the plane is

$$x - 2y + z = 0,$$

and $d = 3/\sqrt{6}$.

4. $\hat{\mathbf{n}} = (3\mathbf{i} + 2\mathbf{j} - \mathbf{k})/\sqrt{14}$; $d = 3/\sqrt{14}$.

5. The line of intersection has the equations

$$\frac{4x - 29}{30} = \frac{y}{1} = \frac{2z + 4}{-5}.$$

The equation of the plane is

$$15x + 2y - 5z = 0.$$

The angle θ between the planes is the angle between their normals $\mathbf{n}_1 = 4\mathbf{i} + 20\mathbf{j} + 20\mathbf{k}$ and $\mathbf{n}_2 = 4\mathbf{i} - 5\mathbf{j} + 10\mathbf{k}$, so

$$\cos\theta = \frac{\mathbf{n}_1 \cdot \mathbf{n}_2}{|\mathbf{n}_1||\mathbf{n}_2|} = \frac{116}{\sqrt{816}\sqrt{141}} = 0.3420 \ (\theta = 70°).$$

6. The lines will intersect if the perpendicular distance d between them is zero. The vectors along the lines are $\mathbf{b}_1 = \mathbf{i} + 2\mathbf{j} + 2\mathbf{k}$ and $\mathbf{b}_2 = 3\mathbf{i} + 4\mathbf{j} + 5\mathbf{k}$, so

$$\hat{\mathbf{n}} = \frac{\mathbf{b}_1 \times \mathbf{b}_2}{|\mathbf{b}_1||\mathbf{b}_2|}$$

is a unit vector normal to both lines, and $\hat{\mathbf{n}} = (2\mathbf{i} + \mathbf{j} - 2\mathbf{k})/3$. The distance d will be the projection of a vector joining a point on each line in the direction of $\hat{\mathbf{n}}$. A point on the first line is $(2, -1, 2)$ and one on the second line is $(1, 1, 2)$, so a vector $\mathbf{a}$ joining a point on each line is $\mathbf{a} = \mathbf{i} - 2\mathbf{j}$. Then $d = \hat{\mathbf{n}} \cdot \mathbf{a} = (2\mathbf{i} + \mathbf{j} - 2\mathbf{k}) \cdot (\mathbf{i} - 2\mathbf{j})/3 = 0$, so the lines intersect. The equation of the plane containing the two lines is $2x + y - 2z = -1$. This follows by using $\hat{\mathbf{n}}$ which is normal to the plane and any point on the plane, say $(2, -1, 2)$.

7. Construct the line through $(0, -1, 0)$ and $(2, 1, -1)$ and the line through $(1, 1, 1)$ and $(3, 3, 0)$ and show the perpendicular distance betwen these lines is zero (see the answer to problem 6).

8. Proceed as in the answer to problem 7. The plane containing the lines has the equation $2x - y + 3z = 1$, and it is found by using $\hat{\mathbf{n}}$ and any one of the given points.

9. The perpendicular distance d of the point $(1, -2, 3)$ from the plane is $1/\sqrt{3}$. The unit vector along the line is $\hat{\mathbf{b}} = (2\mathbf{i} + 3\mathbf{j} - 6\mathbf{k})/7$, and the unit vector normal to the plane is $\hat{\mathbf{n}} = (\mathbf{i} - \mathbf{j} + \mathbf{k})/\sqrt{3}$. Then

$$p|\hat{\mathbf{b}} \cdot \hat{\mathbf{n}}| = d,$$

so

$$p|(2\mathbf{i}+3\mathbf{j}-6\mathbf{k}) \cdot (\mathbf{i}-\mathbf{j}+\mathbf{k})| = 7\sqrt{3}(1/\sqrt{3})$$

and hence $p = 7$.

10. The position vector of R relative to O is $\mathbf{b}-\mathbf{a} = 2\mathbf{i}-\mathbf{j}-4\mathbf{k}$. The vector $\hat{\mathbf{n}} = (2\mathbf{i}+\mathbf{j}+2\mathbf{k})/3$, so $\boldsymbol{\omega} = 9\hat{\mathbf{n}} = 6\mathbf{i}+3\mathbf{j}+6\mathbf{k}$, and hence

$$\mathbf{v} = \boldsymbol{\omega} \times (\mathbf{b}-\mathbf{a}) = -6\mathbf{j}+36\mathbf{j}-12\mathbf{k} \text{ cm/s.}$$

11. For the moment about the origin $\mathbf{r} = \mathbf{i}+\mathbf{j}+\mathbf{k}$, so

$$\mathbf{M} = (\mathbf{i}+\mathbf{j}+\mathbf{k}) \times (\mathbf{i}-\mathbf{j}+3\mathbf{k}) = 4\mathbf{i}-2\mathbf{j}-2\mathbf{k}.$$

For the moment about $(2, 0, -1)$,

$$\mathbf{r} = (\mathbf{i}+\mathbf{j}+\mathbf{k}) - (2\mathbf{i}-\mathbf{k}) = -\mathbf{i}+\mathbf{j}+2\mathbf{k},$$

so

$$\mathbf{M} = (-\mathbf{i}+\mathbf{j}+2\mathbf{k}) \times (\mathbf{i}-\mathbf{j}+3\mathbf{k}) = 5\mathbf{i}+5\mathbf{j}.$$

PROBLEMS 66

1. A right-handed helix. The curve lines on the surface of a cylinder of radius R with its axis along the z-axis. It advances in the z-direction uniformly with t.

2. The curve spirals uniformly outwards with t and advances in the z-direction uniformly with t.

3. (a) $d\mathbf{r}/dt = -6t\mathbf{i}+2\mathbf{j}+2\sin 2t\mathbf{k}$; $d^2\mathbf{r}/dt^2 = -6\mathbf{i}+4\cos 2t\mathbf{k}$;

   (b) $d\mathbf{r}/dt = \mathbf{a}+(2/t^3)\mathbf{b}$; $d^2\mathbf{r}/dt^2 = -(6/t^4)\mathbf{b}$.

4. (a) $d\mathbf{r}/dt = 2\cosh 2t\mathbf{i}+3e^{3t}\mathbf{j}+(\cos t-t\sin t)\mathbf{k}$ so,   when $t = 0$, $d\mathbf{r}/dt = 2\mathbf{i}+3\mathbf{j}+\mathbf{k}$;

   (b) $d\mathbf{r}/dt = (3t^2+2t)\mathbf{i}-2t/[(1+t^2)^2]\mathbf{j}+6t/(1+3t^2)\mathbf{k}$ so, when $t = 0$, $d\mathbf{r}/dt = 0$.

5. $d\mathbf{r}/dt = -\omega\sin\omega t\mathbf{a}-\omega\cos\omega t\mathbf{b}$, $d^2\mathbf{r}/dt^2 = -\omega^2\cos\omega t\mathbf{a}+\omega^2\sin\omega t\mathbf{b}$, so

$$\frac{d^2\mathbf{r}}{dt^2} + \omega^2\mathbf{r} = 0.$$

6. $d\mathbf{r}/dt = \omega e^{\omega t}\mathbf{a}-\omega e^{-\omega t}\mathbf{b}$, $d^2\mathbf{r}/dt^2 = \omega^2 e^{\omega t}\mathbf{a}+\omega^2 e^{-\omega t}\mathbf{b}$, so

$$\frac{d^2\mathbf{r}}{dt^2} - \omega^2\mathbf{r} = 0.$$

7. (a) $\mathbf{r} \cdot \mathbf{s} = 2 \sinh^2 t - 2 \cosh^2 t + te^t = te^t - 2$, so

$$\frac{d}{dt}[\mathbf{r} \cdot \mathbf{s}] = e^t (1 + t);$$

(b) $\mathbf{r} \cdot \mathbf{s} = 4(\sin^2 2t + \cos^2 2t) + 1 = 5$, so

$$\frac{d}{dt}[\mathbf{r} \cdot \mathbf{s}] = 0.$$

8. (a) $d\mathbf{r}/dt = (\mathbf{i} - e^{-t}\mathbf{j} + \cos t\mathbf{k}) \times (\mathbf{i} + t^2\mathbf{j} - \mathbf{k}) + (t\mathbf{i} + e^{-t}\mathbf{j} + \sin t\mathbf{k}) \times 2t\mathbf{j}$

$= (e^{-t} - 2t \sin t - t^2 \cos t)\mathbf{i} + (1 + \cos t)\mathbf{j} + (3t^2 + e^{-t} \cos t)\mathbf{k}$

(alternatively, evaluate the cross product and then differentiate);

(b) $d\mathbf{r}/dt = (2t - \sin t)(\mathbf{i} + 4\mathbf{j} - 6\mathbf{k});$

(c) $d\mathbf{r}/dt = \mathbf{0}.$

9. (a) $d/dt[r] = d/dt[t^2 + t - e^{-t}] = 2t + 1 + e^{-t};$

(b) $d/dt[r] = d/dt[\sin^2 t + \cos^2 t + 1] = d/dt[2] = 0;$

(c) $[(t\mathbf{i} + t^2\mathbf{j}) \times (\mathbf{i} + 3\mathbf{j})] \cdot t\mathbf{k} = t^2(3 - t)$, so

$$dr/dt = 6t - 3t^2.$$

10. (a) $\dfrac{d\mathbf{r}}{dt} = \dfrac{d\mathbf{r}}{du}\dfrac{du}{dt} = \left(\dfrac{2u}{1 + u^2}\mathbf{i} + \mathbf{j} + 3u^2 \sec^2 u^3\mathbf{k}\right)\cos t$

$$= \dfrac{2 \sin t \cos t}{1 + \sin^2 t}\mathbf{i} + \cos t\mathbf{j} + 3 \sin^2 t \cos t \sec^2(\sin^3 t)\mathbf{k};$$

(b) $\dfrac{d\mathbf{r}}{dt} = \dfrac{d\mathbf{r}}{du}\dfrac{du}{dt}$

$$= \left(\dfrac{u}{(1 + u^2)^{1/2}}\mathbf{i} + 2u\mathbf{j} + 2 \sinh (2u + 1)\mathbf{k}\right)\dfrac{1}{1 + t}$$

$$= \dfrac{\ln(1 + t)}{(1 + t)[1 + \ln^2(1 + t)]}\mathbf{i} + \dfrac{2\ln(1 + t)}{1 + t}\mathbf{j} + \dfrac{2 \sinh [2\ln(1 + t) + 1]}{1 + t}\mathbf{k}.$$

11. (a) $\mathbf{r} \times \mathbf{s} = (t + t^2 \sin t)\mathbf{i} + (2 \sin t - 1 - t^2)\mathbf{j} - (2t + t^2 + t^4)\mathbf{k}$, so

$$\frac{d}{dt}[\mathbf{r} \times \mathbf{s}] = (1 + 2t \sin t + t^2 \cos t)\mathbf{i} + (2 \cos t - 2t)\mathbf{j} - (2 + 2t + 4t^3)\mathbf{k};$$

alternatively, but with greater effort, use the fact that

$$\frac{d}{dt}[\mathbf{r} \times \mathbf{s}] = \frac{d\mathbf{r}}{dt} \times \mathbf{s} + \mathbf{r} \times \frac{d\mathbf{s}}{dt};$$

(b) $\mathbf{r} \times \mathbf{s} = (\cos t + e^t \sin t)\mathbf{i} + (e^t \cos t - \sin t)\mathbf{j} - \mathbf{k}$, so

$$\frac{d}{dt}[\mathbf{r} \times \mathbf{s}] = [-\sin t + e^t \sin t + e^t \cos t]\mathbf{i} + [e^t \cos t - e^t \sin t - \cos t]\mathbf{j},$$

or use the alternative approach indicated in (a).

12. $\dfrac{d}{dt}\left[\mathbf{r} \times \dfrac{d\mathbf{r}}{dt}\right] = \dfrac{d\mathbf{r}}{dt} \times \dfrac{d\mathbf{r}}{dt} + \mathbf{r} \times \dfrac{d^2\mathbf{r}}{dt^2} = \mathbf{r} \times \dfrac{d^2\mathbf{r}}{dt^2}$,

because the first vector product is zero.

13. $d\mathbf{r}/dt = (\sin t + t \cos t)\mathbf{i} + 9 \cos t - t \sin t)\mathbf{j}$,

$$d^2\mathbf{r}/dt^2 = (2 \cos t - t \sin t)\mathbf{i} - (2 \sin t + t \cos t)\mathbf{j},$$

$$(d\mathbf{r}/dt) \times (d^2\mathbf{r}/dt^2) = -(t^2 + 2)\mathbf{k} \text{ and } |d\mathbf{r}/dt| = t, \text{ so}$$

$$\kappa = (t^2 + 2)/t^3.$$

14. (a) $\dfrac{-1}{3t^3}\mathbf{i} - \dfrac{1}{2t^2}\mathbf{j} - \dfrac{1}{t}\mathbf{k} + \mathbf{c}$;

(b) $\displaystyle\int_0^\pi (\sin kt\mathbf{a} + \cos kt\mathbf{b})dt = \begin{cases} \dfrac{1}{k}[(1 - \cos k\pi)\mathbf{a} + \sin k\pi\mathbf{b}] & \text{for } k \neq 0 \\ \pi\mathbf{b} & \text{if } k = 0. \end{cases}$

15. $\displaystyle\int (\sinh t\mathbf{i} + e^{-2t}\mathbf{j} + t\mathbf{k}) \times (\mathbf{i} - \mathbf{j} + \mathbf{k})dt = \int [(t + e^{-2t})\mathbf{i} + (t - \sinh t)\mathbf{j}$

$$- (e^{-2t} + \sinh t)\mathbf{k}]dt$$

$$= \frac{1}{2}(t^2 - e^{-2t})\mathbf{i} + \left(\frac{1}{2}t^2 - \cosh t\right)\mathbf{j} + \left(\frac{1}{2}e^{-2t} - \cosh t\right)\mathbf{k} + \mathbf{c},$$

where $\mathbf{c}$ is an arbitrary constant vector.

16. $\dfrac{d\mathbf{r}}{dt} = \displaystyle\int \dfrac{d^2\mathbf{r}}{dt^2}dt = \int \mathbf{a}dt = t\mathbf{a} + \mathbf{c}$,

where $\mathbf{c}$ is an arbitrary constant vector. As $d\mathbf{r}/dt = \mathbf{u}$ when $t = 0$, we have

$$\frac{d\mathbf{r}}{dt} = \mathbf{u} + t\mathbf{a}.$$

A further integration gives

$$\mathbf{r} = \int \frac{d\mathbf{r}}{dt}dt = \int (\mathbf{u} + t\mathbf{a})dt = t\mathbf{u} + \frac{1}{2}t^2\mathbf{a} + \mathbf{d},$$

where $\mathbf{d}$ is an arbitrary constant vector. As $\mathbf{r} = \mathbf{r}_0$, when $t = 0$, it follows that $\mathbf{d} = \mathbf{r}_0$, and thus

$$\mathbf{r} = \mathbf{r}_0 + t\mathbf{u} + \frac{1}{2} t^2 \mathbf{a}.$$

17. $d\mathbf{r}/dt = -\sin t\mathbf{i} + \cos t\mathbf{j} + 2t\mathbf{k}$, so when $t = t_1$,

$$\mathbf{T} = -\sin t_1\mathbf{i} + \cos t_1\mathbf{j} + 2t_1\mathbf{k}.$$

The equation of the plane is

$$\mathbf{r} \cdot \mathbf{T} = \mathbf{a} \cdot \mathbf{T},$$

where $\mathbf{r} = x\mathbf{i} + y\mathbf{j} + z\mathbf{k}$ and $a = \mathbf{i} + 2\mathbf{j} + 3\mathbf{k}$. Thus the Cartesian form of the equation is

$$-x \sin t_1 + y \cos t_1 + 2zt_1 = -\sin t_1 + 2 \cos t_1 + 6t_1.$$

18. $\mathbf{a} = d\mathbf{v}/dt = -\mathbf{i} - 2\mathbf{k}$ and $\mathbf{r} = \int \mathbf{v}dt = \int [-t\mathbf{i} + (1 - 2t)\mathbf{k}]dt$

$$= -\frac{1}{2} t^2 \mathbf{i} + (t - t^2)\mathbf{k} + \mathbf{c},$$

with $\mathbf{c}$ an arbitrary vector constant. As $\mathbf{r} = \mathbf{0}$ when $t = 0$, it follows that $\mathbf{c} = \mathbf{0}$, so

$$\mathbf{r} = -\frac{1}{2} t^2 \mathbf{i} + (t - t^2)\mathbf{k}.$$

The vectors $\mathbf{r}$ and $\mathbf{a}$ will be orthogonal when $\mathbf{r} \cdot \mathbf{a} = 0$, which is equivalent to

$$\frac{1}{2} t^2 - 2(t - t^2) = 0, \quad \text{or} \quad t(3t - 4) = 0.$$

Thus the vectors are orthogonal when $t = 0$ and $t = 4/3$.

19. $\mathbf{r} = \int \mathbf{v}dt = \int (\sin 2t\mathbf{i} + 2 \cos 2t\mathbf{j} + t\mathbf{k})dt$

$$= -\frac{1}{2} \cos 2t\mathbf{i} + \sin 2t\mathbf{j} + \frac{1}{2} t^2 \mathbf{k} + \mathbf{c},$$

where $\mathbf{c}$ is an arbitrary constant vector. As $\mathbf{r} = 3\mathbf{i} + \mathbf{j} - 3\mathbf{k}$ when $t = 0$, it follows that $\mathbf{c} = (7/2)\mathbf{i} + \mathbf{j} - 3\mathbf{k}$, and so

$$\mathbf{r} = \frac{1}{2} (7 - \cos 2t)\mathbf{i} + (1 + \sin 2t)\mathbf{j} + \frac{1}{2} (t^2 - 6)\mathbf{k}.$$

$$\mathbf{a} = d\mathbf{v}/dt = 2 \cos t\mathbf{i} - 4 \sin 2t\mathbf{j} + \mathbf{k},$$

so for orthogonality $\mathbf{v} \cdot \mathbf{a} = 0$, which is equivalent to

$$-6 \sin 2t \cos 2t + t = 0, \text{ or } -3 \sin 4t + t = 0.$$

As $|\sin 4t| \leq 1$, this result can never hold if $t > 3$.

20. $\mathbf{v} = d\mathbf{r}/dt = 3 \sin 3t\mathbf{i} + 3 \cos 3t\mathbf{j} + (2t - 4)\mathbf{k}$,

$$\mathbf{a} = d\mathbf{v}/dt = 9 \cos 3t\mathbf{i} - 9 \sin 3t\mathbf{j} + 2\mathbf{k}.$$

Orthogonality occurs when $\mathbf{r} \cdot \mathbf{a} = 0$, which is equivalent to

$$t^2 - 4t - 5 = 0, \quad \text{or} \quad (t - 5)(t + 1) = 0.$$

Thus the time subsequent to $t = 0$ at which $\mathbf{r}$ and $\mathbf{a}$ are orthogonal is $t = 5$.

PROBLEMS 67

1. The equation of motion is

$$m\frac{d^2\mathbf{r}}{dt^2} = -mg\mathbf{j}, \quad \text{or} \quad \frac{d^2\mathbf{r}}{dt^2} = -g\mathbf{j}.$$

Integrating once gives

$$\mathbf{v} = \frac{d\mathbf{r}}{dt} = -gt\mathbf{j} + \mathbf{a},$$

where $\mathbf{a}$ is an arbitrary constant vector. As $\mathbf{v} = \mathbf{u}$ when $t = 0$ we see that $\mathbf{a} = \mathbf{u}$, and so

$$\mathbf{v} = \mathbf{u} - gt\mathbf{j}.$$

Writing this as

$$\frac{d\mathbf{r}}{dt} = \mathbf{u} - gt\mathbf{j}$$

and integrating gives

$$\mathbf{r} = \mathbf{u}t - \frac{1}{2}gt^2\mathbf{j} + \mathbf{b},$$

where $\mathbf{b}$ is an arbitrary constant vector. As $\mathbf{r} = \mathbf{0}$ when $t = 0$ it follows that $\mathbf{b} = \mathbf{0}$, so

$$\mathbf{r} = \mathbf{u}t - \frac{1}{2}gt^2\mathbf{j}.$$

Setting $\mathbf{u} = u(\cos \alpha\mathbf{i} + \sin \alpha\mathbf{j})$ and equating the $\mathbf{i}$ and $\mathbf{j}$ components shows that

$$x = ut \cos \alpha \quad \text{and} \quad y = ut \sin \alpha - \frac{1}{2}gt^2.$$

After leaving the origin, $y = 0$ when $t = 2(u/g) \sin \alpha$, at which time $x = 2(u^2/g) \sin \alpha \cos \alpha = (u^2/g) \sin 2\alpha$.

2.   Take the x-axis horizontal and the y-axis vertical, so the gravitational force acting on the particle is $-mg\mathbf{j}$. Then the equation of motion becomes

$$m\frac{d\mathbf{y}}{dt} = -mg\mathbf{j} - km\mathbf{v},$$

or

$$\frac{d\mathbf{y}}{dt} + k\mathbf{v} = -g\mathbf{j}.$$

The integrating factor is e^{kt} (as in Example 67.1), so

$$e^{kt}\frac{d\mathbf{y}}{dt} + ke^{kt}\mathbf{v} = -ge^{kt}\mathbf{j},$$

or

$$\frac{d}{dt}[e^{kt}\mathbf{v}] = -ge^{kt}\mathbf{j}.$$

Integrating this result gives

$$e^{kt}\mathbf{v} = \frac{g}{k}e^{kt}\mathbf{j} + \mathbf{a},$$

or

$$\mathbf{v} = -\frac{g}{k}\mathbf{j} + e^{-kt}\mathbf{a},$$

where $\mathbf{a}$ is an arbitrary constant vector. As $\mathbf{v} = \mathbf{v}_0$ when $t = 0$ we have $\mathbf{a} = \mathbf{v}_0 + (g/k)\mathbf{j}$ and so

$$\mathbf{v} = \mathbf{v}_0\,e^{-kt} - (g/k)(1 - e^{-kt})\mathbf{j}.$$

A further integration coupled with the fact that $\mathbf{r} = \mathbf{0}$ when $t = 0$ gives

$$\mathbf{r} = \frac{1}{k}(1 - e^{-kt})\mathbf{v}_0 + \frac{g}{k^2}(1 - e^{-kt})\mathbf{j} - \frac{gt}{k}\mathbf{j}.$$

3.   Proceed as in Example 67.2, but use the fact that now the radical component of $\dot{\mathbf{a}}$ must vanish, giving

$$\dddot{r} - 3\dot{r}\omega^2 = 0,$$

which after an integration becomes

$$\ddot{r} - 2r\omega^2 = \text{const.}$$

4.   As $\dot{\theta} = \omega = \text{const.}$, and $r = a(1 - \cos\theta)$, it follows that

$$\dot{r} = a\omega\sin\theta \quad \text{and} \quad \ddot{r} = a\omega^2\cos\theta = \omega^2(a - r).$$

Thus the radial and transverse components are, respectively,

$$\ddot{r} - r\dot{\theta}^2 = \omega^2(a - 2r) \text{ and } r\ddot{\theta} + 2\dot{r}\dot{\theta} = 2a\omega^2 \sin\theta.$$

5.   The radial velocity is

$$\dot{r} = a\cot\alpha \, e^{\theta \cot\alpha} \, \dot{\theta} = \omega r \cot\alpha,$$

and the transverse velocity is

$$r\dot{\theta} = \omega r,$$

so the velocity

$$\mathbf{v} = \omega r(\cot\alpha \, \hat{\mathbf{e}} + \hat{\mathbf{s}}).$$

If ψ is the angle between the radial unit vector $\hat{\mathbf{e}}$ and $\mathbf{v}$, then

$$\cos\psi = \frac{\hat{\mathbf{e}} \cdot \mathbf{v}}{|\hat{\mathbf{e}}||\mathbf{v}|} = \frac{\omega r \cot\alpha}{1 \cdot \omega r(1 + \cot^2\alpha)^{1/2}} = \cos\alpha,$$

and thus $\psi = \alpha$ (const.). It is for this reason the curve is called an **equiangular spiral**.

PROBLEMS 68

1.   For any $\varphi > 0$ the curve

$$\frac{x^2}{4\varphi} + \frac{y^2}{9\varphi} = 1$$

is an ellipse in the (x, y)-plane with semi-minor axis $2\sqrt{\varphi}$ and semi-major axis $3\sqrt{\varphi}$. The curve is independent of z, so the level surfaces in three-dimensional space are elliptic cylinders (cylinders whose cross-sections are ellipses and whose sides are parallel to the z-axis).

2.   For any $\varphi \neq 0$ the curve

$$\frac{x^2}{\varphi} - \frac{y^2}{\varphi} = 1$$

is an hyperbola with the asymptotes $y = \pm x$. The curve is independent of z, so the level surfaces in three-dimensional space are hyperbolic cylinders (surfaces whose cross-sections are hyperbolas and whose sides are parallel to the z-axis).

3.   For any $\varphi > 0$ the surface

$$x^2 + y^2 + z^2 = \varphi$$

is a sphere of radius $\sqrt{\varphi}$, centred on the origin. Thus for arbitrary $\varphi > 0$ the level surfaces are concentric spheres.

4.   For any φ the surface

$$\varphi = x + y + z$$

is a plane with the normal $\mathbf{n} = \mathbf{i} + \mathbf{j} + \mathbf{k}$ whose perpendicular distance from the origin is $|\varphi/\sqrt{3}|$. Thus for arbitrary constant φ the level surfaces are parallel planes with normal $\mathbf{n}$.

5. $\operatorname{grad} \varphi = 2x\mathbf{i} + 4y\mathbf{j} - 6z\mathbf{k}$ so $(\operatorname{grad} \varphi)_{(1, 2, -1)} = 2\mathbf{i} + 8\mathbf{j} + 6\mathbf{k}$;

$$\hat{\mathbf{n}} = (2\mathbf{i} + 8\mathbf{j} + 6\mathbf{k})/\sqrt{104}.$$

6. $\operatorname{grad} \varphi = y^2 z^3 \mathbf{i} + 2xyz^3 \mathbf{j} + 3xy^2 z^2 \mathbf{k}$ so $(\operatorname{grad} \varphi)_{(1, 1, -1)} = -\mathbf{i} - 2\mathbf{j} + 3\mathbf{k}$;

$$\hat{\mathbf{n}} = (-\mathbf{i} - 2\mathbf{j} + 3\mathbf{k})/\sqrt{14}.$$

7. $\operatorname{grad} \varphi = yz \cos(xyz)\mathbf{i} + xz \cos(xyz)\mathbf{j} + xy \cos(xyz)\mathbf{k}$ so

$$(\operatorname{grad} \varphi)_{(-1, \pi/4, -1)} = -\frac{\pi}{4\sqrt{2}}\mathbf{i} + \frac{\pi}{\sqrt{2}}\mathbf{j} - \frac{\pi}{4\sqrt{2}}\mathbf{k};$$

$$\hat{\mathbf{n}} = \frac{4}{(\pi^2 + 8)^{1/2}}\left(-\frac{\pi}{4\sqrt{2}}\mathbf{i} + \frac{\pi}{\sqrt{2}}\mathbf{j} - \frac{\pi}{4\sqrt{2}}\mathbf{k}\right).$$

8. $\operatorname{grad} \varphi = \dfrac{2x}{x^2 + y^2 + z^2}\mathbf{i} + \dfrac{2y}{x^2 + y^2 + z^2}\mathbf{j} + \dfrac{2z}{x^2 + y^2 + z^2}\mathbf{k}$ so

$$(\operatorname{grad} \varphi)_{(1, 1, 1)} = \frac{2}{3}(\mathbf{i} + \mathbf{j} + \mathbf{k}); \; \hat{\mathbf{n}} = \frac{1}{\sqrt{3}}(\mathbf{i} + \mathbf{j} + \mathbf{k}).$$

9. $\operatorname{grad} \varphi = \sin y\mathbf{i} + (x \cos y + \cos z)\mathbf{j} - y \sin z\mathbf{k}$ so

$$(\operatorname{grad} \varphi)_{(\pi/4, \pi/4, \pi/4)} = \frac{1}{\sqrt{2}}\mathbf{i} + \frac{1}{\sqrt{2}}\left(1 + \frac{\pi}{4}\right)\mathbf{j} - \frac{\pi}{4\sqrt{2}}\mathbf{k};$$

$$\hat{\mathbf{n}} = \frac{4}{(16 + 4\pi + \pi^2)^{1/2}}\left[\frac{1}{\sqrt{2}}\mathbf{i} + \frac{1}{\sqrt{2}}\left(1 + \frac{\pi}{4}\right)\mathbf{j} - \frac{\pi}{4\sqrt{2}}\mathbf{k}\right].$$

10. $\operatorname{grad} \varphi = \dfrac{-2x}{(x^2 + 3y^2 + z^2)^2}\mathbf{i} - \dfrac{6y}{(x^2 + 3y^2 + z^2)^2}\mathbf{j} - \dfrac{2z}{(x^2 + y^2 + z^2)^2}\mathbf{k}$ so

$$(\operatorname{grad} \varphi)_{(1, 0, -1)} = -\frac{1}{2}\mathbf{i} + \frac{1}{2}\mathbf{k}; \; \hat{\mathbf{n}} = -\frac{1}{\sqrt{2}}\mathbf{i} + \frac{1}{\sqrt{2}}\mathbf{k}.$$

11.   Set $\varphi = x^2 + 2xyz + yz^2 - 1$, then the surface has the equation $\varphi = 0$. The point $(-1, 0, 1)$ lies on the surface since $\varphi(-1, 0, 1) = 0$. Thus a vector normal to the surface $\varphi = 0$ is

$$\operatorname{grad} \varphi = (3x^2 + 2yz)\mathbf{i} + (2xz + z^2)\mathbf{j} + (2xy + 2yz)\mathbf{k}.$$

Thus at $(-1, 0, 1)$ a vector $\mathbf{n}$ normal to $\varphi = 0$ is

$$\mathbf{n} = (\operatorname{grad} \varphi)_{(-1, 0, 1)} = 3\mathbf{i} - \mathbf{j}.$$

The equation of the tangent plane at this point is

$$r \cdot n = a \cdot n,$$

where a is the position vector of a point on the plane. Since $(-1, 0, 1)$ lies on the plane, we set $a = -i + k$, and so the equation of the tangent plane is

$$3x - y = -3.$$

12. Argue as in the answer to problem 11. Set $\varphi = x^2 + 3y^2 + 2z^2 - 15$, then $\varphi(1, 2, 1) = 0$ so the point $(1, 2, 1)$ lies on $\varphi = 0$.

$$\text{grad } \varphi = 2xi + 6yj + 4zk.$$

and

$$n = (\text{grad } \varphi)_{(1, 2, 1)} = 2i + 12j + 4k.$$

Setting $a = i + 2j + k$, the equation of the tangent plane at $(1, 2, 1)$ becomes

$$x + 6y + 2z = 15.$$

13. $F = (2x + 2yz)i + 2xzj + (2xy + 3z^2)k$, so

$$(F)_{(1, -1, 1)} = 2j + k \text{ and } |F|_{(1, -1, 1)} = \sqrt{5}.$$

The component of F in the direction of the vector $n = i + j - k$ is

$$F \cdot \hat{n} = (2j + k) \cdot \frac{1}{\sqrt{3}} (i + j - k) = 1/\sqrt{3}.$$

14. Setting $\varphi = x^2 + 4y^2 + z^2 - 6$, we see that the points $(1, 1, 1)$ and $(1, -1, -1)$ both lie on the surface $\varphi = 0$. $\text{grad } \varphi = 2xi + 8yj + 2zk$, so

$$n_1 = (\text{grad } \varphi)_{(1, 1, 1)} = 2i + 8j + 2k \text{ and}$$

$$n_2 = (\text{grad } \varphi)_{(1, -1, -1)} = 2i - 8j - 2k.$$

As n_1 and n_2 are normals to $\varphi = 0$ at $(1, 1, 1)$ and $(1, -1, -1)$, the angle θ between n_1 and n_2 will be the angle between the tangent planes at these points.

Thus

$$\cos \theta = \frac{n_1 \cdot n_2}{|n_1||n_2|} = \frac{-64}{\sqrt{72} \sqrt{72}} = -\frac{8}{9},$$

so $\theta = \arccos(-8/9)$.

15. $\text{grad } \varphi = (3x^2 + 4xy^2z)i + (4x^2yz + 2yz^2)j + (2x^2y^2 + 2y^2z)k$ so a vector normal to the surface $\varphi = 0$ at $(1, 1, 1)$ is $b = 7i + 6j + 4k$. The point $(1, 1, 1)$ lies on the required line, so its vector equation

$$r = a + \lambda b$$

becomes

$$xi + yj + zk = i + j + k + \lambda(7i + 6j + 4k).$$

The Cartesian equations of the line are thus

$$\frac{x-1}{7} = \frac{y-1}{6} = \frac{z-1}{4}.$$

16.   grad $\varphi = 3x^2 i + 4yj - 4zk$, so as the point $(-1, -1, -1)$ lies on the surface $\varphi = 0$ it follows that a vector normal to this surface at $(-1, -1, -1)$ is

$$n = 3i - 4j + 4k.$$

The equation of the plane with this normal through the point with position vector $a = -i - j - k$ is thus

$$3x - 4y + 4z = -3.$$

Thus the perpendicular distance of this plane from the origin is

$$d = \left|\frac{-3}{\sqrt{41}}\right| = \frac{3}{\sqrt{41}}.$$

17.   The directional derivative of a function φ in the direction of a vector a is defined as $\hat{a} \cdot \text{grad } \varphi$, where $\hat{a} = a/|a|$ is the unit vector along a. Here $a = i - 3j + 3k$, so $\hat{a} = (1/\sqrt{19})(i - 3j + 3k)$.

$$\text{grad } \varphi = \frac{(-x^2 + 2y^2 + 3z^2)}{(x^2 + 2y^2 + 3z^2 + 1)^2} i - \frac{4xy}{(x^2 + 2y^2 + 3z^2 + 1)^2} j$$
$$- \frac{6xz}{(x^2 + 2y^2 + 3z^2 + 1)^2} k$$

so

$$\hat{a} \cdot \text{grad } \varphi = \frac{2y^2 + 3z^2 - x^2 + 12xy - 18xz}{\sqrt{19}(x^2 + 2y^2 + 3z^2 + 1)^2}.$$

Thus at the point $(1, -1, -1)$,

$$(\hat{a} \cdot \text{grad } \varphi)_{(1,-1,-1)} = \frac{10}{49}.$$

18. $a \times u = k \times (u_1 i + u_2 j) = u_1 j - u_2 i$ and

$$\text{grad } \varphi = \cos x \sin y i + \sin x \cos y j.$$

Thus $a \times u = \text{grad } \varphi$ becomes

$$u_1 j - u_2 i = \cos x \sin y i + \sin x \cos y j,$$

and hence

$$u_1 = \sin x \cos y \text{ and } u_2 = -\cos x \sin y.$$

As $\mathbf{u} = u_1\mathbf{i} + u_2\mathbf{j}$, it follows that

$$\mathbf{u} = \sin x \cos y\,\mathbf{i} - \cos x \sin y\,\mathbf{j}.$$

19. Set $\varphi = x^2 + 2y^2 + \alpha^2 z^2 - 18$, then the point $(1, 2, 3/\alpha)$ lies on $\varphi = 0$.

$$\operatorname{grad} \varphi = 2x\mathbf{i} + 4y\mathbf{j} + 2\alpha^2 z\mathbf{k},$$

so

$$\mathbf{n} = (\operatorname{grad} \varphi)_{(1, 2, 3/\alpha)} = 2\mathbf{i} + 8\mathbf{j} + 6\alpha\mathbf{k}.$$

Vector $\mathbf{n}$ is along the normal at $(1, 2, 3/\alpha)$ so the equation of the normal is

$$\mathbf{r} = \left(\mathbf{i} + 2\mathbf{j} + \frac{3}{\alpha}\,\mathbf{k} \right) + \lambda(2\mathbf{i} + 8\mathbf{j} + 6\alpha\mathbf{k}).$$

If this is to pass through the point $(0, -2, 8)$, λ and α must be such that

$$-2\mathbf{j} + 8\mathbf{k} = \mathbf{i} + 2\mathbf{j} + \frac{3}{\alpha}\,\mathbf{k} + 2\lambda\mathbf{i} + 8\lambda\mathbf{j} + 6\alpha\lambda\mathbf{k}.$$

Equating $\mathbf{i}$, $\mathbf{j}$ and $\mathbf{k}$ components gives

$$\mathbf{i} : 1 + 2\lambda = 0 \text{ so } \lambda = -\frac{1}{2};$$

$$\mathbf{j} : -2 = 2 + 8\lambda$$

which again gives $\lambda = -1/2$ and so is compatible with the first result;

$$\mathbf{k} : 8 = \frac{3}{\alpha} + 6\lambda\alpha, \text{ or as } \lambda = -1/2,$$

$$3\alpha^2 + 8\alpha - 3 = 0.$$

This has the solutions $\alpha = -3$ and $\alpha = 1/3$.

20. Set $\varphi = 3x^2 - y^2 + 2xyz - 4$, then the points $(1, 1, 1)$ and $(-1, -1, -1)$ both lie on $\varphi = 0$.

$$\operatorname{grad} \varphi = (6x + 2yz)\mathbf{i} + (-2y + 2xz)\mathbf{j} + 2xy\mathbf{k},$$

so

$$\mathbf{n}_1 = (\operatorname{grad} \varphi)_{(1, 1, 1)} = 8\mathbf{i} + 2\mathbf{k}$$

and

$$\mathbf{n}_2 = (\operatorname{grad} \varphi)_{(-1, -1, -1)} = 8\mathbf{i} + 2\mathbf{k}.$$

As the normals at $(1, 1, 1)$ and $(-1, -1, 1)$ have no $\mathbf{j}$ component, the tangent planes at these points must be parallel to the y-axis. If $\mathbf{a}_1 = \mathbf{i} + \mathbf{j} + \mathbf{k}$, the tangent plane at $(1, 1, 1)$ is

$$\mathbf{r} \cdot \mathbf{n}_1 = \mathbf{a}_1 \cdot \mathbf{n}_1, \text{ or } 4x + z = 5.$$

This is seen to be at a perpendicular distance $5/\sqrt{17}$ from the origin, but on the opposite side with respect to the first plane because the constant terms have opposite signs (the other tangent plane is $4x - z = 5$).

PROBLEMS 69

1. (a) order 4, degree 3; (b) order 3, degree 1; (c) order 1, degree 2; (d) order 1, degree 1; (e) order 2, degree 1; (f) order 2, degree 1.

2. (a) order 1 and linear; (b) order 2 and non-linear; (c) order 2 and non-linear; (d) order 2 and linear; (e) order 3 and linear; (f) order 4 and non-linear.

3. $y = \dfrac{1}{6}x^3 + \dfrac{1}{2}Ax^2 + Bx + C.$

4. $y = \dfrac{1}{6}x^3 + \dfrac{1}{24}x^4 + \dfrac{1}{2}Ax^2 + Bx + C.$

5. $y' = \dfrac{1}{3}x^3 + \dfrac{8}{3}$ and $y = \dfrac{1}{12}x^4 + \dfrac{8}{3}x - \dfrac{3}{4}.$

6. $y' = 3 - \cos x$ and $y = 1 + 3x - \sin x.$

7. $y' = \dfrac{1}{2}\cosh 2x + A$ and $y = \dfrac{1}{4}\sinh 2x + Ax^2 + B;$

    $y(0) = 1$ implies $B = 1$ and $y(1) = 4$ implies $A = 3 - \dfrac{1}{4}\sinh 2$, so

    $$y = \frac{1}{4}\sinh 2x + \left(3 - \frac{1}{4}\sinh 2\right)x + 1.$$

8. $y' = \sin x + A$ and $y = -\cos x + Ax + B;$ $y(0) = 0$ implies $B = 1$ and $y(\pi) = 0$ implies $A = -2/\pi$, so

    $$y = 1 - \frac{2}{\pi}x - \cos x.$$

9. $\dfrac{d^2y}{dx^2} + 9y = 0.$

10. $\dfrac{d^2y}{dx^2} - 16y = 0.$

11. $\dfrac{d^2y}{dx^2} - 6\dfrac{dy}{dx} + 9y = 0.$

12. $\dfrac{d^3y}{dx^3} - 4\dfrac{d^2y}{dx^2} - 3\dfrac{dy}{dx} + 18y = 0.$

13. $\dfrac{d^2y}{dx^2} - 6\dfrac{dy}{dx} + 25y = 0.$

14. $\dfrac{d^3y}{dx^3} - 4\dfrac{d^2y}{dx^2} + \dfrac{dy}{dx} - y = 0.$

PROBLEMS 70

1. $y = Cx; \ y = -3x.$

2. $x^2 + y^2 = C^2; \ x^2 + y^2 = 20.$

3. $y = Ce^{1/x}; \ y = 2e^{1/x}.$

4. $y = C \ \exp(\sqrt{x}); \ y = \exp(\sqrt{x} - 3).$

5. $y = \dfrac{1}{2}(C \sin^2 x - 1); \ y = 2\sin^2 x - \dfrac{1}{2}.$

6. $y = \dfrac{Cx^2}{(1+x)^2} - \dfrac{1}{2}; \ y = \dfrac{2x^2}{(1+x)^2} - \dfrac{1}{2}.$

7. $\cot^2 y = \tan^2 x + C.$

8. $\tan y = C(1 - e^x)^2.$

9. $(1 + e^x)(1 + e^y) = C.$

10. $y = \dfrac{1}{2}\ln^2 |x| + C.$

11. $\ln|xy| + x - y = C.$

12. $\dfrac{x+y}{xy} + \ln\left|\dfrac{y}{x}\right| = C.$

13. $\displaystyle\int \dfrac{dy}{4-y} = \int \tan x \, dx,$ so

$$-\ln|4-y| = -\ln|\cos x| - \ln C.$$

This is equivalent to

$$\ln\left|\dfrac{\cos x}{4-y}\right| = -\ln C = \ln(1/C),$$

or to

$$\dfrac{\cos x}{4-y} = \dfrac{1}{C},$$

so the general solution is

$$y = 4 - C \cos x.$$

As $y(0) = -1$ we have $-1 = 4 - C$, so $C = 5$ and $y = 4 - 5 \cos x$.

14. $\displaystyle\int \frac{dy}{1 + \cos 4y} = \int \frac{dx}{x^2}$ or $\displaystyle\frac{1}{2} \int \frac{dy}{\cos^2 2y} = \int \frac{dx}{x^2}.$

Thus $\displaystyle\frac{1}{4} \tan 2y = -(1/x) + C_1$ or $\tan 2y = [C - (4/x)]$ and so

$$y = \frac{1}{2} \arctan [C - (4/x)].$$

As $y(+\infty) = \pi/8$ we have

$$\frac{\pi}{8} = \frac{1}{2} \arctan C,$$

so $C = 1$ and

$$y = \frac{1}{2} \arctan \left(1 - \frac{4}{x}\right).$$

15. In terms of z the equation becomes

$$\frac{dz}{z + 2} + dx = 0,$$

so integration shows the general solution to be

$$\ln |z + 2| + x = \ln C,$$

or

$$z + 2 = Ce^{-x}.$$

Returning to the variables x and y, the general solution becomes

$$y = 2x - 1 + Ce^{-x}.$$

16. In terms of z the equation becomes

$$\frac{dz}{1 - \cos z} = dx$$

so

$$\int \frac{dz}{1 - \cos z} = \int dx.$$

As $1 - \cos z = 2 \sin^2 (z/2)$ this becomes

$$\frac{1}{2} \int \mathrm{cosec}^2 (z/2)dz = \int dx$$

and thus

$$- \cot (z/2) = x - C$$

or

$$z = 2 \, \mathrm{arccot} \, (C - x).$$

Returning to variables x and y shows the general solution to be

$$y = x - 1 - 2 \, \mathrm{arccot} \, (C - x).$$

PROBLEMS 71

1.   The equation of the isoclines is

$$4 - x^2 + y = k,$$

so they are the parabolas

$$y = k - 4 + x^2.$$

Integral curves cutting a parabola do so at an angle $\theta = \arctan k$ to the x-axis. The exact solution is

$$y = x^2 + 2x - 2.$$

n	x_n	y_n	Exact y_n
0	1.0	1.0	1.0
1	1.5	3.1875	3.25
2	2.0	5.8359	6.0
3	2.5	8.9209	9.25
4	3.0	12.4027	13.0

If a step length $h = 0.1$ had been used, the last entry in the table would have become $y(3) = 12.9697$, showing a marked improvement in accuracy.

2.   The equation of the isoclines is

$$\frac{3y}{x} = k,$$

so they are the radial lines through the origin

$$y = \frac{k}{3} x .$$

Integral currves cutting a line do so at an angle $\theta = \arctan k$ to the x-axis. The exact solution is $y = x^3$.

n	x_n	y_n	Exact y_n
0	1.0	1.0	1.0
1	1.5	3.0	3.375
2	2.0	6.7500	8.0
3	2.5	12.8250	15.625
4	3.0	21.8025	27.0
5	3.5	34.2611	42.875
6	4.0	50.7798	64

Clearly the step length $h = 0.5$ is too large to give an accurate result. Had the step length been reduced to $h = 0.1$ the last entry in the table would have become $y(4) = 62.9812$.

3. The equation of the isoclines is

$$k = (x^2 + y^2)/x^2,$$

so the isoclines are the radial lines through the origin

$$y = \pm x \sqrt{(k - 1)} \text{ , with } k \geqslant 1.$$

Integral curves cutting a line do so at an angle $\theta = \arctan k$ to the x-axis. The exact solution is

$$y = \frac{1}{2} x \left[1 + \sqrt{3} \tan \left(\frac{\pi}{6} + \frac{\sqrt{3}}{2} \ln |x| \right) \right].$$

n	x_n	y_n	Exact y_n
0	1.0	1.0	1.0
1	1.5	2.1944	2.3047
2	2.0	4.1153	4.6140
3	2.5	7.4866	9.6012
4	3.0	14.5484	28.5449

Clearly the step length $h = 0.5$ is too large to give an accurate result. Had the step length been reduced to $h = 0.1$ the last entry in the table would have become $y(3) = 26.2089$.

4. The equation of the isoclines is

$$k = 4 - x + y,$$

so the isoclines are the parallel straight lines

$$y = x + k - 4.$$

Integral curves cutting a line do so at an angle $\theta = \arctan k$ to the x-axis. The exact solution is

$$y = 3e^x + x - 3.$$

n	x_n	y_n	Exact y_n
0	0	0	0
1	0.5	2.3750	2.4462
2	1.0	5.9219	6.1548
3	1.5	11.3730	11.9451
4	2.0	19.9187	21.1672
5	2.5	33.4929	36.0475
6	3.0	55.2384	60.2566

Clearly the step length $h = 0.5$ is too large to give an accurate result. Had the step length been reduced to $h = 0.1$ the last entry in the table would have become $y(3) = 59.9777$.

5. The equation of the isoclines is

$$k = 2y/x^2,$$

so the isoclines are the parabolas

$$y = \frac{k}{2} x^2.$$

Integral curves cutting a parabola do so at an angle $\theta = \arctan k$ to the x-axis. The exact solution is

$$y = \exp\left[2\left(\frac{x-1}{x}\right)\right].$$

n	x_n	y_n	Exact y_n
0	1.0	1.0	1.0
1	1.5	1.9444	1.9477
2	2.0	2.7276	2.7183
3	2.5	3.3413	3.3201
4	3.0	3.8240	3.7937

Had the step length been reduced to $h = 0.1$ the last entry in the table would have become $y(3) = 3.7954$.

6. The equation of the isoclines is

$$k = \frac{1}{x(y+2)},$$

so the isoclines are the hyperbolas

$$y = \frac{1}{kx} - 2.$$

All the integral curves cutting a parabola do so at an angle $\theta = \arctan k$ to the x-axis. The exact solution is

$$\frac{1}{2} y^2 + 2y = \ln |x|.$$

n	x_n	y_n	Exact y_n
0	1.0	0	0
1	1.5	0.1991	0.1934
2	2.0	0.3280	0.3208
3	2.5	0.4228	0.4151
4	3.0	0.4973	0.4894

Had the step length been reduced to $h = 0.1$ the last entry in the table would have become $y(3) = 0.4894$.

PROBLEMS 72

1. (a) Homogeneous of degree 2; (b) Homogeneous of degree 3;
    (c) Homogeneous of degree 3; (d) Not homogeneous;
    (e) Homogeneous of degree 1; (f) Not homogeneous.

2. $x = Ce^{-y^2/x^2}$.

3. $x\left(1 - \dfrac{y^2}{x^2}\right) = C;\ x^2 - y^2 + 3x = 0.$

4. $(2x - y)^2 = Cx;\ (2x - y)^2 = 4x.$

5. $x = Ce^{x/y}.$

6. $\sqrt{\dfrac{x}{y}} + \ln |y| = C.$

7. $(x^2 + y^2)^3 (x + y)^2 = C.$

8. $y^2 = Cx\, e^{-x/y}.$

9. $y^2 = x^2 \ln |C/x|.$

10. $2y^2 \ln |Cy| + x^2 = 0.$

11. $(x + y - 1)^3 = C(x - y + 3).$

12. $3x + y + 2 \ln |x + y - 1| = C.$

13. $\ln |4x + 8y + 5| + 8y - 4x = C.$

14. $(y + 1) \exp \left[2 \arctan \left(\dfrac{y + 1}{x - 3} \right) \right] = C.$

15. $10y - 5x + 7 \ln |10x + 5y + 9| = C.$

16. $y = x[3 \ln |Cx|]^{1/3}.$

PROBLEMS 73

1. $x^3 + 2xy^2 + y^2 = C.$

2. $x^2 + xy + y^2 + \cos x + \sin y = C.$

3. $xy + \sqrt{(x^2 + y^2)} = C.$

4. $xye^x + y^2 = C.$

5. $\dfrac{1}{4} x^4 - \dfrac{3}{2} x^2 y^2 + 2x + \dfrac{1}{3} y^3 = C.$

6. $\dfrac{1}{3} x^3 + xy^2 + x^2 = C.$

7. $xy + 2x + y + \sinh (x + 3y) = C.$

8. $x^2 - y^2 = Cy^3.$

9. $\mu = x; \ x^3 y^2 + 3x^2 y^3 = C.$

10. $\mu = x^2 y^2; \ x^4 y^3 + 6x^3 y^5 = C.$

PROBLEMS 74

1. $y = x \ln |A/x|.$

2. $y = \dfrac{1}{x} (A - \cos x).$

3. $y = \dfrac{1}{2} (x + 1)^4 + A(x + 1)^2.$

4. $y = e^x \left(\ln |x| + \dfrac{1}{2} x^2 + A \right).$

5. $y = Ae^{-\cos x} - \cos x + 1.$

6. $y = (1 + x^2)(x + A).$

7. $y = x^2(e^x + A)$.

8. $y = A(x + 1)^2 + \dfrac{1}{2}(x + 1)^4$.

9. $y = (3x - 2)/2$.

10. $y = 2\sqrt{2}\sqrt{(x^2 + 1)} - x - 3$.

11. $y = 2\sin x - \cos x$.

12. $y = x^3(2e + e^x)$.

13. $y = 2(x + 1)/x^3$.

14. $y = (x^3 + 3x - 1)/(3x)$.

15. $y = \dfrac{6x + 2 - 3\pi}{2\sin x}$.

16. $y = \dfrac{x + 1}{\cos x}$.

PROBLEMS 75

1. $y = \dfrac{1}{x \ln |Ax|}$.

2. $y = \dfrac{x}{A - \ln |x|}$.

3. $y = x^4 \left(\dfrac{1}{2} \ln |x| + A \right)^2$.

4. $y = \dfrac{1}{x(x + A)}$.

5. $y^2 = x \ln \left| \dfrac{A}{x} \right|$.

6. $y^2 = \dfrac{1}{x(1 + Ax)}$.

PROBLEMS 76

1. $W = \begin{vmatrix} 1 & x & x^2 & x^3 \\ 0 & 1 & 2x & 3x^2 \\ 0 & 0 & 2 & 6x \\ 0 & 0 & 0 & 6 \end{vmatrix} = 12 \neq 0$.

2. $W = \begin{vmatrix} \sin x & \cos x \\ \cos x & -\sin x \end{vmatrix} = -(\sin^2 x + \cos^2 x) = -1 \neq 0.$

3. $W = \begin{vmatrix} 1 & e^{\lambda x} & e^{\mu x} \\ 0 & \lambda e^{\lambda x} & \mu e^{\mu x} \\ 0 & \lambda^2 e^{\lambda x} & \mu^2 e^{\mu x} \end{vmatrix} = \lambda \mu \, (\mu - \lambda) e^{(\lambda + \mu)x} \neq 0$ if $\lambda \neq \mu.$

4. $W = \begin{vmatrix} e^{\lambda x} \cos \mu x & e^{\lambda x} \sin \mu x \\ \lambda e^{\lambda x} \cos \mu x - \mu \, e^{\lambda x} \sin \mu x & \lambda e^{\lambda x} \sin \mu x + \mu \, e^{\lambda x} \cos \mu x \end{vmatrix} = \mu \, e^{2\lambda x} \neq 0.$

5. $W = \begin{vmatrix} 1 & e^x & xe^x \\ 0 & e^x & (1+x)e^x \\ 0 & e^x & (2+x)e^x \end{vmatrix} = e^{2x} \neq 0.$

6. $W = \begin{vmatrix} x \cos \mu x & x \sin \mu x \\ \cos \mu x - \mu x \sin \mu x & \sin \mu x + \mu x \cos \mu x \end{vmatrix} = \mu \, x^2 \neq 0.$

7. Show that $y_c'' + 9y_c = 0$, and that

$$y_p'' + 9y_p = 9x^2 + 11.$$

8. Show that

$$x^2 y_c'' - 3xy_c' + 3y_c = 0,$$

and that

$$x^2 y_p'' - 3xy_p' + 3y_p = x^4 e^x.$$

The function

$$y(x) = 4x - 5x^3 + x(x-1)e^x$$

is a particular integral, because the terms $4x - 5x^3$ are contained in the complementary function as a special case, and so satisfy the homogenous form of the equation.

PROBLEMS 77

1. $y = Ae^x + Be^{-4x}.$

2. $y = A \cos 4x + B \sin 4x.$

3. $y = Ae^{3x} + Be^{-3x}.$

4. $y = Ae^{-2x} + Be^{-4x}.$

5. $y = A + Be^{-2x}.$

6. $y = (Ax + B)e^{7x}.$

7. $y = (Ax + B)e^{-4x}.$

8. $y = e^{-2x}(A \cos 2x + B \sin 2x)$.

9. $y = e^{3x}(A \cos 6x + B \sin 6x)$.

10. $y = e^x(A \cos 2x + B \sin 2x)$.

11. $y = e^{-x}(A \cos 2x + B \sin 2x)$.

12. $y = e^{2x}(A \cos 3x + B \sin 3x)$.

13. $y = 2e^{3x}$.

14. $y = e^{-x}(\cos 2x + \sin 2x)$.

15. $y = 2(1 - x)e^{5x}$.

16. $y = (2 + 7x)e^{-3x}$.

17. $y = e^x(\cos x + 2 \sin x)$.

18. $y = e^{-x} - 2e^{-2x}$.

19. $y = Ae^x + Be^{-x} + Ce^{2x} + De^{-2x}$.

20. $y = Ae^{2x} + Be^x + Ce^{-x}$.

21. $y = (A + Bx + Cx^2)e^{3x}$.

22. $y = e^{-x}(A \cos \sqrt{2}x + B \sin \sqrt{2}x) + e^x(C \cos \sqrt{2}x + D \sin \sqrt{2}x)$.

23. $y = (Ax + B)e^{2x} + (Cx + D)e^{-2x}$.

24. $y = e^{-x\sqrt{2}}(A \cos \sqrt{2}x + B \sin \sqrt{2}x) + e^{x\sqrt{2}}(C \cos \sqrt{2}x + D \sin \sqrt{2}x)$.

PROBLEMS 78

1. $y = (C_1 + C_2 x)e^{2x} + \dfrac{1}{8}(2x^2 + 4x + 3)$.

2. $y = e^{x/2}\left(A \cos \dfrac{x \sqrt{3}}{2} + B \sin \dfrac{x \sqrt{3}}{2}\right) + x^3 + 3x^2$.

3. $y = Ae^x + Be^{-2x} - \dfrac{2}{5}(3 \sin 2x + \cos 2x)$.

4. $y = (A + Bx)e^x + \dfrac{1}{2}\cos x + \dfrac{x^2}{2}e^x - \dfrac{1}{8}e^{-x}$

   (write $\sinh x = \dfrac{1}{2}(e^x + e^{-x})$).

5. $y = Ae^x + Be^{-2x} - \dfrac{2}{5}(3 \sin 2x + \cos 2x)$.

6. $y = Ae^{2x} + Be^{-3x} + x\left(\dfrac{x}{10} - \dfrac{1}{25}\right)e^{2x}.$

7. $y = Ae^{x} + Be^{-x} + \dfrac{1}{2}\,xe^{x}.$

8. $y = Ae^{-2x} + Be^{4x} - \dfrac{1}{9}\,e^{x} + \dfrac{1}{5}\,(3\cos 2x + \sin 2x).$

9. $y = (A + Bx + Cx^2)e^{-x} + \dfrac{1}{4}\,e^{x}.$

10. $y = A + Be^{3x} - \dfrac{1}{10}\,(\cos x + 3\sin x) - \dfrac{1}{6}\,x^2 - \dfrac{1}{9}\,x.$

11. $y = A\cos 2x + B\sin 2x - \dfrac{x}{4}\,(3\sin 2x + 2\cos 2x) + \dfrac{1}{4}.$

12. $y = Ae^{x} + Be^{-x} + \dfrac{1}{4}\,(x^2 - x)e^{x}.$

13. $y = A + Be^{2x} - 2x\,e^{x} - \dfrac{3}{4}\,x - \dfrac{3}{4}\,x^2.$

14. $y = Ae^{3x} + Be^{-x} + \dfrac{1}{9}\,(2 - 3x) + \dfrac{1}{16}\,(2x^2 - x)e^{3x}.$

15. $y = \cos 2x + \dfrac{1}{3}\,(\sin x + \sin 2x).$

16. $y = \dfrac{1}{8}\,e^{2x}(4x + 1) - \dfrac{1}{6}\,x^3 - \dfrac{1}{4}\,x^2 + \dfrac{1}{4}\,x.$

PROBLEMS 80

1. $x = A\cos t + B\sin t,\ \ y = B\cos t - A\sin t.$

2. $x = (A + Bt)e^{-2t},\ \ y = (B - A - Bt)e^{-2t}.$

3. $x = Ae^{3t} + Be^{-t},\ \ y = Ae^{3t} - Be^{-t}.$

4. $x = (A + Bt)e^{2t},\ \ y = -(A + B + Bt)e^{2t}.$

5. $x = Ae^{t} + Be^{-3t},\ \ y = 3Be^{-3t} - Ae^{t}.$

6. $x = Ae^{-t} + Be^{-3t},\ \ y = Ae^{-t} + 3Be^{-3t} + \cos t.$

7. $x = A\cos t + B\sin t + 1 + 2t,\ \ y = A\sin t - B\cos t - 2 + t;$
   $x = \cos t - \sin t + 1 + 2t,\ \ y = \sin t + \cos t - 2 + t.$

8. $x = A + Be^{-2t} + e^{t},\ \ y = A - Be^{-2t} + e^{t};$
   $x = 1 - Be^{-2t} + e^{t},\ \ y = 1 + e^{-2t} + e^{t}.$

9. $x = A + Bt + 2 \sin t$, $y = -2A - B(1 + 2t) - 3 \sin t - 2 \cos t$;
     $x = 5 - 13t + 2 \sin t$, $y = -10 + 13(1 + 2t) - 3 \sin t - 2 \cos t$.

10. $x = Ae^{t} + Be^{-2t} + 2e^{-t}$, $y = 3Ae^{t} + 2Be^{-2t} + 3e^{-t}$;
     $x = -3e^{t} + 3e^{-2t} + 2e^{-t}$, $y = -9e^{t} + 6e^{-2t} + 3e^{-t}$.

PROBLEMS 81

1. $18/s^{4}$.

2. $4/(s^{2} + 16)$.

3. $1/(s - 5)$.

4. $1/(s - 1)^{2}$.

5. $(s^{2} - 9)/(s^{2} + 9)^{2}$.

6. $5/[(s + 2)^{2} + 25] = 5/(s^{2} + 4s + 29)$.

7. $(s - 1)/[(s - 1)^{2} + 4] = (2 - 1)/(s^{2} - 2s + 5)$.

8. $2/(s^{2} - 4)$.

9. $2/s^{3} + 3s/(s^{2} + 9)$.

10. $1/(s - 2)^{2} + 6/s^{4}$.

11. $(s^{2} - 1)/(s^{2} + 1)^{2} + 4/(s^{2} + 4)$.

12. $(s - 2)/[(s - 2)^{2} + 9] + 3/[(s - 2)^{2} + 9]$.

13. $t^{4}/8$.

14. $\dfrac{5}{4} t \sin 2t$.

15. $\dfrac{1}{3} e^{2t} \sin 3t$.

16. $3 \cosh 3t$.

17. $\dfrac{3}{2} t^{2} + 2e^{-3t}$.

18. $4 \cos 2t + \dfrac{2}{3} \sin 3t$.

19. $e^{4t} + \dfrac{3}{2} t^{2}e^{-t}$.

20. $3 \cos 2t + \dfrac{1}{3} \sin 3t$.

21. $2e^{-4t} + 3e^{t}$.

22. $2\cos 3t - e^{3t}$.

23. $\dfrac{2s+4}{s^2+2s+5} = 2\left(\dfrac{s+1}{(s+1)^2+2^2}\right) + \left(\dfrac{2}{(s+1)^2+2^2}\right)$, so

$$\mathscr{L}^{-1}\left\{\dfrac{2s+4}{s^2+2s+5}\right\} = 2e^{-t}\cos 2t + e^{-t}\sin 2t.$$

24. $\dfrac{4s^2+3s+29}{(s^2+9)(s+2)} = \dfrac{3}{s+2} + \dfrac{1}{s^2+9} + \dfrac{s}{s^2+9}$, so

$$\mathscr{L}^{-1}\left\{\dfrac{4s^2+3s+29}{(s^2+9)(s+2)}\right\} = 3e^{-2t} + \dfrac{1}{3}\sin 3t + \cos 3t.$$

PROBLEMS 82

1. $sY(s) + 6$.

2. $s^2 Y(s) - 2 - s$.

3. $s^2 Y(s) - 3s$.

4. $s^3 Y(s) - 4 + s - 2s^2$.

5. $(s^2 + 3s + 1)Y(s) - 8 - 3s$.

6. $(s^2 - 2s + 3)Y(s)$.

7. $(2s^2 - 3)Y(s) - 4 - 2s$.

8. $(s^2 + 4s + 4)Y(s) - 6 - 2s$.

PROBLEMS 83

5. $(s - 3)/[(s - 3)^2 + 3^2]$.

6. $2/(s + 2)^3$.

7. $2/[(s + 1)^2 - 2^2]$.

8. $2(s - 1)/[(s - 1)^2 + 1]^2$.

9. $[(s - 2)^2 - 2^2]/[(s - 2)^2 + 2^2]^2$.

10. $4(s + 3)/[(s + 3)^2 + 2^2]^2$.

11. $\dfrac{1}{s^2 - 4s + 20} = \dfrac{1}{(s - 2)^2 + 4^2}$, so

$$\mathcal{L}^{-1}\left\{\frac{1}{s^2 - 4s + 20}\right\} = \frac{1}{4}\,e^{2t}\sin 4t.$$

12. $$\frac{5}{s^2 + 4s + 20} = \frac{5}{(s+2)^2 + 4^2} = \frac{5}{4} \cdot \frac{4}{(s+2)^2 + 4^2},\ \text{so}$$

$$\mathcal{L}^{-1}\left\{\frac{5}{s^2 + 4s + 20}\right\} = \frac{5}{4}\,e^{-2t}\sin 4t.$$

13. $$\frac{2(s-1)}{(s^2 - 2s + 10)^2} = \frac{2(s-1)}{[(s-1)^2 + 3^2\,]^2},\ \text{so}$$

$$\mathcal{L}^{-1}\left\{\frac{2(s-1)}{(s^2 - 2s + 10)^2}\right\} = \frac{1}{3}\,e^{t}t\sin 3t.$$

14. $$\frac{s^2 + 2s - 3}{2(s^2 + 2s + 5)^2} = \frac{1}{2}\left\{\frac{(s+1)^2 - 2^2}{[(s+1)^2 + s^2\,]^2}\right\},\ \text{so}$$

$$\mathcal{L}^{-1}\left\{\frac{s^2 + 2s - 3}{2(s^2 + 2s + 5)^2}\right\} = \frac{1}{2}\,e^{-t}t\cos 2t.$$

15.

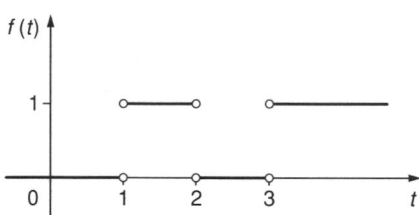

16.

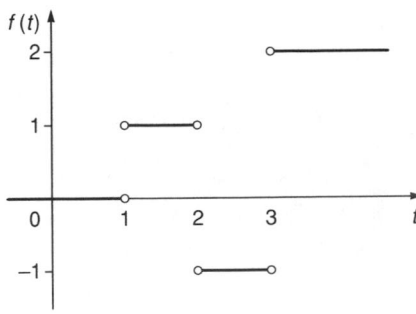

17.

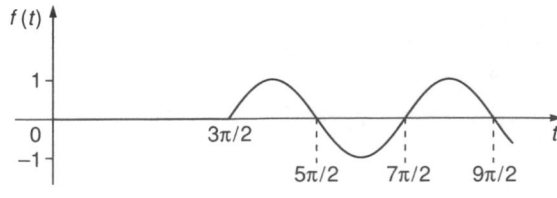

18.

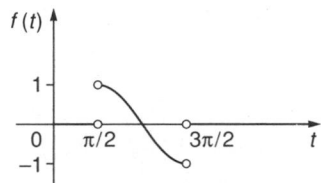

19.

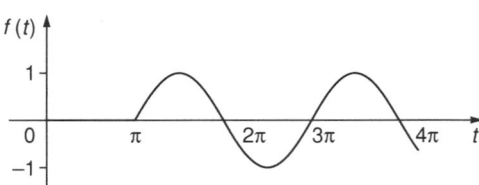

20.

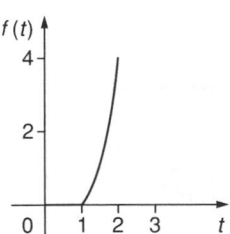

21.

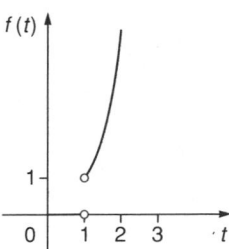

22.

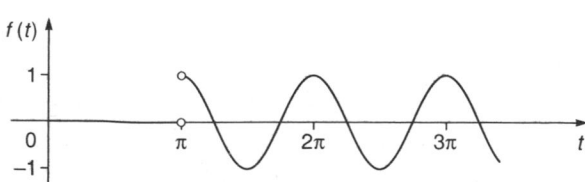

23. $3e^{-\pi s/2}/(s^2 + 9)$.

24. $\left[\dfrac{2}{s^3} + \dfrac{3}{s^2} + \dfrac{4}{5}\right]e^{-s}$.

25. $e^{-2s}/(s^2 - 6s + 10)$.

26. $se^{-s}/(s^2 - 9)$.

27. $u_2(t)\cos[2(t-2)]$.

28. $\dfrac{1}{2}u_1(t)e^{2(t-1)}\sin[2(t-1)]$.

29. $u_4(t)(t-4)\cos[3(t-4)]$.

30. $u_2(t)e^{(t-2)}\cos[3(t-2)]$.

31. $\dfrac{s^2 + 6s - 9}{(s^2 + 9)^2} = \dfrac{s^2 - 9}{(s^2 + 9)^2} + \dfrac{6s}{(s^2 + 9)^2}$, so

$$\mathscr{L}^{-1}\left\{\frac{(s^2 + 6s - 9)e^{-s}}{(s^2 + 9)^2}\right\} = u_1(t)\{(t-1)\cos[3(t-1) + (t-1)\sin[3(t-1)]\}.$$

32. $\dfrac{3s - 8}{s^2 + 4} = 3\left(\dfrac{s}{s^2 + 4}\right) - 4\left(\dfrac{2}{s^2 + 4}\right)$, so

$$\mathscr{L}^{-1}\left\{\frac{(3s - 8)e^{-4s}}{(s^2 + 4)}\right\} = u_4(t)\{3\cos[2(t-4)] - 4\sin[2(t-4)]\}.$$

33. $\dfrac{2s^2 + 3s + 2}{(s^2 + 1)(s - 1)} = \dfrac{2}{s - 1} + \dfrac{3s}{s^2 + 1}$, so

$$\mathscr{L}^{-1}\left\{\frac{(2s^2 + 3s + 2)e^{-3s}}{(s - 1)(s^2 + 1)}\right\} = u_3(t)[2e^{t-3} + 3\cos(t - 3)].$$

34. $\dfrac{6s^2 + 20s + 24}{(s^2 + 4)^3} = \dfrac{6}{s^2 + 4} + \dfrac{20s}{(s^2 + 4)^2}$, so

$$\mathscr{L}^{-1}\left\{\frac{(6s^2 + 20s + 24)e^{-2s}}{(s^2 + 4)^3}\right\} = u_2(t)\{3\sin[2(t-2)] + 5(t-2)\sin[2(t-2)]\}.$$

PROBLEMS 84

1. $Y(s) = 1/(s^2 - 3s + 2) = 1/(s - 2) - 1/(s - 1)$, so

$$y(t) = \mathscr{L}^{-1}\{Y(s)\} = e^{2t} - e^t.$$

2. $Y(s) = (s-1)/(s^2-4) = \dfrac{3}{4}\left(\dfrac{1}{s+2}\right) + \dfrac{1}{4}\left(\dfrac{1}{s-2}\right)$, so

$$y(t) = \mathscr{L}^{-1}\{Y(s)\} = \frac{3}{4}e^{-2t} + \frac{1}{4}e^{2t}.$$

3. $Y(s) = (2s-3)/(s^2-s-2) = \dfrac{5}{3}\left(\dfrac{1}{s+1}\right) + \dfrac{1}{3}\left(\dfrac{1}{s-2}\right)$, so

$$y(t) = \mathscr{L}^{-1}\{Y(s)\} = \frac{5}{3}e^{-t} + \frac{1}{3}e^{2t}.$$

4. $Y(s) = \dfrac{s+2}{(s^2+2s+4)} = \dfrac{s+2}{(s+1)^2+3} = \dfrac{s+1}{(s+1)^2+3} + \dfrac{1}{\sqrt{3}}\dfrac{\sqrt{3}}{(s+1)^2+3}$, so

$$y(t) = \mathscr{L}^{-1}\{Y(s)\} = e^{-t}\cos\sqrt{3}t + \frac{1}{\sqrt{3}}e^{t}\sin\sqrt{3}t.$$

5. $Y(s) = \dfrac{s-4}{(s^2-4s+5)} = \dfrac{s-2}{(s-2)^2+1} - 2\cdot\dfrac{1}{(s-2)^2+1}$, so

$$y(t) = \mathscr{L}^{-1}\{Y(s)\} = e^{2t}\cos t - 2e^{2t}\sin t.$$

6. $Y(s) = -(1+s)/(s^2+2s+10) = -\dfrac{(s+1)}{(s+1)^2+9}$, so

$$y(t) = \mathscr{L}^{-1}\{Y(s)\} = -e^{-t}\cos 3t.$$

7. $Y(s) = \dfrac{3s-6}{(s^2-2s+1)} = \dfrac{3}{s-1} - \dfrac{3}{(s-2)^2}$, so

$$y(t) = \mathscr{L}^{-1}\{Y(s)\} = 3e^{t} - 3te^{t}.$$

8. $Y(s) = \dfrac{s^2-3s+4}{(s^3-3s^2+3s-1)} = \dfrac{2}{(s-1)^3} - \dfrac{1}{(s-1)^2} + \dfrac{1}{s-1}$, so

$$y(t) = \mathscr{L}^{-1}\{Y(s)\} = t^2e^{t} - te^{t} + e^{t}.$$

9. $Y(s) = \dfrac{4(s^2-s-1)}{(s^3-s^2-s+1)} = \dfrac{1}{s+1} - \dfrac{2}{(s-1)^2} + \dfrac{3}{s-1}$, so

$$y(t) = \mathscr{L}^{-1}\{Y(s)\} = e^{-t} - 2te^{t} + 3e^{t}.$$

10. $Y(s) = \dfrac{1}{s^2+1} + \dfrac{3}{(s^2+1)^2} = \dfrac{1}{s^2+1} + \dfrac{3}{2}\left[\dfrac{(s^2+1)-(s^2-1)}{(s^2+1)^2}\right]$

$$= \frac{5}{2}\frac{1}{(s^2+1)} - \frac{3}{2}\frac{(s^2-1)}{(s^2+1)^2}, \text{ so}$$

$$y(t) = \mathscr{L}^{-1}\{Y(s)\} = \frac{5}{2}\sin t - \frac{3}{2}t\cos t.$$

11. $Y(s) = \dfrac{1}{(s-1)} + \dfrac{1}{(s-1)(s^2-1)} - \dfrac{1^{\cdot}}{s^2(s^2-1)}$

$= \dfrac{1}{4}\left(\dfrac{1}{s-1}\right) + \dfrac{3}{4}\left(\dfrac{1}{s+1}\right) + \dfrac{1}{2}\dfrac{1}{(s-1)^2} + \dfrac{1}{s^2}$, so

$$y(t) = \mathcal{L}^{-1}\{Y(s)\} = \dfrac{1}{4}e^t + \dfrac{3}{4}e^{-t} + \dfrac{1}{2}e^t + t.$$

12. $Y(s) = \dfrac{s-3}{(s^2-3s+2)} + \dfrac{3s}{(1+s^2)(s^2-3s+2)}$

$= \dfrac{2}{s-1} - \dfrac{1}{s-2} + \dfrac{3}{10}\left(\dfrac{1}{s^2+1}\right) - \dfrac{9}{10}\left(\dfrac{1}{s^2+1}\right) - \dfrac{3}{2}\left(\dfrac{1}{s-1}\right) + \dfrac{6}{5}\left(\dfrac{1}{s-2}\right)$

$= \dfrac{1}{2}\left(\dfrac{1}{s-1}\right) + \dfrac{1}{5}\left(\dfrac{1}{s-2}\right) + \dfrac{3}{10}\left(\dfrac{s}{s^2+1}\right) - \dfrac{9}{10}\left(\dfrac{1}{s^2+1}\right)$, so

$$y(t) = \mathcal{L}^{-1}\{Y(s)\} = \dfrac{1}{2}e^t + \dfrac{1}{5}e^{2t} + \dfrac{3}{10}\cos t - \dfrac{9}{10}\sin t.$$

13. $Y(s) = \dfrac{1}{(s-1)^4} + \dfrac{1}{(s-1)^6}$, so

$$y(t) = \mathcal{L}^{-1}\{Y(s)\} = te^t + \dfrac{1}{6}t^3 e^t.$$

14. $Y(s) = \dfrac{1}{s^2-4} + \dfrac{1}{s(s^2-4)} + \dfrac{2e^{-s}}{s(s^2-4)}$

$= \dfrac{1}{4}\left(\dfrac{1}{s-2}\right) - \dfrac{1}{4}\left(\dfrac{1}{s+2}\right) + \dfrac{1}{8}\left(\dfrac{1}{s-2}\right) + \dfrac{1}{8}\left(\dfrac{1}{s+2}\right) - \dfrac{1}{4}\left(\dfrac{1}{s}\right)$

$+ \dfrac{1}{4}\left(\dfrac{e^{-s}}{s-2}\right) + \dfrac{1}{4}\left(\dfrac{e^{-s}}{s+2}\right) - \dfrac{1}{2}\left(\dfrac{e^{-s}}{s}\right),$

$= \dfrac{3}{8}\left(\dfrac{1}{s-2}\right) - \dfrac{1}{8}\left(\dfrac{1}{s+2}\right) - \dfrac{1}{4}\left(\dfrac{1}{s}\right) + \dfrac{1}{4}\left(\dfrac{e^{-s}}{s-2}\right) + \dfrac{1}{4}\left(\dfrac{e^{-s}}{s+2}\right) - \dfrac{1}{2}\left(\dfrac{e^{-s}}{s}\right)$, so

$y(t) = \mathcal{L}^{-1}\{Y(s)\}$

$= \dfrac{3}{8}e^{2t} - \dfrac{1}{8}e^{-2t} - \dfrac{1}{4} + u_1(t)\left[\dfrac{1}{4}e^{2(t-1)} + \dfrac{1}{4}e^{-2(t-1)} - \dfrac{1}{2}\right].$

15. $Y(s) = \dfrac{s}{(s^2+1)(s^2+4)} + \dfrac{e^{-\pi s/2}}{s(s^2+1)(s^2+4)}$

$= \dfrac{1}{3}\left(\dfrac{s}{s^2+1}\right) - \dfrac{1}{3}\left(\dfrac{s}{s^2+4}\right) + \dfrac{1}{12}\left(\dfrac{se^{-\pi s/2}}{s^2+4}\right) - \dfrac{1}{3}\left(\dfrac{se^{-\pi s/2}}{(s^2+1)}\right) + \dfrac{1}{4}\left(\dfrac{e^{-\pi s/2}}{s}\right)$, so

$y(t) = \mathcal{L}^{-1}\{Y(s)\}$

$$= \frac{1}{3}\cos t - \frac{1}{3}\cos 2t + u_{\pi/2}(t)\left[\frac{1}{12}\cos[2(t-\pi/2)] - \frac{1}{3}\cos(t-\pi/2) + \frac{1}{4}\right].$$

16. $Y(s) = \dfrac{s^2 + s + 1}{s(s^2 + s - 2)} + \dfrac{e^{-2s}}{s(s^2 + s - 2)}$

$$= \frac{1}{2}\left(\frac{1}{s+2}\right) + \left(\frac{1}{s-1}\right) - \frac{1}{2}\left(\frac{1}{s}\right) + \frac{1}{6}\left(\frac{e^{-2s}}{s+2}\right) + \frac{1}{3}\left(\frac{e^{-2s}}{s-1}\right) - \frac{1}{2}\left(\frac{e^{-2s}}{s}\right),\ \text{so}$$

$y(t) = \mathcal{L}^{-1}\{Y(s)\}$

$$= \frac{1}{2}e^{-2t} + e^t - \frac{1}{2} + u_2(t)\left[\frac{1}{6}e^{-2(t-2)} + \frac{1}{3}e^{(t-2)} - \frac{1}{2}\right].$$

17. $Y(s) = \dfrac{s^2 + 3s + 1}{s(s^2 + 3s + 2)} + \dfrac{e^{-s}}{s(s^2 + 3s + 2)}$

$$= \frac{1}{2}\left(\frac{1}{s}\right) + \frac{1}{s+1} - \frac{1}{2}\left(\frac{1}{s+2}\right) + \frac{e^{-s}}{s+1} - \frac{1}{2}\left(\frac{e^{-s}}{s+2}\right) - \frac{1}{2}\left(\frac{e^{-s}}{s}\right),\ \text{so}$$

$y(t) = \mathcal{L}^{-1}\{Y(s)\}$

$$= \frac{1}{2}e^{-t} - \frac{1}{2}e^{-2t} + u_1(t)\left[e^{-(t-1)} - \frac{1}{2}e^{-2(t-1)} - \frac{1}{2}\right].$$

18. $(s-2)X(s) = 1 + Y(s)$, $(s-4)Y(s) = 3X(s)$; solving for $X(s)$ and $Y(s)$ and finding the inverse Laplace transform gives

$$x(t) = \frac{3}{4}e^t + \frac{1}{4}e^{5t},\ y(t) = -\frac{3}{4}e^t + \frac{3}{4}e^{5t}.$$

19. $(s-1)X(s) = 1 + Y(s)$, $(s-3)Y(s) = 2(1 - X(s))$; solving for $X(s)$ and $Y(s)$ and finding the inverse Laplace transform gives

$$x(t) = e^{2t}(\cos t + \sin t),\ y(t) = 2e^{2t}\cos t.$$

20. $(s-2)X(s) = Y(s)$, $(s-4)Y(s) = -(1 + X(s))$; solving for $X(s)$ and $Y(s)$ and finding the inverse Laplace transform gives

$$x(t) = -te^{3t},\ y(t) = -(1+t)e^{3t}.$$

21. $(s+3)X(s) = 2(1 + Y(s))$, $(s-1)Y(s) = 1 - 2X(s)$; solving for $X(s)$ and $Y(s)$ and finding the inverse Laplace transform gives

$$x(t) = 2(1-t)e^{-t}, y(t) = (1 - 2t)e^{-t}.$$

22. $(s-1)X(s) = 1 + 2Y(s)$, $sY(s) = 1 + X(s) - 5/(s^2 + 1)$; solving for $X(s)$ and $Y(s)$ and finding the inverse Laplace transform gives

$$x(t) = \frac{4}{3}e^{-t} + \frac{2}{3}e^{2t} - \cos t + 3\sin t$$

$$y(t) = -\frac{4}{3}e^{-t} + \frac{1}{3}e^{2t} + 2\cos t - \sin t.$$

23. $sX(s) - 2 = Y(s) - 2/s^2$, $sY(s) - 1 = -X(s) + 1/s^2$; solving for $X(s)$ and $Y(s)$ and finding the inverse Laplace transform gives

$$x(t) = 4\cos t - 2 + t,$$

$$y(t) = -4\sin t + 1 + 2t.$$

PROBLEMS 85

1. Setting $n = 1$ in the theorem gives

$$\mathcal{L}\{-t\} = \frac{d}{ds}\left(\frac{1}{s}\right) = -\frac{1}{s^2},$$

so $\mathcal{L}\{t\} = 1/s^2$. If the result is true for some $n > 1$, then

$$\mathcal{L}\{(-t)t^n\} = \frac{d}{ds}\left(\frac{n!}{s^{n+1}}\right) = -\frac{(n+1)!}{s^{n+2}},$$

which is the result obtained from $\mathcal{L}\{t^n\}$ by replacing n by $n+1$. The result is true for $n = 1$, so it follows by induction that it is true for $n = 1, 2, \ldots$.

2. Setting $n = 1$ in the theorem gives

$$\mathcal{L}\{(-t)e^{at}\} = \frac{d}{ds}\left(\frac{1}{s-a}\right) = -\frac{1}{(s-a)^2},$$

so $\mathcal{L}\{te^{at}\} = 1/(s-a)^2$. If the result is true for some $n > 1$, then

$$\mathcal{L}\{(-t)t^n e^{at}\} = \frac{d}{ds}\left(\frac{n!}{(s-a)^{n+1}}\right) = \frac{-(n+1)!}{(s-a)^{n+2}},$$

which is the result obtained from $\mathcal{L}\{t^n e^{at}\}$ by replacing n by $n+1$. The result is true for $n = 1$, so it follows by induction that it is true for $n = 1, 2, \ldots$.

3. Setting $n = 1$ in the theorem gives

$$\mathcal{L}\{(-t)\sinh at\} = \frac{d}{ds}\left(\frac{a}{s^2-a^2}\right) = \frac{-2as}{(a^2-s^2)^2},$$

so

$$\mathcal{L}\{t\sinh at\} = \frac{2as}{(s^2-a^2)^2}.$$

4.   Setting $n = 1$ in the theorem gives

$$\mathscr{L}\{(-t)\cosh at\} = \frac{d}{ds}\left(\frac{s}{s^2 - a^2}\right) = \frac{-(s^2 + a^2)}{(s^2 - a^2)^2},$$

so

$$\mathscr{L}\{t\cosh at\} = \frac{(s^2 + a^2)}{(s^2 - a^2)^2}.$$

5.   The first result follows from entries 1 and 7 in Table 13, as in Example 85.3. Setting $n = 1$ in the theorem gives

$$\mathscr{L}\{(-t)[1 - \cos at]\} = \frac{d}{ds}\left(\frac{a^2}{s(s^2 + a^2)}\right) = \frac{-a^2(a^2 + 3s^2)}{s^2(s^2 + a^2)^2},$$

so

$$\mathscr{L}\{t - t\cos at\} = \frac{a^2(a^2 + 3s^2)}{s^2(s^2 + a^2)^2}.$$

6.   The first result follows from entries 2 and 6 in Table 13, as in Example 85.3. Setting $n = 1$ in the theorem gives

$$\mathscr{L}\{(-t)[at - \sin at]\} = \frac{d}{ds}\left(\frac{a^3}{s^2(s^2 + a^2)}\right) = \frac{-2a^3(a^2 + 2s^2)}{s^3(s^2 + a^2)^2},$$

so

$$\mathscr{L}\{at^2 - t\sin at\} = \frac{2a^3(a^2 + 2s^2)}{s^3(s^2 + a^2)^2}.$$

7.   The first result follows from entries 6 and 9 in Table 13, as in Example 85.3. Setting $n = 1$ in the theorem gives

$$\mathscr{L}\{(-t)[\sin at + at\cos at]\} = \frac{d}{ds}\left(\frac{2as^2}{(s^2 + a^2)^2}\right) = \frac{-4as(s^2 - a^2)}{(s^2 + a^2)^3},$$

so

$$\mathscr{L}\{t\sin at + at^2\cos at\} = \frac{4as(s^2 - a^2)}{(s^2 + a^2)^3}.$$

8.   The first result follows from entries 12 and 6 in Table 13, as in Example 85.3. Setting $n = 1$ in the theorem gives

$$\mathscr{L}\{(-t)[\sinh at - \sin at]\} = \frac{d}{ds}\left(\frac{2a^3}{(s^4 - a^4)}\right) = \frac{-8a^3s^3}{(s^4 - a^4)^2},$$

so

$$\mathscr{L}\{t\sinh at - t\sin at\} = \frac{8a^3s^3}{(s^4 - a^4)^2}.$$

Reference information

USEFUL IDENTITIES AND CONSTANTS

Trignometric identities

$\sin^2 x + \cos^2 x = 1$

$\sec^2 x = 1 + \tan^2 x$

$\csc^2 x = 1 + \cot^2 x$

$\sin 2x = 2 \sin x \cos x$

$\cos 2x = \cos^2 x - \sin^2 x$

$\qquad = 1 - 2 \sin^2 x$

$\qquad = 2 \cos^2 x - 1$

$\sin^2 x = \frac{1}{2}(1 - \cos 2x)$

$\cos^2 x = \frac{1}{2}(1 + \cos 2x)$

$\sin(x + y) = \sin x \cos y + \cos x \sin y$

$\sin(x - y) = \sin x \cos y - \cos x \sin y$

$\cos(x + y) = \cos x \cos y - \sin x \sin y$

$\cos(x - y) = \cos x \cos y + \sin x \sin y$

$\tan(x + y) = \dfrac{\tan x + \tan y}{1 - \tan x \tan y}$

$\tan(x - y) = \dfrac{\tan x - \tan y}{1 + \tan x \tan y}$

Hyperbolic identities

$\cosh^2 x - \sinh^2 x = 1$

$\operatorname{sech}^2 x = 1 - \tanh^2 x$

$\text{cosech}^2 x = \coth^2 x - 1$

$\sinh 2x = 2 \sinh x \cosh x$

$\cosh 2x = \cosh^2 x + \sinh^2 x$

$\qquad = 1 + 2 \sinh^2 x$

$\qquad = 2 \cosh^2 x - 1$

$\sinh^2 x = \frac{1}{2} (\cosh 2x - 1)$

$\cosh^2 x = \frac{1}{2} (\cosh 2x + 1)$

$\sinh (x + y) = \sinh x \cosh y + \cosh x \sinh y$

$\sinh (x - y) = \sinh x \cosh y - \cosh x \sinh y$

$\cosh (x + y) = \cosh x \cosh y + \sinh x \sinh y$

$\cosh (x - y) = \cosh x \cosh y - \sinh x \sinh y$

$\tanh (x + y) = \dfrac{\tanh x + \tanh y}{1 + \tanh x \tanh y}$

$\tanh (x - y) = \dfrac{\tanh x - \tanh y}{1 - \tanh x \tanh y}$

Complex relationships

$e^{ix} = \cos x + i \sin x$

$\sinh x = \dfrac{e^x - e^{-x}}{2}$

$\sin x = \dfrac{e^{ix} - e^{ix}}{2i}$

$\sin ix = i \sinh x$

$\sinh ix = i \sin x$

$(\cos x + i \sin x)^n = \cos nx + i \sin nx$

$\cosh x = \dfrac{e^x + e^{-x}}{2}$

$\cos x = \dfrac{e^{ix} + e^{-ix}}{2}$

$\cos ix = \cosh x$

$\cosh ix = \cos x$

Constants

$$e = 2.718\ 281\ 828\ 459\ 04$$

$$\pi^2 = 9.869\ 604\ 401\ 089\ 35$$

$$\ln 10 = 2.302\ 585\ 092\ 994\ 04$$

$$\pi = 3.141\ 592\ 653\ 589\ 79$$

$$\log_{10} e = 0.434\ 294\ 481\ 903\ 25$$

Table 14 Basic derivatives and rules

$f(x)$	$f'(x)$	$f(x)$	$f'(x)$
1. x^n	nx^{n-1}	13. $\sinh ax$	$a \cosh ax$
2. e^{ax}	ae^{ax}	14. $\cosh ax$	$a \sinh ax$
3. $\ln x$	$1/x$	15. $\tanh ax$	$a \operatorname{sech}^2 ax$
4. $\sin ax$	$a \cos ax$	16. $\operatorname{cosech} ax$	$-a \operatorname{cosech} ax \coth ax$
5. $\cos ax$	$-a \sin ax$	17. $\operatorname{sech} ax$	$-a \operatorname{sech} ax \tanh ax$
6. $\tan ax$	$a \sec^2 ax$	18. $\coth ax$	$-a \operatorname{cosech}^2 ax$
7. $\operatorname{cosec} ax$	$-a \operatorname{cosec} ax \cot ax$	19. $\operatorname{arc\,sinh} \dfrac{x}{a}$	$1/\sqrt{(x^2 + a^2)}$
8. $\sec ax$	$a \sec ax \tan ax$		
9. $\cot ax$	$-a \csc^2 ax$		$\begin{cases} 1/\sqrt{(x^2 - a^2)} \\ \text{for arc cosh} \dfrac{x}{a} > 0,\ \dfrac{x}{a} > 1. \\ -1/\sqrt{(x^2 - a^2)} \\ \text{for arc cosh} \dfrac{x}{a} < 0,\ \dfrac{x}{a} > 1. \end{cases}$
10. $\operatorname{arc\,sin} \dfrac{x}{a}$	$1/\sqrt{(a^2 - x^2)}$	20. $\operatorname{arc\,cosh} \dfrac{x}{a}$	
11. $\operatorname{arc\,cos} \dfrac{x}{a}$	$-1/\sqrt{(a^2 - x^2)}$		
12. $\operatorname{arc\,tan} \dfrac{x}{a}$	$a/(a^2 + x^2)$	21. $\operatorname{arc\,tanh} \dfrac{x}{a}$	$a/(a^2 - x^2)$

RULES OF DIFFERENTIATION AND INTEGRATION

1. $\dfrac{d}{dx}(u + v) = \dfrac{du}{dx} + \dfrac{dv}{dx}$ (sum)

2. $\dfrac{d}{dx}(uv) = u\dfrac{dv}{dx} + v\dfrac{du}{dx}$ (product)

3. $\dfrac{d}{dx}\left(\dfrac{u}{v}\right) = \left(v\dfrac{du}{dx} - u\dfrac{dv}{dx}\right)\Big/ v^2$ for $v \neq 0$ (quotient)

4. $\dfrac{d}{dx}[f\{g(x)\}] = f'\{g(x)\}\dfrac{dg}{dx}$ (function of a function)

5. $\displaystyle\int (u+v)\,dx = \int u\,dx + \int v\,dx$ (sum)

6. $\displaystyle\int u\,dv = uv - \int v\,du$ and $\displaystyle\int_a^b u\,dv = uv\Big|_a^b - \int_a^b v\,du$ (integration by parts)

SHORT TABLE OF INTEGRALS

Common standard forms

1. $\displaystyle\int x^n\,dx = \dfrac{1}{n+1}x^{n+1} + C,\ n \neq 1$

2. $\displaystyle\int \dfrac{1}{x}\,dx = \ln|x| + C = \begin{cases} \ln x + C, & x>0 \\ \ln(-x) + C, & x<0 \end{cases}$

3. $\displaystyle\int e^{ax}\,dx = \dfrac{1}{a}e^{ax} + C$

4. $\displaystyle\int a^x\,dx = \dfrac{a^x}{\ln a} + C,\ a \neq 1,\ a>0$

5. $\displaystyle\int \ln x\,dx = x\ln x - x + C$

6. $\displaystyle\int \sin ax\,dx = -\dfrac{1}{a}\cos ax + C$

7. $\displaystyle\int \cos ax\,dx = \dfrac{1}{a}\sin ax + C$

8. $\displaystyle\int \tan ax\,dx = -\dfrac{1}{a}\ln|\cos ax| + C$

9. $\displaystyle\int \sinh ax\,dx = \dfrac{1}{a}\cosh ax + C$

10. $\displaystyle\int \cosh ax\,dx = \dfrac{1}{a}\sinh ax + C$

11. $\displaystyle\int \tanh ax\,dx = \dfrac{1}{a}\ln|\cosh ax| + C$

12. $\int \dfrac{1}{\sqrt{(a^2 - x^2)}}\, dx = \arcsin \dfrac{x}{a} + C,\ x^2 \leqslant a^2$

13. $\int \dfrac{1}{\sqrt{(x^2 - a^2)}}\, dx = \operatorname{arcosh} \dfrac{x}{a} + C = \ln \left| x + \sqrt{x^2 - a^2} \right| + C,\ a^2 \leqslant x^2$

14. $\int \dfrac{1}{\sqrt{(a^2 + x^2)}}\, dx = \operatorname{arsinh} \dfrac{x}{a} + C = \ln \left| x + \sqrt{a^2 + x^2} \right| + C$

15. $\int \dfrac{1}{x^2 + a^2}\, dx = \dfrac{1}{a} \arctan \dfrac{x}{a} + C$

16. $\int \dfrac{1}{x^2 - a^2}\, dx = \dfrac{1}{2a} \ln \left| \dfrac{x - a}{x + a} \right| + C = -\dfrac{1}{a} \operatorname{artanh} \dfrac{x}{a} + C,\ a^2 \leqslant x^2$

Algebraic forms

17. $\int (a + bx)^n\, dx = \dfrac{(a + bx)^{n+1}}{b(n + 1)} + C,\ n \neq -1$

18. $\int \dfrac{1}{a + bx}\, dx = \dfrac{1}{b} \ln |a + bx| + C$

19. $\int x(a + bx)^n\, dx = \dfrac{(a + bx)^{n+1}}{b^2} \left[\dfrac{a + bx}{n + 2} - \dfrac{a}{n + 1} \right] + C,\ n \neq -1,\ -2$

20. $\int \dfrac{x}{a + bx}\, dx = \dfrac{x}{b} - \dfrac{a}{b^2} \ln |a + bx| + C$

21. $\int \dfrac{x^2}{a + bx}\, dx = \dfrac{1}{b^3} \left[\dfrac{1}{2} (a + bx)^2 - 2a(a + bx) + a^2 \ln |a + bx| \right] + C$

22. $\int \dfrac{x}{(a + bx)^2}\, dx = \dfrac{1}{b^2} \left[\dfrac{a}{a + bx} + \ln |a + bx| \right] + C$

23. $\int \dfrac{x^2}{(a + bx)^2}\, dx = \dfrac{1}{b^3} \left[a + bx - \dfrac{a^2}{a + bx} - 2a \ln |a + bx| \right] + C$

24. $\int \dfrac{1}{x(a + bx)}\, dx = \dfrac{1}{a} \ln \left| \dfrac{x}{a + bx} \right| + C$

25. $\int \dfrac{1}{x^2 (a + bx)}\, dx = -\dfrac{1}{ax} + \dfrac{b}{a^2} \ln \left| \dfrac{a + bx}{x} \right| + C$

26. $\int \dfrac{1}{x(a + bx)^2}\, dx = \dfrac{1}{a(a + bx)} + \dfrac{1}{a^2} \ln \left| \dfrac{x}{a + bx} \right| + C$

Trigonometric forms

27. $\displaystyle\int \sin ax \, dx = -\frac{1}{a} \cos ax + C$

28. $\displaystyle\int \sin^2 ax \, dx = \frac{x}{2} - \frac{\sin 2ax}{4a} + C$

29. $\displaystyle\int \cos ax \, dx = \frac{1}{a} \sin ax + C$

30. $\displaystyle\int \cos^2 ax \, dx = \frac{x}{2} + \frac{\sin 2ax}{4a} + C$

31. $\displaystyle\int \sin ax \sin bx \, dx = \frac{\sin (a-b)x}{2(a-b)} - \frac{\sin (a+b)x}{2(a+b)}, \quad a^2 \neq b^2$

32. $\displaystyle\int \cos ax \cos bx \, dx = \frac{\sin (a-b)x}{2(a-b)} + \frac{\sin (a+b)x}{2(a+b)}, \quad a^2 \neq b^2$

33. $\displaystyle\int \sin ax \cos bx \, dx = -\frac{\cos (a+b)x}{2(a+b)} - \frac{\cos (a-b)x}{2(a-b)} + C, \quad a^2 \neq b^2$

34. $\displaystyle\int \sin ax \cos ax \, dx = -\frac{\cos 2ax}{4a} + C$

35. $\displaystyle\int x \sin x \, dx = -x \cos x + \sin x + C$

36. $\displaystyle\int x^2 \sin x \, dx = -x^2 \cos x + 2x \sin x + 2 \cos x + C$

37. $\displaystyle\int x \cos x \, dx = x \sin x + \cos x + C$

38. $\displaystyle\int x^2 \cos dx = x^2 \sin x + 2x \cos x - 2 \sin x + C$

39. $\displaystyle\int e^{ax} \sin bx \, dx = \frac{e^{ax}}{a^2 + b^2} (a \sin bx - b \cos bx) + C$

40. $\displaystyle\int e^{ax} \cos bx \, dx = \frac{e^{ax}}{a^2 + b^2} (a \cos bx - b \sin bx) + C$

41. $\displaystyle\int \sec ax \, dx = \frac{1}{a} \ln |\sec ax + \tan ax| + C$

42. $\int \operatorname{cosec} ax \, dx = -\frac{1}{a} \ln |\operatorname{cosec} ax + \cot ax| + C$

43. $\int \cot ax \, dx = \frac{1}{a} \ln |\sin ax| + C$

44. $\int \tan^2 ax \, dx = \frac{1}{a} \tan ax - x + C$

45. $\int \sec^2 ax \, dx = \frac{1}{a} \tan ax + C$

46. $\int \operatorname{cosec}^2 ax \, dx = -\frac{1}{a} \cot ax + C$

47. $\int \cot^2 ax \, dx = -\frac{1}{a} \cot ax - x + C$

Inverse Trignometric Forms

48. $\int \arcsin ax \, dx = x \arcsin ax + \frac{1}{a} \sqrt{(1 - a^2 x^2)} + C, \ a^2 x^2 \leqslant 1$

49. $\int \arccos ax \, dx = x \arccos ax - \frac{1}{a} \sqrt{(1 - a^2 x^2)} + C, \ a^2 x^2 \leqslant 1$

50. $\int \arctan ax \, dx = x \arctan ax - \frac{1}{2a} \ln (1 + a^2 x^2) + C$

Exponential and Logarithmic Forms

51. $\int e^{ax} \, dx = \frac{1}{a} e^{ax} + C$

52. $\int b^{ax} \, dx = \frac{1}{a} \frac{b^{ax}}{\ln b} + C, \quad b > 0, \ b \neq 1$

53. $\int x \, e^{ax} \, dx = \frac{e^{ax}}{a^2} (ax - 1) + C$

54. $\int \ln ax \, dx = x \ln ax - x + C$

Hyperbolic forms

55. $\displaystyle\int \sinh ax \, dx = \frac{1}{a} \cosh ax + C$

56. $\displaystyle\int \sinh^2 ax \, dx = \frac{\sinh 2ax}{4a} - \frac{x}{2} + C$

57. $\displaystyle\int x \sinh ax \, dx = \frac{x}{a} \cosh ax - \frac{1}{a^2} \sinh ax + C$

58. $\displaystyle\int \cosh ax \, dx = \frac{1}{a} \sinh ax + C$

59. $\displaystyle\int \cosh^2 ax \, dx = \frac{\sinh 2ax}{4a} + \frac{x}{2} + C$

60. $\displaystyle\int x \cosh ax \, dx = \frac{x}{a} \sinh ax - \frac{1}{a^2} \cosh ax + C$

61. $\displaystyle\int e^{ax} \sinh bx \, dx = \frac{e^{ax}}{2} \left[\frac{e^{bx}}{a+b} - \frac{e^{-bx}}{a-b} \right] + C, \ a^2 \neq b^2$

62. $\displaystyle\int e^{ax} \cosh bx \, dx = \frac{e^{ax}}{2} \left[\frac{e^{bx}}{a+b} + \frac{e^{-bx}}{a-b} \right] + C, \ a^2 \neq b^2$

63. $\displaystyle\int \tanh ax \, dx = \frac{1}{a} \ln (\cosh ax) + C$

64. $\displaystyle\int \tanh^2 ax \, dx = x - \frac{1}{a} \tanh ax + C$

65. $\displaystyle\int \coth ax \, dx = \frac{1}{a} \ln |\sinh ax| + C$

66. $\displaystyle\int \coth^2 ax \, dx = x - \frac{1}{a} \coth ax + C$

67. $\displaystyle\int \operatorname{sech} ax \, dx = \frac{2}{a} \arctan e^{ax} + C$

68. $\displaystyle\int \operatorname{sech}^2 ax \, dx = \frac{1}{a} \tanh ax + C$

69. $\displaystyle\int \operatorname{cosech} ax \, dx = \frac{1}{a} \ln \left| \tanh \frac{ax}{2} \right| + C$

70. $\displaystyle\int \operatorname{cosech}^2 ax \, dx = -\frac{1}{a} \coth ax + C$

Table 15 Table of Laplace transform pairs

$f(t) = \mathcal{L}^{-1}(F(s))$	$F(s) = \mathcal{L}(f(t))$
1. k	$\dfrac{k}{s}, \; s > 0$
2. t	$\dfrac{1}{s^2}, \; s > 0$
3. t^n, n a positive integer	$\dfrac{n!}{s^{n+1}}, \; s > 0$
4. e^{at}	$\dfrac{1}{s-a}, \; s > 0$
5. $t^n e^{at}$, n a positive integer	$\dfrac{n!}{(s-a)^{n+1}}, \; s > 0$
6. $\sin at$	$\dfrac{a}{s^2 + a^2}, \; s > 0$
7. $\cos at$	$\dfrac{s}{s^2 + a^2}, \; s > 0$
8. $t \sin at$	$\dfrac{2as}{(s^2 + a^2)^2}, \; s > 0$
9. $t \cos at$	$\dfrac{s^2 - a^2}{(s^2 + a^2)^2}, \; s > 0$
10. $e^{at} \sin bt$	$\dfrac{b}{(s-a)^2 + b^2}, \; s > a$
11. $e^{at} \cos bt$	$\dfrac{s-a}{(s-a)^2 + b^2}, \; s > a$
12. $\sinh at$	$\dfrac{a}{s^2 - a^2}, \; s > |a|$
13. $\cosh at$	$\dfrac{s}{s^2 - a^2}, \; s > |a|$
14. Heaviside unit step function $f(t) = u_a(t) = \begin{cases} 0 \text{ for } t < a \\ 1 \text{ for } t > a \end{cases}$	$\dfrac{e^{-as}}{s}, \; s > 0$

TRANSFORMATION OF DERIVATIVES AND THE SHIFT THEOREMS

Transformation of derivatives

When the Laplace transform $Y(s) = \mathcal{L}\{y(t)\}$ exists, then

1. $\mathcal{L}\{dy/dt\} = s\,Y(s) - y(0);$

2. $\mathscr{L}\{d^2y/dt^2\} = s^2 Y(s) - y'(0) - s\, y(0);$

3. $\mathscr{L}\{d^3y/dt^3\} = s^3 Y(s) - y''(0) - s\, y'(0) - s^2\, y(0);$ and, in general,

4. $\mathscr{L}\{d^ny/dt^n\} = s^n Y(s) - y^{(n-1)}(0) - s\, y^{(n-2)}(0) - s^2\, y^{(n-3)}(0) - \ldots - s^{n-1}y(0)\,.$

The first shift theorem

Let $\mathscr{L}\{f(t)\} = F(s)$ for $s > b$, then $\mathscr{L}\{e^{at}f(t)\} = F(s-a)$ for $s-a > b$.

The second shift theorem

If $\mathscr{L}\{f(t)\} = F(s)$ then $\mathscr{L}\{u_a(t)f(t-a)\} = e^{-as}f(s)$ and, conversely, $\mathscr{L}^{-1}\{e^{-as}F(s)\} = u_a(t)f(t-a)$.

Index